NUTRIGENOMICS
AND **NUTRACEUTICALS**
Clinical Relevance and
Disease Prevention

Nutraceuticals: Basic Research/Clinical Applications
Series Editor: Yashwant Pathak, PhD

Nutrigenomics and Nutraceuticals: Clinical Relevance and Disease Prevention
Yashwant V. Pathak, Ali M. Ardekani

Nanotechnology in Nutraceuticals: Production to Consumption
Shampa Sen and Yashwant Pathak

Herbal Bioactives and Food Fortification: Extraction and Formulation
D. Suresh Kumar

Handbook of Metallonutraceuticals
Yashwant V. Pathak and Jayant N. Lokhande

Nutraceuticals and Health: Review of Human Evidence
Somdat Mahabir and Yashwant V. Pathak

Marine Nutraceuticals: Prospects and Perspectives
Se-Kwon Kim

NUTRIGENOMICS AND NUTRACEUTICALS
Clinical Relevance and Disease Prevention

Edited by
Yashwant V. Pathak
Ali M. Ardekani

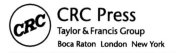

CRC Press
Taylor & Francis Group
Boca Raton London New York

CRC Press is an imprint of the
Taylor & Francis Group, an **informa** business

CRC Press
Taylor & Francis Group
6000 Broken Sound Parkway NW, Suite 300
Boca Raton, FL 33487-2742

© 2018 by Taylor & Francis Group, LLC
CRC Press is an imprint of Taylor & Francis Group, an Informa business

No claim to original U.S. Government works

International Standard Book Number-13: 978-1-4987-6511-4 (Hardback)

This book contains information obtained from authentic and highly regarded sources. Reasonable efforts have been made to publish reliable data and information, but the author and publisher cannot assume responsibility for the validity of all materials or the consequences of their use. The authors and publishers have attempted to trace the copyright holders of all material reproduced in this publication and apologize to copyright holders if permission to publish in this form has not been obtained. If any copyright material has not been acknowledged, please write and let us know so we may rectify in any future reprint.

Except as permitted under U.S. Copyright Law, no part of this book may be reprinted, reproduced, transmitted, or utilized in any form by any electronic, mechanical, or other means, now known or hereafter invented, including photocopying, microfilming, and recording, or in any information storage or retrieval system, without written permission from the publishers.

For permission to photocopy or use material electronically from this work, please access www.copyright.com (http://www.copyright.com/) or contact the Copyright Clearance Center, Inc. (CCC), 222 Rosewood Drive, Danvers, MA 01923, 978-750-8400. CCC is a not-for-profit organization that provides licenses and registration for a variety of users. For organizations that have been granted a photocopy license by the CCC, a separate system of payment has been arranged.

Trademark Notice: Product or corporate names may be trademarks or registered trademarks, and are used only for identification and explanation without intent to infringe.

Library of Congress Cataloging-in-Publication Data

Names: Pathak, Yashwant. | Ardekani, Ali M.
Title: Nutrigenomics and nutraceuticals : clinical relevance and disease prevention / [edited by] Yashwant Pathak and Ali M. Ardekani.
Description: Boca Raton : CRC Press, 2017. | Includes bibliographical references.
Identifiers: LCCN 2017011255 | ISBN 9781498765114 (hardback)
Subjects: LCSH: Nutrition--Genetic aspects. | Functional foods.
Classification: LCC QP144.G45 N84 2017 | DDC 612.3--dc23
LC record available at https://lccn.loc.gov/2017011255

Visit the Taylor & Francis Web site at
http://www.taylorandfrancis.com

and the CRC Press Web site at
http://www.crcpress.com

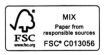

Printed and bound in Great Britain by
TJ International Ltd, Padstow, Cornwall

Dedicated to all the rushies, sages, shamans, medicine men and women, and people of ancient traditions and cultures who contributed to the development of drugs and nutraceuticals worldwide and kept the science of health alive for the past several millennia.

Contents

Series Preface xi

Preface xiii

Contributors xv

1 **Applications of Nutrigenomics for Disease Prevention and Better Health** 1

   Adnan Ali, Ali M. Ardekani, and Yashwant V. Pathak

2 **Omics-Driven Novel Technologies in Food and Nutrition Research** 19

   Rakesh Kumar Tekade, Namrata Soni, Rahul Maheshwari, Neetu Soni, Nidhi Raval, Nagashekhara Molugulu, and Muktika Tekade

3 **Nutrigenomics: The Cutting Edge and Asian Perspectives** 61

   Adela Pilav and Yashwant V. Pathak

4 **Novel Approaches in Food Functions Based on Nutrigenomics Research** 83

   Meenakshisundaram Selvamuthukumaran

vii

5 Recent Trends in Omics-Based Methods and Techniques for Lung Disease Prevention 115

Raisah Salhab and Yashwant V. Pathak

6 Proteomics as a Comprehensive Molecular Means to Understand Dietary Health Effects 135

Jayvadan Patel and Anita Patel

7 Application of Nutritional Metabolomics for Better Health and Healthcare 159

Avipsha Sarkar, Shampa Sen, and Yashwant V. Pathak

8 Facts and Controversies Based on Diet, Genomics, and Cancer 169

Roland Cadet, Charles Preuss, and Yashwant V. Pathak

9 Chronic Degenerative Diseases in Adults and Their Correlation with Childhood Feeding and Genomic Composition 191

Adnan Ali and Yashwant V. Pathak

10 Biology and Optimal Health 201

Amanda Lasher and Yashwant V. Pathak

11 The Role of Pro-Inflammatory Factors and Metabolic Stress in Disease 217

Christopher T. Kaul, Aditya Grover, and Yashwant V. Pathak

12 The Influence of Dietary Components on Gene Expression 227

Hamid Zand, Katayoun Pourvali, Azam Shakeri, and Asieh Mansour

13 Nutrigenomic Aspects of Vitamins 279
Fatemeh Rezaiian, Bahareh Nikooyeh,
and Tirang R. Neyestani

14 Nutrigenomic Aspects of Trace Elements ... 315
Sudabeh Motamed, Bahareh Nikooyeh,
and Tirang R. Neyestani

15 Prenatal Nutrition Exposure Leading to Adult Obesity, Diabetes, and Hypertension 377
Maryam Miraghajani, Hossein Hajianfar,
and Rasoul Salehi

16 Microbiome, Diet, and Health 405
Himaja Nallagatla, Hemalatha Rajkumar,
and Kamala Krishnaswamy

17 Genetic Susceptibility to Common Diseases and Diet Intakes. 423
Jayvadan Patel and Anita Patel

18 Nutrition and Healthy Aging. 451
Manjir Sarma Kataki, Ananya Rajkumari,
and Bhaskar Mazumder

19 The Role of Nutritional Factors in Pathogenesis of Diseases 483
Jayvadan Patel and Anita Patel

20 Gene-Based Dietary Advice and Eating Behavior. 515
Aparoop Das, Manash Pratim Pathak,
Pronobesh Chattopadhyay, and Yashwant V. Pathak

21 Dietary Fats and Cancer **529**
Ananya Rajkumari, Manjir Sarma Kataki,
and Bhaskar Mazumder

Index **557**

Series Preface

- Nutrigenomics is a field that is expanding significantly as the science of nutrition and genomics grows. The terms "Diet, DNA, gene–nutrient interactions, genes, the genome, human genome, metabolome, metabolomics, nutrigenetics, nutrition, nutritional genetics, nutritional genomics, nutritional guidelines, phenotype, polymerase chain reaction (PCR), polymorphisms, proteome, proteomics, single-nucleotide polymorphisms" are widely used by scientists and getting a special attention for solving global health care challenges. In recent years, the incidence of obesity, heart disease, and type 2 diabetes has dramatically increased. Because both diet and genetics are factors in these diseases, scientists are now examining the relationship between nutrients and gene expression.
- Nutrigenomics is looking at research that examines how diet affects gene expression across a person's entire genome. Nutrigenetics is an overlapping field that focuses on individual genes, rather than the entire genome, and how they relate to dietary requirements. A genome is the complete set of genetic material contained in an organism. Genes are the individual units that provide the instructions for proteins that perform all of the functions in the organism.
- Diseases can be classified into two groups: "monogenic" that involve only one gene, while others are "polygenic" that involve several genes. Changes in gene sequence, or mutations, due to many different reasons may cause disease depicted by changing gene expression levels. Because gene expression can also be altered by diet, scientists use both nutrigenomic and nutrigenetic approaches to understand the dietary basis of certain diseases.

- Nutrigenomics research also leads to identification of certain foods and single nutrients that can be consumed for an intended healthy effect on the consumers. Thus, nutraceuticals have a great potential to be used to prevent or treat a number of diseases, leading to better health for consumers.
- The scope of the CRC Press series *Nutraceuticals: Basic Research/ Clinical Applications* aims at bringing out a range of books edited by distinguished scientists and researchers who have significant experience in scientific pursuit and critical analysis. This series will address various aspects of nutraceuticals products, including the historical perspective, traditional knowledge base, analytical evaluations, and green food to processing and applications. The series will be very useful not only for researchers and academicians but will be a valuable reference for personnel in the nutraceuticals and food industries. Previously, we published several books in this series, including *Nutraceuticals and Health: Review of Human Evidence, Handbook of Metallonutraceuticals*, and *Marine Nutraceuticals*, to name a few. This series has been well received by academia as well as the scientific and industrial community in the field of nutraceuticals.

The newest addition to this series is this book, *Nutrigenomics and Nutraceuticals: Clinical Relevance and Disease Prevention*, edited by Dr. Yashwant V. Pathak and Dr. Ali M. Ardekani. This book is a collection of 21 chapters written by leading authorities in this field and covers wide aspects of nutrigenomics and nutraceuticals concerning clinical relevance and disease prevention. This will be a very useful reference book for scientists and academicians, as well as industry people who work in this area.

We welcome new book ideas for this series and enrich the series with your contributions.

Yashwant V. Pathak
University of South Florida

Preface

In the past decade, the evidence has become stronger for a direct link between increased genome/epigenome damage and increased risk for adverse health outcomes during a person's life. Genomics and related areas of research have contributed greatly to efforts to understand the cellular and molecular mechanisms underlying diet–disease relationships.

Environmental exposure to genotoxins is one of the key factors for genome stability; however, it is now exceedingly clear that micronutrients are critical as cofactors for many cellular functions, including DNA repair enzymes, methylation of CpG sequences, DNA oxidation, and/or uracil incorporation into DNA.

The field of nutrigenomics and nutraceuticals in recent years has been the focus of many researchers because it provides an opportunity to apply genomics knowledge to nutrition research, making associations between specific nutrients and gene expression that have significant relevance clinically and can be applied in disease prevention. Nutritional genomics (nutrigenomics) is considered one of the next pioneering research areas in the postgenomic era. Its fundamental premise is that while alterations in gene expression or epigenetic phenomena can subvert a healthy phenotype into manifesting chronic disease, through the introduction of certain nutrients and nutraceuticals, this process can be reversed or modified. Employing state-of-the-art genomic and proteomic investigations that monitor the expression of thousands of genes in response to diet, nutrigenomics investigates the occurrence of relationships between dietary nutrients and gene expression.

Individual differences at the genetic level influence response to diet, and these differences may be at the level of single-nucleotide polymorphisms. Integration and application of genetic and genomics technology

xiii

into nutrition research is, therefore, needed to develop nutrition research programs that are aimed at the prevention and control of chronic disease through genomics-based nutritional interventions.

Understanding how nutrition influences metabolic pathways is very important in our understanding of many human diseases. Because of the wide effects of diet on cellular metabolism and thus many human diseases, bringing the accumulated knowledge in this field to researchers worldwide can serve health communities that are interested in giving dietary advice based on individualized genomic data. The nutraceuticals market is growing significantly and is beneficial for better health for the people.

This book is envisioned to bring a new perspective on disease prevention strategy based on the genomic knowledge and nutraceuticals of an individual and the diet he or she receives. In this book, we bring together a wide spectrum of nutritional scientists worldwide to contribute to the growing knowledge in the field of nutrigenomics and nutraceuticals.

As the title below indicates, our view on this field is comprehensive and we believe that *Nutrigenomics and Nutraceuticals: Clinical Relevance and Disease Prevention* will become a reference book on this matter soon after its publication.

We would like to express our sincere thanks to all the chapter authors who contributed to this book; without their support this book would not have seen daylight. We would also like to express our gratitude to Steve Zollo, Sherry Thomas, Sylvester O'Gilvie, and Todd Perry at CRC Press/ Taylor & Francis Group, as well as Viswanth Prasanna and his team at Datapage, for their diligent efforts with the copyediting, proofreading, and production of this book.

Without our families and their kind support during this endeavor, it would not have been completed.

Last but not least, we have a request to all our readers: if you find any mistakes, kindly inform us. Any suggestions for improving the quality of this book will be greatly appreciated and will be incorporated in the second edition. Those academicians and professors who may use this book as a reference for their programs or classes, kindly do let us know.

Yashwant V. Pathak
University of South Florida

Ali M. Ardekani
Middle-Eastern Association for Cancer Research (MEACR)

Contributors

Adnan Ali, BS
College of Pharmacy
University of South Florida
Tampa, Florida

Ali M. Ardekani, PhD
Division of Medical Biotechnology
The National Institute of Genetic
  Engineering and Biotechnology
  (NIGEB)
Tehran, Iran

and

Middle-Eastern Association for
  Cancer Research (MEACR)
Montreal, Québec, Canada

Roland Cadet, PharmD
College of Pharmacy
University of South Florida
Tampa, Florida

Pronobesh Chattopadhyay
Defence Research Laboratory
Tezpur, India

Aparoop Das, PhD
Department of Pharmaceutical
  Sciences
Dibrugarh University
Dibrugarh, India

Aditya Grover, MD
Morsani College of Medicine
University of South Florida
Tampa, Florida

Hossein Hajianfar, PhD
School of Nursing and Midwifery
Flavarjan Islamic Azad University
Isfahan, Iran

and

School of Nursing and Midwifery
Isfahan Islamic Azad University
Isfahan, Iran

Manjir Sarma Kataki, PhD
Department of Pharmaceutical
  Sciences
Dibrugarh University
Dibrugarh, India

Christopher T. Kaul, MD
Morsani College of Medicine
University of South Florida
Tampa, Florida

**Kamala Krishnaswamy, MD,
FASc, FAPASc, FAMS, FNASc,
FNA, FIUNS, FNAAS, FTWAS**
Former Director
National Institute Nutrition &
    Emeritus Medical Scientist
Indian Council of Medical
    Research (ICMR)
Hyderabad, India

Amanda Lasher, PharmD
College of Pharmacy
University of South Florida,
Tampa, Florida

Rahul Maheshwari, PhD
Department of Pharmaceutics
BM College of Pharmaceutical
    Education & Research
Indore, India

Asieh Mansour, PhD
Cellular and Molecular Nutrition
    Department
Faculty of Nutrition and Food
    Technology
Shahid Beheshti University of
    Medical Sciences
Tehran, Iran

Bhaskar Mazumder, PhD
Department of Pharmaceutical
    Sciences
Dibrugarh University
Dibrugarh, India

Maryam Miraghajani, PhD
Department of Community Nutrition
School of Nutrition and Food Science

and

Food Security Research Center
Isfahan University of Medical
    Sciences
Isfahan, Iran

Nagashekhara Molugulu, PhD
School of Pharmacy
Department of Pharmaceutical
    Technology
International Medical University
Kuala Lumpur, Malaysia

Sudabeh Motamed, PhD
Laboratory of Nutrition Research
National Nutrition and Food
    Technology Research Institute

and

Faculty of Nutrition Sciences and
    Food Technology
Shahid Beheshti University of
    Medical Sciences
Tehran, Iran

Himaja Nallagatla, PhD
Department of Immunology and
    Microbiology
National Institute of Nutrition
    (NIN)
Indian Council of Medical
    Research (ICMR)
Hyderabad, India

Tirang R. Neyestani, PhD
Laboratory of Nutrition Research
National Nutrition and Food
  Technology Research Institute

and

Faculty of Nutrition Sciences and
  Food Technology
Shahid Beheshti University of
  Medical Sciences
Tehran, Iran

Bahareh Nikooyeh, PhD
Laboratory of Nutrition Research
National Nutrition and Food
  Technology Research Institute

and

Faculty of Nutrition Sciences and
  Food Technology
Shahid Beheshti University of
  Medical Sciences
Tehran, Iran

Anita Patel, MPharm, PhD
Faculty of Pharmacy
Sankalchand Patel University
Visnagar, Gujarat, India

Jayvadan Patel, MPharm, PhD, LLB, FICS
Faculty of Pharmacy
Sankalchand Patel University
Visnagar, Gujarat, India

Manash Pratim Pathak, PhD
Department of Pharmaceutical
  Sciences
Dibrugarh University
Dibrugarh, India

Yashwant V. Pathak, MPharm, EMBA, MS (Conflict Management), PhD
College of Pharmacy
University of South Florida
Tampa, Florida

Adela Pilav, PharmD
College of Pharmacy
University of South Florida
Tampa, Florida

Katayoun Pourvali, PhD
Cellular and Molecular Nutrition
  Department
Faculty of Nutrition and Food
  Technology
Shahid Beheshti University of
  Medical Sciences
Tehran, Iran

Charles Preuss, PhD
Morsani College of Medicine
University of South Florida
Tampa, Florida

Hemalatha Rajkumar, MD
Department of Clinical
Immunology and Microbiology
National Institute of Nutrition
Indian Council of Medical
  Research (ICMR)
Hyderabad, India

Ananya Rajkumari, PhD
Department of Pharmaceutical
  Sciences
Dibrugarh University
Dibrugarh, India

Nidhi Raval, PhD
National Institute of
  Pharmaceutical
  Education and Research
  (NIPER)—Ahmedabad
Gandhinagar, India

Fatemeh Rezaiian, PhD
Laboratory of Nutrition Research
National Nutrition and Food
  Technology Research Institute

and

Faculty of Nutrition Sciences and
  Food Technology
Shahid Beheshti University of
  Medical Sciences
Tehran, Iran

Rasoul Salehi, PhD
Department of Genetics and
  Molecular Biology
School of Medicine
Isfahan University of Medical
  Sciences
Isfahan, Iran

Raisah Salhab, PharmD
College of Pharmacy
University of South Florida
Tampa, Florida

Avipsha Sarkar, PhD
Department of Biotechnology
School of Biosciences and
  Technology
VIT University
Vellore, India

**Meenakshisundaram
  Selvamuthukumaran, PhD**
School of Food Science &
  Postharvest Technology
Institute of Technology
Haramaya University
Dire Dawa, Ethiopia

Shampa Sen, PhD
Department of Biotechnology
School of Biosciences and
  Technology
VIT University
Vellore, India

Azam Shakeri, PhD
Cellular and Molecular Nutrition
  Department
Faculty of Nutrition and Food
  Technology
Shahid Beheshti University of
  Medical Sciences
Tehran, Iran

and

Department of Pharmaceutical
  Sciences
Dibrugarh University
Dibrugarh, India

Namrata Soni, PhD
Faculty of Health Sciences
Sam Higginbottom Institute of
  Agriculture, Technology and
  Sciences (Deemed University)
Allahabad, India

Neetu Soni, PhD
Faculty of Health Sciences
Sam Higginbottom Institute of
  Agriculture, Technology and
  Sciences (Deemed University)
Allahabad, India

Muktika Tekade, PhD
TIT College of Pharmacy
Technocrats Institute of
  Technology Campus
Bhopal, India

xviii Contributors

Rakesh Kumar Tekade, PhD
National Institute of
  Pharmaceutical Education and
  Research (NIPER)—Ahmedabad
Gandhinagar, India

and

School of Pharmacy
Department of Pharmaceutical
  Technology
International Medical University
Kuala Lumpur, Malaysia

Hamid Zand, PhD
Cellular and Molecular Nutrition
  Department
Faculty of Nutrition and Food
  Technology
Shahid Beheshti University of
  Medical Sciences
Tehran, Iran

Applications of Nutrigenomics for Disease Prevention and Better Health

Adnan Ali and Yashwant V. Pathak
University of South Florida
Tampa, Florida

Ali M. Ardekani
Middle-Eastern Association for Cancer Research (MEACR)
Montreal, Québec, Canada

Contents

1.1 Nutrigenomics in the genomics and postgenomics age 1
1.2 Nutrigenomics: A brief introduction 2
1.3 A primer on genomics and beyond 3
    1.3.1 Genome-wide association studies 5
    1.3.2 Transcriptomics 5
    1.3.3 Epigenomics 8
1.4 Molecular biology tools for gene editing 10
    1.4.1 Obesity and the *FTO* locus 11
1.5 The microbiome 13
1.6 Conclusion 14
References 14

1.1 Nutrigenomics in the genomics and postgenomics age

The study of nutrition has long preceded the genomics age. Humans, since time immemorial, have been fascinated by how the nutrients we intake influence our health. In the late 1990s and early 2000s, a fundamental shift occurred in nutritional research. Many nutritional researchers, realizing that a fundamental understanding of how nutrition impacts health cannot be achieved without a thorough understanding of how nutritional pathways work on a molecular and genetic level, began to leverage new technologies and experimental data collected from the burgeoning age of sequencing (Müller and Kersten 2003).

With the ever-decreasing cost of DNA sequencing and other molecular biology advances, scientists have now gained an unprecedented ability to not only investigate how genetic variation impacts nutrition and health at a population level but also to dissect the basic molecular mechanisms and systems that integrate to regulate human nutrition. To gain a coherent understanding of nutrigenomics, one must first grasp the basic molecular tools and techniques that are used in modern-day genomics. Here, we will conduct a brief survey of the techniques and theories that underlie modern nutrigenomics. We will then illustrate the powerful uses of these tools through several case studies.

1.2 Nutrigenomics: A brief introduction

Nutrigenomics differs from traditional nutritional studies not only by the genomics-based methods by which it answers questions but also by integrating data from various systems to gain an integrative understanding of the gene–nutrition–disease associations at a mechanistic level, with the overall goal of creating personalized or adaptive nutritional regimes to promote better health and prevent disease. Therefore, nutrigenomics is concerned with both how nutrients impact gene expression or structure and how genetic differences impact the way nutrient response happens. To understand how genetics and nutrition interact, we must first discuss the impacts of the environment and genetics on phenotype. To start, one can write the following simple equation for the phenotype:

$$p = g + e$$

$$var\,(p) = var\,(g) + var\,(e) + 2cov\,(g,e)$$

The first equation states that the phenotype (p) is the sum of genetic (g) and environmental (e) factors. If we want to learn about the phenotypic variability of an individual, we can partition the phenotypic variance into the sum of genetic variation, environmental variation, and covariation between genetics and the environment (Simopoulos, 2010). The notion that a certain proportion of the variance in phenotype can be determined by genetics is encapsulated in the concept of *heritability*, which we can calculate for any phenotype. Heritability can be measured in several different ways, including broad-sense heritability, which is $H^2 = \dfrac{var(g)}{var(p)}$ (Hartl et al. 1997). A narrower definition of heritability, known as *narrow-sense heritability*, only takes into account additive genetic effects and excludes effects from dominance and allele-to-allele effects like epistasis. Narrow-sense heritability is denoted as $h^2 = \dfrac{var(g_{additive})}{var(p)}$. Nutrition itself is strictly an *environmental* effect, and its effects are captured by the portion of the phenotypic variability that is not heritable, in other words, $1 - H^2 = \dfrac{var(e) + 2cov(g,e)}{var(p)}$ (Hartl et al. 1997). It is perhaps illustrative to think about human height, a phenotype that is

2   Nutrigenomics and Nutraceuticals

determined by both genetics and environmental factors, such as nutritional intake. From a recent meta-analysis of many different height heritability studies, we currently estimate that the h^2 of height is at 0.73 ± 0.03 (Polderman et al. 2015). This means that environmental factors and gene–environment interactions impact the remaining 0.27 proportion of phenotypic variance not explained by genetics, of which nutrition and the interaction between genetics and nutrition play a critical role. It is extremely difficult to partition the remaining 0.27 into the proportion that is assigned to environment alone or gene-to-environment interactions. Nutrigenomics itself is primarily concerned with the nutrition–gene interactions and their impact on various important phenotypes, such as disease phenotypes. Although many other systems, such as the microbiome and the epigenome, may change the model we have just postulated, it is important to keep in mind that, depending on the traits, the effects of nutrition on phenotype are primarily exerted at the environment and the gene–environmental interaction levels (Simopoulos, 2010). However, genes alone do not exert any effect. They must be transcribed to mRNA to form the transcriptome, and then they must be translated to proteins to form the proteome before exerting their effects on phenotype. As a result, nutrigenomics is also fundamentally interested in the effects of nutrition at the transcriptomic and proteomic levels as well. Indeed, nutrigenomics takes a *systems-level* approach to understanding the effects of nutrition on the human body (Astley 2007; Müller and Kersten 2003) (Figure 1.1).

By combining genomics, transcriptomics, proteomics, epigenomics, metabolomics, proteomics, and functional genomics with state-of-the-art bioinformatics tools and molecular-biology tools, modern nutrigenomics can not only identify the gene–nutritional interactions but also dissect the mechanistic foundations at a systems level.

1.3 A primer on genomics and beyond

The most basic level at which genetics can influence nutrition is the DNA level. Variation in our DNA—mostly in the form of single nucleotide mutations known as *single nucleotide polymorphisms* (SNPs)—plays a critical role in determining the phenotypic variability in the human population. With advances in sequencing technology, we are now able to interrogate the entire human genome in large cohorts to ascertain the extent of human genetic variation. Large consortium studies such as the HapMap Project and the 1,000 Genomes Project have yielded many insights into the overall diversity of mutations in the human population (Altshuler et al. 2010; Auton et al. 2015). A typical human differs from the reference human genome at about 4.1–5.0 million sites across the genome, affecting over 20 million base pairs, with 99.9% of these sites being SNPs. Only about 2,000 variants per genome are associated with any documented diseases, and only about 24–30 variants per genome are implicated in rare diseases (Auton et al. 2015). Variants themselves can be

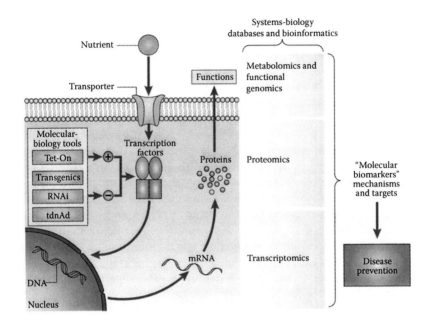

Figure 1.1 The systems-level schema of nutrigenomics. Although a number of tools have changed since the time when this figure was created—such as CRISPR-based systems for gene editing—the overall schema of how nutrigenomics is integrated at the systems level has remained largely the same. (Reproduced from Müller, M. & Kersten, S., Nat. Rev. Genet., 4, 4, 315–322, 2003.)

split between coding and noncoding variants, as coding variants lie directly in the coding regions of genes and may result in a conformational change of the protein, while noncoding variants may affect many other regulatory elements in the genome, including transcription factor binding sites or promoter regions. Assigning functional significance to coding variants is significantly easier than assigning functional impact to noncoding variants. Through resources made possible by the Exome Aggregation Consortium, we are now able to assign functional importance to nearly every coding variant observed in the human population (Lek et al. 2015). It is abundantly clear that many of these variants affect biological processes and pathways that are related to nutrition and especially gene–nutrition interactions. For example, rs671 is a classic missense SNP that produces a defective version of aldehyde dehydrogenase 2 (ALDH2), a key gene in the oxidative pathway of alcohol metabolism. Individuals with either one or two copies of the A-allele will suffer from facial flushing and severe hangovers (Takeuchi et al. 2011; Wang et al. 2013). Recent evidence has shown that rs671 affects more than just alcohol metabolism, as it has been significantly implicated (Sakiyama et al. 2016). The manner by which an individual can avoid the deleterious effects of this variant is simple: consume less alcohol. Indeed, it has been observed that individuals with this variant do in fact consume less alcohol, and when they do consume alcohol, the body is significantly less efficient at metabolizing alcohol (Takeuchi et al. 2011; Wang et al. 2013). This example involving ALDH2 is more of illustrative of *nutrigenetics*—the study of interactions between one gene and one nutrient; however, this term is now becoming increasingly merged together with *nutrigenomics*, as awareness grows that many nutritionally related genes are pleiotropic—one gene affecting multiple phenotypes—or that certain nutritionally related phenotypes are multigenic (Simopoulos 2010).

1.3.1 Genome-wide association studies

In order to ascertain which genetic variants are associated with a certain phenotype, scientists have leveraged the increasingly cheap cost of population-scale sequencing with sophisticated statistical analysis to pinpoint risk variants. Known as a *genome-wide association study* (GWAS), these studies have been critical in unearthing the variants involved in many (Altshuler et al. 2008). By leveraging microarrays (and increasingly, whole-exome or whole-genome sequencing), these studies have allowed massively parallel genotyping of individuals who differ in a particular phenotype (i.e., individuals who are obese versus those who are not obese). These variants can be either coding or noncoding. In Figure 1.2, the schema for a typical GWAS is presented (Kingsmore et al. 2008). In brief, by sequencing large cohorts (with $n > 1,000$ individuals) of cases and controls, scientists can use statistical analysis to identify the SNPs that are most associated with the risk of a certain trait. These studies are now commonplace and are the main bedrocks of modern population genetics. A number of GWAS experiments have focused on various subjects related to nutrition. For example, a massive GWAS of 339,224 individuals identified over 97 loci that accounted for ~2.7% of BMI variation, and on a genome-wide level common variants (alleles with minor allele frequency of more than 1%) accounted for over 20% of the variability in BMI (Locke et al. 2015). This study identified that many of the novel BMI-associated loci harbor genes associated with glutamate receptor activity and synaptic plasticity, leading to the potential environment interactions accounted for earlier. It is likely that many of the risk loci exert additional gene–nutrition effects beyond the gene-only effects studied in this GWAS. Indeed, it is a common trend for GWAS experiments to not factor diet or nutrition into their studies, when such information may be especially illuminating in terms of detailing the nutrition–genetic interactions that are critical to determining phenotype.

1.3.2 Transcriptomics

Although nutrigenetics is a critical part of understanding the effects of nutrients on the body, one must also examine what happens to genes after transcription. By studying the collective mRNA in a cell through technologies such as RNA sequencing (Figure 1.3) or microarray platforms, we can ascertain how nutrients change the expression level of various genes. A number of

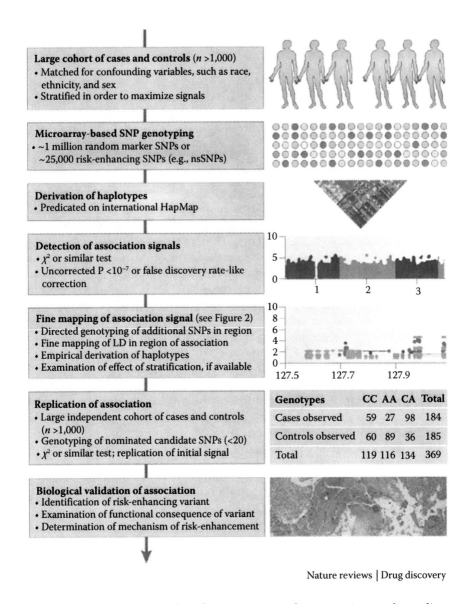

Figure 1.2 The typical workflow for a genome-wide association study to discover genetic variants that influence biological processes. In nutrigenomics, these association studies are typically conducted in search of genetic variation that might impact. (Reproduced from Kingsmore et al., Nat. Rev. Drug Discov., 7, 3, 221–230, 2008.)

key studies in nutrigenomics have analyzed the effects of different nutritional regimes on gene expression in key tissues. For example, Crujeiras et al. investigated whether obese men on or off low-calorie diet had differential gene expression in peripheral blood mononuclear cells. They found that several genes, including IL8, inflammatory genes, and oxidative stress genes, were

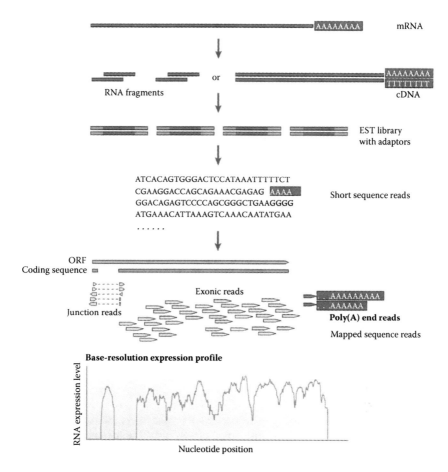

Figure 1.3 *A typical RNA-sequencing experiment. mRNA is typically fragmented and then adapted for shotgun sequencing, typically with Solexa sequencing. By mapping short reads onto a reference genome, we are able to ascertain the expression profiles of genes across the entire genome. (Reproduced from Wang et al., Nat. Rev. Genet., 10, 1, 57–63, 2009.)*

differentially changed when patients had their gene expression measured before and after a 8-week low-calorie diet (Crujeiras et al. 2008). Studies looking at gene expression differences between individuals who are obese and those who are not have been important in identifying the peroxisome proliferator activated receptor (PPAR) gamma as an important gene with profound effects on obesity and weight loss (Vidal-Puig et al. 1997). This gene is a key gene in nutrient sensing, since it binds fatty acids, and similar genes, such as liver X receptor alpha and retinoid X receptor, form a core complement of metabolic sensors diet respond to dietary and nutrient-related signals (Trivedi et al. 2011).

1.3.3 Epigenomics

One major factor in determining what genes are expressed or silenced is the epigenome of a cell. Referring to the complete set of epigenetic modifications—namely DNA methylation and histone modifications—the epigenome plays a key role in regulating the expression of genes in a cell. Although nearly every cell in the human body shares the same genome, different genes are turned on in different tissues. This regulatory framework is mediated by the epigenetic state of the cell. As we enter the postgenomics age, the epigenome plays an important role in nutrigenomics, especially since epigenetic memory is able to retain environmental memory and is critical in gene–environment interactions

The key components that modify the epigenome include DNA methylation and histone modifications. DNA methylation involves adding methyl groups to the fifth carbon in cytosine adjacent to a guanine. This dinucleotide sequence is termed a *CpG dinucleotide*. DNA methylation is carried out by DNA methyltransferases, and methylation typically represses gene expression. In particular, DNA methylation is critical in mammalian development, as key silencing steps—such as turning off pluripotency in early development—requires proper DNA methylation (Smith and Meissner 2013). Methylation is also critical in X-chromosome inactivation, in which one of the two X-chromosomes in human females is silenced, and imprinting, in which gene expression is controlled in a parent of origin-specific manner. DNA methylation can be assessed at the genome level with several different technologies, including bisulfite sequencing (Smith and Meissner 2013).

The other component of the epigenome is the vast array of different modifications of histone tails that can take place. Since the majority of the genome is packaged by histones into nucleosomes, which are then packaged into higher-order chromatin, the relative compactness or openness of the chromatin dictates whether a gene can be accessed or not. Although a variety of marks exist, prominent marks include H3K9me3, H3K27me3, H3K4me3, and H3K27ac. The nomenclature for these marks follows a specific pattern; we will demonstrate by dissecting H3K9me3: (1) we denote which histone subunit a mark is in (H3), (2) which residue the modification lies in (K9), and (3) what type of modification it is, for example, trimethylation (me3) or acetylation (ac). These marks exert various effects on the local chromatin structure; different marks (and combinations of marks) can promote or repress gene expression. By using chromatin immunoprecipitation, which involves using antibodies specific against certain histone marks to target regions of the genome for cross-linking, purification, and then sequencing, scientists have been able to accurately profile a number of histone marks on a genome-scale level. This histone-marking system is complex; however, the combinations of marks gives us a clue as to what each section of the genome is doing, even in noncoding regions (Consortium et al. 2015; Zhou et al. 2011). Chromatin organization can also occur at even higher levels, forming chromatin loops and topologically active domains that involve gene regulatory interactions at a 3D scale. These higher-order structures play a powerful epigenetic role by organizing the genome in a manner suitable for tissue-specific expression (Dixon et al. 2012; Gorkin et al. 2014). A schematic of how the epigenetic marks integrate together is presented in Figure 1.4. Recent work by the Roadmap Epigenome Project has cataloged a number of key epigenetic marks in various human tissues (Consortium et al. 2015). This resource has been critical in understanding the organization of the epigenome in human tissues, and nutrigenomics-related research has already seen the benefit of this research (Claussnitzer et al. 2015).

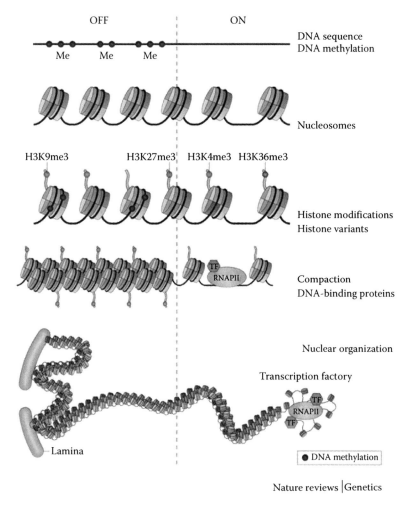

Figure 1.4 Key epigenetic modifications that are involved in gene regulation, as well as the 3D organization of DNA in the nucleus. (Reproduced from Zhou et al., Nat. Rev. Genet., *12, 1, 7–18, 2011.*)

Epigenetics has already played an important role in nutrigenomics, especially in determining the role that early-life (or even prenatal) nutrition has on chronic disorders. Studies have demonstrated that maternal overnutrition may contribute to increased likelihood of obesity in offspring. For example, offspring of rats on a low-protein diet demonstrate different liver gene expression, varying levels of gene promoter methylation, and differential histone modifications at key receptors, such as the previously discussed PPAR-gamma. Later in life, offspring whose parents were on a low-protein diet develop metabolic-related disorders and disorders with cardiovascular functions (Lillycrop et al. 2005). This finding shows the key role that epigenetics plays in nutrigenomics. As epigenomics profiling becomes less expensive, it is clear that such studies will reveal other nutritionally related phenotypes that are heavily influenced by epigenetics.

1.4 Molecular biology tools for gene editing

Although the various profiling experiments can pinpoint various genomic, transcriptomic, or epigenomic features that may influence nutrition, it is also critical to develop the tools to confirm that these feature are causal. Recent developments in genome (and epigenome) engineering tools have allowed scientists to make pinpoint corrections and edits to the genome and epigenome (Cong et al. 2013; Vojta et al. 2016). Recent developments in genome engineering, specifically in the development of CRISPR-Cas9 systems for targeted gene editing, have opened the door for specific edits of the eukaryotic genome by using a bacterial adaptive immune system known as the *CRISPR system*. The CRISPR system involves acquiring DNA elements from invading phages and then transcribing them into CRISPR RNAs (crRNAs) to guide cleavage of RNA or DNA. Several different classes of proteins mediate this guided cleavage process, one of which is Cas9. Cas9 is an RNA-guided nuclease with extremely high specificity, mainly due to Watson–Crick base pairing between the guide RNA and the target DNA site. Scientists have extraordinary freedom to engineer the desired alterations in the genome, by either using donor DNA to promote homology-directed repair or simply letting nonhomologous end joining occur, as depicted in Figure 1.5 (Wang et al. 2015). Scientists have recently realized that Cas9 targeting can be easily reprogrammed by reprogramming the guide RNA, allowing it to be an especially agile tool for DNA editing. Recent advances have improved the accuracy and specificity of CRISPR-based cleavage systems (Zetsche et al. 2015).

Not only can CRISPR systems be used for specific edits at the genome, but they can also be used for editing the epigenome. By using a nuclease-deactivated Cas9 protein fused with epigenetic modulators, such as histone demethylases or DNA demethylases, scientists have demonstrated remarkable accuracy and efficiency in editing the epigenome (Wang et al. 2015). However, epigenomics-based gene editing is still in its infancy, and the most powerful

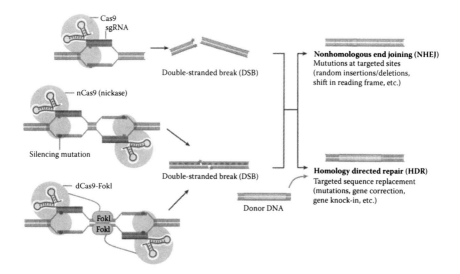

Figure 1.5 The various modes of CRISPR-Cas9–based editing of genomes. By either directing nonhomologous end joining or homology-directed repair, CRISPR-Cas9–based editing can create. (Reproduced from Wang et al., Ann. Rev. Biochem., 85, 227–264, 2015.)

uses of CRISPR have been as a genomics-based tool. CRISPR-based technology is more powerful as a screening role in determining the key functioning genes involved in a biological process. Recent developments in combinatorial CRISPR-based screening techniques have allowed high-throughput and massively parallel screening of key genes or known variants involved in a key biological process (Wong et al. 2016). Although it has only been applied to screening for cancer-inhibiting small molecules, one can easily imagine that such a tool can be used to screen for key genes involved in nutritional sensing or metabolic pathways.

1.4.1 Obesity and the FTO locus

The developments in epigenomics and transcriptomics sequencing and profiling technologies have led many scientists to state that we are now in a "postgenomics era." In order to demonstrate how these technologies can be integrated together to powerfully dissect the biological pathways involved in obesity, one can review the story of the *FTO* locus (a region that contains multiple genes). Obesity itself has been a key focus of nutrigenomics studies in recent years, due to its status as the most prevalent nutritional disorder in the developed world (Kussmann et al. 2006). As discussed earlier, the phenotypic variability that can be explained by common variants alone is around 20% (Locke et al. 2015), which suggests that nutrition and gene-to-nutrition interactions play a large role. Early studies, including ones by Frayling et al., demonstrated that a common variant in the *FTO* gene, rs9939609, was significantly associated with BMI and a predisposition to type 2 diabetes. Individuals who have the rs9939609 allele have decreased insulin sensitivity, generally low physical inactivity, and preferences for high caloric density in foods (Frayling et al. 2007; Simopoulos 2010). In fact, individuals with the risk genotypes at rs9939609 consumed between 125 and 280 kcal more than nonrisk individuals, even though there was no significant difference between energy expenditures between individuals with or without the risk allele (Speakman et al. 2008).

However, rs9939609 was not alone in being associated with obesity and BMI; soon, other studies implicated the entire *FTO* locus—a number of SNPs that also lie outside of the coding regions of the *FTO* gene—in type 2 diabetes and obesity. It was not until recently that a study published in the *New England Journal of Medicine* showed that one of the key *FTO*-associated noncoding variants plays a key role in adipocyte browning, lipid storage, and fatty acid oxidation (Claussnitzer et al. 2015).The authors of this study first used GWAS data to pinpoint several SNPs that were known to be highly associated with BMI. Next, they used epigenomics data from human cell lines to determine which of the SNPs are likely to be causal. By using bioinformatics tools, they were able to determine that rs1421085 T-to-C mutation, a noncoding variant, changed the binding of a transcription factor known as ARID5B, which represses two genes known as IRX3 and IRX5. Both IRX3 and IRX5 are key genes in adipocyte development and differentiation. By disrupting these repressive genes, adipocytes tend to shift away from a browning program to a whitening program; in other words, the adipocytes tend to lose mitochondrial thermogenesis, leading to greater lipid buildup (Figure 1.6). They also lose sensitivity to other thermogenic stimuli, such as exercise, exacerbating the effect. By repairing the allele to its nonrisk state in patient-derived primary adipocyte with CRISPR-Cas9, they were able to restore the browning expression program and restore thermogenesis, by a factor 7. Since this risk allele increases adipocyte fat storage programs, individuals with the risk allele

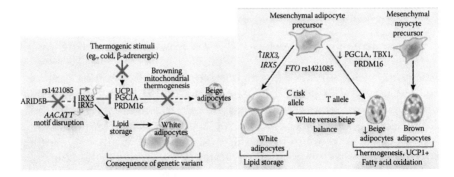

Figure 1.6 *On the left, the pathways leading from ARID5B to adipocyte browning. On the right, the overall biological network at play with rs1421085. (Reproduced from Claussnitzer et al., New Engl. J. Med., 373, 10, 895–907, 2015.)*

should avoid a high-fat diet. Although this nutrigenomics prediction was not explicitly tested in the study, it is reasonable to extrapolate this outcome from this study. However, this study illustrates the power of combining the genetic, epigenetic, and novel gene-editing tools to dissect a regulatory pathway that is critical to influencing metabolism and nutrition. This model can be applied to both coding and noncoding variants alike, hopefully leading to further discoveries in nutrigenomics that integrate the powerful developments of the genomics and postgenomics era.

1.5 The microbiome

What does the future hold for nutrigenomics? Given current advances in genomics, transcriptomics, and epigenomics, it is clear that more biological pathways and factors involved in nutritional response will be discovered in the future. However, it is clear that several other rapidly developing fields may influence the development of nutrigenomics. Chief among them is the study of the microbiome, which consists of the trillions of microbial microorganisms that inhabit our body. Of special concern is the gut microbiome, which has been shown to play an important role in determining our responses to various foods and dietary habits. In order to profile the gut microbiome, scientists can sequence the 16s portion of the ribosome, which yields an abundance of various microbial species. By sequencing the 16s portion of the ribosome, scientists can rapidly discern an abundance of various microbial clades in a population (Human Microbiome Project Consortium 2012). When placed on different diets, individuals' gut microbiomes undergo irreversible in their composition. These microorganisms provide essential functions to human health, such as synthesizing numerous amino acids that we cannot produce (David et al. 2014). A recent study by Zeevi and colleagues illustrates the power that the microbiome can possess in controlling nutritional response (Zeevi et al. 2015). By studying 800 people across 46,898 meals and collecting various physiological measurements, blood parameters, and gut microbiota samples, they were able to build a machine learning algorithm that was able to predict postprandial (postmeal) glycemic response (PPGR). High PPGR itself is a risk factor for various conditions linked with obesity, including diabetes and cardiovascular disease (Gallwitz 2009). Their model was validated on a held-out set of over 100 study participants, and it was demonstrated to be effective. Finally, they demonstrated that not only their algorithm is predictive but it can also suggest interventions in the form of personalized diets based on initial readings of a person's microbiome and physiological status. These personalized diets were successful in generating lower PPGR, showing that the microbiome plays an important predictive role in determining a personalized nutritional regime.

An even more striking study regarding the gut microbiome involves transplanting human fecal microbiota from twins with differing body mass into germ-free mice. The fecal bacteria were able to transmit obesity-associated metabolic phenotypes into the mice, and, even more strikingly, co-housing mice from the obese and thin donors prevented the development of obesity-associated phenotypes in the obese-transplanted mice (Ridaura et al. 2013). This prevention was associated with the invasion of members of the Bacteroidales order from the thin-transplanted mice into the obese-transplanted mice. This result shows that the gut microbiota plays a causal role in determining the body's response to nutrition, and it is clear that further research into the gut microbiota is necessary to understand why.

Is the study of the gut microbiome part of nutrigenomics? Regardless of whether or not the study of the microbiome itself is classified as nutrigenomics, it is clear that human genetics plays an important role in determining the composition of the gut microbiota. A recent GWAS was conducted with an isolated human population with the phenotype as the composition of their gut microbiota. This study found several associations between genes, such as *PLD1*, a gene previously associated with BMI, with microbiome composition (Davenport et al. 2015). Results such as this show that interactions between the microbiome and the genome (and the epigenome) no doubt play an important role in the regulation of the body's response to nutrition. Moreover, several disorders, such as inflammatory bowel disease, possess both microbiome-related signatures and gene-associated signatures (Cho and Brant 2011; Dicksved et al. 2008; Ferguson 2010). Deciphering the interactions between the host genome and the microbiome will play an important role not only in nutrigenomics but also in our understanding of the human health.

1.6 Conclusion

There are also other avenues of research not discussed at length here. Single-cell transcriptomics has begun revealing the hitherto-unnoticed heterogeneity in many human tissues; these discoveries, especially with regard to the gut, will no doubt play an important role in the development of nutrigenomics (Shapiro et al. 2013). Also not discussed at length here is the development of metabolomics and proteomics, two important fields that can (and should) be integrated with the previously discussed areas to build a systems-level understanding of the effects of nutrition. It is our hope that this review will introduce the readers to the basics of modern genomics and the wonderful opportunities it offers. It is clear that we are only at the beginning of working out the science behind nutrigenomics, and with the rapid development of novel technologies and theories, far more will be discovered in the coming decades regarding nutrigenomics.

References

Altshuler, D., Daly, M. J., & Lander, E. S. (2008). Genetic mapping in human disease. *Science, 322*(5903), 881–888. http://doi.org/10.1126/science.1156409

Altshuler, D. M., Gibbs, R. A., Peltonen, L., Dermitzakis, E., Schaffner, S. F., Yu, F., et al. (2010). Integrating common and rare genetic variation in diverse human populations. *Nature, 467*(7311), 52–58. http://doi.org/10.1038/nature09298

Astley, S. B. (2007). An introduction to nutrigenomics developments and trends. *Genes & Nutrition, 2*(1), 11–13. http://doi.org/10.1007/s12263-007-0011-z

Auton, A., Abecasis, G. R., Altshuler, D. M., Durbin, R. M., Abecasis, G. R., Bentley, D. R., et al. (2015). A global reference for human genetic variation. *Nature, 526*(7571), 68–74. http://doi.org/10.1038/nature15393

Cho, J. H., & Brant, S. R. (2011). Recent insights into the genetics of inflammatory bowel disease. *Gastroenterology, 140*(6), 1704–1712. http://doi.org/10.1053/j.gastro.2011.02.046

Claussnitzer, M., Dankel, S. N., Kim, K.-H., Quon, G., Meuleman, W., Haugen, C., et al. (2015). FTO obesity variant circuitry and adipocyte browning in humans. *New England Journal of Medicine, 373*(10), 895–907. http://doi.org/10.1056/NEJMoa1502214

Cong, L., Ran, F. A., Cox, D., Lin, S., Barretto, R., Habib, N., et al. (2013). Multiplex genome engineering using CRISPR/Cas systems. *Science, 339*(6121), 819–823. http://doi.org/10.1126/science.1231143

Consortium, R. E., Kundaje, A., Meuleman, W., Ernst, J., Bilenky, M., Yen, A., et al. (2015). Integrative analysis of 111 reference human epigenomes. *Nature, 518*(7539), 317–330. http://doi.org/10.1038/nature14248

Crujeiras, A. B., Parra, D., Milagro, F. I., Goyenechea, E., Larrarte, E., Margareto, J., et al. (2008). Differential expression of oxidative stress and inflammation related genes in peripheral blood mononuclear cells in response to a low-calorie diet: A nutrigenomics study. *OMICS: A Journal of Integrative Biology, 12*(4), 251–261. http://doi.org/10.1089/omi.2008.0001

Davenport, E. R., Cusanovich, D. A., Michelini, K., Barreiro, L. B., Ober, C., & Gilad, Y. (2015). Genome-wide association studies of the human gut microbiota. *PLoS One, 10*(11), e0140301. http://doi.org/10.1371/journal.pone.0140301

David, L. A, Maurice, C. F., Carmody, R. N., Gootenberg, D. B., Button, J. E., Wolfe, B. E., et al. (2014). Diet rapidly and reproducibly alters the human gut microbiome. *Nature, 505*(7484), 559–63. http://doi.org/10.1038/nature12820

Dicksved, J., Halfvarson, J., Rosenquist, M., Järnerot, G., Tysk, C., Apajalahti, J., et al. (2008). Molecular analysis of the gut microbiota of identical twins with Crohn's disease. *The ISME Journal, 2*(7), 716–727. http://doi.org/10.1038/ismej.2008.37

Dixon, J. R., Selvaraj, S., Yue, F., Kim, A., Li, Y., Shen, Y., et al. (2012). Topological domains in mammalian genomes identified by analysis of chromatin interactions. *Nature, 485*(7398), 376–380. http://doi.org/10.1038/nature11082

Ferguson, L. R. (2010). Nutrigenomics and inflammatory bowel diseases. *Expert Review of Clinical Immunology, 6*(4), 573–583. http://doi.org/10.1586/eci.10.43

Frayling, T. M., Timpson, N. J., Weedon, M. N., Zeggini, E., Freathy, R. M., Lindgren, C. M., et al. (2007). A common variant in the FTO gene is associated with body mass index and predisposes to childhood and adult obesity. *Science, 316*(5826), 889–894. http://doi.org/10.1126/science.1141634

Gallwitz, B. (2009). Implications of postprandial glucose and weight control in people with type 2 diabetes: Understanding and implementing the International Diabetes Federation guidelines. *Diabetes Care, 32*(Suppl 2), S322–S325. http://doi.org/10.2337/dc09-S331

Gorkin, D. U., Leung, D., & Ren, B. (2014). The 3D genome in transcriptional regulation and pluripotency. *Cell Stem Cell, 14*(6), 762–775. http://doi.org/10.1016/j.stem.2014.05.017

Hartl, D. L., Clark, A. G., & Clark, A. G. (1997). *Principles of Population Genetics* (Vol. 116). Sinauer associates, Sunderland.

Human Microbiome Project Consortium. (2012). Structure, function and diversity of the healthy human microbiome. *Nature, 486*(7402), 207–214. http://doi.org/10.1038/nature11234

Kingsmore, S. F., Lindquist, I. E., Mudge, J., Gessler, D. D., & Beavis, W. D. (2008). Genome-wide association studies: Progress and potential for drug discovery and development. *Nature Reviews. Drug Discovery, 7*(3), 221–230. http://doi.org/10.1038/nrd2519

Kussmann, M., Raymond, F., & Affolter, M. (2006). OMICS-driven biomarker discovery in nutrition and health. *Journal of Biotechnology, 124*(4), 758–787. http://doi.org/10.1016/j.jbiotec.2006.02.014

Lek, M., Karczewski, K., Minikel, E., Samocha, K., Banks, E., Fennell, T., et al. (2015). Analysis of protein-coding genetic variation in 60,706 humans. *bioRxiv*. Retrieved from http://biorxiv.org/content/early/2015/10/30/030338.abstract

Lillycrop, K. A., Phillips, E. S., Jackson, A. A., Hanson, M. A., & Burdge, G. C. (2005). Dietary protein restriction of pregnant rats induces and folic acid supplementation prevents epigenetic modification of hepatic gene expression in the offspring. *Journal of Nutrition, 135*(6), 1382–1386. http://doi.org/135/6/1382 [pii]

Locke, A. E., Kahali, B., Berndt, S. I., Justice, A. E., Pers, T. H., Day, F. R., et al. (2015). Genetic studies of body mass index yield new insights for obesity biology. *Nature, 518*(7538), 197–206. http://doi.org/10.1038/nature14177

Müller, M., & Kersten, S. (2003). Nutrigenomics: Goals and strategies. *Nature Reviews Genetics, 4*(4), 315–322. http://doi.org/10.1038/nrg1047

Polderman, T. J. C., Benyamin, B., de Leeuw, C. A., Sullivan, P. F., van Bochoven, A., Visscher, P. M., et al. (2015). Meta-analysis of the heritability of human traits based on fifty years of twin studies. *Nature Genetics, 47*(7), 702–709. http://doi.org/10.1038/ng.3285

Ridaura, V. K., Faith, J. J., Rey, F. E., Cheng, J., Duncan, A. E., Kau, A. L., et al. (2013). Gut microbiota from twins discordant for obesity modulate metabolism in mice. *Science, 341*(6150), 1241214–1241214. http://doi.org/10.1126/science.1241214

Sakiyama, M., Matsuo, H., Nakaoka, H., Yamamoto, K., Nakayama, A., Nakamura, T., et al. (2016). Identification of rs671, a common variant of ALDH2, as a gout susceptibility locus. *Scientific Reports, 6*, 25360. http://doi.org/10.1038/srep25360

Shapiro, E., Biezuner, T., & Linnarsson, S. (2013). Single-cell sequencing-based technologies will revolutionize whole-organism science. *Nature Reviews. Genetics, 14*(9), 618–30. http://doi.org/10.1038/nrg3542

Simopoulos, A. P. (2010). Nutrigenetics/Nutrigenomics. *Annual Review of Public Health, 31*(1), 53–68. http://doi.org/10.1146/annurev.publhealth.031809.130844

Smith, Z. D., & Meissner, A. (2013). DNA methylation: Roles in mammalian development. *Nature Reviews Genetics, 14*(3), 204–220. http://doi.org/10.1038/nrg3354

Speakman, J. R., Rance, K. A., & Johnstone, A. M. (2008). Polymorphisms of the FTO gene are associated with variation in energy intake, but not energy expenditure. *Obesity, 16*(8), 1961–1965. http://doi.org/10.1038/oby.2008.318

Takeuchi, F., Isono, M., Nabika, T., Katsuya, T., Sugiyama, T., Yamaguchi, S., et al. (2011). Confirmation of ALDH2 as a major locus of drinking behavior and of its variants regulating multiple metabolic phenotypes in a Japanese population. *Circulation Journal : Official Journal of the Japanese Circulation Society, 75*(4), 911–8.

Trivedi, R., Patel, P. N., Jani, H. J., & Trivedi, B. A. (2011). Nutrigenomics: From molecular nutrition to prevention of disease. *BioTechnology: An Indian Journal, 5*(2), 112–116. http://doi.org/10.1016/j.jada.2006.01.001

Vidal-Puig, A. J., Considine, R. V, Jimenez-Liñan, M., Werman, A., Pories, W. J., Caro, J. F., et al. (1997). Peroxisome proliferator-activated receptor gene expression in human tissues. Effects of obesity, weight loss, and regulation by insulin and glucocorticoids. *Journal of Clinical Investigation, 99*(10), 2416–2422. http://doi.org/10.1172/JCI119424

Vojta, A., Dobrinić, P., Tadić, V., Bočkor, L., Korać, P., Julg, B., et al. .. (2016). Repurposing the CRISPR-Cas9 system for targeted DNA methylation. *Nucleic Acids Research, 44*(12), 5615–5628. http://doi.org/10.1093/nar/gkw159

Wang, H., La Russa, M., & Qi, L. S. (2015). CRISPR/Cas9 in genome editing and beyond. *Annual Review of Biochemistry, 85,* 227–264. http://doi.org/10.1146/annurev-biochem-060815-014607

Wang, Y., Zhang, Y., Zhang, J., Tang, X., Qian, Y., Gao, P., et al. (2013). Association of a functional single-nucleotide polymorphism in the ALDH2 gene with essential hypertension depends on drinking behavior in a Chinese Han population. *Journal of Human Hypertension, 27*(3), 181–186. http://doi.org/10.1038/jhh.2012.15

Wang, Z., Gerstein, M., & Snyder, M. (2009). RNA-Seq: A revolutionary tool for transcriptomics. *Nature Reviews Genetics, 10*(1), 57–63. http://doi.org/10.1038/nrg2484

Wong, A. S. L., Choi, G. C. G., Cui, C. H., Pregernig, G., Milani, P., Adam, M., et al. (2016). Multiplexed barcoded CRISPR-Cas9 screening enabled by CombiGEM. *Proceedings of the National Academy of Sciences, 113*(9), 2544–2549. http://doi.org/10.1073/pnas.1517883113

Zeevi, D., Korem, T., Zmora, N., Israeli, D., Rothschild, D., Weinberger, A., et al. (2015). Personalized nutrition by prediction of glycemic responses. *Cell, 163*(5), 1079–1094. http://doi.org/10.1016/j.cell.2015.11.001

Zetsche, B., Gootenberg, J. S., Abudayyeh, O. O., Slaymaker, I. M., Makarova, K. S., Essletzbichler, P., et al. (2015). Cpf1 Is a single RNA-guided endonuclease of a class 2 CRISPR-cas system. *Cell, 163*(3), 759–771. http://doi.org/10.1016/j.cell.2015.09.038

Zhou, V. W., Goren, A., & Bernstein, B. E. (2011). Charting histone modifications and the functional organization of mammalian genomes. *Nature Reviews Genetics, 12*(1), 7–18. http://doi.org/10.1038/nrg2905

2

Omics-Driven Novel Technologies in Food and Nutrition Research

Rakesh Kumar Tekade
National Institute of Pharmaceutical Education and Research (NIPER)
Ahmedabad, Gandhinagar, India
and
International Medical University
Kuala Lumpur, Malaysia

Namrata Soni and Neetu Soni
Sam Higginbottom Institute of Agriculture, Technology and
Sciences (Deemed University), Allahabad, India

Rahul Maheshwari
BM College of Pharmaceutical Education & Research
Indore, India

Nidhi Raval
National Institute of Pharmaceutical Education and Research (NIPER)
Ahmedabad, Gandhinagar, India

Nagashekhara Molugulu
International Medical University
Kuala Lumpur, Malaysia

Muktika Tekade
TIT College of Pharmacy
Bhopal, India

Contents

2.1 Introduction 20
    2.1.1 What is omics technology? 20
    2.1.2 History of omics 22
    2.1.3 "Ome" and "omics" 22
2.2 Omics techniques applied in the field of nutrition 23
    2.2.1 Nutritional genomics or nutrigenomics 23
        2.2.1.1 Genomics (gene analysis) 25
        2.2.1.2 Proteomics (protein expression analysis) 26
        2.2.1.3 Transcriptomics (gene expression analysis) 29
        2.2.1.4 Metabolomics (metabolite profiling) 30
2.3 Effect of food on gene 32
    2.3.1 Effect of alcohol 33
    2.3.2 Effect of caffeine 36
    2.3.3 Effect of dietary fat 37
    2.3.4 Effect of fruits and vegetables 38
2.4 Food safety, quality, and traceability with MS-based
"omics" approaches 39
    2.4.1 Assessment of exogenous food contaminants 39
    2.4.2 Assessment of food allergens 41
    2.4.3 Assessment of pathogens and microbiological toxins 44
    2.4.4 Consequences of genetic modifications 47
2.5 Future trends of omics technology in food and nutrition 48
2.6 Conclusion 49
2.7 Acknowledgments 49
References 49

2.1 Introduction

2.1.1 What is omics technology?

Over the last few decades, much attention has been gained by nano-based medicines (Dhakad et al. 2013; Maheshwari et al. 2012) and omics-based technologies, although the nano delivery of drugs using different techniques (Maheshwari et al. 2015; Tekade and Chougule 2013) and omics developments are two different aspects. In recent times, "omics"-based sciences have been attaining momentous attraction by the scientific community. Nowadays, the impact of diet and dietary constituents on human health has been revealed, and the areas related to it are nutrition, nutrient–gene interaction, and nutritional biomarkers. In addition, some non-essential nutrients and bioactive food components are also altering genetic and epigenetic events in the human body (Xu 2017).

Recent advances in pharmaceutical technology allow the monitoring of multiple molecules (small/macro) with simultaneous monitoring of intracellular and extracellular pathways. RNA (transcriptome), proteins (proteome), and

20   **Nutrigenomics and Nutraceuticals**

intermediary metabolites (metabolome) are part of the cellular molecular family and are measured by new "global" techniques called "omics" technologies (Meyer et al. 2013). These omics technologies are capable of characterizing most of the members of the molecular family in a single cycle of analysis. Omics is half-way between biology and technology, which is utilized to explore the system in a wide spectrum of biology and medicine (Ning and Lo 2010).

Interestingly, omics covers all the parameters and provides vital information on nutritional status. Omics technologies consider the nature of the human biological system and its response to particular stimuli and also the interaction network between nutrients and molecules in the biological system. Advances in omics technologies have also made possible the characterization of functional aspects of biological processes and genetic sequence alterations within individuals and genus, which were not possible with older technologies (Kussmann et al. 2006).

Evaluating and assessing the importance of the interrelationship between biological food elements with the physiological system of the body in the context of omics (genomics, transcriptomics, proteomics, and metabolomics) will be of great help in understanding the disease pattern and its prevention. At the present time, the huge availability of omics data accounts for the tremendous developments in systems biology. Stakeholders in the pharma and other related industries are required to explore on this omics information in-depth to improve their research methodology. Systems biology has all such tools that enable to improve innovation in omics by providing the methodology, computational qualifications, and interdisciplinary capabilities (Kakoti et al. 2015).

Genetics discovered that a single gene is responsible for genetic variation in biological response and adverse reactions (to drugs) in individual. The term "omics" includes whole genome, drug response, and drug development efforts (Goetz et al. 2004). Omics medication is of vital significance in personalized medicine, which involves comprehensive and preventative diagnosis and treatment of the disorder using genomic, transcriptomic, proteomic, and metabolomic data (Meyer et al. 2012).

Business opportunities are growing tremendously as various pharma majors, including biotechnology research organizations, start to collect and connect several types of omics data into a more sound computational system. Apart from that, many bioinformatics-based companies are coming with the rising interest towards offering systems biology solutions to drug manufacturers and analytical companies. Omics approaches have much significance and potential, and they can be used to increase the conceptual basics of normal physiological responses in addition to disease physiology and play a crucial part in the prediction, etiology, and diagnosis of diseases (Xu 2017).

The Omics technology is increasingly employed in molecular discovery and evaluation of adverse effects and clinical efficacy. The interface between genomics and pharmacology is pharmacogenomics, and an investigation of the function of inheritance in an individual variation in drug response can be significantly employed to individualize and optimize medication efficacy. Omics technology is of vital significance in the treatment of cancer, because of the associated high rate of undesirable side effects and severe systemic toxicity. Advances in omics strategies, especially in various forms of metastasis, blood-related disorders, and obesity, provide the opportunity to select new targets for therapy and drug development. Systems biology utilizes novel strategies that will be predictive, preventive, and personalized, as a futuristic approach. Ongoing advances in obstetrics and gynecology are reaping the benefits of omics technological potential (Davis et al. 2017).

2.1.2 History of omics

The term "omics" was invented by Hans Winkler in 1920 and derived from the term genome (hence "genomics"). The term, even if the use of "ome" is older, signifies the "collectivity" of a set of things. The word *genomics* is said to come into existence in the 1980s and became widely used in the 1990s. The first genome was completely sequenced by Sanger in Cambridge, UK, in the 1970s. The genome is the most fundamental part of many omics. The suffix "-om-" originated as a back-formation from "genome," a word formed in analogy with "chromosome." The word "chromosome" comes from the Greek stems meaning "color" and "body" (Pirih and Kunej 2017; Eisen 2012).

The word genomics implies some hidden network among genetic elements. This network is regulated by many other omics such as proteomics, transcriptomics, metabolomics, and physiomics. It was Brennan who first demonstrated the term nutrigenetics in 1975 and came out with the idea of "nutrigenetics as a new concept for relieving hypoglycemia." Since that time, nutrigenetics has been used as structural frame for the improvement of genotype-dependent novel foods for health management and diagnosis of chronic disorders (Cozzolino and Cominetti 2013). There are general dietary protocols available for the management of genetic variation on dietary responses (Davis et al. 2017).

2.1.3 "Ome" and "omics"

The suffix *–ome* is the main suffix behind the terms "ome" and "omics." Its long history links this suffix to a lot of already existing terminologies with either speculative or tangible meaning, such as genome, proteome, transcriptome, and metabolome. Omics technologies enable a complete analysis of the cell or body of an organism. The primary function of omics technologies is the collective detection of genes, mRNA, metabolites, and proteins (Figure 2.1) in a particular biosample with a nontargeted and nonbiased approach. Adding to omics technology, systems biology is nothing but the high-dimensional biological integration of these techniques (Stepczynska et al. 2016).

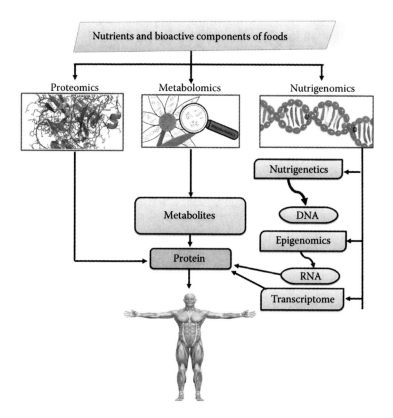

Figure 2.1 Relationship between nutrigenomics and the human body.

2.2 Omics techniques applied in the field of nutrition

From the perspective of foodomics, proteomics, metabolomics, and transcriptomics are the optimized diagnostic platform implemented in the measurement of proteins and metabolites in gene expression (Kussmann et al. 2006). Omics methodologies were developed to recognize the outcomes of cells, tissues, or organs, which in turn emerged as a novel discipline termed systems biology (Hood et al. 2004). Therefore, it is considered an integrated strategy to understand biological processes at cellular or organ level by using, estimating, and analyzing genomic, proteomic, and metabolic statistics (Raqib and Cravioto 2009). Wide knowledge of nutrigenomics is a first prerequisite to understanding healthy phenotypes.

2.2.1 Nutritional genomics or nutrigenomics

Since Hippocrates, it has been well recognized that nutrition plays a very significant role in health maintenance and people have been recommended to consider "food intake as a real medicine." Modern science suggested that the intake of not only specific nutrients but also specific quantities of each and every nutrient is important and essential for an optimal condition of health maintenance (McKenzie et al. 2017). It has been accounted that nutrition can directly contribute to disease manifestation (nutrients/food generally interact with the genes in a "benign" way, but in some circumstances, this interaction can also have fatal consequences) (Kaput 2004). Human health is affected by both environmental factors (diet, smoking, education, physical activity, etc.) and heredity factors, and both factors should be given the same consideration, for the maintenance of the state of health (Castle 2008).

Nutrigenomics involves the understanding of the effect of food on our genes and the way we respond to nutrients considering individual genetic variations. It also involves genetic variation as a consequence of the interaction between diet and disease (Zeisel 2007). In our daily diet, general dietary elements affect our health and nutrigenomics enables us to analyze the genetic perceptive in context. Genetic predisposition is believed to participate in a key function in analyzing every single issue of developing a definite health problem.

Nutrigenomics provides the source for personalized diet management based on the individual's genetic arrangement, and this strategy has been implemented since many years for certain diseases caused by a single gene and for common complex disorders, and to fabricate tools to diagnose genetic predisposition and to treat common disorders decades before their manifestation (Braicu et al. 2017). Nutrigenomics has gained a lot of attention recently because of its potential for treating, diagnosing, and curing severe disease including cancers, through small but highly informative dietary changes (Kornman et al. 2004).

Nutritional genomics cover the response to bioactive food components, the changes induced by nutrients on DNA methylation, chromatin alterations (Ross 2007), and nutrients-induced gene expression (nutritional transcriptomics). Nutrigenomics and nutrigenetics are an emerging area of development carrying huge possibilities for future treatment therapies, for example, for certain diseases such as degenerative diseases that increase with DNA impairment, which is also attributed to nutritional status. Nutrigenomics mainly involves an identified interaction among food and inherited genes known as an "inborn error of metabolism." One example is phenylketonuria (inborn metabolic error of the amino acid phenylalanine), produced by an alteration in an individual gene. Currently, the primary results involving gene–diet interactions for blood-related disorders, obesity, diabetes, inflammatory bowel disease, and cancer are encouraging, but most of them are uncertain (Ferguson 2013). Therefore, much attention is required in this field with special focus on integration of diverse fields and exhaustive studies designed to appropriately investigate gene–environment interactions (Oommen et al. 2005).

Despite the multifaceted challenges, initial level outcomes strongly indicate that the concept of nutrigenomics will be functional and able to exploit information contained in genetic makeup to attain successful aging using

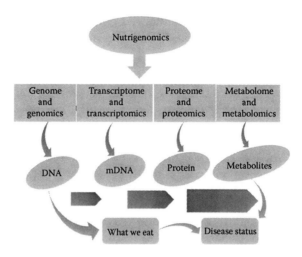

Figure 2.2 *Different field of nutrigenomics.*

behavioral alterations; nutrition will be the basis of this endeavor. The different fields of nutrigenomics are depicted in Figure 2.2. The area of nutrigenomics has exploited various fields and involves dietary impact on genome stability, epigenome changes (DNA methylation), RNA and micro-RNA expression (transcriptomics), protein expression (proteomics), and metabolite modifications (metabolomics). All of these can be investigated independently (Cooney et al. 2002).

2.2.1.1 Genomics (gene analysis)

Genomics is the study of an organism's genome or genetic material. It is the latest area to study the diverse, biological manifestation of the genome where novel technologies were employed to expose the static sequences of genes (Carlson et al. 2004). The "genomic" perspective of nutrigenomics is to impart a great deal of interest and its alterations in the nucleotide sequence of genes under the influence of diets. These alterations are identified as single-nucleotide polymorphisms (SNPs), which are able to alter characteristics of individuals like susceptibility to some lifestyle-based diseases, nutrient requirements, and sensitivity to insufficient diet composition (Hirschhorn and Daly 2005).

One of the most prominent techniques for measuring SNPs is DNA microarray estimation. DNA microarrays are miniaturized, sequenced arrangements of nucleic acid fragments of individual genes positioned in definite places with strong support, and they can detect alterations in the expression of multiple of genes simultaneously by specific hybridization in multiple samples in parallel and identify the effect of different nutrients (Clarke et al. 2013). Tanaka et al. (2016) reported that in recent times, whole-genome sequencing technologies have appeared as innovative and enhanced output schemes to estimate gene expression, epigenetic changes, and DNA–protein binding.

Ushiama et al. reported a gene expression analysis of energy metabolism-associated genes in the livers of rats by DNA microarray technology. The rats were permitted to feed for 6.0 h prior to fasting, and the results were different in the rats those fasted for 18.0 versus 24.0 h. In addition, refeeding mimicked regulation of the genes coding immunoproteasome components (Ushiama et al. 2010). The wide-ranging advantage of DNA microarray measurement and SNPs of multiple of sites can be estimated at once. The data inferred from SNP estimation may then be implemented to tailor-made nutrition, which is also known as order-made or individualized nutrition. Van der Lee et al. analyzed the effect of calorie restriction by DNA microarray technique. They showed that increase in the durability of calorie restriction varied the expression of genes like those associated with DNA disturbance, metabolic imbalance, and protein over expression (Tibshirani et al. 2015). The investigation was further explored many times to demonstrate the effects of calorie restriction on gene expression profiles in many tissues in a multiple of animal species.

2.2.1.2 Proteomics (protein expression analysis)

The proteome is regarded as the total protein component of an individual cell. Proteomics measurement permits modification in protein expression prototypes and their character to be exhibited and analyzed together (Wu et al. 2012). The global total protein component analysis of the genome expressed in an individual cell, in plasma or in serum, comprises its potential to identify biomarkers that work in response to alteration in diet or to therapy, which may have analytical means of modeling responses. Proteomics has functionalized nutritional investigations on a vast scale; in addition, it is also beneficial over transcriptome profiling methodologies, in which it directly evaluates biological processes (Gouw et al. 2010).

Currently, mass spectroscopy (MS) technology has potential to analyze, identify, and quantify hundreds of proteins in an individual test sample. It also has the potential to characterize post-translational changes and protein response numbers (Domon and Aebersold 2010; Walther and Mann 2010). An example of the technique that commonly involves digesting proteins in the sample into peptides is trypsin and its identification and extraction of small fractions of the peptides. Most of these techniques depend on a bottom-up proteomic strategy, more accurately, in coalition of the classical 2-DE fractionation of proteins and MS analysis of the in-gel digested proteins. Further, the peptides are subjected to ionization and then the mass-to-charge ratio is analyzed.

Frequently, a combination of mass analyzers are used in sequence separation after fragmentation and this step is known as tandem MS or MS/MS, and the spectra produced by it can be used in resolving the amino acid sequence. This is how proteins are evaluated by employing bioinformatics tools.

26   Nutrigenomics and Nutraceuticals

Norheim et al. (2011) successfully demonstrated tandem MS technique in analyzing the skeletal muscle secretome. The peptides that secrete myokines from the skeletal muscle in response to muscle contractions exert a paracrine/endocrine effect. These myokines might have a mediating role in the advantageous effects of physical exercise. The excreted proteins of cultured human myotubes were recognized by liquid chromatography mass spectroscopy (LC-MS) measurement of the conditioned cell culture media. However, 236 proteins were identified, of which almost 15 proteins were excreted and had increased mRNA expression in biopsies of healthy individuals from their *m. vastus lateralis* and/or *m. trapezius* after less than 3 months of strength training.

The virtual or precise measurement of peptides can be done by using MS, either by the approach of applied labelling of peptides or by using label-free techniques before MS investigation based on spectral characters. On the contrary, the stable isotopes such as isobaric tags for relative and absolute quantitation are covalently complexed all peptides in a sample (Unwin et al. 2010). In the metabolic labelling approach, the cells and their proteomes are marked by developing them in heavy or light isotopes of an essential amino acid media, which is known as stable isotope labelling with amino acids in cellular culture (SILAC) (Ong et al. 2002). Heavy isotope-labelled model organisms, for example, rodents, are also accessible, permitting systemic studies (Gouw et al. 2010). These labelling approaches have generally differentially labelled samples that are pooled and peptides are sequenced and quantified simultaneously.

Using the SILAC technique, Forner et al. (2009) studied the mitochondrial proteomes of two differently colored adipose tissues in mice. They compared each tissue to a SILAC-labelled control fragment from cultured cells, and the outcomes revealed many exciting differences. Another study reported a label-free approach to measure transformation in protein composition in a skeletal muscle concerned with insulin resistance, and it revealed a decreased profusion of mitochondrial proteins as compared to the muscle tissue of healthy volunteers (Hwang et al. 2010).

Schwer et al. (2009) also utilized a label-free technique and revealed dramatic, tissue-specific changes for the measurement of lysine acetylation of mitochondrial proteins during energy restriction, as studied in mice. The acetylation of mitochondrial proteins was initially controlled in brown adipose tissue and liver. The MS was employed to determine particular proteins with modified acetylation, and 72 candidate proteins involved in metabolic processes were demonstrated in the liver. Selected reaction monitoring is a targeted mass spectrometry approach that is an innovative tool in the area of metabolomics and proteomics as well as a complement to untargeted shotgun techniques (Picotti and Aebersold 2012). This approach is specifically advantageous when premeasured pairs of proteins, like those involved in the composition of cellular networks or sets of candidate biomarkers, are required to be analyzed in a number of samples in a precise manner.

Currently, there is a tremendous technological outbreak in the area of proteomics. Utilization of tryptic digestion, chromatography, MS, antibodies, and bioinformatics together with biological methods creates several novel opportunities for futuristic nutritional research.

Bioinformatics and the science of proteomics with computing and restructuring is an innovative novel technique to learn various patterns of gene/protein expression and have predominant value in drug discovery (Petricoin et al. 2002), in biotechnology (Washburn and Yates 2000), and in pathological advancement including diagnosis of cancer cells (Mariani 2003; Rai and Chan 2004). However, unfortunately, only a few reports on nutritional proteomics were found so far, and many of them used rodents as the animal model or human cells as the culture media (Fuchs et al. 2005; Wenzel et al. 2004). In another study, Dieck et al. correlated an enhanced liver fat content with impaired fatty acid metabolism, which was generally seen as a Zn deficiency in the rat by the combined application of microarray and proteome measurement methods. Herzog et al. (2004) and Wenzel et al. (2004) characterized the target proteins of flavonoid action in colonic metastasis by the use of proteome determination (Dieck et al. 2005). Fuchs et al. (2005) revealed the putative anti-atherosclerotic actions of genistein in endothelial culture stressed with oxidized low-density lipoprotein or homocysteine with proteome determination. A two-dimensional (2D) gel electrophoresis technique was explored by Gianazza et al. to find out the effect of cobalamin deficiency on the proteome of cerebrospinal fluid in different rat models. In this study, they found that in total gastrectomized rats, there was an enhancement in absolute protein in cerebrospinal fluid, which reached a peak 4 months after the surgery (Gianazza et al. 2003). In rats kept in a cobalamin-deficient state by dietary depletion, a similar peak was observed 6 months after the introduction of the diet. The 4-month peak in protein concentration was related to a particular elevation in a 1-antitrypsin and the *de novo* appearance of thiostatin and haptoglobin-b, nonetheless all of these alterations were corrected by the addition of cobalamin.

Linke et al. (2004) demonstrated the utilization of proteomics to plasma samples from rats with differing retinol status. Plasma samples were measured directly employing surface-enhanced laser desorption/ionization–time-of-flight (SELDI-TOF) MS. Prefractionation of the samples by anion-exchange chromatography, using 96-well filter plates, was exhibited to significantly upregulate the total number of peptides and proteins diagnosed by this technique. Some proteins with a molecular mass ranging from 10,000 to 20,000 were revealed to be present at decreased concentration in the plasma of retinol-deficient rats, and the investigators concluded that their technique provides a novel means of tracing alterations in nutritional status at the whole-body level.

Park et al. (2004) also described the use of proteomic methods to exhibit the importance of atherogenic diets on hepatic protein expression in C57BL/6J mice

(B6, atherosclerosis-susceptible strain) and C3H/HeJ mice (C3H, atherosclerosis-resistant strain); both strains were fed atherogenic diets and revealed a different prototype of both plasma lipids and intracellular lipid droplets.

2.2.1.3 Transcriptomics (gene expression analysis)

The absolute assortment of gene transcripts in cells or tissues at a specified time is called as transcriptomics, and it may be applied in the investigation of gene transcription in response to dietary alterations (Misra et al. 2007). Transcriptomic investigations cover the transition of information from DNA to RNA. Transcriptomics presents much wide information about nutrition status and metabolic responses to diet. Transcriptomics is widely explored for three different rationales in nutrition research: (1) in providing information on a mechanism underlying the effects of a definite nutrient or diet; (2) in identifying genes, proteins, or metabolites that are modified in a pre-disease state and as molecular biomarkers; (3) in identifying and distinguishing different pathways controlled by nutrients (Li et al. 2008).

The consequences of dietary involvements at the global level of gene expression determined by transcriptomic data are primarily generated using cDNA microarrays. It would represent one aspect of the nutrigenomic approach considering this as the analysis of how dietary elements react with genes to change phenotype and conversely metabolize these constituents into nutrients, anti-nutrients, and biologically active compounds. De Fourmestraux et al. (2004) observed transcript profiling in mice that revealed differential metabolic adaptation with ISRN Nutrition 17 to a high fat, and it was observed that the diet was related to change in liver to muscle lipid fluxes.

Furthermore, the nature and extent of transcript variation differ from cell to cell in every single or among individuals in part because of cardiac output, with hormone signaling immune response, androgen regulation, lipid metabolism, social stress, extracellular matrix, or epigenetic programming. Du et al. (2010) revealed this variation among genetically identical mice when treated with diets of high glucose content and also found the modified expressions of genes associated with thiol redox, peroxisomal fatty acid oxidation, and cytochrome P450 in C57BL/6J mice, contributing to enhance oxidative stress by the use of transcriptome technique. Watanabe et al. reported that rats fed with a 20% maple syrup diet for 11 days revealed potentially lower values of hepatic function markers than those fed with a 20% sugar mix syrup diet. A DNA microarray measurement suggested that the expression of genes for the enzymes of ammonia formation was silenced in the liver of the maple syrup diet (Watanabe et al. 2011).

The nuclear hormone receptors are the most essential group of nutrient sensors and are the superfamily of transcription factors that influence gene expression. Many nuclear hormone receptors, such as retinoid X receptor, peroxisome proliferator-activated receptor (PPARs), and liver X receptor, connect to the nutrients and result in conformational alterations, which lead to the coordinated dissociation of corepressors and regeneration of co-activator proteins to facilitate transcription stimulation. Human dietary intervention findings have been promptly implicated in transcriptomics to illustrate that diet induced changes in gene expression. In human transcriptomics investigations, the most vital problem is the inaccessibility of human tissues. On the contrary, blood, subcutaneous adipose tissue, and skeletal muscle can be obtained easily. Therefore, animal investigations can replace better compared to human investigations supplements to comprehend that nutrients alter gene expression in several tissues (Gravouil et al. 2017).

Caesar and colleagues studied the effect of expanding mesenteric adipose tissue in a murine model. In this study, microarray measurement on mesenteric, subcutaneous, and epididymal adipose tissues was carried up to 3 months maintaining high-fat feeding. Surprisingly, they revealed that high-fat feeding induced a decrease in subcutaneous and mesenteric adipose tissue, that is, *de novo* lipogenesis, whereas the gene regulation in epididymis adipose tissue was unaltered. Further measurements with targeted lipidomics and biochemical estimation depicted that *de novo* lipogenesis was down-regulated in the distal epididymis adipose tissue, and this tissue is responsible in promoting the elongation and desaturation of some essential polyunsaturated fatty acids (PUFA) for spermatogenesis (Ide 2017).

2.2.1.4 Metabolomics (metabolite profiling)

The type and amount of all metabolites in a biochemical sample are regarded as metabolomics. Metabolomics gains great attention in the field of nutrition innovation. These are particular products of genomic, transcriptomic, and proteomic pathways of the host or external organisms in addition to intrinsic and extrinsic influence. The features and concentrations of all tiny molecules like water offer a potential for measuring flux across significant biochemical pathways and thus permit comprehensive understanding of how metabolites react with tissue elements of functional importance (Zhang et al. 2012).

The biomarkers for the intake of specialized nutrients and health are also diagnosed by metabolomics. A recent example has been shown in a meta-analysis that blood concentrations of carotenoids, a biomarker for fruit and vegetable intake, are more tightly connected with decreased breast cancer threat than are carotenoids demonstrated in dietary surveys. Preferably, metabolomics should have the ability to give a complete picture of biological pathways at any specific point in time. In nutritional research, such technique may give a break to characterize alterations in metabolic processes induced by nutrients or other lifestyle aspects; to explore relationships between environmental factors, health and disease; and to find out novel biomarkers (Lodge et al. 2010). Owing to the different chemical nature of low-molecular metabolites, lipids, amino acids, peptides, nucleic acids, organic acids, vitamins, thiols, and carbohydrates, the global, untargeted measurement represents a tough problem. Even if an expansion of analytical platforms facilitates separation, detection, identification, and quantification of a huge number of metabolites from only minimal amounts of biochemical samples, targeted metabolomics is most frequently employed (Griffiths et al. 2010).

In the targeted estimation, a pre-defined set of metabolites are available, and they may be employed for the evaluation of single nutrients or metabolites and analysis of subsets of metabolites, including lipids, inflammatory markers, or oxidative damage (German et al. 2007). The lipid profiling has emerged into its own field of lipidomics, and as negatively altered lipid metabolism is an underlying factor in a number of human chronic diseases, lipidomics has turned into a significant tool to quantify the emerging molecular targets (Puri et al. 2012; Wood et al. 2012).

Moreover, the implication of pattern-recognition methods is important for revealing innovative molecules that may function as biomarkers. In addition, the data sets based on metabolomics are generally vital and multidimensional. The metabolomics data should be accumulated along with data on transcriptomics and proteomics, supporting a much extensive application of bioinformatics including multivariate measurements. Because of the identified and vital intra-individual differences, there is a requirement for the standardization of study design, use of large study cohorts, and homogenous study populations based on preliminary phenotyping of study subjects (Griffiths et al. 2010).

Metabolomics is supposed to be more advanced with the emergence of new MS interfaces for which sample preparation is hardly required (Chen et al. 2006; Huang et al. 2007). The innovative expansion in separation methods is a comprehensive multidimensional technique that involves GCxGC or LCxLC, which will be applied in metabolomics investigations in the near future. Along with providing the increased resolution and a sharpness in peak number, these techniques also offer an enhancement in selectivity and sensitivity as compared to conventional separation methodologies. For example, comprehensive GCxGC coupled to TOF MS is a novel tool for metabolic profiling (Pasikanti et al. 2008).

The ideal tools for metabolomics are capillary electrokinetic methods and their conjugation to mass spectrometry (CE and CE-MS) because of their low sample-preparation prerequisites, a broad range of applications, increased efficiency and resolution, and minimum sample utilization. Although CE and CE-MS have not been commonly employed in foodomics (Herrero et al. 2010), they have been identified as the most recognized tools for metabolomics investigations (Oh et al. 2010). Simo et al. (2010) used these techniques in the investigation of substantial equivalence of transgenic and conventional soybean from their peptide profiles with a shot-gun method.

2.3 Effect of food on gene

Nutrigenomics involved the identification of the dynamics of how nutrients alter the genes expression and function and how genes are related to the diet (eating behavior of an individual). It covers the very broad range of research techniques from basic cellular to molecular biology to clinical trials, epidemiology, and population health, which permit a more accurate and redefined knowledge of nutrient-genome reactions in both health and disease. In addition, it also gives rise to knowledge about genetic of how diet, nutrients, or other food elements alter the balance between health and disease by changing the expression and/or structure of an individual's genome. Diet and dietary tools can change the risk of disease progression by redefining several pathways concerned with the onset, incidence, development, and/or severity. These components highly effect on the genetic makeup of individual, in direct or indirect ways, which in turn affect the gene regulation and gene products. The way of gene and nutrients interaction is depicted in Figure 2.3.

The most profound basis for all health and diseases resides in the interaction between the multiple mechanisms, which happens between genetics, environment, nature, and nurture as illustrated in Figure 2.4 and Table 2.1. Some diseases flow from generation to generation, such as ischemic heart disease, blood-related disorders, up- and down-regulated sugar level, metastasis, and many more chronic severities because families share both genes and environment.

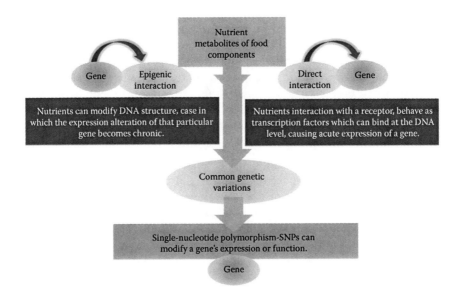

Figure 2.3 Different modes of interaction between gene and nutrition.

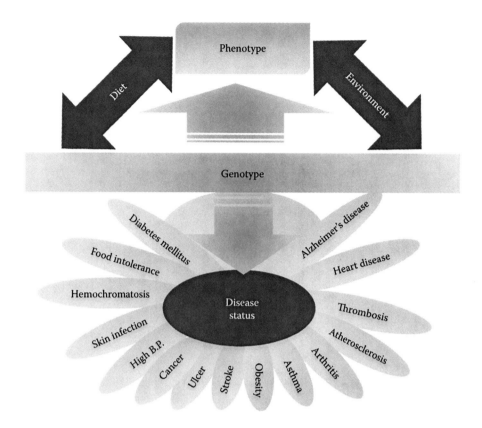

Figure 2.4 Interaction of diet and environment on genotype and its effect on disease status.

There are numerous different types of genetic variations, including SNPs, which are alterations in a single nucleotide (Ordovas 2008). Moreover, specific dietary foods such as alcohol, caffeine, fat, fruits, and vegetable also affect the genetic environment of an individual.

2.3.1 Effect of alcohol

Many studies were correlated and well connected with the effects of alcohol on the particular health outcome based on the observation that interaction between dietary element and health problem was affected by the functional variants in genes involved in the metabolism of the dietary elements. The above fact can be exemplified by the consumption of alcohol drinks, which moderately initiate and relate to the risk of heart disease. The association between alcohol consumption and genetic changes is directly or indirectly influenced by the levels of high-density lipoprotein (HDL), which is responsible for many severe complications (Shiffman et al. 2005). In another finding, it was evident that a dose response decrease in heart disease as certain

Table 2.1 Tabular Representation of Different Diseases and Accountable Diet

Name of Diseases	Responsible Gene	Symptoms	Causing Agents	Diet Suggested	References
Atherosclerosis	FADS1/FADS2	Rise in intima-media thickness among carriers of two variant alleles	High fat diet	High omega-3 fatty acids intake and low omega-6 fatty acids intake	(Garcia-Rios et al. 2013)
Alzheimer	APOE4, ACELRP1	Progressive deterioration of neurons in the brain, affecting memory and behavior	Age, Alcohol consumption, high cholesterol levels	Lower calorie intake and lipid intake	(Kidd 2008)
Brest cancer	BRCA1/BRCA2	–	Tobacco, overweight/ obesity High alcohol consumption	High omega-3 fatty acids intake and low omega-6 fatty acids intake increase consumption of fruits and vegetables, and legumes, whole grains	(Chiuve et al. 2012)
Prostate Cancer	ALOX5AP/ COX-2	Intraprostatic urine reflux, or diet Inflammation may result from bacterial or viral infections,	Tobacco, overweight/ obesity High alcohol consumption	High omega-3 fatty acids intake and low omega-6 fatty acids intake increase consumption of fruits and vegetables, and legumes, whole grains	(Carter et al. 2002)
Colon cancer	FAP, 5-LOX and COX-2	–	Preserved meat and red meat, cigarette smoke	Dietary fibre, increase consumption of fruits and vegetables, and legumes, whole grains	(Soumaoro et al. 2006)
Haemochromatosis	HFE	Iron metabolism and affected damage organs such as the liver, Pancreas and heart	Iron overload	Limited Fe diet/red meat consumption	(Beutler et al. 2002)
Cardiovascular disorder	EAPOE2, APOE3, and APOE4 Cholesterol Ester Transfer Protein (CETP)	Increase in intima-media thickness of coronary artery	High caloric and lipid intake	High omega-3 fatty acids intake and low omega-6 fatty acids intake	(Lloyd-Jones et al. 2009)

(Continued)

Table 2.1 *(Continued)* Tabular Representation of Different Diseases and Accountable Diet

Name of Diseases	Responsible Gene	Symptoms	Causing Agents	Diet Suggested	References
High Blood pressure	Angiotensinogen gene AGT)	Raise blood pressure and Influence the salt sensitivity of the blood pressure	Obesity, sodium, chloride, alcohol, low potassium, low calcium, low omega-3 fatty acid intake, stress, physical inactivity)	Control obesity, low sodium, chloride, alcohol withdrawal, high potassium, high calcium, high omega-3 fatty acid intake, low stress, high physical inactivity	(Dahlöf et al. 2005)
Milk	LCT (lactase)	Vomiting and diarrhea	Milk intake	Avoid milk intake	(Malek et al. 2013)
Alcohol	ALDH2	Facial flushing, nausea and dizziness	Alcohol consumption	Avoid alcohol	
Type 2 diabetes mellitus	PPAR-γ	Obesity, hypertension, dyslipidemia, hyperinsulinemia, insulin resistance, and hyperglycemia	High caloric and lipid intake	Physical Exercise, Low calorie intake and lipid intake low limit the intake of free sugars;	(Pavo et al. 2003)

genotypes will result in slowing down alcohol metabolism. In a study by Hines et al. (2001), 86% reduction in heart disease risk was reported in subjects with the slow-alcohol-metabolizing capacity who consumed at least one alcoholic drink per day.

On the contrary, protective action of moderate alcohol consumption is because of some confounding lifestyle factors concerned with moderate alcohol intake that differs from abstainers or heavy drinkers.

Alcohol is oxidized in the presence of the enzyme alcohol dehydrogenase 1C (ADH1C), also called alcohol dehydrogenase type 3 (ADH3), forming acetaldehyde. The oxidized alcohol possesses two different polymorphic types along with different kinetic properties: *ADH1C*1* allele produces γ1 and the *ADH1C*2* allele produces γ2. Thus, if there is a general protective effect of moderate alcohol on risk of heart disease, this effect would be expected to be stronger in individuals with the slow *ADH1C* genotype compared to those with a faster metabolism.

2.3.2 Effect of caffeine

Apart from alcohol, caffeine is also one of the dietary foods explored in nutrigenomics in relation to certain health outcomes. Being most abundant in coffee, caffeine has a potential impact on the origin of several complications. Some studies have also determined how a response to coffee by a specific genotype can be advantageous or harmful based on the disease under examination. Caffeine is metabolized by the cytochrome P450-1A2 (CYP1A2) enzyme, and a polymorphism in the *CYP1A2* gene determines whether individuals are "rapid" caffeine metabolizers (those who are homozygous for the –163 A allele) or "slow" caffeine metabolizers (carriers of the –163 C allele).

However, for individuals those metabolize caffeine at a slower pace, the consumption of coffee is related with an enhanced risk of myocardial infarction (MI) (Cornelis et al. 2006), indicating that caffeine elevates the risk of MI since it is the only major compound in coffee that is known to be detoxified by CYP1A2. This coffee–*CYP1A2* genotype interaction has since been supported by a prospective investigation that described the effect of coffee consumption on the risk of developing blood pressure problems in individuals stratified by *CYP1A2* genotype (Palatini et al. 2009). In addition, epinephrine and norepinephrine estimated in the urine of the subjects and the level of catecholamine have been shown to increase after caffeine administration in humans. Among slow caffeine metabolizers, urinary epinephrine was found to be drastically increased due to enhanced sympathetic activity that is considered as an important mechanism through which caffeine raises blood pressure.

Researchers also correlated the effect of coffee on breast cancer by isolating subjects into *CYP1A2* genotypes and determined the defensive effect of coffee against the risk of breast cancer (Nkondjock et al. 2006; Yaghjyan et al. 2017), because it involves a diet–gene relation. Unlike the studies on the risk of MI and hypertension where slow caffeine metabolizers were at increased risk from drinking coffee, in this study coffee was associated with a lower risk of breast cancer among slow caffeine metabolizers (Kotsopoulos et al. 2007). Among fast caffeine metabolizers, no protective effect was observed, which implicates caffeine as the defensive component of coffee and is consistent with findings from animal studies that caffeine restrains the development of mammary tumors (Yang et al. 2004).

2.3.3 Effect of dietary fat

Research has been devoted significantly to studying the effect of dietary fat on chronic disease, such as concentrations of blood lipids and their relation to biomarkers. The recent research provides evidence that an individual's unique genetic profile depends on the dietary fat intake in optimal amount and its type (Ordovas 2008). Plourde et al. (2009) found that apoE ε4 modulated the response of plasma omega 3 fatty acid to the intake of an omega 3 fatty acid supplement, but not by the common *PPAR-α* L162V polymorphism. Only non-carriers of ε4 had amplified omega-3 in their plasma after supplementation. Lindi et al. (2003) reported that changes in cholesterol, including HDL cholesterol concentrations, were similar among the *PPAR-α* L162V genotypes after a 3-month supplementation with 3.6 g of omega 3 fatty acids/day (containing 2.4 g of ecosapentanoic acid and decosahexanoic acid) or placebo capsules containing olive oil.

In a further study, subjects pursued a low-fat diet for a period of 8 weeks and thereafter were supplemented every day with 5 g of fish oil for a period of 6 weeks; the decrease in plasma triglyceride concentrations was equivalent for both *PPAR-α* L162V genotype groups, although for the plasma C-reactive protein a considerable diet–gene interaction perceived (Caron-Dorval et al. 2008). Due to small sample sizes and short durations to assess physiological changes, such clinical studies are often limited, and such limitations could be overcome by partnerships and collaborations among researchers (McCabe-Sellers et al. 2008).

A vital step towards personalized nutrition is the diet–gene interactions replication, because it reinforces the confirmation that will be applied to drawing clinical trials and successive nutrition advices based on genotype. It is extensively documented that nutrigenomics offers the industry with an inducement to expand functional foods and novel nutritional foodstuffs. For the prevention of chronic disease, the functional foods created may incorporate bioactive compounds, such as PUFA, without considering the interaction with genetic polymorphisms (Plourde et al. 2009). There may be a lag between the science where diet–gene interactions are well established and the evidence-based improvement and encouragement of functional foods optimized to certain genotypes. For example, the utilization of a food with PUFA could lead to an assortment of responses from important benefit to an adverse effect in individuals (Ferguson 2009).

2.3.4 Effect of fruits and vegetables

Since fruits and vegetables are sources of water, fiber, vitamins, minerals, and numerous phytochemicals, they can persuade a variety of pathways and biological processes in the human body. High fruit and vegetable intake is linked with a reduced risk of various cancers, which has been confirmed from various epidemiological studies (Kim and Park 2009), as well as cardiovascular disease (He et al. 2006). This may be due to general challenges associated with performing long-lasting clinical trials or due to variations in dietary management and controls. On the contrary, the human genetic variation could also be one of the factors modifying an effect to plant foods and their constituents.

It has been notified that dietary ingestion of a phytochemical might not necessarily result in comparable exposure levels in the circulation or target tissues of interest. The observed heterogeneity in transversely diverse study populations may vary according to the response of the individual. Evaluating how genetic aspect amends the sound effects of a high plant-based diet or definite elements in plant foods on human health result could explain how plant foods persuade disease risk and facilitate to recognize populations that might assist the majority from high fruit and vegetable intake. The absorption, distribution, utilization, biotransformation, and excretion of phytochemical are affected by variations in genes, which potentially influence nutrient experience at the tissue level (Lampe 2009). For the case in hand, the protein expression and action of numerous nutrient metabolizing enzymes are transformed by several compounds, as well as by the substrates they act on. Consequently, genetic variations in the pathways and the action of these compounds could modify biological reaction to dietary factors.

Some studies have explored that the effects of genetic variation in biotransformation enzymes such as glutathione S-transferases (GSTs) lead to genetic differences (Lampe et al. 2000; Probst-Hensch et al. 1998). The genetic variation can also persuade our food preferences and digestive behaviors and determine how an individual respond to an ingested amount of a specific dietary bioactive. The genes involved in general polymorphisms for flavor perception may report for differences in food preferences and dietary habits (Eny and El-Sohemy 2010). The choices of food could have been affected by this variability, which may influence health status and the risk of chronic disease (Garcia-Bailo et al. 2009). For instance, there are several vegetables that have been associated with enhanced health results which are immensely bitter in taste due to two structurally similar bitter substances called phenylthiocarbamide (PTC) and 6-n-propylthiouracil (PROP), which are not found in foods detected by the taste receptor 2 member 50 (*TAS2R38* receptor) (El-Sohemy et al. 2007). The PAV haplotype carriers have been classified as "super-tasters" because they have a higher sensitivity to PTC and PROP in contrast to individuals homozygous for AVI (Drayna 2005; Wooding et al. 2004). *TAS2R50* has been linked with the risk of MI, which has been hypothesized to be due

38 Nutrigenomics and Nutraceuticals

to differences in dietary preferences for bitter foods that appear to offer cardiovascular protection (Shiffman et al. 2005).

A genetic basis for food likes and dislikes establishment may somewhat give details of the unpredictability among epidemiologic studies involving diet to the risk of chronic diseases since the nutritional exposure of interest could be confounded by the genetic makeup of a group of individuals. Fruit and vegetables are consumed by all, usually established as healthy foods. Conversely, it may be advantageous for definite individuals, based on genetics, to focus on specific fruits and vegetables. For example, genotypes linked with more favorable metabolism of carcinogens may be linked with fewer favorable metabolism of phytochemicals. The outcomes of research to date propose an intricate union among utilization of several vegetables and biotransformation enzyme activities in humans (Lampe et al. 2000). The nutrient absorption, transport, utilization and excretion, taste preference, and food tolerance all potentially influence the effect of plant-based diets on the risk of disease, which are affected by genetic variation in pathways.

2.4 Food safety, quality, and traceability with MS-based "omics" approaches

The safety of food is nowadays a tough task in which recent analytical chemistry must present perfect, precise, and robust methods for the estimation of any deleterious elements or organisms that might be present in minute amount in foodstuff. The employment of foodomics and MS technologies has a very significant impact on the safety of food and develops permeable limits demanded by food safety legislation. Strict maximum residue levels, known as the maximum quantity of a specific compound that might enter in the final foodstuff, were imposed by the legislation of different countries for limiting and controlling the utilization of deleterious compounds to protect the health of the consumers (Bohm et al. 2009). Hence, the applications of these compounds do not pretense a hazard to human health by the establishment of this limit, while the employment of a few of them is severely prohibited (Bohm et al. 2009). The different approaches for maintenance of food quality and safety are shown in Figure 2.5.

2.4.1 Assessment of exogenous food contaminants

The exogenous contaminants estimation is a vital measure in the field of safety of food stuff. The MS applications joined to new analytical techniques, mostly separation techniques, permit the estimation of contaminants in foodstuff in simultaneous and sensitive manner. The analytical device is selected independently, and in MS/MS analyses, two product-ions are frequently preferred for every precursor-ion for these estimations (in Commission decision 2002/657/EC).

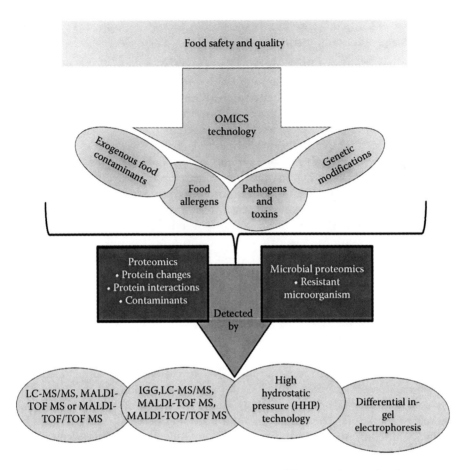

Figure 2.5 *Different approaches for maintenance of food quality and safety.*

Besides the ionization source settings, the collision-induced dissociation (CID) should be carefully optimized, and its parameters for the in-source CID fragmentation are of great consequence; since they have an intense persuasion on the sensitivity for obtaining precise and reproducible results, the blend of LC with an electrospray interface (ESI) and triple quadrupole analyzers is the most commonly used technique along with the coupled analytical techniques employed for these applications. For the estimation of pesticides in fruits (Wong et al. 2010), vegetables (Chung and Chan 2010), wines (Economou et al. 2009), milk (Dagnac et al. 2009), or meat (Carretero et al. 2008), this technique has been beneficially employed. For example, the most employed sample pretreatment methods are solid-phase extraction or QuEChERS (referred as Quick, Easy, Cheap, Effective, Rugged, and Safe). With LC-MS/MS, values of limit of quantitation as low as minute mg kg^{-1} are generally reached, and also the analyses are comparatively fast.

Approximately 58 antibiotics were estimated in milk in less than 15 min (Gaugain-Juhel et al. 2009). Still, the careful estimation of the triple quadrupole analyzers permits the precise analysis of partly isolated compounds. Indeed, in approximately the equivalent analysis time (approximately 15 min), more than 190 pesticide residues were estimated from different fruits (Wong et al. 2010a). Taylor et al. (2008) employed ultra-high pressures in LC-MS/MS, MALDI-TOF MS, or MALDI-TOF/TOF MS for analysis of more than 100 pesticides in strawberry samples in less than 5 min. In addition, gas chromatography (GC) is another most employed tool, which in combination with triple quadrupole analyzer is used to measure food contaminants due to restricted use of organic solvents or higher electrical field.

Furthermore, Wong et al. (2010a) studied that GC-MS/MS methods allowed comparable greater throughput, (e.g., quantification and identification of >160 pesticide residues in vegetables, which is attainable with the detection capacity) than those obtained with LC-MS/MS. Apart from that, investigators also designed large-volume injections to further improve the GC-MS performance. In addition, authors suggested SIM mode to trace and identify the contaminants (because of greater accessibility to an individual quadrupole instrument). Working mechanism was also demonstrated which shows how the application of GC-MS/MS tremendously enhances the specificity, sensitivity, resolution, and reliability of the technique. In addition, comprehensive 2D GC (GCxGC) was introduced for quantitative determination of >100 pesticide residues by coupling GCxGC to TOF MS (Van der Lee et al. 2008).

2.4.2 Assessment of food allergens

The identification of food allergen is of pivotal importance for food safety. Food allergens might stimulate undesired effects in susceptible individuals and are naturally present in some foods. Thus, allergic patients are needed to outreach from the expenditure of the allergen, even in minute concentrations. This is the basis for the strict legislation by food control agencies (Food and Drug administration, European food and safety authority, etc.), in order to maintain clarity in the food labels for the illustration of the generally used food allergens. Many proteins have been identified as food allergens in several food products, like milk and related products, eggs, soybeans, peanuts, cereals, fish, seafood, and processed food (Mahler and Goodman 2017).

To quantify the allergens in food products, MS-based proteomics such as food blotting and high-resolution mass spectrometry has become a very useful tool. Proteomic measurements revealed different contents of these allergens in various peanut varieties and also the presence of different fragments of these proteins (Schmidt et al. 2009). In this regard, proteomics techniques are broadly employed for the identification of food allergens and strategy involved protein digestion to fabricate a set of peptides obtained from the various proteins contained in the sample and their detection as a part of a specific protein. Stevenson et al. (2009) found that these proteins are deficient in genetically engineered peanut seeds. In subsequent *in silico* modelling, high homology between epitopes of known allergens from walnut (Mills et al. 2004), cashew nut (Teuber et al. 2002), and buckwheat (Yoshioka et al. 2004) was found. Further proteomic analyses of plant proteomes were performed to detect allergens in wheat and maize flour (Mahler and Goodman 2017; Fasoli et al. 2009).

Chaissaigne et al. (2007) studied a proteomic methodology, for instance, to join capillary LC with Q-TOF MS to pick a series of peptides as markers for the presence of three main peanut allergens (Ara-h1, Ara-h2, and Arah3) in food products independently of the use of raw or roasted peanuts. Careri et al. (2007) detected concentrations of peanut allergen proteins as low as 1 mg/g in complex food products, like rice crispy/chocolate-based snacks by use of proteomic methods.

Additionally, Krishnan et al. (2009) demonstrated the use of MS to characterize intact allergen proteins that were earlier identified with immunoblotting with sera from allergic patients and proved to be useful to detect that the a- and b-subunits of b-conglycinin were also potential soybean allergens. Martín-Pedraza et al. (2016) suggested that the combination of immunoassays with MS has also demonstrated higher potential for the characterization of food allergens. They applied IgE immunoblotting technique to unveil the potential allergens in tomato fruits and seeds, while a multidimensional protein fractionation strategy and LC-MS/MS were employed for the precise molecular determination of the allergens.

Hsieh et al. (2002) demonstrated the SELDI microarrays for the characterization of novel food allergens and observed that it is an effective tool not only as the traditional Western blot but also faster. The same procedure was employed to detect and identify allergens in banana. Nevertheless, it is also useful to identify known allergens, such as lysozyme in cheeses.

The stability of the protein in an acidic environment in the presence of stomach protease pepsin causes risk of food antigenicity. The *in vitro* and *in vivo* binding assays to human immunoglobulin E (IgE) were performed and no adverse reactions were found. But some residual risk after long-term consummation of such food still remains, and further studies regarding the allergenic potential of genetically modified (GM) plants were performed.

In a subsequent proteomic study, Ahsan et al. (2016) compared GM versus non-modified soybean samples and identified two new potential allergens. In a short-term study, none of the individuals tested reacted differently to the GM versus non-modified samples. After a long-term consumption of GM crops, a residual risk of allergies still remains. Food of animal origin, especially seafood and milk products, can also cause allergies. Moreover, proteomics techniques have only been sparingly implicated in the research of allergens in these products. It is recognized that during the production process, mainly heating, changes such as carboxylation in the key milk protein casein (Scaloni et al. 2002) or forming of covalent bonds between casein micelles and b-lacto globulin (Henry et al. 2002) and modification of other proteins (Casado et al. 2009) can cause stimulation of allergies to milk products (Gardini et al. 2006).

It was also revealed that metabolomics can be efficiently applied for the study of different disruptive metabolic reaction in cattle after the use of anabolic steroids (Dumas et al. 2005). Numerous biomarkers were detected in the urine of cattle treated with anabolic steroids, and these urinary biomarkers such as trimethylamine-N-oxide, dimethylamine, hippurate, creatine, and creatinine characterize the biological fingerprint of anabolic treatment. Pineiro et al. (2003) used proteomics as a tool for the investigation of allergens in seafood and other marine products. However, there are still only a few studies in this field. Taka et al. (2000) characterized an allergenic parvalbumin from frog by the use of LC-ESI-MS. The main crustacean allergens are proteins tropomyosin and arginine kinase. Tropomyosin is a myofibrillar protein of 35–38 kDa, and proteins from six species of crustaceans have also been cloned (Ishikawa et al. 2001; Motoyama et al. 2007).

In some commercially relevant shrimp species, arginine kinase was obtained and characterized by the use of proteomic methods (Ortea et al. 2009). Some additional shrimp allergens such as sarcoplasmatic calcium-binding protein have also been noticed by proteomic technique (Shiomi et al. 2008). If not inactivated or degraded during processing, some food components such as plant lectins constitute a possible risk, since consumption of raw or incorrectly processed beans can cause severe side reactions such as gastroenteritis, nausea, diarrhea, and even more. Lectins such as concanavalin A, phytohemagglutinin, pea lectin, and flavin are present in quite high levels and accumulate in vacuoles in cotyledons.

Generally, lectins demonstrate high specificity to distinct sugars, but they also have an extensive homology in primary structure, also from unrelated species. Conversely, a plant species such as castor bean may contain structurally similar lectins with different toxicity. Castor bean lectin ricin shows a very high toxicity for humans, and animals cause relatively weak agglutination; *Ricinus communis* agglutinin is weakly toxic, but strong agglutinin. Ricin and *Phaseolus vulgaris* lectin are two most common lectins that cause food poisoning. The quantitative analysis of proteomic strategies of potentially harmful lectins in raw and processed food in dietary preparations includes the use of chromatographic or electrophoretic strategies combined with mass spectrometry (LC-MS/MS, MALDI-TOF MS, or MALDI-TOF/TOF MS).

Nasi et al. (2009) used lectin-enriched fraction that can be further separated by cation-exchange chromatography, followed by tryptic digestion and protein identification by mass spectrometry. Hsieh et al. (2002) demonstrated microarrays efficient technique for the identification of new food allergens in banana, which is not only prominent as a traditional Western blot but also faster. Xu et al. (2010) employed principal component analysis to detect valuable regions in the GC-MS chromatogram that resulted from the profile of volatile organic compounds from natural spoiled pork and pork contaminated with *Salmonella typhimurium.*

MALDI-TOF MS has been utilized to detect and quantify low molecular weight proteins obtained from intact bacterial cells or even ribosomal proteins. From reference, it was likely to differentiate among the various bacterial species and genera under MS fingerprints (from 2,000 to 10,000 Da). Kassim et al. (2017) studied phyllo-proteomic correlation based on the MS data statistically and provided the similar clustering than the phylogenetic determination based on the 16S rRNA gene; those data revealed the usefulness and adoptability of the method. Besides, the comparison of the reference profiles and the profiles collected from seafood samples permitted the appropriate application of this technology to track unknown bacterial strains. In addition, Li et al. (2010) employed inductive coupled plasma MS with an immunoassay with antibody-conjugated gold nanoparticles for analysis of the concentration of *E. coli* available in a sample. Other novel strategies include use of an extraction mechanism, followed by a high-resolution separation step coupled to MS. The QuEChERS method was widely used for the simultaneous extraction and determination of relatively wide groups of toxins in which triple quadrupole analyzers provide a limit of detection (LOD) of few mg kg^{-1}, while ultra-performance liquid chromatography (UPLC) proved as a superior separation method (Rasmussen et al. 2010; Zachariasova et al. 2010).

Furthermore, the high-resolution mass spectrometers coupled with UPLC, such as orbitrap (reduction in sample treatment and handling, and enhanced the sample yield), potentially uplift the accuracy of the analysis and maintained comparable LOD to those attained with a TOF MS instrument. The mass accuracy revealed by orbital analyzers is higher than general tandem mass analyzers. However, it is practically not possible so far to reach the number of identification points needed for the current EU legislation for the analysis of mycotoxins (Commission decision 2002/657/EC), because accuracy is not considered in the identification points system implemented by the EU (Commission decision 2002/657/EC).

2.4.3 Assessment of pathogens and microbiological toxins

Foodborne illnesses cause numbers of hospitalizations and even deaths. In the USA, about 325,000 hospitalizations and 5,000 deaths caused by food poisoning are registered each year. The recognition, confirmation, and quantification of bacteria and bacterial toxins in food are significant analytical problems. The most common bacteria that cause food poisoning are *Staphylococcus aureus, Campylobacter jejuni,* some *Salmonella,* and *Staphylococcus* species, some

Bacillus strains and *Escherichia coli* O157:H7 strain. Ochoa and Harrington (2005) suggested that the careful monitoring of microbial contamination in the final product and the monitoring of the production process and cleaning and sanitation are one of the most crucial factors of the manufacturing process in food technology and biotechnology.

For the detection of bacteria and their toxins, well-established and sensitive methods are available, predominantly based on immunochemical methods. For the identification of microbial food contaminants and their toxins, and for monitoring of cleaning and sanitation, proteomics and genomics technologies present additional, more sensitive and specific methods (Willerslev-Olsen et al. 2016; Dupuis et al. 2008). The use of high hydrostatic pressure (HHP) technology is a new method for food preservation which follows changes of proteomics of contaminating bacteria during food processing and equipment sanitation.

Smeller et al. (2002) reported that proteins are known to be the most important target of high pressure in living organisms, and Smelt et al. (2001) suggested that HHP hinders the growth of microorganisms by inactivating key enzymes that are involved in DNA replication and transcription enzymes and modifying both microbial cell walls and membranes. However, some bacteria such as *Bacillus cereus* can survive HHP treatment. Martínez-Gomariz et al. (2009) analyzed changes in the proteome of this *Bacillus cereus* during the HHP treatment. They found quantitative differences and identified some of differently expressed proteins.

As expected, Samuel et al. (2017) followed proteomic changes in whey samples from a group of cows before and 18 h after the infection with *E. coli*. Due to decreased milk production and quality, discarded milk and cattle mortality, such infections can cause mastitis, which is the costliest disease that affects the dairy industry. The purpose of that study was the identification of biomarkers for the evaluation of the efficacy of adjunctive therapies in decreasing inflammation connected with mastitis. Higher expression of some acute-phase proteins such as transthyretin and complement C3 was found in whey samples 18 h after bacterial infection, but some antimicrobial peptides and further acute phase a-1-acid glycoprotein were also detected, and such proteins are candidate biomarkers for future research into the effect of bacterial inflammation during mastitis.

During the design of cleaning of stainless containers and other surfaces in food processing facilities, biofilm formation is an important fact that has to be taken into consideration. In biofilms, some microorganisms such as sporogen bacterium *Bacillus cereus*, the Gram-positive bacterium *Listeria monocytogens,* and some pathogenic *E. coli* strains can survive on the surface of stainless steel containers and other surfaces in the manufacturing facility, even under cleaning and sanitizing conditions.

Planchon et al. (2009) reported that biofilm-forming bacteria, such as *Staphylococcus* species, can survive food processing and cause human and animal infection. Incorporation of microorganisms is a kind of usual means for their immobilization, and the high density of biofilms gives them not only better ability to survive aggressive treatment but also a substantial bio-catalytic potential.

Junter et al. (2002) discussed the use of physiological and genomic analyses; proteomic analysis of biofilm-forming microbial cells gives important information about their behavior during food processing and storage, symbiosis, possible infection and potential food poisoning, their defense against antimicrobial agents, and the potential to survive the cleaning and sanitation process.

Some bacterial species are gaining popularity as food additives due to their health-promoting properties, and these are colonizing the human gastrointestinal tract, which have been documented in clinical trials. Kailasapathy and Chin (2000) reported that bifidobacteria and lactobacilli are added as live bacteria to food preparations under the generic name of probiotics. Vitali et al. (2005) first performed the proteomic map of *Bifidobacterium longum,* a strict fermentative anaerobe, about 5 years ago.

The deposition of an abnormal conformation (PrPSc) of a normal cellular protein (PrPC) in neural tissues in humans and animals is known as prion disease or transmissible spongiform encephalopathy (TSE). PrPC is relatively soluble and protease sensitive, while PrPSc is relatively insoluble and protease resistant. TSEs include scrapie in sheep and goats and bovine spongiform encephalopathy (mad cow disease or BSE).

Ramljak et al. (2008) reported that the human form of this disease is infectious Creutzfeldt-Jakob disease (CJD) caused by the consumption of meat and meat products of prion-infected animals. The outbreaks of BSE and infectious variant CJD have prompted the need for reliable screening methods for prion infections as part of the safety control for meat and meat products. Strom et al. (2006) identified prion proteins by use of immune affinity techniques, combined with one- and 2D electrophoresis and mass spectrometry. Although those are reliable biomarkers for prion infection, detection of prion-binding proteins did not give further revealing information about the biology of prions and the pathogenesis of TSE.

Steinacker et al. (2010) suggested that ubiquitin is a potential biomarker candidate which could be identified in the cerebrospinal fluid of CJD patients. Herbst et al. (2009) used a multidisciplinary approach to identify *ante mortem* markers for prion disease. This rather complex strategy combines matrix-assisted laser desorption/ionization Fourier transform mass spectrometry (MALDI-FTMS), mass fingerprinting, and bioinformatics for the identification of candidate biomarkers in prion-infected animals. Again, results of this study are still rather limited, and the true positive rate was relatively low. Nomura et al. (2009) reported the detection of autoantibodies in the sera of cattle with bovine spongiform encephalopathy. These autoantibodies were directed against glial fibrillary acidic proteins and could be detected only in the serum of TSE-infected

46   Nutrigenomics and Nutraceuticals

animals. Tsiroulnikov et al. (2004) presented a method for decontamination of meat and bone meal by use of bacterial proteolytic enzymes.

Hsu et al. (2009) used nattokinase from *Bacillus subtilis* for fermentation of boiled soybeans, which is also able to degrade prion proteins and potentially prevent prion infection (Nomura et al. 2009). However, it is still a safety risk, if such contaminated animal food is used, and prion detection and elimination of diseased animals and contaminated meat is a much safer way to prevent these kinds of foodborne diseases.

2.4.4 Consequences of genetic modifications

Improvement of productiveness, quality, enhancement of tolerance to herbicides, or inducing production of new substances and removal of some harmful or allergenic proteins can be executed by genetic modifications by the introduction of exogenous DNA fragments into the genome of the host organism (Uzogara et al. 2000). However, proteins in the living cell are in permanent interaction, and an introduction of a foreign gene product, change in concentration, or complete removal of another cellular protein can persuade complex and possibly unexpected changes in complete cellular proteome (Dombre et al. 2017).

The agronomic and phenotypic characteristics are very sensitive indices of alterations and also robust indicators for the comparison between GM and non-GM crops. The GM food has been in use internationally for over 10 years, and until now, no verifiable unintended toxic or nutritional effects as a result of consumption of GM products have been registered (Kok and Kuiper 2003). The consequence of GM can be identified by the only use of proteomics technology as complex changes in a proteome.

Ruebelt et al. (2006) compared proteomes of GM and non-GM seeds of the model plant *Arabidopsis thaliana*. In this extensive series of studies, authors performed an analytical validation of the method such as comparative 2D electrophoresis and assessments of both natural variability and unintended effects. Although the methods such as differential in-gel electrophoresis (DIGE) (Martínez-Gomari et al. 2009), isotope labelling techniques (Schmidt et al. 2005), and gel-free, label-free quantitative approaches have recently been developed, they are faster and more effective, so they can be used as fundaments for further quality assessment of GM crops. Maize, tomato, and soybean are intensively used for proteomic studies and are considered as GM crops.

Erny et al. (2007) uses capillary electrophoresis method followed by mass spectrometry for the study of alcohol-soluble endosperm proteins, so-called zein proteins from corn of GM and non-GM maize. Different maize lines including the transgenic one were analyzed by proteomic finger printing. Miernyk et al. (2016) used comparative 2D electrophoresis for the analysis of GM and non-GM soybean seeds, and eight differently expressed proteins were identified, and one of them is an allergen known as Gly m Bd 28k fragment.

Allergens were already identified in GM soybean seeds and further careful monitoring of these foods is still necessary.

2.5 Future trends of omics technology in food and nutrition

In recent years, omic technology has gained much attention in the area of nutritional biology similar to the advancement noted in the field of nano-technology (Tekade et al. 2009, 2015a, 2015b). On the contrary, MS has been established as a stand-alone tool or in combination with 2-DE, liquid chroma-tography or capillary gel electrophoresis for the precise detection of various dietary foods and is a promising technology to avoid potential hurdles of optimal operation in foodomics in the non-distant future. However, in proteomics, there is an urgent requirement of technological increment (e.g., protein microarrays) to make more easy and reproducible routine analysis for proteome research, as well as improvements in the resolution of peptides to promote protein coverage. Schittmayer and Birner-Gruenberger (2009) studied the use of functional proteomics in foodomics.

However, MS is a constantly growing and essential technique for carrying systematic research in proteomics for detection and treatment of more-sophisticated samples, but sometimes it is combined with other tools like sophisticated and compact mass spectrometers with two or more analyzers which in turn support the more precise proteomic profiling. Gilad et al. (2010) demonstrated new applications of proteomics technologies that are expected in the investigation of microbial flora in the gut, although MS-based proteomics is a well-reputed and valuable technique for the quantification, characterization, and detection of food allergens (Chen et al. 2006; Huang et al. 2007).

The widespread multidimensional techniques, such as GCxGC or LCxLC, are also an innovative improvement in separation techniques that will be implemented in metabolomics studies in the near future. In comparison with conventional separation techniques, they might provide not only an enhanced resolution and a large increase in the peak number, but also an increase in selectivity and sensitivity.

As an example, comprehensive GCxGC coupled to TOF MS is a promising tool for metabolic profiling (Pasikanti 2008). Due to their minimal sample-preparation requirements, wide range applications, great efficiency, and resolution, and low sample consumption, the capillary electrokinetic techniques and their coupling to mass spectrometry (CE and CE-MS) are ideal tools for metabolomics profiling. Although CE and CE-MS have not been widely used in foodomics (Herrero et al. 2010), they have already been identified as a very promising tool for metabolomics studies (Oh et al. 2010). This knowledge can be better generated with multidisciplinary approaches that consider international consortia and working on foodomics based on extensive populations. By considering the two different approaches, foodomics can also be important in terms of public health. It involves the clinical application to treat metabolic alterations, such as diabetes, considered at short term, and at long term, more related to the public primary prevention—which means to hinder the development of disease before it appears.

2.6 Conclusion

The new "-omic" technology is a global method of measuring families of cellular molecules, such as DNA, RNA, proteins, and intermediary metabolites. In nutrigenomics, it includes the expansion of new transgenic foods with molecular tools; the genomic/transcriptomic/proteomic and/or metabolomic represents characteristics, and the complex interaction between genome and food/nutrient (nutritional phenotype) should represent the evaluation basis of the nutritional status of a person. The study of omics technology for compound profiling/authenticity and/or biomarkers analysis related to food quality, new investigations on food bioactivity and its effect on human health, development of global omics strategies to investigate food safety issues are some of the steps. The advancement of omics technologies in nutritional field improves consumer's welfare health and confidence. Omic techniques based on MS are gradually used more for management of food quality and food safety. The use of proteomics in food technology is available, particularly for characterization and standardization of raw materials, process development, and detection of batch-to-batch variations and quality control of the final product. Nutrigenomics/nutrigenetics in this century is an exciting field of research, new information being obtained almost every day regarding the way in which the interaction between lifestyle and genotype contributes to the preservation of the state of health or, on the contrary, to disease appearance.

2.7 Acknowledgments

The authors acknowledge the support by Fundamental Research Grant (FRGS) scheme of Ministry of Higher Education, Malaysia, to support research on gene delivery. We also acknowledge internal grants to Dr Tekade from the IMU-JC support to our research group. The authors would like to acknowledge NIPER, Ahmedabad, for providing research support for research on cancer and arthritis.

References

Ahsan, N., Rao, R. S. P., Gruppuso, P. A., Ramratnam, B. & Salomon, A. R. 2016. Targeted proteomics: Current status and future perspectives for quantification of food allergens. *J Proteomics*, 143:15–23.

Beutler, E., Felitti, V. J., Koziol, J. A., Ho, N. J. & Gelbart, T. 2002. Penetrance of 845G → A (C282Y) HFE hereditary haemochromatosis mutation in the USA. *The Lancet*, 359:211–218.

Bohm, B.A, C.S. Stachel, P. Gowik, 2009. Multi-method for the determination of antibiotics of different substance groups in milk and validation in accordance with Commission Decision 2002/657/EC. *J Chromatogr A*, 1216:8217–8223.

Braicu, C., Mehterov, N., Vladimirov, B., Sarafian, V., Nabavi, S., Atanasov, A. G. & Berindan-Neagoe, I. Nutrigenomics in cancer: revisiting the effects of natural compounds. *Seminars in Cancer Biology*, 2017. Elsevier.

Careri M, A. Costa, L. Elviri, J.B. Lagos, A. Magia, M. Terenghi, A. Cereti, L.P. Garoffo, 2007. Use of specific peptide biomarkers for quantitative confirmation of hidden allergic peanut proteins Ara h 2 and Ara h 3/4 for food control by liquid chromatography-tandem mass spectrometry. *Anal Bioanal Chem*, 389:1901–1907.

Carlson, C.S., M.A. Eberle, L. Kruglyak, D.A. Nickerson, 2004. Mapping complex disease loci in whole-genome association studies. *Nature*, 429:446–452.

Caron-Dorval, D., P. Paquet, A.M. Paradis, I. Rudkowska, S. Lemieux, P. Couture, M. C. Vohl, 2008. Effect of the PPAR-Alpha L162V polymorphism on the cardiovascular disease risk factor in response to n-3 polyunsaturated fatty acids. *J Nutrigenet Nutrigenomics*, 1(4):205–212.

Carretero, V, C., Blasco, Y. Picó, 2008. Multi-class determination of antimicrobials in meat by pressurized liquid extraction and liquid chromatography-tandem mass spectrometry. *J Chromatogr A*, 1209:162–173.

Carter, H. B., Walsh, P. C., Landis, P. & Epstein, J. I. 2002. Expectant management of nonpalpable prostate cancer with curative intent: preliminary results. *J Urol*, 167:1231–1234.

Casado, B., M. Affolter, M. Kussmann, 2009. OMICS-rooted studies of milk proteins, oligosaccharides and lipids. *J Proteomics*, 73:196–208.

Castle, D., 2008. Genomic nutritional profiling: Innovation and regulation in nutrigenomics. *Minn J Law Sci Technol*, 9(1):37–60.

Chaissaigne, H., J.V. Norgaard, A.J. van Hengel, 2007. Proteomics-based approach to detect and identify major allergens in processed peanuts by capillary LC-Q-TOF (MS/MS). *J Agric Food Chem*, 55:4461–4473.

Chen, H., Z. Pan, N. Talaty, D. Raftery, R.G. Cooks, 2006. Combining desorption electrospray ionization mass spectrometry and nuclear magnetic resonance for differential metabolomics without sample preparation. *Rapid Commun Mass Spectrom*, 20:1577–1584.

Chiuve, S. E., Fung, T. T., Rimm, E. B., Hu, F. B., Mccullough, M. L., Wang, M., Stampfer, M. J. & Willett, W. C. 2012. Alternative dietary indices both strongly predict risk of chronic disease. *The Journal of nutrition, jn*. 111.157222.

Chung, S.W.C., B.T.P. Chan, 2010. Validation and use of a fast sample preparation method and liquid chromatography-tandem mass spectrometry in analysis of ultra-trace levels of 98 organophosphorus pesticide and carbamate residues in a total diet study involving diversified food types. *J Chromartogr A*, 1217:4815–4824.

Clarke, W.E., I.A. Parkin, H.A. Gajardo, D.J. Gerhardt, E. Higgins, C. Sidebottom, A.G. Sharpe, R.J. Snowdon, M.L. Federico, F.L. Iniguez-Luy, 2013. Genomic DNA enrichment using sequence capture microarrays: A novel approach to discover sequence nucleotide polymorphisms (SNP) in *Brassica napus* L. *PLoS One*, 8(12):e81992.

Cooney, C.A., A.A. Dave, G.L. Wolff, 2002. Maternal methyl supplements in mice affect epigenetic variation and DNA methylation of offspring. *J Nutr*, 132(8 Suppl):2393S–2400S.

Cornelis, M.C., A. El-Sohemy, E.K. Kabagambe, H. Campos, 2006. Coffee, CYP1A2 genotype, and risk of myocardial infarction. *JAMA*, 295(10):1135–1141.

Cozzolino, S., C. Cominetti, 2013. *Biochemical and Physiological Bases of Nutrition in Different Stages of Life in Health and Disease*. Monole, Sao Paulo, Brazil.

Dagnac, T, M. Garcia-Chao, P. Pulleiro, C. Garcia-Jares, M. Llompart, 2009. Dispersive solid-phase extraction followed by liquid chromatography-tandem mass spectrometry for the multi-residue analysis of pesticides in raw bovine milk. *J Chromatogr A*, 1216:3702–37093.

Dahlöf, B., Sever, P. S., Poulter, N. R., Wedel, H., Beevers, D. G., Caulfield, M., Collins, R., Kjeldsen, S. E., Kristinsson, A. & Mcinnes, G. T. 2005. Prevention of cardiovascular events with an antihypertensive regimen of amlodipine adding perindopril as required versus atenolol adding bendroflumethiazide as required, in the Anglo-Scandinavian Cardiac Outcomes Trial-Blood Pressure Lowering Arm (ASCOT-BPLA): a multicentre randomised controlled trial. *The Lancet*, 366:895–906.

Davis, A. P., Grondin, C. J., Johnson, R. J., Sciaky, D., King, B. L., Mcmorran, R., Wiegers, J., Wiegers, T. C. & Mattingly, C. J. 2017. The comparative toxicogenomics database: update 2017. *Nucleic Acids Research*, 45:D972–D978.

De Fourmestraux, V., H. Neubauer, C. Poussin, P. Farmer, L. Falquet, R. Burcelin, M. Delorenzi, B. Thorens, 2004. Transcript profiling suggests that differential metabolic adaptation of mice ISRN Nutrition 17 to a high fat diet is associated with changes in liver to muscle lipid fluxes. *J Biol Chem*, 279(49): 50743–50753.

Dhakad, R.S., R.K. Tekade, N.K. Jain, 2013. Cancer targeting potential of folate targeted nanocarrier under comparative influence of tretinoin and dexamethasone. *Curr Drug Deliv*, 10:477–491.

Dombre, C., Guyot, N., Moreau, T., Monget, P., Da Silva, M., Gautron, J. & Réhault-Godbert, S. Egg serpins: The chicken and/or the egg dilemma. *Seminars in cell & developmental biology*, 2017. Elsevier, 120–132.

Domon, B., R. Aebersold, 2010. Options and considerations when selecting a quantitative proteomics strategy. *Nat Biotechnol*, 28:710–721.

Drayna, D., 2005. Human taste genetics. *Annu Rev Genomics Hum Genet*, 6:217–235.

Du, D., Y.-H. Shi, G.-W. Le, 2010. Oxidative stress induced by high-glucose diet in liver of C57BL/6J mice and its underlying mechanism. *Mol Biol Rep*, 37(8):3833–3839.

Dumas M.E., C. Canlet, J. Vercauteren, F. André, A. Paris, 2005. Homeostatic signature of anabolic steroids in cattle using 1H-13C HMBC NMR metabolomics. *J Proteome Res*, 4:1493–1502.

Dupuis, A., J.A. Hennekinne, J. Garin, V. Brun, 2008. Protein standard absolute quantification (PSAQ) for improved investigation of staphylococcal food poisoning outbreaks. *Proteomics*, 8:4633–4636.

Eisen, J.A., 2012. Badomics words and the power and peril of the ome-meme. *Gigascience*, 1(1):6.

El-Sohemy, A., L. Stewart, N. Khataan, B. Fontaine-Bisson, P. Kwong, S. Ozsungur, M.C. Cornelis, 2007. Nutrigenomics of taste—Impact on food preferences and food production. *Forum Nutr*, 60:176–182.

Eny, K.M., A. El-Sohemy, 2010. Genetic determinants of ingestive behaviour: Sensory, energy homeostasis and food reward aspects of ingestive behaviour. In: *Obesity Prevention: The Role of Brain and Society on Individual Behavior*, John W. Erdman, Jr., Ian A. MacDonald, Steven H. Zeisel (Eds.), Elseiver, NY, 149–160.

Erny, G.L., M.L. Marina, A. Cifuentes, 2007. Capillary electrophoresis-mass spectrometry of zein proteins from conventional and transgenic maize. *Electrophoresis*, 28:4192–4201.

Fasoli, E., E.A. Pastorello, L. Farioli, J. Scibilia, G. Aldini, M. Carini, A. Marocco, E. Boschetti, P.G. Righetti, 2009. Searching for allergens in maize kernels via proteomic tools. *J Proteomics*, 72:501–510.

Ferguson, L.R. 2009. Nutrigenomics approaches to functional foods. *J Am Diet Assoc*, 109(3):452–458.

Ferguson, L.R. ed., 2013. *Nutrigenomics and Nutrigenetics in Functional Foods and Personalized Nutrition*. CRC Press, Boca Raton, FL.

Forner, F., C. Kumar, C.A. Luber, T. Fromme, M. Klingenspor, M. Mann, 2009. Proteome differences between brown and white fat mitochondria reveal specialized metabolic functions. *Cell Metab*, 10:324–335.

Fuchs, D., S. De Pascual-Teresa, G. Rimbach, F. Virgili, R. Ambra, R. Turner, H. Daniel, U. Wenzel, 2005. Proteome analysis for identification of target proteins of genistein in primary human endothelial cells stressed with oxidized LDL or homocysteine. *Eur J Nutr*, 44:95–104.

Garcia-Bailo, B., C. Toguri, K.M. Eny, A. El-Sohemy, 2009. Genetic variation in taste and its influence on food selection. *OMICS*, 13(1):69–80.

Garcia-Rios, A., Delgado-Lista, J., Alcala-Diaz, J. F., Lopez-Miranda, J. & Perez-Martinez, P. 2013. Nutraceuticals and coronary heart disease. *Current Opinion in Cardiology*, 28:475–482.

Gardini, G., P. Del Boccio, S. Colombatto, G. Testore, D. Corpillo, C. Di Illio, A. Urbani, C. Nebbia, 2006. Proteomic investigation in the detection of the illicit treatment of calves with growth-promoting agents. *Proteomics*, 6:2813–2822.

Gaugain-Juhel, M., B. Delépine, S. Gautier, M.P. Fourmond, V. Gaudin, D. Hurtaud-Pessel, E. Verdon, P. Sanders, 2009. Validation of a liquid chromatography-tandem mass spectrometry screening method to monitor 58 antibiotics in milk: A qualitative approach. *Food Addit Contam Part A Chem Anal Control Expo Risk Assess*, 26:1459–1471.

German, J.B., L.A. Gillies, J.T. Smilowitz, A.M. Zivkovic, S.M. Watkins, 2007. Lipidomics and lipid profiling in metabolomics. *Curr Opin Lipidol*, 18:66–71.

Gianazza, E, D. Veber, I. Eberini, F.R. Buccellato, E. Mutti, L. Sironi G. Scalabrino, 2003. Cobalamin (vitamin B12)-deficiency-induced changes in the proteome of rat cerebro-spinal fluid. *Biochem J*, 374:239–246.

Gilad, O., S. Jacobsen, B. Stuer-Lauridsen, M.B. Pedersen, C. Garrigues, B. Svensson, 2010. Combined transcriptome and proteome analysis of *Bifidobacterium animalis* subsp. lactis BB-12 grown on xylo-oligosaccharides and a model of their utilization. *Appl Environ Microb*, 76:7285–7291.

Goetz, M.P., M.M. Ames, R.M. Weinshilboum, 2004. Primer on medical genomics: Part XII: pharmacogenomics—General principles with cancer as a model. *Mayo Clin Proc*, 79:376–384.

Gouw, J.W., J. Krijgsveld, A.J. Heck, 2010. Quantitative proteomics by metabolic labeling of model organisms. *Mol Cell Proteomics*, 9:11–24.

Gravouil, K., Ferru-Clément, R., Colas, S., Helye, R., Kadri, L., Bourdeau, L., Moumen, B., Mercier, A. & Ferreira, T. 2017. Transcriptomics and Lipidomics of the Environmental Strain Rhodococcus ruber Point out Consumption Pathways and Potential Metabolic Bottlenecks for Polyethylene Degradation. *Environmental Science & Technology*, 51:5172–5181.

Griffiths, W.J., T. Koal, T., Y. Wang, M. Kohl, D.P. Enot, H.P. Deigner, 2010. Targeted metabolomics for biomarker discovery. *Angew Chem Int Ed Engl*, 49:5426–5445.

He, F.J., C.A. Nowson, G.A. MacGregor, 2006. Fruit and vegetable consumption and stroke: Meta-analysis of cohort studies. *The Lancet*, 367(9507):320–326.

Henry, G., D. Mollé, F. Morgan, J. Fauquant, S. Bouhallab, 2002. Heat-induced covalent complex between casein micelles and b-lactoglobulin from goat's milk: Identification of an involved disulfide bond. *J Agric Food Chem*, 50:185–191.

Herbst, A., S. McIlwain, J.J. Schmidt, J.M. Aiken, C.D. Page, L. Li, 2009. Prion disease prognosis by proteomic profiling. *J Proteome Res*, 8:1030–1036.

Herrero, M, V. García-Cañas, C. Simo, A. Cifuentes, 2010. Recent advances in the application of CE methods for food analysis and Foodomics. *Electrophoresis*, 31:205–228.

Herzog, A., S. Kuntz, H. Daniel, U. Wenzel, 2004. Identification of biomarkers for the initiation of apoptosis in human preneoplastic colonocytes by proteome analysis. *Int J Cancer*, 109:220–229.

Hines, L.M., M.J. Stampfer, J. Ma, J.M. Gaziano, P.M. Ridker, S.E. Hankinson, F. Sacks, E.B. Rimm, and D.J. Hunter, 2001. Genetic variation in alcohol dehydrogenase and the beneficial effect of moderate alcohol consumption on myocardial infarction. *N Engl J Med*, 344(8):549–555.

Hirschhorn, J.N., M.J. Daly, 2005. Genome-wide association studies for common diseases and complex traits. *Nat Rev Genet*, 6:95–108.

Hood, L., J.R. Health, M.R. Phelps, B. Lin, 2004. Systems biology and new technologies enable predictive and preventative medicine. *Science*, 306:640–643.

Hsieh, L.S., R. Moharram, A. Akasawa, J. Slater, B.M. Martin, 2002. Banana allergen detection and identification using SELDI technology. *J Allergy Clin Immunol*, 1:S305.

Hsu, R.L., K.T. Lee, J.T. Wang, L.Y.L. Lee, R.P.Y. Chen, 2009. Amyloid-degrading ability of nattokinase from *Bacillus subtilis natto*, *J Agric Food Chem*, :503–508.

Huang, Z, Y. Li, B. Chen, S. Yao, 2007. Simultaneous determination of 102 pesticide residues in Chinese teas by gas chromatography-mass spectrometry. *J Chromatogr B Analyt Technol Biomed Life Sci*, 856:154–162.

Hwang, H., B.P. Bowen, B.P., N. Lefort, C.R. Flynn, E.A. de Filippis, C. Roberts, C.C. Smoke, C. Meyer, K. Hojlund, Z. Yi, L.J. Mandarino, 2010. Proteomics analysis of human skeletal muscle reveals novel abnormalities in obesity and type 2 diabetes. *Diabetes*, 59:33–42.

Ide, T. 2017. Physiological activities of the combination of fish oil and α-lipoic acid affecting hepatic lipogenesis and parameters related to oxidative stress in rats. *European Journal of Nutrition*, 1–17.

Ishikawa, M., K. Shiomi, F. Suzuki, M. Ishida, Y. Nagashima, 2001. Identification of tropomyosin as a major allergen in the octopus *Octopus vulgaris* and elucidation of its IgE binding epitopes. *Fish Sci*, 67:934–942.

Junter, G.A., L. Coquet, S. Vilain, T. Jouenne, 2002. Immobilized-cell physiology: Current data and the potentialities of proteomics. *Enzyme Microb Technol*, 31:201–212.

Kailasapathy, K., J. Chin, 2000. Survival and therapeutic potential of probiotic organisms with reference to *Lactobacillus acidophilus* and *Bifidobacterium* spp. *Immunol Cell Biol*, 78:80–88.

Kakoti, B, A. Anjali Hirani, V. Sutariya, Y. Pathak, 2015. Omics driven trends in nutrition, disease prevention and better health. *J Bioinform, Genomics, Proteomics*, 1(1):1001, 1–4.

Kaput, J., 2004. Diet-disease gene interactions. *Nutrition*, 20:26–31

Kassim A, Pflüger V, Premji Z, Daubenberger C, Revathi G. Comparison of biomarker based Matrix Assisted Laser Desorption Ionization-Time of Flight Mass Spectrometry (MALDI-TOF MS) and conventional methods in the identification of clinically relevant bacteria and yeast. *BMC Microbiology*, 2017; 17:128.

Kidd, P. M. 2008. Alzheimer's disease, amnestic mild cognitive impairment, and age-associated memory impairment: current understanding and progress toward integrative prevention. *Alternative Medicine Review*, 13:85.

Kim, M.K., J.H. Park, 2009. Conference on "Multidisciplinary approaches to nutritional problems." Symposium on "Nutrition and health." Cruciferous vegetable intake and the risk of human cancer: Epidemiological evidence. *Proc Nutr Soc*, 68(1):103–110.

Kok, E.J., H.A. Kuiper, 2003. Comparative safety assessment for biotech crops. *Trends Biotechnol*, 21:439–444.

Kornman, K.S., P.M. Martha, G.W. Duff, 2004. Genetic variations and inflammation: A practical nutrigenomics opportunity. *Nutrition*, 20:44–49.

Kotsopoulos, J., P. Ghadirian, A. El-Sohemy, H.T. Lynch, C. Snyder, M. Daly, S. Domchek, et al., 2007. The CYP1A2 genotype modifies the association between coffee consumption and breast cancer risk among BRCA1 mutation carriers. *Cancer Epidemiol Biomarkers Prev*, 16(5):912–916.

Krishnan, H.B., W.S. Kim, S. Jang, M.S. Kerley, 2009. All three subunits of soybean b- conglycinin are potential food allergens. *J Agric Food Chem*, 57:938–943.

Kussmann, M., F. Raymond, M. Affolter, 2006. OMICS-driven biomarker discovery in nutrition and health. *J Biotechnol*, 124:758–787.

Lampe, J.W., 2009. Interindividual differences in response to plant-based diets: Implications for cancer risk. *Am J Clin Nutr*, 89(5):1553S–1557S.

Lampe, J.W., C. Chen, S. Li, J. Prunty, M.T. Grate, D.E. Meehan, K.V. Barale, D.A. Dightman, Z. Feng, and J.D. Potter, 2000. Modulation of human glutathione S-transferases by botanically defined vegetable diets. *Cancer Epidemiol Biomarkers Prev*, 9(8):787–793.

Li, F., Q. Zhao, C. Wang, X. Lu, X.F. Li, C. Le, 2010. Detection of *Escherichia coli* O157:H7 using gold nanoparticle labelling and inductively coupled plasma mass spectrometry. *Anal Chem*, 82:3399–3403.

Li, H., Z. Xie, J. Lin, H. Song, Q. Wang, K. Wang, M. Su, et al., 2008. Transcriptomic and metabolomic profiling of obesity-prone and obesity-resistant rats under high fat diet. *J Proteome Res*, 7(11):4775–4783.

Lindi, V., U. Schwab, A. Louheranta, M. Laakso, B. Vessby, K. Hermansen, L. Storlien, G. Riccardi, and A.A. Rivellese, 2003. Impact of the Pro12Ala polymorphism of the PPAR-gamma2 gene on serum triacylglycerol response to n-3 fatty acid supplementation. *Mol Genet Metab*, 79(1):52–60.

Linke T, A.C. Ross, E.H. Harrison, 2004. Profiling of rat plasma by surface enhanced laser desorption/ionization time-of-flight mass spectrometry, a novel tool for biomarker discovery in nutrition research. *J Chromatogr A*, 1043:65–71.

Lloyd-Jones, D., Adams, R., Carnethon, M., De Simone, G., Ferguson, T. B., Flegal, K., Ford, E., Furie, K., Go, A. & Greenlund, K. 2009. Heart disease and stroke statistics—2009 update. *Circulation*, 119:e21–e181.

Lodge, J.K., 2010. Symposium 2: Modern approaches to nutritional research challenges: Targeted and non-targeted approaches for metabolite profiling in nutritional research. *Proc Nutr Soc*, 69:95–102.

Maheshwari R., M. Tekade, P.A. Sharma, R.K. Tekade, 2015. Nanocarriers assisted siRNA gene therapy for the management of cardiovascular disorders. *Curr Pharm Des*, 21:4427–4440.

Maheshwari, R.G., R.K. Tekade, P.A. Sharma, G. Darwhekar, A. Tyagi, R.P. Patel, D.K. Jain, 2012. Ethosomes and ultradeformable liposomes for transdermal delivery of clotrimazole: A comparative assessment. *Saudi Pharm J*, 20:161–170.

Mahler, V. & Goodman, R. 2017. Definition and design of hypoallergenic foods. *Molecular Allergy Diagnostics*. Springer.

Malek, A. J., Klimentidis, Y. C., Kell, K. P. & Fernández, J. R. 2013. Associations of the lactase persistence allele and lactose intake with body composition among multiethnic children. *Genes & Nutrition*, 8:487–494.

Mariani, S.M., 2003. Clinical proteomics: New promises for early cancer detection. *MedGenMed*, 5:23.

Martínez-Gomariz, M., M.L. Hernáez, D. Gutiérrez, P. Ximénez-Embún, G. Préstamo, 2009. Proteomic analysis by two-dimensional differential gel electrophoresis (2D DIGE) of a high-pressure effect in *Bacillus cereus*. *J Agric Food Chem*, 57:3543–3549.

Martín-Pedraza, L., González, M., Gómez, F., Blanca-López, N., Garrido-Arandia, M., Rodríguez, R., Torres, M. J., Blanca, M., Villalba, M. & Mayorga, C. 2016. Two nonspecific lipid transfer proteins (nsLTPs) from tomato seeds are associated to severe symptoms of tomato-allergic patients. *Molecular Nutrition & Food Research*, 60:1172–1182.

McCabe-Sellers, B., D. Lovera, H. Nuss, C. Wise, B. Ning, C. Teitel, B.S. Clark, T. Toennessen, B. Green, M.L. Bogle, J. Kaput, 2008. Personalizing nutrigenomics research through community based participatory research and omics technologies. *OMICS*, 12(4):263–272.

Mckenzie, A. L., Hallberg, S. J., Creighton, B. C., Volk, B. M., Link, T. M., Abner, M. K., Glon, R. M., McCarter, J. P., Volek, J. S. & Phinney, S. D. 2017. A Novel Intervention Including Individualized Nutritional Recommendations Reduces Hemoglobin A1c Level, Medication Use, and Weight in Type 2 Diabetes. *JMIR Diabetes*, 2:e5.

Meyer, U.A., 2012. Personalized medicine: A personal view. *Clin Pharmacol Ther*, 91(3):373–375.

Meyer, U.A., Zanger, U.M. Schwab, M. 2013. Omics and drug response. *Ann Rev Pharmacol Toxicol*, 53:475–502.

Miernyk, J. A., Jett, A. A. & Johnston, M. L. 2016. Analysis of soybean tissue culture protein dynamics using difference gel electrophoresis. *J Proteomics*, 130:56–64.

Mills, E.N., J.A. Jenkins, M.J. Alcocer, P.R. Shewry, 2004. Structural, biological, and evolutionary relationships of plant food allergens sensitizing via the gastrointestinal tract. *Crit Rev Food Sci Nutr*, 44:379–407.

Misra, J., I. Alevizos, D. Hwang, G. Stephanopoulos, G. Stephanopoulos, 2007. Linking physiology and transcriptional profiles by quantitative predictive models. *Biotechnol Bioeng*, 98(1):252–260.

Motoyama, K., Y. Suma, S. Ishizaki, Y. Nagashima, K. Shiomi, 2007. Molecular cloning of tropomyosins identified as allergens in six species of crustaceans. *J Agric Food Chem*, 55:985–991.

Nasi, A., G. Picariello, P. Ferranti, 2009. Proteomic approaches to study structure, functions, and toxicity of legume seeds lectins. Perspectives for the assessment of food quality and safety. *J Proteomics*, 72:527–538.

Ning, M., E.H. Lo, 2010. Opportunities and challenges in Omics. *Transl Stroke Res*, 1:233–237.

Nkondjock, A., P. Ghadirian, J. Kotsopoulos, J. Lubinski, H. Lynch, C. Kim-Sing, D. Horsman, et al., 2006. Coffee consumption and breast cancer risk among BRCA1 and BRCA2 mutation carriers. *Int J Cancer*, 118(1):103–107.

Nomura S., T. Miyasho, N. Maeda, K. Doh-Ura, H. Yokota, 2009. Autoantibody to glial fibrillary acidic protein in the sera of cattle with bovine spongiform encephalopathy, *Proteomics*, 9:4029–4035.

Norheim, F., T. Raastad, B. Thiede, A.C. Rustan, C.A. Drevon, F. Haugen, 2011. Proteomic identification of secreted proteins from human skeletal muscle cells and expression in response to strength training. *Am J Physiol Endocrinol Metab*, 301:E1013–E1021.

Ochoa, M., P.B. Harrington, 2005. Immunomagnetic isolation of enterohemorrhagic Escherichia coli O157:H7 from ground beef and identification by matrix-assisted laser desorption/ionization-time-of-flight mass spectrometry and database searches. *Anal Chem*, 77:5258–5267.

Oh, E, M.N. Hasan, M. Jamshed, S.H. Park, H.M. Hong, E.J. Song, Y.S. Yoo, 2010. Growing trend of CE at the omics level: The frontier of systems biology. *Electrophoresis*, 31:74–92.

Ong, S.E., B. Blagoev, I. Kratchmarova, D.B. Kristensen, H. Steen, A. Pandey, M. Mann, 2002. Stable isotope labeling by amino acids in cell culture, SILAC, as a simple and accurate approach to expression proteomics. *Mol Cell Proteomics*, 1:376–386.

Oommen, A.M., J.B. Griffin, G. Sarath, J. Zempleni, 2005. Roles for nutrients in epigenetic events. *J Nutr Biochem*, 16:74–7.

Ordovas, J.M. 2008. Genotype-phenotype associations: Modulation by diet and obesity. *Obesity (Silver Spring)*, 16 Suppl 3:S40–S46.

Ortea, I., B. Cañas, J.M. Gallardo, 2009. Mass spectrometry characterization of species-specific peptides from arginine kinase for the identification of commercially relevant shrimp species. *J Proteome Res*, 8:5356–5362.

Palatini, P., G. Ceolotto, F. Ragazzo, F. Dorigatti, F. Saladini, I. Papparella, L. Mos, G. Zanata, M. Santonastaso, 2009. CYP1A2 genotype modifies the association between coffee intake and the risk of hypertension. *J Hypertens*, 27(8):1594–1601.

Park, J.Y., J.K. Seong, and Y.K. Paik, 2004. Proteomic analysis of diet-induced hypercholesterolemic mice. *Proteomics* 4, 514–523.

Pasikanti, K.K., P.C. Ho, E.C. Chan, 2008. Gas chromatography/mass spectrometry in metabolic profiling of biological fluids. *J Chromatogr B Analyt Technol Biomed Life Sci*, 871:202–211.

Pavo, I., Jermendy, G. R., Varkonyi, T. T., Kerenyi, Z., Gyimesi, A., Shoustov, S., Shestakova, M., Herz, M., Johns, D. & Schluchter, B. J. 2003. Effect of pioglitazone compared with metformin on glycemic control and indicators of insulin sensitivity in recently diagnosed patients with type 2 diabetes. *The Journal of Clinical Endocrinology & Metabolism*, 88:1637–1645.

Petricoin, E.F., K.C. Zoon, E.C. Kohn, J.C. Barrett, L.A. Liotta, 2002. Clinical proteomics: Translating benchside promise into bedside reality. *Nat Rev Drug Discov*, 1:683–695.

Picotti, P. R. Aebersold, 2012. Selected reaction monitoring-based proteomics: Workflows, potential, pitfalls and future directions. *Nat Methods*, 9:555–566.

Pineiro, C., J. Barros-Velázquez, J. Vázquez, A. Figueras, J.M. Gallardo, 2003. Proteomics as a tool for the investigation of seafood and other marine products. *J Proteome Res*, 2:127–135.

Pirih, N. & Kunej, T. 2017. Toward a taxonomy for multi-omics science? Terminology development for whole genome study approaches by omics technology and hierarchy. *OMICS: A Journal of Integrative Biology*, 21:1–16.

Planchon, S., M. Desvaux, I. Chafsey, C. Chambon, S. Leroy, M. Hébraud, R. Talon, 2009. Comparative subproteome analyses of planktonic and sessile *Staphylococcus xylosus C2a*: New insight in cell physiology of a coagulase-negative Staphylococcus in biofilm. *J Proteome Res*, 8:1797–1809.

Plourde, M., M.C. Vohl, M. Vandal, P. Couture, S. Lemieux, S.C. Cunnane, 2009. Plasma n-3 fatty acid response to an n-3 fatty acid supplement is modulated by apoE epsilon4 but not by the common PPAR-alpha L162V polymorphism in men. *Br J Nutr*, 102(8):1121–1124.

Probst-Hensch, N.M., S.R. Tannenbaum, K.K. Chan, G.A. Coetzee, R.K. Ross, M.C. Yu, 1998. Absence of the glutathione S-transferase M1 gene increases cytochrome P4501A2 activity among frequent consumers of cruciferous vegetables in a Caucasian population. *Cancer Epidemiol Biomarkers Prev*, 7(7):635–638.

Puri, R., M. Duong, K. Uno, Y. Kataoka, S.J. Nicholls, 2012. The emerging role of plasma lipidomics in cardiovascular drug discovery. *Expert Opin Drug Discov*, 7:63–72.

Rai, A.J., D.W. Chan, 2004. Cancer proteomics: Serum diagnostics for tumor marker discovery. *Ann N Y Acad Sci*, 1022:286–294.

Ramljak, S., A.R. Asif, V.W. Armstrong, A. Wrede, M.H. Groschup, A. Buschmann, W. Schulz-Schaeffer, W. Bodemer, I. Zerr, 2008. Physiological role of the cellular prion protein (PrPC): Protein profiling study in two cell culture systems. *J Proteome Res*, 7:2681–2695.

Raqib, R, A. Cravioto, 2009. Nutrition, immunology, and genetics: Future perspectives. *Nutr Rev*, 67:227–236.

Rasmussen, R.R., I.M. Stom, P.H. Rasmussen, J. Smedsgaard, K.F. Nielsen, 2010. Multimycotoxin analysis of maize silage by LC-MS/MS. *Anal Bioanal Chem*, 397:765–776.

Ross, S.A., 2007. Nutritional genomic approaches to cancer prevention research. *Exp Oncol*, 29(4):250–256.

Ruebelt, M.C., M. Lipp, T.L. Reynolds, J.D. Astwood, K.H. Engel, K.D. Jany, 2006. Application of two-dimensional gel electrophoresis to interrogate alterations in the proteome of genetically modified crops. 2. Assessing natural variability. *J Agric Food Chem*, 54:2162–2168.

Samuel, M., Chisanga, D., Liem, M., Keerthikumar, S., Anand, S., Ang, C.-S., Adda, C. G., Versteegen, E., Jois, M. & Mathivanan, S. 2017. Bovine milk-derived exosomes from colostrum are enriched with proteins implicated in immune response and growth. *Scientific Reports*, 7.

Scaloni, A., V. Perillo, P. Franco, F. Fedele, R. Froio, L. Ferrara, P. Bergamo, 2002. Characterization of heat-induced lactosylation products in caseins by immunoenzymatic and mass spectrometric methodologies. *Biochim Biophys Acta*, 1598:30–39.

Schittmayer, M., R. Birner-Gruenberger, 2009. Functional proteomics in lipid research: Lipases, lipid droplets and lipoproteins. *J Proteom*, 72:1006–1018.

Schmidt, A., J. Kellermann, F. Lottspeich, 2005. A novel strategy for quantitative proteomics using isotope-coded protein labels. *Proteomics*, 5:4–15.

Schmidt, H., C. Gelhaus, T. Latendorf, M. Nebendahl, A. Petersen, S. Krause, M. Leippe, W.M. Becker, O. Janssen, 2009. 2-D DIGE analysis of the proteome of extracts from peanut variants reveals striking differences in major allergen contents. *Proteomics*, 9:3507–3521.

Schwer, B., M. Eckersdorff, Y. Li, J.C. Silva, D. Fermin, M.V. Kurtev, C. Giallourakis, M.J. Comb, F.W. Alt, D.B. Lombard, 2009. Calorie restriction alters mitochondrial protein acetylation. *Aging Cell* 8:604–606.

Shiffman, D., S.G. Ellis, C.M. Rowland, M.J. Malloy, M.M. Luke, O.A. Iakoubova, C.R. Pullinger, et al., 2005. Identification of four gene variants associated with myocardial infarction. *Am J Hum Genet*, 77(4):596–605.

Shiomi, K., Y. Sato, S. Hamamoto, H. Mita, K. Shimakura, 2008. Sarcoplasmatic calcium-binding proteIn: identification as a new allergen of the black tiger shrimp *Penaeus monodon*. *Int Arch Allergy Immunol*, 146:91–98.

Simo, C, E. Domínguez-Vega, M.L. Marina, M.C. García, G. Dinelli, A. Cifuentes, 2010. CE-TOF MS analysis of complex protein hydrolyzates from genetically modified soybeans-A tool for foodomics. *Electrophoresis* 31:1175–1183.

Smeller, L., 2002. Pressure-temperature phase diagram molecules. *Biochem Biophys Acta*, 1595(1):11–29.

Smelt, J.P.P.M, J.C. Hellemons, M.F. Patterson, 2001. Effects of high pressure on vegetative microorganisms. In: *Ultra HighPressure Treatments of Foods*, M.E.G. Hendrickx, D. Knorr (Eds.), Kluwer Academic, New York, pp. 55–76.

Soumaoro, L. T., Uetake, H., Takagi, Y., Iida, S., Higuchi, T., Yasuno, M., Enomoto, M. & Sugihara, K. 2006. Coexpression of VEGF-C and Cox-2 in human colorectal cancer and its association with lymph node metastasis. *Diseases of the Colon & Rectum*, 49:392–398.

Steinacker, P., W. Rist, M. Swiatek-de-Lange, S. Lehnert, S. Jesse, A. Pabst, H. Tumani, et al., 2010. Ubiquitin as potential cerebrospinal fluid marker of Creutzfeldt-Jakob disease. *Proteomics*, 10:81–89.

Stepczynska, A., Schanstra, J. P. & Mischak, H. 2016. Implementation of CE-MS-identified proteome-based biomarker panels in drug development and patient management. *Bioanalysis*, 2016;8(5):439–455.

Stevenson S.E., Y. Chu, P. Ozias-Akins, J.J. Thelen, 2009. Validation of gel-free, label-free quantitative proteomics approaches: Applications for seed allergen profiling. *J Proteomics*, 72:555–566. 83.

Strom, A., S. Diecke, G. Hunsmann, A.W. Stuke, 2006. Identification of prion protein binding proteins by combined use of far-Western immunoblotting, two dimensional gel electrophoresis and mass spectrometry. *Proteomics*, 6:26–34.

Taka, H., N. Kaga, T. Fujimura, R. Mineki, M. Imaizumi, Y. Suzuki, R. Suzuki, M. Tanokura, N. Shindo, K. Murayama, 2000. Rapid determination of parvalbumin amino acid sequence from *Rana catesbeiana* (pI 4.78) by combination of ESI mass spectrometry, protein sequencing, and amino acid analysis. *J Biochem*, 127:723–729.

Tanaka, M., G. Wang, Y.P. Pitsiladis, 2016. Advancing sports and exercise genomics: Moving from hypothesis-driven single study approaches to large multi-omics collaborative science. *Physiol Genomics*, 48(3):173–174.

Taylor, M.J., G.A. Keenan, K.B. Reid, D.U. Fernandez, 2008. The utility of ultraperformance liquid chromatography/electrospray ionisation time-of-flight mass spectrometry for multi-residue determination of pesticides in strawberry. *Rapid Commun Mass Spectrom*, 22:2731–2746.

Tekade, R.K., M.B. Chougule, 2013. Formulation development and evaluation of hybrid nanocarrier for cancer therapy: Taguchi orthogonal array based design. *Biomed Res Int*, 2013:712678.

Tekade, R.K., P.V. Kumar, N.K. Jain, 2009. Dendrimers in oncology: An expanding horizon. *Chem Rev*, 109:49–87.

Tekade, R.K., R.G. Maheshwari, P.A. Sharma, M. Tekade, A.S. Chauhan, 2015a. siRNA therapy, challenges and underlying perspectives of dendrimer as delivery vector. *Curr Pharm Des*, 21:4614–36.

Tekade, R.K, M. Tekade, M. Kumar, A.S. Chauhan, 2015b. Dendrimer-stabilized smart-nanoparticle (DSSN) platform for targeted delivery of hydrophobic antitumor therapeutics. *Pharm Res*, 32:910–928.

Teuber, S.S., S.K. Sathe, W.R. Peterson, K.H. Roux, 2002. Characterization of the soluble allergenic proteins of cashew nut (*Anacardium occidentale* L.). *J Agric Food Chem*, 50:6543–6549.

Tibshirani, R., T. Hastie, M. Elsen, D. Rose, D. Bostatin, P. Brown, 2015. *Clustering Methods for Analysis of DNA Microarray Data. Technical Report*, Department of statistics.

Tsiroulnikov, K., H. Rezai, E. Bonch-Osmolovskaya, P. Nedkov, A. Goustrova, V. Cueff, A. Godfroy, et al., 2004. Hydrolysis of the amyloid prion protein and nonpathogenic meat and bone meal by anaerobic thermophilic prokaryotes and *Streptomyces* subspecies. *J Agric Food Chem*, 52:6353–6360.

Unwin, R.D., J.R. Griffiths, A.D. Whetton, 2010. Simultaneous analysis of relative protein expression levels across multiple samples using iTRAQ isobaric tags with 2D nano LC-MS/MS. *Nat Protoc*, 5:1574–1582.

Ushiama, S., T. Nakamura, T. Ishijima, T. Misaka, K. Abe, Y. Nakai, 2010. The hepatic genes for immunoproteasome are upregulated by refeeding after fasting in the rat. *Biosci Biotechnol Biochem*, 74(6):1320–1323.

Uzogara, S.G., 2000. The impact of genetic modification of human foods in the 21st century: A review. *Biotechnol Adv*, 18:179–206.

Van der Lee, M.K., G. van der Weg, W.A. Traag, H.G.J. Mol, 2008. Qualitative screening and quantitative determination of pesticides and contaminants in animal feed using comprehensive two-dimensional gas chromatography with time-of-flight mass spectrometry. *J Chromatogr A*, 1186:325–339.

Vitali, B., V. Wasinger, P. Brigidi, M. Guilhaus, 2005. A proteomic view of *Bifidobacterium infantis* generated by multi-dimensional chromatography coupled with tandem mass spectrometry. *Proteomics*, 5:1859–1867.

Walther, T.C., M. Mann, M, 2010. Mass spectrometry-based proteomics in cell biology. *J Cell Biol*, 190:491–500.

Washburn, M.P. and J.R. Yates, 3rd, 2000. Analysis of the microbial proteome. *Curr Opin Microbiol*, 3:292–297.

Watanabe, Y., A. Kamei, F. Shinozaki, T. Ishijima, K. Iida, Y. Nakai, S. Arai, K. Abe, 2011. Ingested maple syrup evokes a possible liver-protecting effect-physiologic and genomic investigation with rats. *Biosci Biotechnol Biochem*, 75(12):2408–2410.

Wenzel, U, A. Herzog, S. Kuntz, H. Daniel, 2004. Protein expression profiling identifies molecular targets of quercetin as a major dietary flavonoid in human colon cancer cells. *Proteomics*, 4:2160–2174.

Willerslev-Olsen, A., Krejsgaard, T., Lindahl, L. M., Litvinov, I. V., Fredholm, S., Petersen, D. L., Nastasi, C., Gniadecki, R., Mongan, N. P. & Sasseville, D. 2016. Staphylococcal enterotoxin A (SEA) stimulates STAT3 activation and IL-17 expression in cutaneous T-cell lymphoma. *Blood*, 127:1287–1296.

Wong, J, C. Hao, K. Zhang, P. Yang, K. Banerjee, D. Hayward, I. Iftakhar, et al., 2010. Development and interlaboratory validation of a QuEChERS-based liquid chromatography-tandem mass spectrometry method for multiresidue pesticide analysis. *J Agric Food Chem*, 58:5897–5903.

Wood, P.L., 2012. Lipidomics of Alzheimer's disease: Current status. *Alzheimers Res Ther*, 4:5.

Wooding, S., U.K. Kim, M.J. Bamshad, J. Larsen, L.B. Jorde, and D. Drayna, 2004. Natural selection and molecular evolution in PTC, a bitter-taste receptor gene. *Am J Hum Genet*, 74(4):637–646.

Wu, Q., H. Yuan, L. Zhang, and Y. Zhang, 2012. Recent advances on multidimensional liquid chromatography-mass spectrometry for proteomics: From qualitative to quantitative analysis—A review. *Anal Chim Acta*, 731:1–10.

Xu, Y.-J. 2017. Foodomics: a novel approach for food microbiology. *TrAC Trends in Analytical Chemistry*.

Xu, Y, W. Cheung, C.L. Winder, R. Gooacre, 2010. VOC-based metabolic profiling for food spoilage detection with the application to detecting Salmonella typhimurium-contaminated pork. *Anal Bioanal Chem*, 397:2439–2449.

Yaghjyan, L., Colditz, G., Rosner, B., Gasparova, A. & Tamimi, R. 2017. Associations of coffee consumption and caffeine intake with mammographic breast density. AACR.

Yang, H., J. Rouse, L. Lukes, M. Lancaster, T. Veenstra, M. Zhou, Y. Shi, Y.G. Park, and K. Hunter, 2004. Caffeine suppresses metastasis in a transgenic mouse model: A prototype molecule for prophylaxis of metastasis. *Clin ExpMetastasis*, 21(8):719–735.

Yoshioka, H., T. Ohmoto, A. Urisu, Y. Mine, T. Adachi, 2004. Expression and epitope analysis of the major allergenic protein Fag e 1 from buckwheat. *J Plant Physiol*, 161:761–767.

Zachariasova, M, O. Lacina, A. Malachova, M. Kostelanska, J. Poutska, M. Godula, J. Hajslova, 2010. Novel approaches in analysis of Fusarium mycotoxins in cereals employing ultra-performance liquid chromatography coupled with high resolution mass spectrometry. *Anal Chim Acta*, 662:51–61.

Zeisel, S.H., 2007. Nutrigenomics and metabolomics will change clinical nutrition and public health practice: Insights from studies on dietary requirements for choline. *Am J Clin Nutr*, 86(3):542–548.

Zhang, A., H. Sun, P. Wang, Y. Han, X. Wang, 2012. Modern analytical techniques in metabolomics analysis. *Analyst*, 137:293–300.

Nutrigenomics
The Cutting Edge and Asian Perspectives

Adela Pilav and Yashwant V. Pathak
University of South Florida
Tampa, Florida

Contents

3.1 Introduction 61
3.2 Nutrigenomics: Omics 63
3.3 Cutting-edge research in the field of cardiovascular disease states 66
3.4 Homeopathic and ayurvedic medicine 72
3.5 Cancer 74
3.6 Conclusion 79
References 80

3.1 Introduction

With the advent of the Human Genome Project (HGP), the link between nutrition and genetics opened like a sluice gate. Out came pouring a number of omics-based fields of research, such as transcriptomics, metabolomics, proteomics, and more. As cultures that have practiced medicine and nutrition for centuries, the Asian and Middle Eastern populations have had ample amounts of research flooding the scientific realm regarding nutrigenomics in recent years. The respective cultures contain diversity in their diets, due to economic, agricultural, and taste preference differences over centuries past. Furthermore, genome differences between cultures reflect contrasts with regard to nutrient bioavailability, an inherited aspect. In this chapter, we will discuss novel, cutting-edge nutrigenomics research in Asia and the Middle East (Fenech et al. 2011).

Nutrigenomics is the study of the manner in which one's nutritional intake affects one's genetic expression. The multiple mechanisms by which the diet may regulate gene expression include transcriptomics, proteomics, and metabolomics. The HGP and genome-wide association studies (GWAS) have enabled an array of research studies to inspect the manner in which an individual's diet or drug use may affect the transcription of RNA molecules, the subsequent protein expression and activity, and the overall metabolic processes of the body in response to diet and drugs (Figure 3.1). Overall, nutrigenetics and nutrigenomics have three major spearheading hypotheses for future research and development (Fenech et al. 2011; Riscuta 2016).

The first fundamental hypothesis is that nutrition may enact a specific effect on the expression of genes in such a way as to alter metabolic pathways and/or to exert genetic mutation indirectly. Genetic mutation may occur at a base sequence level or at a chromosomal level, resulting in changes in gene expression. The second fundamental hypothesis is that the health outcomes of specific nutrients may depend on an individual's inherited genes. Among such genes are genetic variants that are likely to modify uptake and subsequent

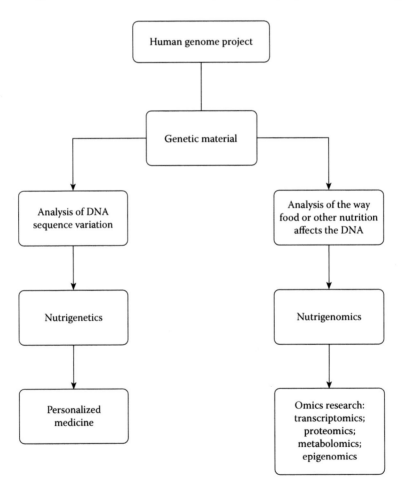

Figure 3.1 Flowchart illustrating the opportunities of the Human Genome Project. Future developments may lead to personalized medicine and omics-based research, which may also result in individualized treatments for patients.

metabolism of nutrients. Furthermore, genetic variants may modify the manner in which enzymes interact with nutrient cofactors, resulting in specific effects. The third fundamental hypothesis of nutrigenomics and nutrigenetics is that the customization of nutritional requirements may lead to improved health outcomes. This may be enhanced with proper analysis of an individual's genetic characteristics, as well as factors such as age, health status, and even preferences in diet (Fenech et al. 2011).

Nutrigenetics, the study of how the genes interact with nutritional intake, involves polymorphisms, or polymorphic variants, which are differences in genetic material within 1% of any population. A major propulsive discovery in the field of nutrigenetics is the single nucleotide polymorphism (SNP), an occurrence in which a DNA building block, a nucleotide base, is replaced with another. This action has been thought to alter the synthesis of proteins and thus alter their function, creating discrepancies in nutritional requirements as well as the metabolism of bioactive components (Ferguson et al. 2016).

Other structural DNA alterations, such as translocations, deletions, insertions, and copy number variations, may occur, yielding unusual protein synthesis and behavior. These novel discoveries have allowed nutrigenetics to flourish with studies aimed at understanding why genetic material interacts with nutrients in a specific manner. However, although *nutrigenomics* and *nutrigenetics* are often terms used interchangeably, nutrigenomics strives to pinpoint the actions of ingested biomolecules upon the genetic material of an individual. As shown in Figure 3.2, nutrigenomics includes omics-based fields such as transcriptomics, proteomics, epigenomics, metabolomics, and more. This chapter will highlight the many aspects of each type of omics-based field, as well as discuss novel research performed in cutting-edge Asian studies within each omics-based field (Fenech et al. 2011; Ferguson et al. 2016).

3.2 Nutrigenomics: Omics

Included under the umbrella term *nutrigenomics* is the study of the transcriptome, the entire set of RNA transcripts within the body. Transcriptomics can be performed by providing altered nutrient sources or specific nutrients to experimental animals via food, water, or injection. Subsequent excision of the target organ then allows for DNA microarray analysis to carefully inspect the RNA samples between control and experimental animal subjects. Transcriptomics can also be carried out by modifying culture cell composition, with subsequent DNA microarray analysis, as with the animal subjects (Ferguson et al. 2016; Merdad et al. 2015).

Transcription and genetic variation are the driving forces of the presence of metabolites, making metabolites direct indicators of the metabolomic phenotype gleaned from one's diet. Therefore, understanding the metabolic pathways may reflect different metabolite levels and patterns between individuals

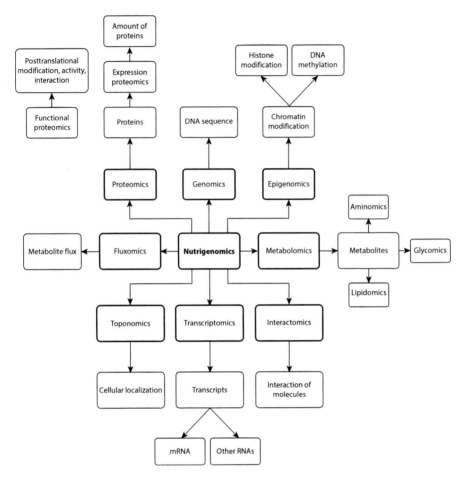

Figure 3.2 *Map outlining the branches of nutrigenomics. The major branches of nutrigenomic research include genomics, proteomics, epigenomics, transcriptomics, metabolomics, interactomics, toponomics, and fluxomics.*

with differing diets and genetic variation. The metabolic profile may include an abundance of different metabolites, ranging from contrasting polarities, sizes, functions, and concentrations. Due to genetic variation uncovered by Mendelian randomization studies, inherited components may result in differences of metabolite concentrations. Specifically, researching the association between an SNP and the concentrations of a metabolite may open doors to study the manner in which this particular SNP is associated with a disease state (Ferguson et al. 2016).

The vast array of metabolites to study poses a difficulty for modern technologies, but nuclear magnetic resonance spectroscopy and mass spectrometry combined with gas and liquid chromatography remain prevailing methodologies in the efforts to scrutinize metabolic profiles. Although approximately

5,000 metabolites have been detected in human serum, technological advancements must be made in order to effectively establish a metabolome map (Ferguson et al. 2016).

Along with transcriptomics, the umbrella terms *nutrigenetics* and *nutrigenomics* also cover the field of epigenomics. Epigenomic mechanisms include the modification of genetic material in a variety of ways, such as altering the chromatin structure and DNA without directly sullying the genetic sequences. These processes can be accomplished by hydroxymethylation of the DNA, as well as modification of the histone constituents. DNA methylation typically involves methyltransferases, which combine a methyl functional group with a cytosine base, thus sterically blocking the binding between the DNA sequence and transcription factors. DNA can also be acetylated, ubiquitinated, and phosphorylated. These blockades on the DNA silence the underlying sequence, preventing transcription. In contrast to this, histone modifications, including methylation, acetylation, phosphorylation, and ubiquitination, all effectively compress the molecule and deter access for transcription regulators to bind parts of the DNA (Ferguson et al. 2016).

Biomarkers that have been deemed as candidates for epigenomics are those that are causal to disease mechanisms, those that are byproducts of the disease itself, and the initial byproducts of the disease, which result in signs and symptoms as the disease progresses later. With the rise of cardiovascular disease in Asian cultures, biomarkers such as mRNA and proteins are a current focus of novel research (Fenech et al. 2011)

Classic targets of epigenomics are methyl-donating nutrients such as folate, vitamin B, zinc, and methionine, all of which promote the creation of S-adenosyl methionine. This compound is a metabolite of the pathway that provides methyl functional groups for DNA and histone methylation. Studies performed *in vivo* have concentrated on this set of nutrients and have shown that deficiency or excessive supplementation may lead to dysfunction of this pathway, resulting in epigenomic activity. Prior studies have induced in obesity in mice using high-fat diets, promoting methylation alterations of DNA and histones. Although the link between cardiometabolic disease states and epigenomics has been studied, future research may further expound upon the mechanisms behind these alterations of DNA and histones. Future observations may usher in novel treatments and preventions against cardiovascular disease and its risk factors, as outlined in a later section of this chapter about cardiometabolic disease states (Fenech et al. 2011; Ferguson et al. 2016).

Mass spectrometry is also utilized to examine lipid profiles in lipidomics, which is closely related to metabolomics. Like metabolites, lipids in the serum can be intricate in their molecular structure and composition, belonging to a wide array of lipid classes. Recent *in vivo* studies have used dietary precursors to construct lipid species, allowing lipidomics to act as a promising endeavor in the field of nutrigenomics, particularly due to studies finding associations between lipid profiles and cardiometabolic disease states (Ferguson et al. 2016).

One of the more complex branches of nutrigenomics is proteomics, which involves the modification of proteins post-translation. Advanced technology has allowed the use of mass spectrometry coupled with liquid chromatography in order to scrutinize an array of biomarkers and related disease states. Proteomics will be delved into in later sections of this chapter, as it is a novel subject in the discoveries regarding nutrition and genes (Ferguson et al. 2016).

3.3 Cutting-edge research in the field of cardiovascular disease states

In the 1950s, ecological research formulated a connection between the consumption of saturated fat and cardiovascular disease mortality. The discovery of this link triggered a movement towards the study of nutrition and its effect on the body. Factors such as smoking, exercise, stressors, diet, and medication use are all aspects that may affect the way the human body functions. Diet is one of the most prevalent exogenous factors to which human beings are exposed on a daily basis. With this knowledge, the Cohorts for Heart and Aging Research in Genomic Epidemiology (CHARGE) Consortium has developed initiatives to discover the links between genes and diet. To do this, CHARGE utilizes GWAS in order to facilitate meta-analyses focused on possible gene–diet links. Observational studies have indicated associations between genes and cardiovascular disease, or phenotypes related to cardiovascular disease, such as severe hypertension, diabetes mellitus, and dyslipidemia. However, because these studies were observational and thus limited compared to experimental studies, the future path towards genetic research would benefit from experimental deductions. Some recent examples of experimental studies in Asia and the Middle East have utilized cardiovascular disease–related end points to elucidate conclusions derived from the research. Although prior studies promoted primary prevention against cardiovascular disease, recent experimental studies in the field of genomics have merit in possibly being useful for future advancements towards personalized medicine (Ferguson et al. 2016; Teschke et al. 2016).

The goal of new research based in the Asian continent and cultures is to pinpoint candidates related to cardiometabolic functions. Global profiling of transcription may yield more profound measurements of RNA expression before and after applied dietary changes. This will promote the discovery of genes responsive to nutrients, which will thus facilitate the discovery of genes responsive to interventions (Cheng et al. 2017; Ferguson et al. 2016).

An example of this type of link between nutrition and genetics can be found in an Asian study exploring the association between foods introduced after industrialization and metabolic disorders such as obesity and type 2 diabetes. The main proponent studied was fructose, which had been shown in prior studies to reduce memory in the hippocampus of human subjects and exacerbate

66   Nutrigenomics and Nutraceuticals

brain disorders in rodent subjects. Another main feature in this study is docosahexaenoic acid (DHA), previously shown to counteract the effects of fructose on brain structure and function. Rodent subjects were assigned to three subject groups of different diets including or excluding fructose and omega-3 fatty acid, or in the case of the control, neither. The rats' brains were excised, and two compartments were investigated: the hypothalamus (the regulator of metabolism) and the hippocampus (the driving force of cognition) (Cheng et al. 2017).

Using the emerging technique of RNA-Seq, study outcomes (see Figure 3.3) illustrated that fructose was capable of DNA methylation; alternative splicing; and disorganization of genes located in the brain related to cell metabolism, cell communication, immunity, inflammation, and more. Fructose was able to affect the critical genes responsible for the synthesis and/or function of processes like insulin, transforming growth factor beta (TGF-β), PDGF signaling pathways, and more, clearly signifying a link to metabolic disorders such as type 2 diabetes, as well as brain disorders. When compared to human GWAS, the genes perturbed by the effect of fructose overlapped with genes involved in a number of brain disorders including but not limited to attention deficient hyperactivity disorder, depression, Alzheimer's disease, Parkinson's disease, and addictive behaviors. Other genes affected by fructose were

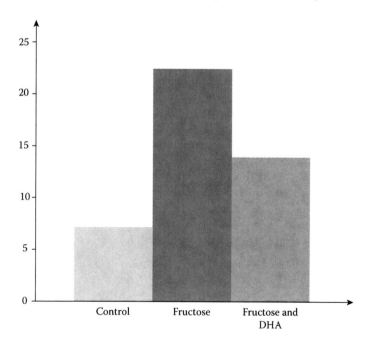

Figure 3.3 Bar graph reflecting the results of a study on the effects of fructose and docosahexaenoic acid (DHA) on properties of cardiometabolic diseases. It is shown that the insulin resistance index is highest with high consumption of fructose, while DHA has been shown to reduce the insulin-resistant effects of fructose.

compared to human GWAS genes for metabolic disorders and were found to overlap with genes associated with obesity, type 2 diabetes, dyslipidemia, and hypertension (Cheng et al. 2017).

In contrast, the study showed that DHA reversed the deleterious effects of fructose by stimulating transcriptional regulators and network regulators, offering insight to the beneficial potential of omega-3 fatty acid consumption. These outcomes shed light on the significance of personalized medicine— patients diagnosed with metabolic disorders or brain disorders may be intolerant to prescription medications, or have contraindications, or may simply prefer nutraceutical alternatives. In many cultures, such as in parts of Asia and the Middle East, the preference for nutraceuticals and healthy eating is a major societal attribute. Therefore, the insights gleaned from recent studied regarding diet and nutrition may offer more personalized methods towards treatment and health (Cheng et al. 2017).

With the knowledge gleaned in recent years regarding high-fat and high-carbohydrate diets, type 2 diabetes mellitus is an important area of focus. Type II diabetes mellitus is becoming increasingly prevalent on the Asian continent, spurring research intertwined with GWAS, as in the aforementioned study. In recent years, Asia and the Middle East have seen a significant cultural move from traditional foods rich in vegetables grown from personal or local gardens to a modern industrial diet of processed sugars and fats. Studies are exponentially aggregating new information regarding the effects of post-industrialism diets. Diets abundant in fats and sugars have been shown to deter the metabolism of both fatty acids and carbohydrates, as has been discussed in this chapter so far. Several studies have found that the hindered metabolism of fatty acids and carbohydrates spurred inflammatory attributes in adipose tissue and decreased oxidation of fatty acids. Insulin signaling has been shown to be impaired in cases of high fatty-acid influx, subsequent to a diet excessive in carbohydrates and fat. One study performed in 2015 in Thailand strived to discover a dietary source with nutritional value that could counteract the harmful effects of processed carbohydrates and fats. What they utilized in this study was rice, a staple of nutrition on the Asian continent and all over the world. The outer layer of rice grain, known as *rice bran*, is easily accessible as a byproduct from rice milling and has been found, in prior experiments, to protect the body against diabetes and dyslipidemia, *in vivo* and *in vitro* (Boonloh et al. 2015; Soldati et al. 2015; Yilmaz et al. 2016).

The study focused on the protein hydrolysates of rice bran and their effects on glucose regulation, lipid regulation, insulin resistance, and several other factors related to metabolic syndrome. To investigate these hydrolysates, rat subjects with metabolic syndrome were initially given high-carbohydrate, high-fat diets. After several weeks, the rats were then separated into a group receiving rice bran and a positive control group receiving pioglitazone, which is in the class of thiazolidinedione antidiabetic drugs, capable of hypoglycemic effect.

HOMA-IR elucidated that the high-carbohydrate, high-fat diet indeed augmented the serum levels of both glucose and insulin (Boonloh et al. 2015).

Rice bran appeared to suppress the genes *Srebf1* and *fasn*, which are involved in stimulating lipogenesis during conditions of stress, such as high carbohydrate intake, which exacerbates insulin resistance. Therefore, the suppression of *Srebf1* and *fasn* by rice bran ameliorates dyslipidemia. As in previous studies, this study confirmed that a high-carbohydrate, high-fat diet results in increased gene expression of *Tnf-α*, *Il-6*, and *Nos2*, all of which are not only proinflammatory but also are able to downregulate the insulin signaling pathways within hepatocytes and skeletal muscle cells. Rice bran is able to suppress the expression of these genes, exemplifying an insulin-sensitizing feature (Boonloh et al. 2015).

There are a great number of nutrient-responsive genes encoding for transcription factors. The peroxisome proliferator activated receptor (PPAR) has been recognized for its association with cardiovascular disease. The high-carbohydrate and high-fat diet provided to the laboratory rats appeared to reduce the expression of the gene *Ppar-γ*, which, when elevated, enhances insulin sensitivity, improves metabolism of glucose, and decreases inflammation. Rice bran, unlike the carbohydrate- and fat-rich diet provided for the rat subjects, stimulated the up-regulation of the gene, thus suggesting that rice bran possibly ameliorates insulin resistance. As rice is a traditional and modern staple in homes of the Asian continent, the positive effects on fat and glucose metabolism enacted by rice bran may imply that the traditional dietary habits in Asian cultures reverse and protect against the deleterious effects of excessive processed carbohydrates and fat. In addition to its therapeutic effect in working against insulin resistance and metabolic syndrome, the outcome of this Thai study conveys that patients with metabolic syndrome worldwide may benefit from rice bran in their diets. This type of knowledge may be utilized in future research regarding cardiometabolic disease states and may possibly revolutionize the manner in which a mere rice milling by-product may be used by the industrial world (Boonloh et al. 2015; Ferguson et al. 2016).

Due to the manner in which industrialization has altered the collective dietary habits of humanity worldwide, it is safe to say that another indirect aspect of diet may be immigration (Figure 3.4). One study examined the effects of urbanization on a South Asian immigrant community in Canada. This specific population, in other studies, reported a decreased intake of fruits and vegetables, while also reporting increased consumption of fats and carbohydrates. The diet to which they had been introduced consisted of sugary drinks, red meat, and fried foods. In this study, more than 400 South Asian immigrants in Canada were recruited and asked to complete culturally tailored self-report surveys of background information, as well as food screenings, which included outlines of modern diets as well as traditional South Asian meals (Kandola et al. 2016).

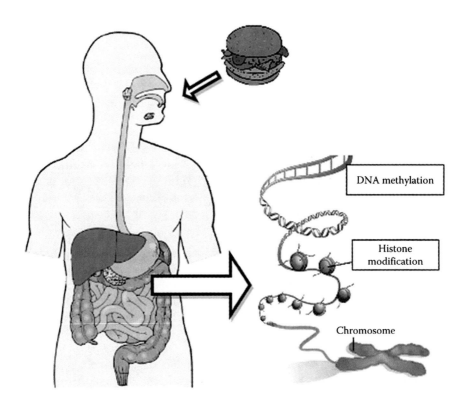

Figure 3.4 *Effect of nutrition upon one's genetic material. In this case, certain foods may result in epigenomic changes known as* DNA methylation *and* histone modification.

Multiple linear regression adjusted for age, sex, income, employment, education, and marital status. Of the sample of South Asian individuals who partook in the self-report surveys, almost 33% did not consume fruit daily, and about 66% reported eating vegetables three times or less per week. These results reflected the results of a study regarding Indian immigrant subjects, of whom only 26% reported abiding by a diet similar to or identical to Canada's nutrition guidelines. Despite this, these participants reported having more access to a greater variety of fruits and vegetables in Canada compared to their respective South Asian nation of birth, suggesting that population alterations in diet may be due to accessibility of high-fat and high-carbohydrate foods, rather than due to acclimating to the more urbanized foods of Western society (Kandola et al. 2016; Phani et al. 2016).

Large-population epidemiological studies have shown that individuals of Indian descent have greater central obesity, which may increase the incidence of those of Indian origin developing type 2 diabetes mellitus a decade earlier than, and at a BMI lower than, Caucasians. Furthermore, GWAS studies have illustrated that Indian populations are more inclined towards insulin resistance and diabetes mellitus, genetically, when compared to Caucasians. The predisposition to insulin resistance among individuals of this population is known as the *Asian–Indian phenotype*, which promotes the need for research regarding this population in association with diabetes mellitus (Phani et al. 2016; Sittig et al. 2016).

In a 2016 study, case cohorts were performed on more than 1,000 Indian participants, who were genotyped for nine SNPs, alongside normal glucose-tolerant controls. Logic regression was utilized, along with multifactor dimensionality reduction analysis, to examine gene-to-gene interactions. Using results gleaned from GWAS, selected SNPs were those with associations with type 2 diabetes mellitus. Among the selected SNPs was SLC30A8 and TCF7L2. The latter was, in past studies, the SNP most predominantly linked to diabetes among an array of ethnicities. This study had the same outcome, conveying that there was a positive association between type 2 diabetes mellitus and the TCF7L2 polymorphism among individuals of Indian origin (Phani et al. 2016; Sittig et al. 2016).

Computational analysis of loci identified to be related to type 2 diabetes mellitus showed that the overexpression of TCF7L2, which is a regulator of insulin production, increased one's risk for diabetes mellitus. Additionally, it was indicated that the silencing of the *Tcf7l2* gene causes decreased mRNA expression of the gene *Slc30a8*, which encodes a zinc transporter known as ZnT8. This β-cell transporter's role is packaging and subsequently storing insulin. These discoveries are rich with opportunity, as not only could these genes be mapped more clearly for pharmacogenomics, but the triad of genes, nutrition, and even societal diets between nations could be connected to propagate research towards personalized medicine (Phani et al. 2016).

Among the ample research uncovering the negative aspects of paradigm shifts in diet, there are quite a few that highlight the benefits particular nutrients have on genetic material. For example, researchers in Iran have delved into investigating cardiovascular disease, which is the leading causes of death in the eastern countries of the Mediterranean, including Iran. In a 2013 study, researchers focused on the effects vitamin A has on atherosclerosis, which is a chronic inflammation of the arterial walls of the cardiovascular system. This inflammation causes T lymphocytes to proliferate, allowing both adaptive and innate immune responses to promote the progression of the disease state. Cytokines influx occurs, allowing accumulation of lymphocytes, further propagating atherosclerotic development. Vitamin A, also known as retinoic acid, is able to regulate the immune system by suppressing autoimmune behavior. Furthermore, it illustrates transcriptomic activities by enhancing histone acetylation of Foxp3 promoter sites, causing Foxp3 expression to increase. Another component, TGF-β, to which vitamin A has been shown to act as a cofactor, induces Foxp3 expression as well, generating a trickling effect of augmented Foxp3 expression. Heightened expression of both components was shown to stabilize atherosclerotic lesions, therefore deterring the development of atherosclerosis (Mottaghi et al. 2012).

The study utilized a group of subjects taking retinyl palmitate once a day for 4 months, along with a control group taking a placebo for 4 months. Real-time polymerase chain reaction allowed the researchers to observe T-cell expression. The data showed that Foxp3 expression was elevated in patients taking vitamin A, as opposed to the control group, while TGF-β was also increased in those receiving vitamin A. The plaque stabilization enacted by TGF-β, along with its anti-inflammatory effects, are indicators that the use of vitamin A may slow the progression of atherosclerosis (Mottaghi et al. 2012).

3.4 Homeopathic and ayurvedic medicine

As a region known for its natural and ayurvedic medicine, as well as a preference for herbal alternatives, Asia has an abundance of history behind these preferences. For centuries past, nutraceuticals have been widely utilized among entire populations, ethnicities, and cultures in the Asian continent. Among the many natural remedies are plant-based medicines, which many believed to have a multitude of uses. A significant opportunity for future development is regarding the plant Krishna tulsi, studied in an Indian-based transcriptomics study. The herb tulsi, known scientifically *Ocimum tenuiflorum*, is regarded as a significant plant in places of worship in India, but it is also used to produce essential oils, which are metabolites possessing antifungal, antioxidant, anticancer, and anti-inflammatory activity. Therefore, in places where *O. tenuiflorum* has grown naturally, such as in warm temperate or tropical regions, the tulsi plant has been known to be utilized as treatment for diarrhea, bronchitis, malaria, and dysentery. While previous studies have isolated and analyzed a number of terpenoids and phenylpropanoids from the *Ocimum* genus, a 2015 India-based study aimed to construct the genome of the Krishna tulsi subtype, to be examined with transcriptomics via RNA-Seq (Upadhyay et al. 2015).

As the genomic material of Krishna tulsi was investigated in the study, several enzymes were discovered. These enzymes are involved in the biosynthesis of various metabolites, each of which are related to an array of disease states. Flavonoids such as apigenin and luteolin have both been implicated in protective attributes against cancer. The phenylpropanoids discovered, such as rosmarinic acid, eugenol, and methylchavicol, had various properties: anticancer effects, antioxidant effects, anti-infective effects, antifungal effects, and antiparasitic effects. An opportunity for future research arises from phenylpropanoids, not only in the field of oncology, but also in the field of infectious diseases, such as bacteria, fungi, and parasites. Eugenol, in particular, was confirmed in this study with mass spectrometry, possibly propagating study of this metabolite for future medicine. A sesquiterpene known as ursolic acid, involved with the enzyme cytochrome P450 monooxygenase, was also

72   Nutrigenomics and Nutraceuticals

associated with battling cancer cells and was, like eugenol, confirmed using mass spectrometry, indicating that this data could be used and reproduced to innovate cancer treatment (Upadhyay et al. 2015).

Overall, the tulsi plant, which has been utilized as a significant and sacred plant in Hinduism, may contain properties with which future medicine may be improved. The use of this plant in natural home remedies is significant because the people of India have often considered the Tulsi plant as being useful for a number of indications. Technology is now able to map its genome, and we may be able discover if and how this nutraceutical is capable of facilitating medical innovations (Upadhyay et al. 2015).

One example of a significant nutraceutical is that of *Antrodia camphoratus*, a fungus containing active constituents of steroids, fatty acids, lignans, polysaccharides, triterpenoids, and more. The fungus is traditionally used in Chinese medicines with indications for treating digestive issues, hypertension, and even pain. The plant has also been traditionally believed by Asian populations, from China to Taiwan, to combat inflammation and cancer, while acting as an antioxidant. The traditional uses are not without merit; recent studies have indicated that *A. camphoratus* conveys protection of the liver against the many deleterious effects of oxidative stress. One of the more recent studies of this traditional medicine, however, has focused on the fungus' effects on osteoporosis (Liu et al. 2016).

This study by Chinese investigators was performed by deriving culture from the *A. camphoratus* fungus and concentrating it with alcohol extract to create *A. camphoratus* alcohol extract (ACAE). The investigators hypothesized that ACAE would balance bone remodeling and, thus, trigger bone recovery (Figure 3.5). The study utilized the significant *in vivo* technique of senescence accelerated mouse prone 8 (SAMP8), as well as *in vitro* preosteoblast cells, both of which were treated with ACAE. The ACAE proved to be slightly cytotoxic to preosteoblasts, signifying anticancer effects as well as stimulating osteogenesis. Furthermore, osteogenic gene expression was vastly upregulated, resulting in an increased ratio of OPG to RANKL biomolecules. This modification illustrates inhibition of the osteoclastic pathway, therefore signifying maintenance of bone matrix. Alizarin Red S was used to stain the preosteoblasts treated with ACAE, further ensuring mineralization (Liu et al. 2016).

Bisphosphonates are currently the first-line pharmacological products used to treat osteoporosis, and they may reduce fractures while preventing bone loss. However, bisphosphonates carry the risk of a variety of adverse events, ranging from upset stomach to esophageal erosion and more. This class of drugs also carries contraindications for decreased renal function, while ACAE in contrast has shown signs of hepatoprotective attributes. With such an outcome, it is clear that the growing field of transcriptomics has provided alternatives within the world of nutraceuticals, illustrated the effects of diet on the development of cancer, and signified the dangers that arise in our genetic material when faced with environmental toxicities (Liu et al. 2016).

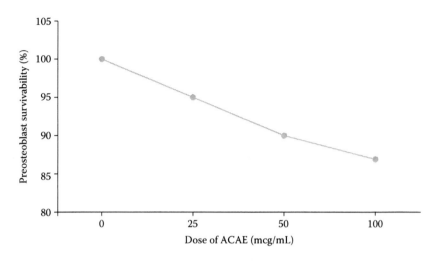

Figure 3.5 *Results of a study performed by Chinese investigators, who studied the effects of* Antrodia camphoratus *alcohol extract (ACAE) on osteoporosis. The line graph conveys the manner in which ACAE was able to reduce the viability of preosteoblasts.*

3.5 Cancer

As global cancer rates rise, developing and developed countries are facing a dire need for more effective treatments. Due to the association between age and cancer, Asian studies have spearheaded the analysis of how nutrition may affect not only aging but also tumor development. Nutrigenomics, as stated before, is defined primarily by the goal to understand the influence bioactive components in food have upon the human genome. The effect of nutrition may be enacted in direct or indirect ways, resulting in possible alterations of gene expression. As a result, modification of cellular processes may occur. Among such cellular processes may be aging, as well as the onset and progression of diseases such as cancer. An individual's genetic material may also affect the manner in which health consequences of one's diet manifest, causing some individuals to be more prone to certain disease states, such as cancer, due to inherited genes (Riscuta 2016).

As the field of transcriptomics grows, Asia and the Middle East, as cultures with diverse genetic polymorphisms and focused interest in nutritional background, have developed a number of research studies to discuss the effect of nutrients upon the RNA biomolecule within the body. A particularly striking example is that of a study performed in Saudi Arabia, in response to an increasing incidence rate of breast cancer in Saudi Arabian females. While the median age of breast cancer incidence among females in the United States and Western Europe is 68 at presentation, the median age is currently 48 for females in Saudi Arabia (Merdad et al. 2015; Riscuta 2016).

With the advent of genetic expression profiling, a great deal of links made between specific genes and breast cancer have followed. However, a number of risk factors seen in Caucasian females appear to be closely linked to breast cancer, according to some studies. These risk factors include nulliparity (the status of not having or having had any children), low parity (the status of having less children than the average female within one's population), late-age first-time pregnancy, and having no history of breastfeeding. These risk factors are not prevalent in the female population of Saudi Arabia, despite the median age of breast cancer being much lower in the Saudi Arabian population than in Caucasian females in Western Europe and the United States. Furthermore, a study in Taiwan presented an inverse correlation between breast cancer and factors such as having more than three full-term pregnancies, having children before age 30, and 3 or more years of breastfeeding, all factors common to the Saudi Arabian culture and therefore factors that should be providing protection against breast cancer for this population (Merdad et al. 2015; Riscuta 2016).

Therefore, as risk factors regarding pregnancy and breastfeeding did not appear to be the cause, Saudi Arabian researchers turned to genetic analysis aimed at discovering a disease–gene association, as well as finding biomarkers available for drug targeting. Transcriptomic profiling was performed upon the breast tumor tissue of 45 patients, more than two-thirds of whom were either obese or overweight, contrasted against the breast tissue of eight nontumor control samples. Analysis of the microarray data obtained showed that metabolism of lipids, endocrine, and drugs were significantly downregulated in the Saudi Arabian female subjects with breast cancer. Most downregulated, however, were the genes involved in lipid metabolism, which include genes for fatty-acid-binding protein, adipocytes, adinopectin, and retinol-binding protein. This indicates impairment of cardiovascular development and function and production of energy, as well as the synthesis of small biomolecules (Merdad et al. 2015).

It was concluded that the lipid metabolism pathway was in many ways intertwined with the pathogenesis of breast cancer cases of the Saudi Arabian population. As more than two-thirds of the sample of Saudi Arabian females with breast cancer were either obese or overweight, it was also concluded that the cultural shift towards an unhealthy diet and obesity has resulted in risk factors for breast cancer in women and that further education regarding nutrition in this region of the Middle East should be emphasized. This study highlighted the importance and effect of nutrition upon the genetic makeup within the body, facilitating future research regarding breast cancer and possibly other types of cancer, such as the incidence of cervical cancer in Indian women (Merdad et al. 2015).

As the second leading cause of cancer mortality in women across the globe, cervical cancer and its risk factors have recently been studied in nutrigenomic research. One such study was performed regarding Indian women, whose cooking habits may intervene with proper intake of folate, a nutrient shown to be effective in deterring the presence of HPV-related dysplasia in females. Some cultural

Indian cooking methods involve extensive time periods of heating food in open containers, as well as removing remaining water after food has finished cooking. Both practices may destroy or discard necessary folate supplement and thus may cause folate deficiency if these practices are regularly performed. Deficiency in vitamin B12 has also been shown to be involved in the mechanisms of cervical cancer. However, Indian society abides by a predominantly vegetarian lifestyle, and deficiencies due to diet may not always be the primary factor in cervical cancer incidence of this culture (Ragasudha et al. 2012).

This study deemed it necessary to focus on the methylene tetrahydrofolate reductase (MTHFR) gene, which may influence the metabolism of folate and vitamin B12 in the event of an SNP. Polymorphism in the MTHFR gene results in the translated protein, methylene tetrahydrofolate reductase, becoming thermolabile, or easily decomposed by heat. With a lack of enzyme to metabolize folate, a deficiency in folate will occur, which will subsequently result in an accumulation of homocysteine, an event further enhanced by vitamin B12 deficiency (Ragasudha et al. 2012).

In the study, 322 female subjects of similar socioeconomic background from Kerala, South India, were picked and separated into a control group, as well as groups varying in severity of cervical cancer. Peripheral blood was obtained from all subjects, as well as serum folate, vitamin B12, and homocysteine levels. This nutrigenomic study utilized chemiluminescence assay for folate and vitamin B12 detection and enzyme immunoassay for homocysteine detection. Furthermore, DNA was extracted from cervical biopsies, with which they applied the technique of polymerase chain reaction to detect the presence of HPV genotype (Ragasudha et al. 2012).

The results of the research showed that reduced levels of vitamin B12 were associated with abnormally high homocysteine levels. When combined with the MTHFR allele A1298C, the deficiency of vitamin B12 elucidates the interaction an individual's genes and nutrition may have on the risk of cervical cancer (Ragasudha et al. 2012).

This study, therefore, signifies the importance of proper diet. Despite the predominantly vegetarian population in India, particularly in the region of Kerala, it was noted that the women of Kerala rarely incorporate raw vegetables or salads into their meals. The presence of the MTHFR polymorphism results in the body's inability to effectively metabolize folate ingested, and with little folate present in the body a folate deficiency will be exacerbated. It was further noted in the study that, while folate deficiency may have possible links with cervical cancer, the synergistic effect of folate deficiency and vitamin B12 deficiency increases the risk of cancer (Ragasudha et al. 2012).

Another Asian study covering the field of epigenetics involved a focus on prostate cancer and the epigenetic effect of phenethyl isothiocyanate (PEITC). PEITC is a derivative of glucosinolate, which is a bioactive compound rich in sulfur, and is often found in cruciferous vegetables such as kale, broccoli, cauliflower, and cabbage. Due to the common quality of the vegetarian lifestyle in many Asian countries, it may be vital to analyze the correlations between diet and prostate cancer, which is one of the most commonly diagnosed cancers in the United States. PEITC has been a target of prior studies, with conclusions addressing the possible antitumor effects in prostate cancer cells and possibly altering DNA via methylation and histone modification. Growing evidence illustrates that PEITC exerts a chemopreventive ability by inducing antioxidant and cytoprotective enzymes, inhibiting excessive inflammatory responses, and regulating a wide array of signaling pathways, such as proliferation, epithelial–mesenchymal transition, cancer stem cell renewal, and apoptosis (Zhang 2016; Yacoubian et al. 2016).

In the 2016 study, miRNA expression was evaluated in prostate cancer cells subsequent to treatment with PEITC. Using an oligonucleotide microarray, it was discovered that PEITC significantly decreases MMP2 and MMP9 levels, thus subsequently yielding inhibition of invading prostate cancer cells. Furthermore, it was found that treatment of cells with PEITC upregulated gene expression of miR-194, which normally acts as a tumor suppressor in liver cancer, gastric cancer, and non-small cell lung cancer, making it a prime target among microRNA profiling candidates. As a suppressor, its elevated levels due to PEITC may be the triggering factor for inhibition of prostate cancer cell invasion. Overall, the effect PEITC has on miR-194 may result in an amplified effect on multiple mRNA molecules and may even induce the expression of p53 protein, known to suppress tumors. Therefore, the importance of a vegetable-rich diet is yet again implicated in this study, propagating a deeper look into the effects of vegetable-derived bioactive compounds (Zhang 2016; Nagao et al. 2017; Yacoubian et al. 2016).

However, diet is not the only constituent of the nutrition portion in nutrigenomics. As a culture historically known for natural medicines and home remedies, Chinese researchers are studying the benefits of herbal medicines in cancer treatment. Among them is a study delving into the reasoning behind why the plant *Bolbostemma paniculatum* has for so long been utilized in Chinese culture. Prostate cancer is not only the second leading cause of cancer-related death in males but also includes various treatment options such as surgery, chemotherapy, radiation therapy, and hormone therapy. The leading treatment is androgen deprivation therapy. However, despite being seemingly successful initially, this therapy frequently falters as a treatment in the advanced stages of cancer and often results in onset of castration-resistant prostate cancer (CRPC). Due to radiation therapy and surgery of the prostate being limited treatment options for localized prostate cancer, CRPC is deemed virtually impossible to treat. Although chemotherapy, such as use of docetaxel and cabazitaxel, is utilized for advanced-stage prostate cancer, the disease prognosis is poor (Yacoubian et al. 2016; Yang et al. 2016).

Due to these challenges, Chinese researchers in a 2016 study isolated tubeimoside-1 from the *B. paniculatum* plant. Tubeimoside-1 is a triterpenoid saponin that has illustrated cytotoxic activity against an array of cancer cells, including but not limited to ovarian cancer SKOV-3, cervical cancer HeLa, lung carcinoma A549, and esophageal squamous cell carcinoma EC109. Therefore, this study's goal was to examine the effect of tubeimoside-1 on prostate cancer cells. Human prostate cancer cells, DU145 and PC3, were isolated and purified and were then treated with several different concentrations of tubeimoside-1 for 24 hours each (Yang et al. 2016).

It was discovered that tubeimoside-1 inhibited prostate cancer cell proliferation (Figure 3.6). This inhibition of cancer cells appeared in a dose-dependent manner. Furthermore, prostate cancer cells illustrated severe morphological changes: among the overall decreased cell number, cells showed shrinkage and rounding. Pretreatment of cells using a pancaspase inhibitor significantly reduced apoptosis induced by tubeimoside-1, conveying that the effects of tubeimoside-1 are due to caspase-dependent apoptosis. Tubeimoside also induced significant condensation of chromatin and fragmentation of nuclei in a dose-dependent manner (Yang et al. 2016).

Additionally, data showed that tubeimoside-1 resulted in cell cycle arrest at the G_0/G_1 phase, performing this in both a time-dependent and dose-dependent manner. What is particularly interesting at this point is that a tumor-suppressor protein, p53, had been shown in previous studies to regulate progression at the G_0/G_1 phase, and downstream, induce the expression

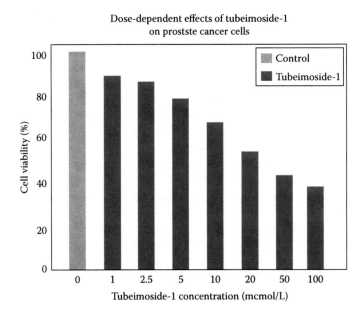

Figure 3.6 Bar graph illustrating the manner in which tubeimoside-1, a component of the plant species Bolbostemma paniculatum, causes decreases in prostate cancer cell survivability, in a dose-dependent manner.

of p21 protein. When an assay was performed in this study to examine the expression of both p53 and p21, it appeared that tubeimoside-1 increased the expression of both proteins in a dose-dependent manner, promoting the suppression of tumor cells. Tubeimoside-1 was also shown to phosphorylate Thr845 in a dose-dependent manner, inducing the activation of apoptosis signal-regulating kinase 1 (ASK-1). ASK-1 is an oxidative stress-induced mitogen-activated protein kinase with downstream target proteins, JNK and p38. Tubeimoside-1 appeared to induce intracellular generation of reactive oxygen species (ROS) and dissipated mitochondrial membrane potential, which are both signs of mitochondrial apoptosis (Yang et al. 2016; Nagao et al. 2017).

Overall, this study appeared to convey that the natural medicine in question, *B. paniculatum*, carries a component, tubeimoside-1, that activates mitochondria within cells. This activation propagates intrinsic apoptosis in cancer cells of the prostate. Prior research on mitochondria has shown that augmented levels of ROS promotes cancer cell survival and proliferation. However, increasing the ROS levels above a threshold that is toxic destroys cancer cells selectively, an experiment reproduced *in vitro* and *in vivo* in past studies. This action results in the activation of upstream proteins such as JNK, p38, and ASK-1, which are mediated by oxidative stress to activate the mitochondrial apoptosis pathway. This study appeared to conclude that the use of this particular home remedy, *B. paniculatum*, is an opportunity to develop targets of interest in the fight against cancer, all the while providing insight into the possible protective power of herbal medicines in the field of oncology (Riscuta 2016; Yang et al. 2016).

3.6 Conclusion

In recent times, societies in Asia and the Middle East have deviated from traditional dietary habits, such as regular consumption of vegetables, due to industrialization. However, current perspectives in these cultures are such that individuals are not only receptive to the idea of personalized natural medicine and diet but also motivated to adopt these lifestyle changes. Although nutrigenomic research currently utilizes optimal methodologies to isolate and examine biomarkers with links to genetic material, future endeavors would further benefit from using large, randomized, controlled studies (Fenech 2011; Teschke and Andrade 2016).

Nevertheless, the field of nutrigenomics is deterred by a number of limitations. For example, the vastness of interactions between components of the diet can alter or muffle the examination of one nutrient's effects on the genes. Oftentimes, studies focused on associations between disease states and biomarkers do not include the effect of a patient's diet, while in contrast, studies regarding dietary components are not equipped to develop omics-based profiles. Therefore, future achievements will result from intertwining nutritional expertise and omics expertise, possibly promoting a novel stage in which nutrigenomics may be efficiently implemented in studies involving human subjects (Ferguson et al. 2016; Riscuta 2016).

Overall, despite the limitations hindering the field of nutrigenomics, Asian and Middle Eastern studies have ample research to propagate and encourage future discoveries regarding genetics and disease states. Cooperation between nutrition-based research, genetics-based research, and disease state research can ameliorate gaps of information and reveal biomarker candidates with which personalized medicine and individualized dietary changes may become a reality.

References

Boonloh, K, et al. Rice bran protein hydrolysates improve insulin resistance and decrease pro-inflammatory cytokine gene expression in rats fed a high c-high fat diet. *Nutrients.* 2015, 7, 6313–6329. doi: 10.3390/nu7085292

Cheng, M, et al. Computational analyses of type 2 diabetes-associated loci identified by genome-wide association studies. *J Diabetes.* 2017, 9, 362–377. doi: 10.1111/1753-0407.12421

Fenech, M, et al. Nutrigenetics and nutrigenomics: Viewpoints on the current status and applications in nutrition research and practice. *J Nutrigenet Nutrigenomics.* 2011, 4, 69–89. doi: 10.1159/000327772

Ferguson, J, et al. Nutrigenomics, the microbiome, and gene-environment interactions: New directions in cardiovascular disease research, prevention, and treatment. *Circ Cardiovasc Genet.* 2016, 9, 291–313. doi: 10.1161/HCG.0000000000000030

Kandola, K, et al. Immigration and dietary patterns in South Asian Canadians at risk for diabetes. *J Diabetes Complications.* 2016, 30, 1462–1466. doi: 10.1016/j.jdiacomp.2016.08.003

Liu, H, et al. Osteoporosis recovery by antrodia camphorata alcohol extracts through bone regeneration in SAMP8 mice. *Evid Based Complement Alternat Med.* 2016, 1–9. doi: 10.1155/2016/2617868

Meng, Q, et al. Systems nutrigenomics reveals brain gene networks linking metabolic and brain disorders. *EBioMedicine* 2016, 7, 157–166. doi: 10.1016/j.ebiom.2016.04.008

Merdad, A, et al. Transcriptomics profiling study of breast cancer from Kingdom of Saudi Arabia revealed altered expression of Adiponectin and Fatty Acid Binding Protein4: Is lipid metabolism associated with breast cancer? *BMC Genomics.* 2015, 16(Suppl 1), S11. doi: 10.1186/1471-2164-16-S1-S11

Mottahgi, A, et al. The influence of vitamin A supplementation on Foxp3 and TGF-β gene expression in atherosclerotic patients. *J Nutrigenet Nutrigenomics.* 2012, 5, 314–326. doi: 10.1159/000341916

Nagao, T, et al. p53 and ki67 as biomarkers in determining response to chemoprevention for oral leukoplakia. *J Oral Pathol Med.* 2017, 46(5), 346–352. doi: 10.1111/jop.12498

Phani, N, et al. Replication and relevance of multiple susceptibility loci discovered from genome wide association studies for type 2 diabetes in an Indian population. *PLoS One.* 2016, 11(6), e0157364. doi: 10.1371/journal.pone.0157364

Ragasudha, P, et al. A case-control nutrigenomic study on the synergistic activity of folate and vitamin B12 in cervical cancer progression. *Nutr Cancer.* 2012, 64(4), 550–558. doi: 10.1080/01635581.2012.675618

Riscuta, G. Nutrigenomics at the interface of aging, lifespan, and cancer prevention. *J Nutr.* 2016, 146, 1–9. doi: 10.3945/jn.116.235119

Santini, A, et al. Nutraceuticals: A paradigm of proactive medicine. *Eur J Pharm Sci.* 2017, 96, 53–61. doi: 10.1016/j.ejps.2016.09.003

Sittig, LJ, et al. Genetic background limits generalizability of genotype-phenotype relationships. *Neuron.* 2016, 91, 1253–1259. doi: 10.1016/j.neuron.2016.08.013

Soldati, L, et al. State of art and science advances on nutrition and nutrigenetics in nutrition-related non-communicable diseases in Middle East. *J Transl Med.* 2015, 13, 40. doi: 10.1186/s12967-015-0390-7

Teschke, R, Andrade R. Drug, herb, and dietary supplement hepatotoxicity. *Int J Mol Sci.* 2016, 17(9), E1488. doi: 10.3390/ijms17091488

Upadhyay, A, et al. Genome sequencing of herb Tulsi (Ocimum tenuiflorum) unravels key genes behind its strong medicinal properties. *BMC Plant Biology.* 2015, 15, 212. doi: 10.1186/s12870-015-0562-x

Yacoubian, A, et al. Overview of dietary supplements in prostate cancer. *Curr Urol Rep.* 2016, 17(11), 78. doi: 10.1007/s11934-016-0637-8

Yang, JB, et al. Tubeimoside-1 induces oxidative stress-mediated apoptosis and $G0/G_1$ phase arrest in human prostate carcinoma cells *in vitro. Acta Pharmacol Sin.* 2016, 37, 950–962. doi: 10.1038/aps.2016.34

Yilmaz, Z, et al. Supplements for diabetes mellitus: A review of the literature. *J Pharm Pract.* 2016, 11, 0897190016663070.

Zhang, C, et al. Phenethyl isothiocyanate (PEITC) suppresses prostate cancer cell invasion epigenetically through regulating microRNA-194. *Mol Nutr Food Res.* 2016, 60, 1427–1436. doi: 10.1002/mnfr.201500918

Novel Approaches in Food Functions Based on Nutrigenomics Research

Meenakshisundaram Selvamuthukumaran
Haramaya University
Dire Dawa, Ethiopia

Contents

4.1 Nutrigenomics: Introduction 83
4.2 Nutrigenomics: Measuring nutrition responsive genome activity 84
    4.2.1 Transcriptomics 84
        4.2.1.1 Advances in transcriptomics 85
    4.2.2 Proteomics 90
        4.2.2.1 Advances in proteomics 91
    4.2.3 Metabolomics 96
        4.2.3.1 Advances in metabolomics 97
    4.2.4 Analytical techniques in metabolomics 98
        4.2.4.1 Mass spectrometry approaches 99
        4.2.4.2 NMR approaches 99
4.3 Systems biology 100
4.4 Use of the nutrigenomics approach in nutrition research 102
4.5 Future prospects 108
References 109

4.1 Nutrigenomics: Introduction

Nutrition and genetics both play an important role in human health as well as the development of chronic diseases such as cancer, osteoporosis, diabetes, and cardiovascular disease. Nutritional genomics, or *nutrigenomics*, is the study of how food and genes interact, and it aims to understand the effects of diet on an individual's genes and health. It attempts to study the genome-wide influences of nutrition, to identify the genes that influence the risk of diet-related diseases on a genome-wide scale, and to understand the mechanisms that underlie these genetic predispositions (Muller and Kersten 2003).

It describes a scientific approach that integrates nutritional sciences and genomics and includes the application of other high-throughput omics technologies, such as transcriptomics, proteomics, and metabolomics, to investigate the effects of nutrition on health.

Nutrigenomics examines how nutrients affect genes (i.e., influence gene expression and function) and how genes affect diet (i.e., what an individual eats and how an individual responds to nutrients), with the latter sometimes being referred to as *nutrigenetics*. Nutrigenomics can include the full spectrum of research strategies, from basic cellular and molecular biology to clinical trials, epidemiology, and population health. These different experimental approaches can be used to improve our understanding of how nutrition affects various health outcomes. Current trends in personalized nutrition have focused on the role of genetic variation to understand why some individuals respond differently than others to the same nutrients consumed.

Nutrigenomics aims to determine the influence of common dietary ingredients on the genome and attempts to relate the resulting different phenotypes to differences in the cellular and/or genetic response of the biological system (Mutch et al. 2005). More practically, nutrigenomics describes the use of functional genomic tools to probe a biological system following a nutritional stimulus that will permit an increased understanding of how nutritional molecules affect metabolic pathways and homeostatic control.

Nutrigenomics will unravel the optimal diet from within a series of nutritional alternatives, whereas nutrigenetics will yield critically important information that will assist clinicians in identifying the optimal diet for a given individual, that is, personalized nutrition.

4.2 Nutrigenomics: Measuring nutrition responsive genome activity

Nutrigenomics is the science that examines the response of individuals to dietary compounds, foods, and diets using postgenomic and related technologies, that is, genomics, transcriptomics, proteomics, and metabolomics. It studies the genome-wide influences of nutrition or dietary compounds on the transcriptome, proteome, and metabolome of cells, tissues, or organisms at a given time.

4.2.1 Transcriptomics

The transcriptome is the complete set of RNA that can be produced from the genome. Transcriptomics is the study of the transcriptome, that is, gene expression at the level of the mRNA. Using either cDNA or oligonucleotide microarray technology, it describes the approach in which gene expression (mRNA) is analyzed in a biological sample at a given time under specific conditions. It is the most widely used of the omics technologies.

Regulation of the rate of transcription of genes by food components represents an intriguing site for regulation of an individual's phenotype (Trujillo et al. 2006). A host of essential nutrients and other bioactive food components can serve as important regulators of gene expression patterns.

Macronutrients, vitamins, minerals, and various phytochemicals can modify gene transcription and translation, which can alter biological responses such as metabolism, cell growth, and differentiation, all of which are important in the disease process. Genome-wide monitoring of gene expression using DNA microarrays allows the simultaneous assessment of the transcription of thousands of genes and of their relative expression between normal cells and diseased cells or before and after exposure to different dietary components. This information should assist in the discovery of new biomarkers for disease diagnosis and prognosis prediction and of new therapeutic tools.

4.2.1.1 Advances in transcriptomics

In the expression process of genomic information, several steps may be regulated by nutrients and other bioactive compounds in food. Consequently, the analysis of changes in mRNA expression by nutrients and bioactive food constituents is often the first step in studying the flow of molecular information from the genome to the proteome and metabolome and one of the main goals in nutrigenomics research (Muller and Kersten 2003). For years, the expression of individual genes has been determined by quantification of mRNA with northern blotting. This classical technique has gradually been replaced by more sensitive techniques such as real-time PCR.

In contrast, the analysis of global gene expression may offer better opportunities to identify the effect of bioactive food constituents on metabolic pathways and homeostatic control and how this regulation is potentially altered in the development of certain chronic diseases (Hu and Kong 2004). In the past decade, two conceptually different analytical approaches have emerged to allow quantitative and comprehensive analysis of changes in the mRNA expression levels of hundreds or thousands of genes. One approach is based on microarray technology, and the other group of techniques is based on DNA sequencing (Morozova and Marra 2008).

4.2.1.1.1 Gene expression microarray technology

During recent years, owing to extensive optimization and standardization, gene expression microarrays have become a leading analytical technology in nutrigenomics research for the investigation of the interactions between nutrients and other bioactive food compounds and genes (Anderle et al. 2004; Gaj et al. 2008). Typically, DNA microarrays are collections of oligonucleotides or probes, representing thousands of genes, attached to a substrate, usually a glass slide, at predefined locations within a grid pattern. This technique is based on specific nucleic acid hybridization, and it can be used to measure the relative quantities of specific mRNAs in two or more samples for thousands of genes simultaneously.

Regardless of the platform used for the analysis, the typical experimental procedure is based on the same analytical steps: RNA is extracted from a source of interest (tissue, cells, or other materials), labeled with a detectable marker (typically, fluorescent dye), and allowed to hybridize to the microarrays, with individual DNA sequences hybridizing to their complementary gene-specific probes on the microarray. Once hybridization is complete, samples are washed and imaged using a confocal laser scanner (Figure 4.1). Theoretically, the fluorescent signal of derivatized nucleic acids bound to any probe is a function of their concentration. The relative fluorescence intensity for each gene is extracted and transformed to a numeric value (Storhoff et al. 2005). Certain bioactive food constituents have also been investigated by microarray technology. A summary of some representative applications of microarrays in the field of nutrigenomics is given in Table 4.1.

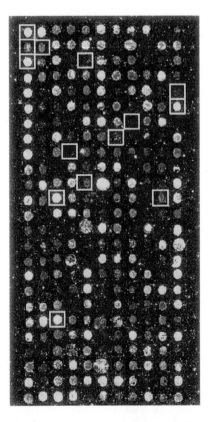

Figure 4.1 Scanned image of a microarray composed of a total of 250 kinases and phosphatases showing the expression profile obtained from human prostate carcinoma LNCaP cells treated with 12 mM epigallocatechin gallate or water only for 12 h (Modified from Wang and Mukhar, Cancer Lett. 182: 43–51, 2002.)

Table 4.1 Applications of DNA Expression Microarrays in Nutrigenomics Research

Bioactive Compound/ Food Ingredient	Food/Beverage	Study Model	Expected Effect/Target Illness	Analytical Methodology	References
Anthocyanins C3G and cyanidin Cy	Fruits, vegetables, red wine	Human adipocyte cells	Regulation of adipocyte function	Affymetrix Human Genome microarray	Tsuda et al. (2006)
Astaxanthin	Fish, algae	Mice	Regulation of oxidative phosphorylation and oxidative stress	Affymetrix Mouse Expression microarray	Naito et al. (2006)
Chlorella algae intake	Diet	Healthy men (blood cells)	Regulation of fat and glucose metabolism Modulation of glucose sensitivity in humans	Custom diabetes-related microarray (Hitachi)	Mizoguchi et al. (2008)
Epicatechin	Cocoa	Human colon adenocarcinoma Caco-2 cells	Prevention of the oxidative DNA damage, reduction of inflammatory response	Clontech Human Haematology microarray	Noe et al. (2004)
Epigallocatechin-3 gallate	Green tea	Human bronchial epithelial 21BES cells Human prostate carcinoma LNCaP cells Human HT 29 colon carcinoma cells	Chemopreventive agent in cancer Antiproliferative action Antiproliferative action	Custom printed human microarray cDNA microarray Affymetrix Human Genome microarray	Vittal et al. (2004); Wang and Mukhar (2002); Mcloughlin et al. (2004)
Genistein	Soybean	Postmenopausal women (peripheral lymphocytes)	Regulation camp signalling and cell differentiation	Human oligo microarrays	Niculescu et al. (2007)
High-cholesterol intake	Diet	Rats	Effects in cardiovascular disease	Custom-printed cDNA microarray	Puskas et al. (2004)

(Continued)

Table 4.1 *(Continued)* Applications of DNA Expression Microarrays in Nutrigenomics Research

Bioactive Compound/ Food Ingredient	Food/ Beverage	Study Model	Expected Effect/Target Illness	Analytical Methodology	References
High-protein/high-carbohydrate intakes	Dairy-based breakfasts	Healthy men (blood cells)	Regulation of glycogen metabolism and protein biosynthesis	Affymetrix Human Genome microarray	Van-Erk et al. (2006)
Long chain polyunsaturated fatty acids	Fish oil	Mice	Regulation of hepatic beta-oxidation and gluconeogenesis	Affymetrix Murine Genome microarray	Berger et al. (2002)
Low-calorie intake	Diet	Obese men (blood cells)	Regulation of oxidative stress and inflammation	Agilent Human Oligo microarray	Parra et al. (2008)
Omega-3 fatty acid	Fish oil	Human colon adenocarcinoma Caco-2 cells	Chemopreventive agent in cancer	Clontech Human Atlas Glass Arrays	Narayanan et al. (2003)
Quercetin	Fruits and vegetables	CO115 colon-adenocarcinoma cells	Chemopreventive agent in cancer	Affymetrix Human Genome microarray	Murtaza et al. (2006)
Sulforaphane	Cruciferous vegetables	Mice	Chemopreventive agent in cancer	Affymetrix Murine Genome microarray	Thimmulappa et al. (2002)

4.2.1.1.2 Sequencing-based technologies

In contrast to microarray technology, sequencing-based techniques consist of counting tags of DNA fragments to provide "digital" representation of gene expression levels using sequencing. These techniques include serial analysis of gene expression (SAGE) (Velculescu et al. 1995) and some of its variants, including long SAGE (Saha et al. 2002), cap analysis of gene expression (Shiraki et al. 2003), and gene identification signature (Ng et al. 2005). In SAGE-based methods, the abundance of a particular mRNA species is estimated from the count of tags derived from one of its ends. First, restriction enzymes are used to obtain short tags of 14–21 bp, usually derived from one end of an mRNA, which are then concatenated, cloned, and sequenced to determine the expression profiles of their corresponding RNAs. Despite greater statistical robustness and less stringent standardization and replication requirements than those used for microarrays, the size of the sample tags should be increased in order to improve the precision and accuracy for detecting rare mRNAs (Wang 2007). Unfortunately, most of these methods are based on the expensive Sanger sequencing method and, therefore, a sequenced SAGE library rarely exhibits the saturated tag counts that would indicate complete representation of the cellular transcriptome (Brenner et al. 2000). An additional limitation of these techniques GE tags is shared by the transcripts from different genes, which can complicate gene identification (Tuteja 2008). Moreover, the many PCR amplifications, cloning and bacterial cell propagations that these techniques involve may result in a quantitative bias for different tags (Nielsen et al. 2006). Massively parallel signature sequencing (MPSS) is a more sophisticated "clone-and-count" technique that also generates small tags of each mRNA species; moreover, it uses a different strategy that involves neither propagation in bacteria nor Sanger sequencing (Brenner et al. 2000). Nevertheless, MPSS technology has been restricted to only a few specialized laboratories (Nielsen et al. 2006).

4.2.1.1.3 Bioinformatics and gene ontology database

As mentioned, high-throughput technologies in transcriptomics usually generate large lists of differentially expressed genes as the final output. However, the biological interpretation of such results is very challenging. Over the last several years, the biological knowledge accumulated in public databases by means of bioinformatics has allowed us to systematically analyze large gene lists in an attempt to assemble a summary of the most enriched and significant biological aspects. The principle behind enrichment analysis is that if a certain biological process occurs in a given study, the co-functioning genes involved should have a higher (enriched) potential to be selected as a relevant group by high-throughput screening technologies. This approach increases the probability for researchers to identify the correct biological processes pertinent to the biological mechanism under study (Huang et al. 2009). Thus, a variety of high-throughput enrichment tools (e.g., DAVID, Onto-Express, FatiGO, GOminer, EASE, ProfCom, etc.) have been developed since 2002 in order to assist the microarray end user to understand the biological mechanisms behind the large set of regulated genes. These bioinformatics resources systematically map the list of interesting (differentially expressed) genes to the associated biological annotation terms and then statistically examine the enrichment of gene members for each of the terms by comparing them to a control (or reference). Leong et al. (2006) showed the potential of exploiting bioinformatics tools for extracting valuable biological information from microarray experiments. In their work, use of the Affymetrix microarray platform and stringent data analysis provided interesting insights into a homeostatic mechanism, based on arginine-sensitive regulation that coordinates aspects related to nutrient availability in hepatic cells.

Enrichment analysis would not be possible without appropriately structured databases such as Gene Ontology (Gene Ontology Consortium 2008). More specifically, Gene Ontology provides a systematic and controlled language, or ontology, for the consistent description of attributes of genes and gene products, in three key biological domains that are shared by all organisms: molecular function, biological process, and cellular components. Thus, standard biological phrases, referred to as *terms*, which are applied to genes and proteins, are then linked or associated with other Gene Ontology terms by trained curators at genome databases (Ashburner et al. 2000). Niculescu et al. (2007) studied the effects of soy isoflavones, based on gene expression microarray data. They revealed potential mechanisms of action for genistein by the combined use of GoMiner as the enrichment tool, the Gene Ontology database, and information from the Dragon Estrogen Responsive Genes Database.

4.2.2 Proteomics

Dietary components can also modify the translation of RNA to proteins and post-translational events, which can affect protein activity (Trujillo et al. 2006). Just as the genome is the entire set of genes, the proteome is the set of proteins produced by a species. However, unlike the genome, the proteome is dynamic and varies according to the cell type and the functional state of the cell. The complexity of a proteome is overwhelming. While the human genome comprises "only" >25,000 genes, the human proteome is estimated to encompass several hundred thousand proteins and an order of magnitude more protein forms and variants.

Proteomics is the study of the proteome, and it addresses three categories of biological interest: protein expression, structure, and function (Kussmann et al. 2006). It attempts to characterize all proteins in a biological sample, including their relative abundance, distribution, post-translational modifications, functions, and interactions with other biological molecules. Proteomics is technically very challenging and the presence/absence of protein is not necessarily indicative of metabolic change. Currently, the most widely used technologies for proteomics are two-dimensional gel electrophoresis (2DE) to separate the proteins in a complex mixture isolated from cells or tissues and specialized mass spectrometry (MS) techniques as protein identification tools (Fuchs et al. 2005; Kussmann et al. 2006). This is a rapidly developing field, and new and improved techniques continue to emerge.

The potential value of proteomics for the nutritional sciences has been recognized for some years. However, in contrast to the techniques for large-scale transcriptome analysis that are already used by the nutrition research community and that have led to numerous published studies, only a very few reports have described the use of proteome analysis as a tool in nutrition research. Most of them have involved the use of rodent models or human cells in culture (Fuchs et al. 2005).

4.2.2.1 Advances in proteomics

The proteome is the set of expressed proteins at a given time under defined conditions; it is dynamic and varies according to the cell type and functional state. In the case of a nutrigenomic study, the proteome provides a "picture" of the impact of specific bioactive nutrients and diets on a certain organism, tissue, or cell in a particular moment. Thus, the importance of proteomics as a tool to understand the effect of diet on health has already been recognized by several researchers (Moresco et al. 2008; Ovesna et al. 2008; Schweigert 2007).

One of the main differences when working with proteins is that there is not an amplification methodology for proteins comparable to PCR. The physical and chemical diversity of proteins are also higher than for nucleic acids. They differ among individuals, cell types, and within the same cell depending on cell activity and state. In addition, there are hundreds of different types of post-translational modifications (PTMs), which will obviously influence the chemical properties and functions of proteins. PTMs are key to the control and modulation of many processes inside the cell. The analytical strategy selected for the detection of PTMs will depend on the type of modification: acetylation, phosphorylation, ubiquitination, sumoylation, glycosylation, etc. It is already known that dietary components can also modify the translation of RNA to proteins and the post-translational procedures (Knowles and Milner 2000). Thus, dietary components such as diallyl disulfide, a compound found in processed garlic, have been shown to post-translationally modify proteins (Knowles and Milner 2000). In other cases, post-translational regulation of proteins by dietary components can involve the modification of their thiol groups (Dinkova-Kostova 2002).

Although proteomics has been scarcely applied to study the effect of nutrients on health, two fundamental analytical strategies can be employed: the bottom-up approach and the top-down approach. Both methodologies differ on the separation requirements and the type of MS instrumentation.

4.2.2.1.1 Bottom-up approach

The bottom-up approach is the most widely used in proteomics, since it can apply conventional or modern methodologies. In a conventional approach, large-scale analyses of proteomes are accomplished by the combination of 2DE followed by MS analysis (Wittmann-Liebold et al. 2006). 2DE is the methodology that currently provides the highest protein species resolution capacity with the lowest instrumentation cost. However, 2DE is laborious, time-consuming, and presents low sensitivity, depending strongly on staining and visualization techniques. 2DE has also some limitations to separate highly hydrophobic biomolecules or proteins with extreme isoelectric point or molecular weight values.

Moreover, one of the major sources of error in 2DE is gel-to-gel variation. In this sense, the introduction of difference gel electrophoresis (DIGE), in which gel variation is eliminated by loading different samples in the same gel (Marouga et al. 2005), has brought about an important improvement. DIGE methodology is based on the use of novel ultrahigh-sensitivity fluorescent dyes (typically, Cy3, Cy5, and Cy2) to label up to three different protein samples that will be separated in the same 2DE run. After image analysis of the 2DE gels, the protein spots of interest are subsequently submitted to an in-gel digestion step with a protease enzyme. MS and databases of protein sequences are then used in different ways for protein identification, (i) following the peptide mass fingerprint approach using MS data, in which the molecular masses of the peptides from the protein digest are compared with those simulated for already-sequenced proteins, or (ii) by tandem MS in a sequence tag search in which a few peptide sequences obtained from MS/MS analysis (using collisional activation or some other energy deposition process) can be used to search protein databases. The main limitation of the bottom-up approach is that the information obtained is related to a fraction of the protein, losing information about PTMs. There have been limited studies of the effect of specific natural compounds, nutrients, or diets on the proteome, most of which were based on the bottom-up approach, more precisely in classical two-dimensional electrophoresis mass spectrometry (2DEMS), although liquid chromatography–mass spectrometry (LC-MS)/MS has also been applied for this purpose; these studies are summarized in Table 4.2.

Shotgun proteomics is an advanced bottom-up approach in which a complex protein mixture is digested with endoproteinases of known specificity (Nesvizhskii and Aebersold 2005), providing a comprehensive, rapid, and automatic identification of complex protein mixtures. In spite of the higher sample complexity due to the huge number of peptidic species obtained from the protein mixture hydrolysate, peptides are in general better separated and analyzed by MS than proteins.

To carry out shotgun proteomics, most efforts have focused on the development of online combinations of various chromatography and/or electrokinetic separation methods, as well as on multidimensional protein identification

Table 4.2 Applications of Proteomics in Nutrigenomics Research

Bioactive Compound/ Food Ingredient	Food/Beverage	Study Model	Expected Effect/Target Illness	Analytical Methodology	References
Quercetin	—	Human SW480 colon carcinoma cells	Colorectal cancer prevention	2DE, MALDI-TOF-MS	Mouat et al. (2005)
Fatty acids	Dietary fish oil	Leiden transgenic mice	Lipid and glucose metabolism study	2DE, MALDI-TOF-MS	De-Roos et al. (2005)
Genistein and daidzein isoflavones	Soy extract	Human endothelial cells	Atherosclerosis-preventive activities	2DE, MALDI-TOF-MS	Fuchs et al. (2005, 2006, 2007)
Isoflavones	Cereal bars	Human peripheral blood mononuclear cells	Atherosclerosis-preventive activities	2DE, MALDI-TOF-MS	Fuchs et al. (2007)
Monacolin K	Fungus	Caco-2 cells	Chemopreventive agent in cancer	2DE, MALDI-TOF/TOF-MS	Lin et al. (2006)
Volatile compounds	Coffee bean	Rat brain	Antioxidant and stress relaxation	2DE, MALDI-TOF-MS, MALDI-Q-TOF-MS/MS	Seo et al. (2008)
Polyphenols	Green tea	Human lung adenocarcinoma A549 cells	Anticancer activity	2DE, nLC-ESI-Q-TOF-MS/MS	Lu et al. (2007)
No specific bioactive compound	Diets with different % of vegetable	Mouse colon mucosal cells	Colorectal cancer prevention	2DE, MALDI-TOF-MS	Breikers et al. (2006)
Iso flavones	Soyfoods	Human serum	Vascular protection	DIGE, LC-MS/MS	Wong et al. (2008)
Vitamin A	—	Rat plasma	Changes in nutritional status	SELDI-TOF	Linke et al. (2004)

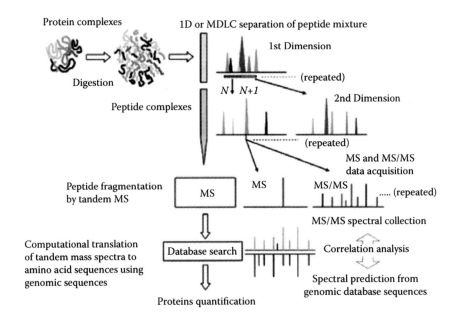

Figure 4.2 *Workflow of multidimensional separation–MS/MS-based shotgun proteomics strategy. N is the sample fraction (Modified from Motoyama and Yates* Anal. Chem. 80: 7187–7193, 2008).

technology, coupled with MS or tandem MS (Fournier et al. 2007) (Figure 4.2). The vast majority are based on the combination of ion-exchange chromatography and reversed-phase (RP) chromatography. This has also been described as the great potential of monolithic compared to particle-based columns, because monolithic columns can be used together with higher flows and gradients (Wu et al. 2008). This is of special interest in a multidimensional chromatography setup, where the separation and identification of a vast number of analytes in a short time is mandatory, mainly in the second dimension. Other novel couplings have been described, as for instance those based on hydrophilic interaction LC (Boersema et al. 2008). The capabilities of multidimensional systems involving online combination of capillary isoelectric focusing with nano-reversed phase liquid chromatography have also been demonstrated to be effective in the analysis of proteins and peptides (Guo et al. 2006), creating new and encouraging perspectives in the discovery of biomarkers in nutrigenomics studies.

4.2.2.1.2 Top-down approach

A growing number of researchers are focusing on the use of top-down proteomics, a relatively new approach compared to bottom-up, in which the structure of proteins is studied through measurement of their intact mass followed by direct ion dissociation in the gas phase (Breuker et al. 2008). The main advantages over the bottom-up approach are that higher sequence coverage is obtained, it permits the study of PTMs, and it makes it possible to discern between biomolecules with a high degree of sequence identity.

Today, Fourier transform ion cyclotron resonance (FTICR) MS offers the highest mass resolution, resolving power, accuracy, and sensitivity among present MS technologies (Bogdanov and Smith 2005). Nevertheless, its high purchase and maintenance costs, mostly derived from the expensive super-conducting magnet and liquid helium supply required, precludes its general use. Thus, use of a variety of instruments suitable for routine top-down proteomics, such as MALDI-TOF/TOF (matrix-assisted laser desorption–ionization/time of flight), ESI-Q/TOF (electrospray ionization–quadruple/time of flight), electrospray ionization–ion trap (ESI-IT), and the novel OrbitrapTM, has been reported (Macek et al. 2006). In those cases in which the molecular mass of proteins exceeds the analytical power of the mass spectrometer, they can be subjected to a limited proteolysis to produce large polypeptides that are then analyzed employing top-down proteomic approaches. This has been called the *middle-down approach*, maintaining the advantages of high sequence coverage and PTM information.

A key to the top-down approach is the capacity to fragment intact proteins inside the mass spectrometer. Usually, low-energy multiple collision-induced dissociation is used, although ultraviolet photo dissociation (Morgan et al. 2005), infrared multiphoton dissociation (Raspopov et al. 2006), and black body infrared radiative dissociation have also been used by various researchers (Gea et al. 2001). Alternative dissociation techniques such as electron capture dissociation (ECD) represent one of the most recent and significant advances in tandem MS (Sweet and Cooper 2007). This alternative technique is based on the fragmentation of multiply charged protein cations due to interaction with low-energy electrons. A newer dissociation method similar to ECD is electron transfer dissociation (ETD), which also uses charge reduction by electron transfer (Wiesner et al. 2008). Both charge-reduction dissociation techniques, ECD and ETD, initially used in FTICR-MS and now extended to hybrid linear ion trap (LTQ Orbitrap Instruments) provide more extensive sequence fragments over the entire protein backbone, preserving the PTM after cleavage, resulting in easier identification of the modification sites.

Top-down proteomics approaches are usually limited to simple protein mixtures, since very complex spectra are usually generated by multiple charged proteins. In general, a protein isolate from a previous fractionation or purification step is directly infused to the high-resolution MS. In this regard, due to the capabilities of capillary electrophoresis (CE) for complex protein separation, CE coupled with high-resolution MS is one of the most promising methodologies in top-down studies (Simpson et al. 2006). However, improved ECD and ETD speed will be needed for future high-throughput CE-MS (and also LC-MS) applications in top-down proteomics.

4.2.3 Metabolomics

One of the newest omics technologies in nutrition is metabolomics. It focuses on the analysis of metabolites—the metabolome. It tries to measure the levels of all substances (other than DNA, RNA, or protein) present in a sample; the metabolome comprises the complete set of metabolites synthesized by a biological system (Gibney et al. 2005; Harland 2005).

Such a system can be defined by the level of biological organization, such as organism, organ, tissue, cell, or cell compartment levels. Biologically relevant samples can easily be obtained from blood, urine, saliva, and fecal water. Metabolomics is a useful tool for generating individual metabolite profiles, such as complete plasma lipid (i.e., cholesterol, triglycerides) and vitamin profiles. Metabolomics examines the whole metabolism, which ultimately reflects the behavior of different patterns of genes. It investigates metabolic regulation and flux in individual cells or tissues, in response to specific environmental changes. In common with transcriptomics and proteomics, it involves the nontargeted determination of all metabolites present under specific environmental conditions. Analysis and interpretation of the data that is derived from the comparison of different cell conditions is achieved by the use of bioinformatics. Some researchers use the term *metabolomics* to refer to both simple (cellular) and complex (whole tissue or organism) systems; others distinguish between metabolomics studies, which are simple system only, and metabonomics, in complex systems (Harland 2005; Whitfield et al. 2004). In metabonomics, systematic biochemical profiles and regulation of functions are determined in whole organisms by analyzing biofluids and tissues.

Metabolomics has been making great advances in this complex approach to nutrition research (German et al. 2004; Rochfort 2005). This is partly because nuclear magnetic resonance (NMR) and MS are established techniques but also because the application of pattern recognition statistics, such as principle component analysis, is conventional in this field. Metabolomics also has the advantage of offering more immediate information about our metabolism, which is not presented by changes in gene transcription or protein expression, since both can occur without apparent metabolic consequences.

At the present time, there is a limited number of researchers with the facilities required to do such specific studies. Until now there have been only few reported examples of metabolomics studies in human subjects. Most examples have involved the metabolic profiling of individuals, where large-scale analyses of body fluids have been used to diagnose metabolic disorders or exposure to xenobiotics (Harland 2005; Whitfield et al. 2004). In contrast to transcriptomics, proteomics and metabolomics are not yet routine and standardized procedures. It is not yet possible to measure the whole proteome or metabolome, and it is not known how many endogenous metabolites exist or how many exogenous food-derived metabolites can be measured in human samples.

There is currently no single technology capable of comprehensively assessing all of the metabolites in a biological sample. Metabolomics continues to face challenges such as sample preparation, technological sensitivity, lack of standardized statistical methods, and public databases.

Nevertheless, their potential benefits for health management are undisputed and have fueled current efforts to assess, utilize, interpret, and ultimately integrate these global technologies in order to define a phenotype characterizing health status.

4.2.3.1 Advances in metabolomics

As defined by Trujillo et al. (2006), the metabolome can be described as the full set of endogenous or exogenous low-molecular-weight metabolic entities of approximately <1,000 Da (metabolites) and the small pathway motifs that are present in a biological system (cell, tissue, organ, organism, or species). The most common metabolites are amino acids, lipids, vitamins, small peptides, or carbohydrates. Metabolites are the real end points of gene expression and of any physiological regulatory processes. Any change in metabolite concentration may better describe the biochemical state of a biological system than proteomic or transcriptomic variations. The objective of metabolomics within the frame of nutrigenomics is to investigate the metabolic alterations produced by the effect of nutrients or bioactive food constituents in the different metabolic pathways. Its importance not only lies in the information obtained about the molecular events involved in nutrition and how the body adapts through metabolic pathways to different nutrient fluxes but also in the identification of certain metabolites such as cholesterol or glucose as biomarkers for health or disease status (Kussman et al. 2008).

There are three basic approaches used in metabolomic research: target analysis, metabolic profiling, and metabolic fingerprinting. Target analysis aims at the quantitative measurement of selected analytes, such as a specific biomarker or reaction product. Metabolic profiling is a nontargeted strategy that focuses on the study of a group of related metabolites or a specific metabolic pathway. It is one of the basic approaches to phenotyping, as the study of metabolic profiles of a cell gives a more accurate description of a phenotype (Wai-Nang et al. 2005). Meanwhile, metabolic fingerprinting does not aim to identify all metabolites but to compare patterns of metabolites that change in response to the cellular environment (Fiehn 2002).

Metabolomics has diverse applications such as biomarker discovery, determination of the metabolic effects of environmental changes in the body, and early disease detection (Walsh et al. 2008). The most relevant application of metabolomics in nutrigenomics is the possible health benefits provided by ingestion of functional compounds. In this regard, the effects of phytochemicals on human health are the most studied. Some examples are the potential benefits of flavones in heart diseases, of stanols in cholesterol metabolism, and soy-based estrogen analogues in cancer (Cassidy and Dalais 2003). Because of the extensive consumption of polyphenols and its association with health benefits, the biological activity of these compounds is an important topic of investigation in nutrigenomics (Lambert et al. 2005).

4.2.4 Analytical techniques in metabolomics

Unlike transcriptomics or proteomics, which intend to determine a single chemical class of compounds (mRNA or proteins), metabolomics has to deal with very different compounds of very diverse chemical and physical properties. Moreover, the relative concentration of metabolites in biofluids varies from the millimolar level (or higher) to picomolar, making it easy to exceed the linear range of the analytical technique employed. As no single technique can be expected to meet all these requirements, many metabolomics approaches can employ several analytical techniques (Koulman 2008).

Metabolomics is an emerging technology, so new analytical techniques and methods are continuously being developed and will continue to be developed in the near future in order to achieve its goals. So far, metabolomics is proving to be very useful for the analysis of metabolic patterns and changes in the metabolism derived from different situations in the cellular environment. This is certainly interesting in the nutrition field, as it can determine variations in different metabolic pathways due to the consumption of different compounds in the diet.

In order to gain detailed knowledge of human metabolism by means of metabolomic tools, the ideal steps should be first to elucidate the nature and concentration of the searched metabolites and second to share the information in accessible databases (Astle et al. 2007) (Figure 4.3). The two most common analytical techniques used so far in metabolomics are NMR and MS.

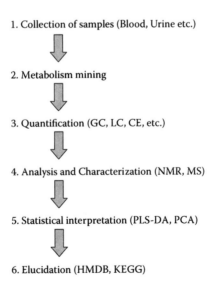

Figure 4.3 Metabolomics workflow in nutrigenomics research (Modified from Garcia-Canas et al. J. Pharm. Biomed. Anal. *51:* 290–304, 2010).

4.2.4.1 Mass spectrometry approaches

MS can be used as a standalone technique or most commonly combined with a preliminary chromatographic separation technique, either gas chromatography, high-performance chromatography with MS (HPLC-MS), or CE-MS (Koulman 2008). Direct injection is performed for metabolomics with high or ultra-high resolution mass analyzers such as TOF-MS (mass accuracy <10 ppm) or FTICR-MS, which provides a mass accuracy <1 ppm and detection limits lower than the attomole or femtomole levels. These characteristics make them ideal tools for metabolomic studies as shown by Rosello-Mora et al. (2008), who stated that different strains of *Salinibacter ruber* could be differentiated by some characteristic metabolites. Hybrid analyzers, as, for example, Q-TOF, have the advantages of mass accuracy given by a TOF analyzer combined with the possibility to fragment the ions and thus provide information about the structure of the detected metabolites (Dettmer et al. 2007).

These kinds of analyzers should lead metabolomic studies in the near future. As for proteomics, the most usual ionization techniques are the ones that use atmospheric pressure ionization, especially ESI interfaces, as they can work with a wide range of polarities (Werner et al. 2008).

The most recent introduction into the field of separation techniques with enormous potential in metabolomics research is ultra-performance liquid chromatography coupled to MS (UPLCTM-MS) technology. UPLCTM-MS has been used in the determination of metabolic profiles in human urine (Guy et al. 2008). The small particle size and the high pressure allow reduction of analysis time by approximately ten times with respect to conventional LC, while increasing efficiency and maintaining resolution.

4.2.4.2 NMR approaches

NMR is a high-reproducibility technique that has demonstrated its great potential in metabolomics studies (Dumas et al. 2006). Using this analytical technique, Wang et al. (2005) studied the relationship between the consumption of chamomile tea and some human biological responses. Statistical differences were found in three different excreted metabolites between high-resolution 1H NMR analyses of urine samples taken before and after chamomile tea consumption (Wang et al. 2005). In another study, the metabolic profiling approach using high resolution 1H NMR spectroscopy was applied to study metabolite changes in human feces after intake of grape juice and ethanol-free wine extracts (Jacobs et al. 2008) (Figure 4.4). This study showed changes in the levels of isobutyrate when the mixture of juice and wine was taken but could not find any difference in the metabolic profile due to the intake of juice. This could be explained through the modulation of the microbial gut metabolism produced by the polyphenols present in wine. Metabolic profiling after dietary intervention with soy isoflavones was also determined by 1H NMR differences in lipoprotein, amino acids, and carbohydrate levels in

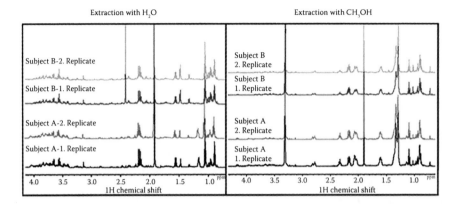

Figure 4.4 Nuclear magnetic resonance profiles of feces from different subjects using two different extraction methods (water and methanol) (Modified from Jacobs et al. NMR Biomed. *21: 615–626, 2008*).

plasma from five healthy premenopausal women, thus suggesting a metabolic alteration due to soy consumption (Solanky et al. 2003). In another 1H NMR study on the effect of soy isoflavones, an improvement in renal function and an increase in the urinary excretion of the osmolyte trimethylamine-N oxide was proven (Solanky et al. 2005). A summary of the main metabolomic applications in the nutrigenomics field is listed in Table 4.3.

4.3 Systems biology

The long-term aim of nutrigenomics is to understand how the whole body responds to real foods using an integrated approach termed *systems biology*. Systems biology is an approach to studying biological systems that analyzes multiple macromolecular species (DNA polymorphisms, RNA, protein, metabolites, etc.) in one experiment. It is a holistic approach to studying biological systems. In the relation between nutrition and health (unlike the relation between nutrition and disease), it is necessary to develop a new concept for biomarkers (van Ommen and Stierum 2002). The biomarker needs to reflect subtle changes in homeostasis and the efforts of the body to maintain this homeostasis. Also, it should preferably take into account a wide variety of biological actions. Furthermore, both efficacy and safety aspects should be monitored simultaneously. Single nutrients may have multiple known and unknown biochemical targets and physiological actions, which may not be easily addressed with classical biomarkers (i.e., the single gene, protein, or metabolite approach), usually under nonphysiological conditions. In addition, the efficacy assessment of the health effects of nutritional components is even further complicated by the fact that single dietary constituents are hardly consumed as separate entities but are part of a dietary mixture.

An important challenge in the development of functional foods for the prevention of complex (multifactorial) diseases is to obtain a better and improved overview (holistic) picture of the early phases of the process (Van-Ommen and

Table 4.3 Metabolomics Applications in Nutrigenomics Research

Bioactive Compound/Food Ingredient	Food/Beverage	Study Model	Expected Effect/Target Illness	Analytical Methodology	References
Phytochemicals	Low and standard phytochemical diet	Human urine samples	Acute effects in urinary metabolism	1H NMR and HPLC-ESI-Q-TOF	Walsh et al. (2007)
Flavonoids/phenolic compounds	Red wine/red grape juice/tea	Human urine, plasma and fecal samples	Reduced risk of cardiovascular disease via study of the gut microbial impact in polyphenols	GC-TOF-MS	Grun et al. (2008)
Polyphenols	Chamomile Tea	Human urine samples	Increased excretion of hippurate and glycine and depleted of creatinine	1H NMR	Wang et al. (2005)
Polyphenols	Wine/grape juice	Human fecal samples	Modulation of the gut microflora to prevent inflammatory bowel	1H NMR	Jacobs et al. (2008)
Isoflavones	Soy-enriched diets	Human plasma samples	Changes in carbohydrate and energy metabolism	1H NMR	Solanky et al. (2003)
Isoflavones	Soy-enriched diets	Human urine samples	Improved glomerular function or general kidney function	1H NMR	Solanky et al. (2005)

Stierum 2002). The concept of systems biology relates to the integration of all information at the different levels of genomic expression (mRNA, protein, metabolite). Thus, systems biology generates pathway information and provides the capacity to measure (small) perturbations of the pathway resulting from nutritional influences. The challenge here is not so much on a technological level, as enormous progress is being made in the omics technologies. Instead, it is the bioinformatics side (data processing, clustering, dynamics, integration of the various omics levels, and so on) that will have to produce major breakthroughs in order for systems biology for nutrition to mature.

Nutrition is chronic, constantly varying, and composed of a very large amount of known and unknown bioactive compounds. Furthermore, nutrition touches the core of metabolism by supplying the vast majority of ingredients (both macro and micronutrients) for maintaining metabolic homeostasis. Thus, nutrition by its nature needs to be studied in an integrated way (Corthésy-Theulaz et al. 2005).

These analytical platforms are now widely used by both the pharmaceutical and nutritional communities alike; however, whereas pharmaceuticals have a targeted approach aimed at restoring health, diet is a multiparametric approach to preserving and/or optimizing health. Indeed, the diet is comprised of a multitude of nutritional and chemical molecules, each capable of regulating disparate biological processes, and thus cannot use an approach similar to the pharmaceutical industry, that is, the "one drug, one target" paradigm. Hence, nutrition is a true integrative science that is well positioned to benefit from the exploitation of novel technologies capable of assessing biological networks rather than single end points (Mutch et al. 2005). Despite the powerful analytical platforms available for the analysis of genes, proteins, and metabolites, few examples have used a comprehensive and integrative approach to understand the influences of nutritional factors on metabolism. Rather, the great majority of intervention studies performed to date are platform specific. In as much as each of these analytical platforms provides increasingly accurate information describing a given phenotype, it is the integration of these technologies that provides the optimal means to unravel the effects of a biological challenge on an organism, thus the concept of systems biology (or integrated metabolism). The integrated metabolism approach yields an attracting and exciting future for both the pharmaceutical and nutritional communities and their quest to ameliorate health and prevent disease. Currently, few examples exist in which an integrated approach has been used to examine the influences of exogenous factors on metabolism (Mutch et al. 2005), yet even these eloquent examples have only provided the genomic and metabolomic profiles of a single organ. Nevertheless, an underlying theme has begun to emerge with these studies.

4.4 Use of the nutrigenomics approach in nutrition research

Several studies have been conducted to research the application of omics technologies to investigation of the effects of nutrients, phytochemicals, foods, or diets in human models. The following studies highlight the effects of a nutrient on the chosen model by various researchers.

A weight-loss intervention trial was carried out to investigate effects on inflammation-related genes in the adipose tissue of obese subjects (Clement et al. 2004). The gene expression profiles of subcutaneous white adipose tissue were analyzed from 29 obese subjects during very low calorie diet (VLCD) using cDNA microarray and reverse transcription quantitative PCR. The patterns of expression were compared with those of 17 nonobese subjects. The study showed that gene expression profiling identified 100 inflammation-related transcripts that are regulated in obese individuals when eating a 28-day VLCD but not a 2-day VLCD. Cluster analysis showed that the pattern of gene expression in obese subjects after a 28-day VLCD was closer to the profile of lean subjects than to the pattern of obese subjects before VLCD. Weight loss improved the inflammatory profile of obese subjects through a decrease in pro-inflammatory factors and an increase in anti-inflammatory molecules. The genes were expressed mostly in the stromal vascular fraction of adipose tissue, which was shown to contain numerous macrophages. The researchers concluded that the beneficial effect of weight loss on obesity-related complications may be associated with the modification of the inflammatory profile in adipose tissue.

The other trial was carried out to study the changes in adipose tissue gene expression with different energy-restricted diets in obese women (Dahlman et al. 2005). Forty obese women were randomly assigned to a moderate fat, moderate carbohydrate diet or a low fat, high carbohydrate hypoenergetic (600 kcal/d) diet for 10 weeks. Subcutaneous adipose tissue samples were obtained before and after the diet period. High-quality RNA samples were obtained from 23 women at both time points, and these samples were hybridized to microarrays containing the 8,500 most extensively described human genes. The results were confirmed by separate messenger RNA measurements. Both diets resulted in weight losses of approximately 7.5% of baseline body weight. A total of 52 genes were significantly upregulated and 44 were downregulated as a result of the intervention, and no diet-specific effect was observed. No major effect on lipid-specific transcription factors or genes regulating signal transduction, lipolysis, or synthesis of acylglycerols was observed. Most changes were modest (<25% of baseline), but all genes regulating the formation of polyunsaturated fatty acids from acetyl CoA and malonyl CoA were markedly downregulated (35%–60% decrease). The authors concluded that macronutrients have a secondary role in changes in adipocyte gene expression after energy-restricted diets. The most striking alteration after energy restriction was a coordinated reduction in the expression of genes regulating the production of polyunsaturated fatty acids.

Di-Caro et al. (2005) investigated the influence of *L rhamnosus GG* on the genetic expression patterns in the small bowel mucosa. Six male patients with endoscopically proven esophagitis were enrolled. All patients were treated for

1 month with esomeprazole and randomized to receive *L rhamnosus GG* or placebo. After 1 month of treatment, upper endoscopy was repeated. Biopsies of the duodenal mucosa were taken prior to and after the treatment, and the gene expression patterns were assessed using a GeneChip Human U133A array. Genes with significant expression changes were selected and analyzed to identify specific cellular pathways modified by *L rhamnosus GG*. To support the array data, 10 target genes were studied using SYBR Green PCR. Microarray analysis showed that *L rhamnosus GG* administration determined the up- and downregulation of 334 and 92 genes, respectively. Real-time PCR confirmed the reliability of the analysis. *L rhamnosus GG* mainly affected the expression of genes involved in immune response and inflammation (transforming growth factor-beta (TGF-beta) and tumor necrosis factor (TNF) family members, cytokines, nitric oxide synthase 1, and defensin alpha 1), apoptosis, cell growth and cell differentiation (cyclins and caspases, oncogenes), cell–cell signaling (ICAMs and integrins), cell adhesion (cadherins), signal transcription, and transduction. The data indicated that administration of *L rhamnosus GG* is associated with a complex genetic response of the duodenal mucosa, reflected by the up- and downregulation of several genes involved in specific cellular pathways.

Van Erk et al. (2006) evaluated the potential of gene expression profiling in blood cells collected in a human intervention study that investigated the effect of a high-carbohydrate (HC) or a high-protein (HP) breakfast on satiety. Blood samples were taken from eight healthy men before and 2 h after consumption of an HP or HC breakfast. Both breakfasts contained acetaminophen for measuring the gastric emptying rate. Analysis of the transcriptome data focused on the effects of the HP or HC breakfast and of acetaminophen on blood leukocyte gene expression profiles. Breakfast consumption resulted in differentially expressed genes, 317 for the HC breakfast and 919 for the HP breakfast. Immune response and signal transduction, specifically T-cell receptor signaling and nuclear transcription factor kappa B signaling, were the overrepresented functional groups in the set of 141 genes that were differentially expressed in response to both breakfasts. Consumption of the HC breakfast resulted in differential expression of glycogen metabolism genes, and consumption of the HP breakfast resulted in differential expression of genes involved in protein biosynthesis. Gene expression changes in blood leukocytes corresponded with and may be related to the difference in macronutrient content of the breakfast, meal consumption as such, and acetaminophen exposure. This study illustrated the potential of gene expression profiling in blood to study the effects of dietary exposure in human intervention studies.

Considerable research efforts have been devoted to studying dietary fat in relation to biomarkers of chronic disease such as concentrations of blood lipids. There is growing evidence that the optimal amount and type of dietary fat intake depends, in part, on an individual's unique genetic profile (Ordovas 2008). A major focus has been placed on epidemiological diet–gene interaction studies, but clinical dietary trials that examine the difference in response to treatment among genotypes have also been conducted based on the findings from observational studies. For example, plasma omega-3 fatty acid response to an omega-3 fatty acid supplement was found to be modulated by apoE ε4 but not by the common *PPAR-α* L162V polymorphism (Plourde et al. 2009). After supplementation, only noncarriers of E4 had increased omega-3 in their plasma (Plourde et al. 2009). After 3 months of supplementation with 3.6 g of omega-3 fatty acids per day (containing 2.4 g of eicosapentaenoic acid and docosahexaenoic acid) or placebo capsules containing olive oil, changes in cholesterol, including high-density lipoprotein (HDL) cholesterol concentrations, were similar among the *PPAR-α* L162V genotypes (Lindi et al. 2003).

In another study, subjects followed a low-fat diet for 8 weeks and then were supplemented daily with 5 g of fish oil for 6 weeks. The decrease in plasma triglyceride concentrations was comparable for both *PPAR-α* L162V genotype groups, although a significant diet–gene interaction was observed for plasma C-reactive protein (Caron-Dorval et al. 2006). The replication of diet–gene interactions is an important step towards personalized nutrition because it strengthens the evidence that will be used to design clinical trials and subsequent nutrition recommendations based on genotype.

Fruits and vegetables can affect multiple pathways and biological processes in the human body because they are sources of water, fiber, vitamins, minerals, and numerous phytochemicals. Evidence derived from epidemiological studies has suggested that high fruit and vegetable intake is associated with a reduced risk of a variety of cancers (Kim and Park 2009) as well as cardiovascular disease (He et al. 2006).

However, human genetic variation could also be one of the factors modifying response to plant foods and their constituents. It has been observed that dietary intake of a phytochemical might not necessarily result in comparable exposure levels in the circulation or target tissues of interest (Lampe 2009). This variation in individual response may explain, in part, the observed heterogeneity across different study populations. Characterizing how genetic factors modify the effects of a high-plant-based diet or specific components in plant foods on human health outcome could clarify how plant foods influence disease risk and help to identify populations that might benefit most from high fruit and vegetable intake.

Variations in genes affecting phytochemical absorption, distribution, utilization, biotransformation, and excretion potentially influence nutrient exposure at the tissue level (Lampe 2009). For example, the protein expression and activity of many nutrient-metabolizing enzymes are modulated by several compounds, including the substrates they act on. Therefore, genetic variations in the pathways that these compounds act on could alter biological response to dietary factors. Although few studies have addressed these potential genetic differences (Lampe 2009), some studies have explored the effects of genetic variation in biotransformation enzymes such as glutathione S-transferases (Lampe et al. 2000; Probst-Hensch et al. 1998).

In addition to determining how an individual responds to an ingested amount of a specific dietary bioactive, genetic variation can also influence our food preferences and ingestive behaviors. Flavor, including taste, is an important determinant of how much a food is liked or disliked and subsequently eaten or not. Common polymorphisms in genes involved in flavor perception may account for differences in food preferences and dietary habits (Eny and El-Sohemy 2010). This variability could affect food choices, which may influence health status and the risk of chronic disease (Garcia-Bailo et al. 2009). For example, there are several vegetables that are disliked by many because they are experienced as tasting extremely bitter, yet many of these vegetables are rich sources of nutrients that have been associated with improved health outcomes. The *TAS2R38* receptor is known to detect two bitter substances called *phenylthiocarbamide* (PTC) and *6-n-propylthiouracil* (PROP) (El-Sohemy et al. 2007; Kim et al. 2003), which are not found in foods but have structural similarities to bitter compounds in certain foods. Carriers of the PAV haplotype have been classified as "super tasters" because they have a higher sensitivity to PTC and PROP in comparison to individuals homozygous for AVI (Drayna 2005; Wooding et al. 2004). *TAS2R50* has been associated with risk of myocardial infarction (MI), which has been hypothesized to be due to differences in dietary preferences for bitter foods that appear to offer cardiovascular protection (Shiffman et al. 2005).

Establishing a genetic basis for food likes and dislikes may partially explain some of the inconsistencies among epidemiologic studies relating diet to risk of chronic diseases, because the genetic makeup of a group of individuals could be a confounder to the nutritional exposure of interest. Additionally, polymorphisms strongly associated with taste perception may potentially be useful as surrogate markers of dietary exposure in gene–disease association studies where information on dietary habits is not available. Finally, an understanding of the genetics of taste perception may lead to the development of realistic personal and public health strategies for providing dietary advice.

Fruit and vegetables are generally regarded as healthy foods to be consumed by all. However, it may be beneficial for certain individuals, based on genetics, to focus on specific fruits and vegetables. For example, genotypes associated with more favorable metabolism of carcinogens may be associated with less favorable metabolism of phytochemicals (Lampe 2009). Research findings to date suggest a complex association between consumption of several vegetables and biotransformation enzyme activities in humans (Lampe et al. 2000). Genetic variation in pathways affecting nutrient absorption, transport, utilization, and excretion; taste preference; and food tolerance all potentially influence the effect of plant-based diets on the risk of disease.

Knowledge gained by incorporating genetic variation into a nutrition study not only provides a more rational basis for giving personalized dietary advice but will also improve the quality of evidence used for making population-based dietary recommendations for the prevention of specific diseases. This can be illustrated by considering studies that explore the effects of caffeine on certain health outcomes (Cornelis et al. 2006). These studies have helped pinpoint caffeine as the bioactive compound in coffee that affects certain diseases. These studies have also identified how a response to coffee by a specific genotype can be beneficial or detrimental depending on the disease being examined. Caffeine is metabolized primarily by the cytochrome P450 1A2 (CYP1A2) enzyme, and a polymorphism in the *CYP1A2* gene determines whether individuals are rapid caffeine metabolizers (those who are homozygous for the Minus 163 A allele) or slow caffeine metabolizers (carriers of the Minus 163 C allele). Intake of coffee is associated with an increased risk of MI only among individuals with slow caffeine metabolism (Cornelis et al. 2006), suggesting that caffeine increases risk of MI, since it is the only major compound in coffee that is known to be detoxified by CYP1A2. Furthermore, a protective effect of moderate coffee consumption was observed among the fast metabolizers, suggesting that other components of coffee might be protective and their effects are "unmasked" in those who eliminate caffeine rapidly. This coffee–*CYP1A2* genotype interaction has since been supported by a prospective study investigating the effect of coffee intake on the risk of developing hypertension in individuals stratified by *CYP1A2* genotype (Palatini et al. 2009). That study also measured epinephrine and norepinephrine in the urine of the subjects, because these catecholamines have been shown to increase after caffeine administration in humans. Urinary epinephrine was significantly higher in coffee drinkers than abstainers, but only among slow caffeine metabolizers, which is of interest because increased sympathetic activity is considered an important mechanism through which caffeine raises blood pressure.

A similar concept was utilized in an observational study of coffee and breast cancer (Kotsopoulos et al. 2007). By dividing subjects into *CYP1A2* genotypes, this study aimed to determine if caffeine was the compound in coffee that explains the protective effect that had previously been observed between coffee and risk of breast cancer (Baker et al. 2006; Nkondjock et al. 2006). Indeed, a diet–gene interaction was present. However, unlike the studies on risk of MI and hypertension in which slow caffeine metabolizers were at increased risk from drinking coffee, in this study coffee was associated with a lower risk of breast cancer among slow metabolizers (Kotsopoulos et al. 2009). No protective effect was observed among fast metabolizers, implicating caffeine as the protective component of coffee. This is consistent with findings from animal studies showing that caffeine inhibits the development of mammary tumors (Wolfrom et al. 1991; Yang et al. 2004).

Incorporating data on genetic variability into a nutrition study can clarify whether or not a specific dietary compound is linked to a particular health outcome. This diet–disease connection is made by the observation of whether the association between the disease and the dietary factor is influenced by functional variants in genes involved in the metabolism of the dietary factor. For example, moderate alcohol consumption has been associated with a lower risk of heart disease. The primary mechanism proposed for this association is the higher levels of HDL cholesterol found among moderate drinkers. However, it is possible that the protective effect of moderate alcohol consumption is due to some confounding lifestyle factor associated with moderate alcohol intake that differs from abstainers or heavy drinkers.

The enzyme alcohol dehydrogenase 1C (ADH1C), also known as *alcohol dehydrogenase type 3* (ADH3), oxidizes alcohol to acetaldehyde. It has two polymorphic forms with distinct kinetic properties. The *ADH1C*1* allele produces ɣ1 and the *ADH1C*2* allele produces ɣ2. The rate of alcohol metabolism (ethanol oxidation) in ɣ1 ɣ1 individuals is more than twice as high as in ɣ2 ɣ2 individuals, with heterozygous individuals metabolizing alcohol at an intermediate rate. Therefore, if there is a causal protective effect of moderate alcohol on the risk of heart disease, this effect would be expected to be stronger in individuals with the slow *ADH1C* genotype compared to those with fast metabolism. An early gene–diet interaction study examined data from the Physicians' Health Study and the Nurses' Health Study to determine whether the effect of moderate alcohol consumption on HDL levels and the risk of MI varies according to ADH3 genotype (Hines et al. 2001). The study reported evidence of a dose–response decrease in heart disease as alcohol metabolism slows according to genotype, for a marked 86% reduction in heart disease risk in subjects with the slow-alcohol-metabolizing genotype who consumed at least one alcoholic drink per day (Hines et al. 2001). The polymorphism was also associated with higher levels of HDL.

The finding of an effect of the functional *ADH1C* polymorphism on the relation between alcohol consumption and the risk of heart disease suggests that the protective effect is due to the alcohol and not some associated lifestyle factor, since those with the slow-alcohol-metabolizing genotype who did not consume alcohol were not at a lower risk. A key step in nutrigenomics research is to identify the subset(s) of the population that have different reactions to dietary factors. In the case of alcohol, those groups were identified based on genetic differences in alcohol metabolism. The extent to which this knowledge is being or will be incorporated into nutrition practice remains unknown.

4.5 Future prospects

Dietary recommendations are based on epidemiological, clinical, and experimental studies that have investigated biochemical, physiological, and anthropometric outcomes of various populations. During the past two to three decades the development of new noninvasive or mildly invasive methods has been assisting in studying mechanisms in humans. Recent years have also brought nutrigenomics as part of the acknowledged nutritional research and made it evident that nutrients and other bioactive compounds in food interact with genetic factors, which either modify the effects of these compounds or determine the way they function. This interplay is based on individual genetic makeup, and the development of omics methods has opened an avenue for studying it.

Systems biology or nutrigenomics aims to understand physiology and disease by integrating and considering molecular pathways, regulatory networks, cells, tissues, organs, and ultimately the whole organism. Nutrigenomic research will yield long-term benefits to human health by revealing novel nutrient–gene interactions, developing new diagnostic tests for adverse responses to diets, and by identifying specific populations with special nutrient needs.

In short, nutrigenomics is expected to deliver biomarkers for health, deliver early biomarkers for disease disposition, differentiate dietary responders from nonresponders, and discover bioactive food components.

References

Anderle, P., Farmer, P., Berger, A. and Roberts, M.A. 2004. Nutrigenomic approach to understanding the mechanisms by which dietary long-chain fatty acids induce gene signals and control mechanisms involved in carcinogenesis. *Nutrition* 20: 103–108.

Ashburner, M., Ball, C.A., Blake, J.A., Botstein, D., Butler, H., Cherry, J.M., Davis, A.P., et al. 2000. Gene ontology: Tool for the unification of biology. *Nat. Genet.* 25: 25–29.

Astle, J., Ferguson, J.T., German, J.B., Harrigan, G.G., Kelleher, N.L., Kodadek, T., Parks, B.A., Roth, M.J., Singletary, K.W., Wenger, C.D. and Mahady, G.B. 2007. Characterization of proteomic and metabolomic responses to dietary factors and supplements. *J. Nutr.* 137: 2787–2793.

Baker, J.A., Beehler, G.P., Sawant, A.C., Jayaprakash, V., McCann, S.E. and Moysich, K.B. 2006. Consumption of coffee, but not black tea, is associated with decreased risk of premenopausal breast cancer. *J. Nutr.* 136: 166–171.

Boersema, P.J., Mohammed, S. and Heck, A.J.R. 2008. Hydrophilic interaction liquid chromatography (HILIC) in proteomics. *Anal. Bioanal. Chem.* 391: 151–159.

Bogdanov, B. and Smith, R.D. 2005. Proteomics by FTICR mass spectrometry: Top down and bottom up. *Mass Spectrom. Rev.* 24: 168–200.

Brenner, S., Johnson, M., Bridgham, J., Golda, G., Lloyd, D.H., Johnson, D., Luo, S. et al. 2000. Gene expression analysis by massively parallel signature sequencing (MPSS) on microbead arrays. *Nat. Biotechnol.* 18: 630–634.

Breuker, K., Jin, M., Han, X., Jiang, H. and McLafferty, F.W. 2008. Top-down identification and characterization of biomolecules by mass spectrometry. *J. Am. Soc. Mass Spectrom.* 19: 1045–1053.

Cassidy, A. and Dalais, F.S. 2003. Phytochemicals. In: *Nutrition and Metabolism*, Gibney, M.J., Macdonald, I.A., Roche, H.M., (Eds.). Oxford: Blackwell Publishing, pp. 307–317.

Clement, K., Viguerie, N., Poitou, C., Carette, C., Pelloux, V., Curat, C.A., Sicard, A., et al. 2004. Weight loss regulates inflammation related genes in white adipose tissue of obese subjects. *FASEB J.* 18: 1657–1669.

Cornelis, M.C., El-Sohemy, A., Kabagambe, E.K. and Campos, H. 2006. Coffee, CYP1A2 genotype, and risk of myocardial infarction. *JAMA.* 295: 1135–1141.

Corthesy-Theulaz, I., Den-Dunnen, J.T., Ferre, P., Geurts, J.M.W., Muller, M., Van-Belzen, N. and Van-Ommen, B. 2005. Nutrigenomics: The impact of biomics technology on nutrition research. *Ann. Nutr. Metab.* 49: 355–365.

Dahlman, I., Linder, K., Arvidsson-Nordstrom, E., Andersson, I., Liden, J., Verdich, C., Sorensen, T.I. and Arner, P. 2005. Changes in adipose tissue gene expression with energy restricted diets in obese women. *Am. J. Clin. Nutr.* 81: 1275–1285.

Dettmer, K., Aronov, P.A. and Hammock, B.D. 2007. Mass spectrometry-based metabolomics. *Mass Spectrom. Rev.* 26: 51–78.

Di-Caro, S., Tao, H., Grillo, A., Elia, C., Gasbarrini, G., Sepulveda, A.R. and Gasbarrini, A. 2005. Effects of Lactobacillus GG on genes expression pattern in small bowel mucosa. *Dig. Liver Dis.* 37: 320–329.

Dinkova-Kostova, A.T. 2002. Protection against cancer by plant phenylpropenoids: Induction of mammalian anticarcinogenic enzymes. *Mini Rev. Med. Chem.* 2: 595–610.

Drayna, D. 2005. Human taste genetics. *Annu. Rev. Genomics Hum. Genet.* 6: 217–235.

Dumas, M.E., Maibaum, E.C., Teague, C., Ueshima, H., Zhou, B., Lindon, J.C., Nicholson, J.K., Stamler, J., Elliot, P., Chan, Q. and Holmes, E. 2006. Assessment of analytical reproducibility of 1H NMR spectroscopy based metabonomics for large-scale epidemiological research: The INTERMAP study. *Anal. Chem.* 78: 2199–2208.

El-Sohemy, A., L. Stewart, N., Khataan, B., Fontaine-Bisson, P., Kwong, S., Ozsungur, and Cornelis, M.C. 2007. Nutrigenomics of taste – impact on food preferences and food production. *Forum Nutr.* 60:176–182.

Eny, K.M. and El-Sohemy, A. 2010. The genetic determinants of ingestive behavior: Sensory, energy homeostasis and food reward aspects of ingestive behavior. In: L. Dube, A.D. Bechara, A. Drewnowski, J., LeBel, P. James, R.Y., Yada and M.C. Laflamme-Sanders (eds) *Obesity Prevention: The Role of Brain and Society on Individual Behavior.* Amsterdam: Elsevier. pp. 149–160.

Fiehn, O. 2002. Metabolomics—The link between genotypes and phenotypes. *Plant Mol. Biol.* 48: 155–171.

Fournier, M.L., ilmore, J.M., Martin-Brown, S.A. and Washburn, M.P. 2007. Multidimensional separations-based shotgun proteomics. *Chem. Rev.* 107: 3654–3686.

Fuchs, D., Winkelmann, I., Johnson, I.T., Mariman, E., Wenzel, U. and Daniel, H. 2005. Proteomics in nutrition research: Principles, technologies and applications. *Br. J. Nutr.* 94: 302–314.

Gaj, S., Eijssen, L., Mensink, R.P. and Evelo, C.T. 2008. Validating nutrient-related gene expression changes from microarrays using RT2 PCR-arrays. *Genes Nutr.* 3: 153–157.

Garcia-Bailo, B., Toguri, C., Eny, K.M. and El-Sohemy, A. 2009. Genetic variation in taste and its influence on food selection. *OMICS.* 13: 69–80.

Garcia-Canas, V., Simo, C., Leon, C. and Cifuentes, A. 2010. Advances in nutrigenomics research: Novel and future analytical approaches to investigate the biological activity of natural compounds and food functions. *J. Pharm. Biomed. Anal.* 51: 290–304.

Gea, Y., Horna, D.M. and McLafferty, F.W. 2001. Blackbody infrared radiative dissociation of larger (42 kDa) multiply charged proteins. *Int. J. Mass Spectrom.* 210–211: 203–214.

Gene Ontology Consortium. The Gene Ontology Consortium. 2008. The gene ontology project in 2008. *Nucl. Acids Res.* 36: D440–D444.

German, J.B., Bauman, D.E., Burrin, D.G., Failla, M.L., Freake, H.C., King, J.C., Klein, S., Milner, J.A., Pelto, G.H., Rasmussen, K.M. and Zeisel, S.H. 2004. Metabolomics in the opening decade of the 21st century: Building the roads to individualized health. *J. Nutr.* 134: 2729–2732.

Gibney, M.J., Walsh, M., Brennan, L., Roche, H.M., German, B., Van-Ommen, B. 2005. Metabolomics in human nutrition: Opportunities and challenges. *Am. J. Clin. Nutr.* 82: 497–503.

Guo, T., Lee, C.S., Wang, W., De-Voe, D.L. and Balgley, B.M. 2006. Capillary separations enabling tissue proteomics-based biomarker discovery. *Electrophoresis* 27: 3523–3532.

Guy, P.A., Tavazzi, I., Bruce, S.J., Ramadan, Z. and Kochhar, S. 2008. Global metabolic profiling analysis on human urine by UPLC-TOFMS: Issues and method validation in nutritional metabolomics. *J. Chromatogr. B* 871: 253–260.

Harland, J.I. 2005. *Nutrition and Genetics: Mapping Individual Health. Monograph Series.* Belgium: ILSI Europe Publisher. pp. 1–32.

He, F. J., Nowson, C.A. and Macgregor, G.A. 2006. Fruit and vegetable consumption and stroke: Meta-analysis of cohort studies. *The Lancet.* 367(9507): 320–326.

Hines, L. M., Stampfer, M.J., Ma, J., Gaziano, J.M., Ridker, P.M., Hankinson, S.E., Sacks, F., Rimm, E.B. and Hunter, D.J. 2001. Genetic variation in alcohol dehydrogenase and the beneficial effect of moderate alcohol consumption on myocardial infarction. *N. Engl. J. Med.* 344: 549–555.

Hu, R. and Kong, A.N. 2004. Activation of MAP kinases, apoptosis and nutrigenomics of gene expression elicited by dietary cancer-prevention compounds. *Nutrition* 20: 83–88.

Huang, D.W., Sherman, B.T. and Lempicki, R.A. 2009. Bioinformatics enrichment tools: Paths toward the comprehensive functional analysis of large gene lists. *Nucl. Acids Res.* 37:1–13.

Jacobs, D.M., Deltimple, N., Van-Velzen, E., Van-Dorsten, F.A., Bingham, M., Vaughan, E.E. and Van-Duynhoven, J. 2008. (1)H NMR metabolite profiling of feces as a tool to assess the impact of nutrition on the human microbiome. *NMR Biomed.* 21: 615–626.

Kim, M.K. and Park, J.H. 2009. Conference on "Multidisciplinary approaches to nutritional problems." Symposium on "Nutrition and Health." Cruciferous vegetable intake and the risk of human cancer: Epidemiological evidence. *Proc. Nutr. Soc.* 68: 103–110.

Kim, U.K., Jorgenson, E., Coon, H., Leppert, M., Risch, N. and Drayna, D. 2003. Positional cloning of the human quantitative trait locus underlying taste sensitivity to phenylthio-carbamide. *Science.* 299(5610): 1221–1225.

Knowles, L.M. and Milner, J.A. 2000. Diallyl disulfide inhibits p34 (cdc2) kinase activity through changes in complex formation and phosphorylation. *Carcinogenesis.* 21: 1129–1134.

Kotsopoulos, J., Ghadirian, P., El-Sohemy, A., Lynch, H. T., Snyder, C., Daly, M., Domchek, S., Randall, S., Karlan, B., Zhang, P., Zhang, S., Sun, P., and Narod, S. A. 2007. The CYP1A2 genotype modifies the association between coffee consumption and breast cancer risk among BRCA1 mutation carriers. *Cancer Epidemiol Biomarkers Prev.* 16 (5):912–916.

Kotsopoulos, J., Ghadirian, P., El-Sohemy, A., Lynch, H.T., Snyder, C., Daly, M., Lampe, J. W. 2009. Interindividual differences in response to plant-based diets: Implications for cancer risk. *Am. J. Clin. Nutr.* 89:1553S–1557S.

Koulman, A. and Volmer, D.A. 2008. Perspectives for metabolomics in human nutrition: An overview. *Nutr. Bull.* 33: 324–330.

Kussmann, M., Raymond, F. and Affolter, M. 2006. OMICS driven biomarker discovery in nutrition and health. *J. Biotechnol.* 124: 758–787.

Kussman, M., Rezzi, S. and Danelore, H. 2008. Profiling techniques in nutrition and health research. *Curr. Opin. Biotechnol.* 19: 83–99.

Lambert, J.D., Hong, J., Yang, G., Liao, J. and Yang, C. 2005. Inhibition of carcinogenesis by polyphenols: Evidence from laboratory investigations. *Am. J. Clin. Nutr.* 81: 284S–291S.

Lampe, J. W. 2009. Interindividual differences in response to plant-based diets:implications for cancer risk. Am J Clin Nutr 89 (5):1553S–1557S.

Lampe, J. W., King, I.B., Li, S., Grate, M.T., Barale, K.V., Chen, C., Feng, Z. and Potter, J.D. 2000. Brassica vegetables increase and apiaceous vegetables decrease cytochrome P450 1A2 activity in humans: Changes in caffeine metabolite ratios in response to controlled vegetable diets. *Carcinogenesis.* 21: 1157–1162.

Leong, H.X., Simkevich, C., Lesieur-Brooks, A., Lau, B.W. and Fugere, E. 2006. Short-term arginine deprivation results in large-scale modulation of hepatic gene expression in both normal and tumor cells: Microarray bioinformatic analysis. *Nutr. Metab. (Lond).* 3: 37–49.

Lindi, V., Schwab, U., Louheranta, A., Laakso, M., Vessby, B., Hermansen, K., Storlien, L., Riccardi, G. and Rivellese, A. 2003. Impact of the Pro12Ala polymorphism of the PPAR-gamma2 gene on serum triacylglycerol response to n-3 fatty acid supplementation. *Mol. Genet. Metab.* 79: 52–60.

Macek, B., Waanders, L.F., Olsen, J.V. and Mann, M. 2006. Top-down protein sequencing and MS3 on a hybrid linear quadrupole ion trap-orbitrap mass spectrometer. *Mol. Cell. Proteomics.* 5: 949–958.

Marouga, R., David, S. and Hawkins, E. 2005. The development of the DIGE System: 2D fluorescence difference gel analysis technology. *Anal. Bioanal. Chem.* 382: 669–678.

Moresco, J.J., Dong, M.Q. and Yates, J.R. 2008. Quantitative mass spectrometry as a tool for nutritional proteomics. *Am. J. Clin. Nutr.* 88: 597–604.

Morgan, J.W., Hettick, J.M. and Russell, D.H. 2005. Peptide sequencing by MALDI 193-nm photodissociation TOF MS. *Methods Enzymol.* 402: 186–209.

Morozova, O. and Marra, M.A. 2008. Applications of next-generation sequencing technologies in functional genomics. *Genomics.* 92: 255–264.

Motoyama, A. and Yates, J.R. 2008. Two modes of separation coupled with MS enable researchers to study complicated biological structures. *Anal. Chem.* 80: 7187–7193.

Muller, M. and Kersten, S. 2003. Nutrigenomics: Goals and strategies. *Nat. Rev. Gen.* 4: 315–322.

Mutch, D.M., Wahli, W. and Williamson, G. 2005. Nutrigenomics and nutrigenetics: The emerging faces of nutrition. *FASEB J.* 19: 1602–1616.

Nesvizhskii, A.I. and Aebersold, R. 2005. Interpretation of shotgun proteomic data: The protein inference problem. *Mol. Cell. Proteomics.* 4: 1419–1440.

Ng, P., Wei, C.L., Sung, W.K., Chiu, K.P., Lipovich, L., Ang, C.C., Gupta, S., Shahab, A., Ridwan, C.H. and Wong. 2005. Gene identification signature (GIS) analysis for transcriptome characterization and genome annotation. *Nat. Methods* 2: 105–111.

Niculescu, M.D., Pop, E.A., Fischer, L.M. and Zeisel, S.H. 2007. Dietary isoflavones differentially induce gene expression changes. *J. Nutr. Biochem.* 18: 380–390.

Nielsen, K.L., Hogh, A.L. and Emmergen, J. 2006. DeepSAGE—Digital transcriptomics with high sensitivity, simple experimental protocol and multiplexing of samples. *Nucl. Acids Res.* 34: e133.

Nkondjock, A., Ghadirian, P., Kotsopoulos, J., Lubinski, J., Lynch, H., Kim-Sing, C., Horsman, D., et al. 2006. Coffee consumption and breast cancer risk among BRCA1 and BRCA2 mutation carriers. *Int. J. Cancer.* 118: 103–107.

Ordovas, J.M. 2008. Genotype-phenotype associations: Modulation by diet and obesity. *Obesity* 16: S40–S46.

Ovesna, J., Slaby, O., Toussaint, O., Kodicek, M., Marsik, P., Pouchova, V. and Vanek, T. 2008. High throughput omics approaches to assess the effects of phytochemicals in human health studies. *Br. J. Nutr.* 99: ES127–ES134.

Palatini, P., Ceolotto, G., Ragazzo, F., Dorigatti, F., Saladini, F., Papparella, I., Mos, L., Zanata, G. and Santonastaso, M. 2009. CYP1A2 genotype modifies the association between coffee intake and the risk of hypertension. *J. Hypertens.* 27: 1594–1601.

Plourde, M., Vohl, M.C., Vandal, M., Couture, P., Lemieux, S. and Cunnane, S.C. 2009. Plasma n-3 fatty acid response to an n-3 fatty acid supplement is modulated by apoE epsilon4 but not by the common PPAR-alpha L162V polymorphism in men. *Br. J. Nutr.* 102: 1121–1124.

Probst-Hensch, N. M., Tannenbaum, S.R., Chan, K.K., Coetzee, G.A., Ross, R.K. and Yu, M.C. 1998. Absence of the glutathione S-transferase M1 gene increases cytochrome P4501A2 activity among frequent consumers of cruciferous vegetables in a Caucasian population. *Cancer Epidemiol. Biomarkers Prev.* 7: 635–638.

Raspopov, S.A., El-Faramawy, A., Thomson, B.A. and Siu, K.W.M. 2006. Infrared multiphoton dissociation in quadrupole time-of-flight mass spectrometry: Top-down characterization of proteins. *Anal. Chem.* 78: 4572–4577.

Rochfort, S. 2005. Metabolomics reviewed: A new omics platform technology for systems biology and implications for natural products research. *J. Nat. Prod.* 68: 1813–1820.

Rosello-Mora, R., Lucio, M., Pea, A., Brito-Echeverria, J., Lopez-Lopez, A., Valens-Vadell, M., Frommberger, M., Anton, J. and Schmitt-Kopplin, P. 2008. Metabolic evidence for biogeographic isolation of the extremophilic bacterium Salinibacter ruber. *ISME J.* 2: 242–253.

Saha, S., Sparks, A.B., Rago, C., Akmaev, V., Wang, C.J., Vogelstein, B., Kinzler, K.W. and Velculescu, V.E. 2002. Using the transcriptome to annotate the genome. *Nat. Biotechnol.* 20: 508–512.

Schweigert, F.J. 2007. Nutritional proteomics: Methods and concepts for research in nutritional science. *Ann. Nutr. Metab.* 51: 99–107.

Shiffman, D., Ellis, S.G., Rowland, C.M., Malloy, M.J., Luke, M.M., Iakoubova, O.A., Pullinger, C.R., et al. 2005. Identification of four gene variants associated with myocardial infarction. *Am. J. Hum. Genet.* 77: 596–605.

Shiraki, T., Kondo, S., Katayama, S., Waki, K., Kasukawa, T., Kawaji, H., Kodzius, R., Watahiki, A., et al. 2003. Cap analysis gene expression for high-throughput analysis of transcriptional starting point and identification of promoter usage. *Proc. Natl. Acad. Sci. U.S.A.* 100: 15776–15781.

Simpson, D.C., Ahn, S., Pasa-Tolic, L., Bogdanov, B., Mottaz, H.M., Vilkov, A.N., Anderson, G.A., Lipton, M.S. and Smith, R.D. 2006. Using size exclusion chromatography-RPLC and RPLC-CIEF as two-dimensional separation strategies for protein profiling. *Electrophoresis.* 27: 2722–2733.

Solanky, K.S., Bailey, N.J., Beckwith-Hall, B.M., Bingham, S., Davis, A., Holmes, E., Nicholson, J.K. and Cassidy, A. 2005. Biofluid 1H NMR-based metabonomic techniques in nutrition research—metabolic effects of dietary isoflavones in humans. *J. Nutr. Biochem.* 16: 236–244.

Solanky, K.S., Bailey, N.J., Beckwith-Hall, B.M., Davis, A., Bingham, S., Holmes, E., Nicholson, J.K. and Cassidy, A. 2003. Application of biofluid 1H nuclear magnetic resonance-based metabonomic techniques for the analysis of the biochemical effects of dietary isoflavones on human plasma profile. *Anal. Biochem.* 323: 197–204.

Storhoff, J.J., Marla, S.S., Garimella, V., and Mirkin, C.A. 2005. *Microarray Technology and its Applications.* Heidelberg: Springer-Verlag. pp. 147–180.

Sweet, S.M. and Cooper, H.J. 2007. Electron capture dissociation in the analysis of protein phosphorylation. *Expert Rev. Proteomics.* 4: 149–159.

Trujillo, E., Davis, C. and Milner, J. 2006. Nutrigenomics, proteomics, metabolomics, and the practice of dietetics. *J. Am. Diet Assoc.* 106: 403–413.

Tuteja, R. 2008. *Bioinformatics: A Practical Approach.* Boca Raton, FL: Chapman and Hall. pp. 189–218.

Van-Erk, M.J., Blom, W.A., Van-Ommen, B. and Hendriks, H.F. 2006. High protein and high carbohydrate breakfasts differentially change the transcriptome of human blood cells. *Am. J. Clin. Nutr.* 84: 1233–1241.

Van-Ommen, B. and Stierum, R. 2002. Nutrigenomics: Exploiting systems biology in the nutrition and health arena. *Curr. Opin. Biotechnol.* 13: 517–521.

Velculescu, V.E., Zhang, L., Bofelstein, B. and Kinzler, K.W. 1995. Serial analysis of gene expressions. *Science* 270: 484–487.

Wai-Nang P. Lee and Vay Liang W. Go. 2005. Nutrient-Gene Interaction: Tracer-Based Metabolomics. *J. Nutr.* 135 (12): 3027S–3032S.

Walsh, M.C., Nugent, A., Brennan, L. and Gibney, M.J. 2008. Understanding the metabolome— Challenges for metabolomics. *Nutr. Bull.* 33: 316–323.

Wang, S.I. and Mukhar, H. 2002. Gene expression profile in human prostate LNCaP cancer cells by (–) epigallocatechin-3-gallate. *Cancer Lett.* 182: 43–51.

Wang, S.M. 2007. Understanding SAGE data. *Trends Genet.* 23: 42–50.

Wang, Y., Tang, H., Nicholson, J.K., Hylands, P.J., Sampson, J. and Holmes, E. 2005. A metabonomic strategy for the detection of the metabolic effects of chamomile (Matricaria recutita L.) ingestion. *J. Agric. Food Chem.* 53: 191–196.

Werner, E., Heilier, J.F., Ducruix, C., Ezan, E., Junot, C. and Tabet, J.C. 2008. Mass spectrometry for the identification of the discriminating signals from metabolomics: Current status and future trends. *J. Chromatogr. B Analyt. Technol. Biomed. Life Sci.* 871: 143–163.

Whitfield, P.D., German, A.J. and Nobel, P.J. 2004. Metabolomics: An emerging post genomic tool for nutrition. *Br. J. Nutr.* 92: 549–555.

Wiesner, J., Premsler, T. and Sickmann, A. 2008. Application of electron transfer dissociation (ETD) for the analysis of posttranslational modifications. *Proteomics.* 8: 4466–4483.

Wittmann-Liebold, B., Graack, H. R. and Pohl, T. 2006. Two-dimensional gel electrophoresis as tool for proteomics studies in combination with protein identification by mass spectrometry. *Proteomics.* 6: 4688–4703.

Wolfrom, D.M., Rao, A.R. and Welsch, C.W. 1991. Caffeine inhibits development of benign mammary gland tumors in carcinogen-treated female Sprague-Dawley rats. *Breast Cancer Res. Treat.* 19: 269–275.

Wooding, S., Kim, U.K., Bamshad, M.J., Larsen, J., Jorde, L.B. and Drayna, D. 2004. Natural selection and molecular evolution in PTC, a bitter-taste receptor gene. *Am. J. Hum. Genet.* 74: 637–646.

Wu, R., Hu, L., Wang, F., Ye, M. and Zou, H. 2008. Recent development of monolithic stationary phases with emphasis on microscale chromatographic separation. *J. Chromatogr. A* 1184: 369–392.

Yang, H., Rouse, J., Lukes, L., Lancaster, M., Veenstra, T., Zhou, M., Shi, Y., Park, Y.G. and Hunter, K. 2004. Caffeine suppresses metastasis in a transgenic mouse model: A prototype molecule for prophylaxis of metastasis. *Clin. Exp. Metastasis.* 21: 719–735.

5

Recent Trends in Omics-Based Methods and Techniques for Lung Disease Prevention

Raisah Salhab and Yashwant V. Pathak
University of South Florida
Tampa, Florida

Contents

5.1 Transcriptomics 115
5.2 Proteomics 119
5.3 Metabolomics.. 123
5.4 Breathomics.. 126
5.5 Lipidomics 129
    5.5.1 Phosphatidylcholine 130
    5.5.2 Phosphatidylglycerol 130
    5.5.3 Sphingolipids.. 131
References 132

5.1 Transcriptomics

As the use of engineered nanoparticles (ENMs) in the manufacturing environment and consumer products has increased, the concern over human exposure to ENMs has also increased. Due to the varying physical and chemical characteristics of ENMs, the level of toxicity varies based on the shape, size, solubility, surface area, and surface charges of the ENM that is synthesized. However, with the lack of reference materials and inconsistent protocols, the validation of novel methods in order to determine toxicity has been deemed challenging; thus, there is an inability to make an accurate assessment based on the human health risk assessment (HHRA) of environmental chemicals when exposure has occurred (Labib et al. 2015). Also, current methods for chemical risk assessments are not without additional limitations, as their high cost and the reliance on observing the effects of toxicity in animals has led to very few assessments done on chemicals that are in use in manufacturing (Bourdon-Lacombe et al. 2015). With the use of toxicogenomics, there is the ability to determine the level of toxicity that is associated with certain properties of ENMs as well as to assist in the identification of potential health hazards (Bourdon-Lacombe et al. 2015; Nikota et al. 2015). DNA microarray, large-scale real-time quantitative polymerase chain reaction, and RNA sequencing are among the most commonly used technologies within toxicogenomics (Bourdon-Lacombe et al. 2015).

Measurement of gene expression using a DNA microarray is done through the binding of complimentary DNA to probes attached to the array in order to detect mRNA. This then allows the comparison of the levels of gene expression. Although this method is well validated and has the ability to measure gene expression of large numbers of genes, there is still the disadvantage that the number of genes measured is fixed (Bourdon-Lacombe et al. 2015).

Gene expression profiling has been utilized in studies in order to explore either lung injury or lung disease caused by exposure to ENMs, specifically if nanoTiO2, carbon black, or multiwalled carbon nanotubes (MWCNTs) present an association with the development of certain lung diseases. As a result of their wide use in commercial and biomedical applications, carbon nanotubes (CNTs) and their effects on pulmonary pathology have been studied. After exposure to CNTs, more particularly MWCNTs, rodents experienced effects on their lungs such as pulmonary inflammation, granulomas, and lung fibrosis. Certain features of MWCNTs, such as persistence in lung tissue after exposure, being composed of fiber-like structures, and chemical groups found on their surface, may lead to the development of pulmonary fibrosis. However, the underlying mechanism of how MWCNTs cause pulmonary fibrosis has yet to be understood and has proven to be challenging (Labib et al. 2015). Data from other studies have shown that MWCNTs have the potential to induce fibrosis through Th2-mediated signaling. Analyses of microarray studies have shown that the initial response to MWCNTs is similar to the response of exposure to substances such as bleomycin or bacterial challenge. Bleomycin exposure models exhibit an initial response characterized by the disruption of innate immune mechanisms, which progresses to the activation of CD4+ T cells, triggering Th2 cytokines. Th2 cytokines, when upregulated, engage in the development of fibrosis (Labib et al. 2015). There is also a difference in a later response as compared to the initial response; later response to MCWNT exposure is similar to Th2 response after exposure to allergens, as altered Th2 gene expression of chemokines, cytokines, and growth factors play a role in lung fibrosis (Nikota et al. 2015). Unlike MWCNTs, which were classified by Nikota et al. as potentially disease-causing ENMs, nano-TiO2 and carbon black were not classified as such, although exposure to both ENMs can induce lung inflammation as well as change the expression of inflammatory genes. However, the instance of change in the expression of genes through exposure to nano-TiO2 and carbon black were lower as well as reversible. Compared to MWCNTs that had multicell-type involvement in inflammation, nano-TiO2 and carbon black exposure exhibited less inflammation with primarily neutrophil cell involvement.

The concept of RNA sequencing is that there is the ability to count how many times a transcript has been sequenced, which then provides the level of expression of each exon in a gene. RNA sequencing can also detect both known and unknown transcripts that have low signal–noise ratio as well as a high degree of sensitivity, unlike microarray technology (Pathak and Vrushank 2014). Due to its reliance on counting transcripts, this method becomes more quantitative and can theoretically measure any potential transcripts. However, it is not as validated as microarrays due to the continuing evolution of RNA sequencing technology (Bourdon-Lacombe et al. 2015).

RNA sequencing has been used to exhibit the differences between the transcriptomic profile of *in vivo* whole human endobronchial biopsies between patients with asthma and healthy nonatopic controls. Between asthma patients and controls, 46 genes were differentially expressed and a number of those genes were shown to have differing effects on biological processes such as mRNA degradation and translation, which go on to affect cellular functions, such as STAU2 and WARS, within the airways. When the phrase "differentially expressed" is used, it means that the number of copies of the gene's transcript is increased (upregulated) or decreased (downregulated). The number of genes that are differentially expressed presents information on the magnitude of a transcriptional response (Bourdon-Lacombe et al. 2015). Pendrin, BCL2, and periostin were among the 46 genes that were differentially expressed. From the genes that were differentially expressed, a large number have yet to be linked to asthma, thus there is the potential for novel disease-related genes (Yick et al. 2013). Due to the complexity of asthma, as well as the difference in the biological processes between patients that have asthma and subjects who are healthy as exhibited by this study, these findings may be pertinent to the pathogenesis of asthma.

Gene expression profiling with the use of RNA-sequencing of lung tissues was also done to understand the molecular mechanisms that take part in the pathogenesis of COPD. Lung tissue samples were acquired from patients who required resection for lung cancer, and total RNA was isolated from lung tissue that was away from the area with lung cancer. The subjects were made up of 98 patients with COPD and 91 control subjects. Genes that had expression levels that were found to be related to COPD status by RNA-seq was validated using TaqMan real-time PCR. A total of 2,312 genes were identified as differentially expressed between the lung tissues of COPD patients and control subjects. MICAL2 and NOTCH2 were upregulated in the resected lung tissue of patients with COPD, while S100A6 and genes encoding ribosomal proteins had lower expression in the COPD group compared to the control subjects (Kim et al. 2015). The expression of these genes was also reduced in the small airway epithelium of smokers, as previously shown by RNA-seq. The protein catabolism pathway and ubiquitination–proteasome pathway were impaired in the lung tissues of patients with COPD. There was also downregulation of genes that are related to the 20S proteasome such as *PSMA2*, *PSMB1*, *PSMC5*, *PSMD4*, and *PSMD13*. The genes for chromatin modification, an important mechanism in epigenetics, were found to be upregulated in the lung tissue of COPD patients. The findings of this study may help in the understanding of the mechanistic implications of COPD as oxidative phosphorylation, protein degradation, and chromatin modification were the most altered pathways in COPD lung tissues (Kim et al. 2015).

Quantitative reverse transcription PCR, or RT-qPCR, is a method that is as well validated as microarray but is more sensitive. Due to the fact that analyses are done separately, the drawback lies in that a finite number of genes can be examined at a time. RT-qPCR was used in order to validate microarray results when assessing if miRNA expression was altered in the sputum of patients who had active pulmonary tuberculosis. Other studies have shown that miRNA is present in sputum and there is alteration of unique miRNA signatures in lung diseases such as COPD. To understand the role of miRNA in active pulmonary TB, the study showed that there were 95 differentially expressed miRNAs; 43 miRNAs were overexpressed and 52 miRNAs were underexpressed in the tuberculosis group as compared to the control. In order to validate microarray results, miR-19b-2*, miR-3179, and miR-147 were chosen, due to results showing that miR-19b-2* was the most underexpressed, miR-3179 was the most overexpressed, and miR-147 was both overexpressed and is a negative regulator of inflammatory response. With use of RT-qPCR for validation of microarray results, the results were consistent with microarray showing that miR-147 was overexpressed in the tuberculosis group as compared to the control group (Yi et al. 2012).

With the concern that the microbial microenvironment relates to the development of pulmonary diseases, RT-qPCR has also been used to study the potential relationship of TLR4 and endothelial PAS domain-containing protein 1, a key regulator of COPD. Bronchoalveolar fluid was collected from 55 patients who had COPD and 25 healthy subjects. The detection of the expression levels of TLR4 and TLR5 was done with the use of RT-qPCR. In the lower respiratory track of COPD patients, the expression of TLR4 was significantly increased, as well as the levels of neutrophils, lymphocytes, and macrophages. Associated with the increase in TLR4 expression, EPAS1 mRNA was decreased while EPAS1 promoter methylation was increased in COPD. Thus, the study suggests that overexpression of TLR4 leads to decreased expression in EPAS1 expression, leading to the progression of COPD (Li et al. 2016).

The innate immunity of COPD patients who were stable was investigated using RT-qPCR. Patients were divided into four groups based on risk and symptoms exhibited. Patients were also classified based on sputum cellularity. If sputum neutrophil count was ≥76%, then the patient was classified as having a neutrophilic phenotype. Subjects who were healthy did not display any respiratory symptoms or airway responsiveness. The expression of IL-29 was positive in 16 of the 51 COPD patients, as well as in 9 out of 35 healthy subjects. IFN-β was found in 6 of the 51 COPD patients, while 2 out of the 35 healthy patients had IFN-β detected in sputum samples.

Interferon-stimulated genes were expressed in both patients with COPD and healthy subjects. In terms of the severity of airway obstruction, there was no difference detected in the expression of IL-29 or IFN-β between the two groups, but patients who had severe COPD did exhibit lower expression of OAS. OAS is an enzyme that activates the latent form of RNaseL, which leads to viral and host RNA degradation. Compared to patients with mild to moderate COPD, patients with severe COPD had low expression of interferon-stimulated genes. The results showed a correlation between MxA and OAS expression and postbronchodilator FEV_1/FVC ration, demonstrating that the expression of interferon-stimulated genes is lowered as airway obstruction progresses (Hilzendeger et al. 2016).

5.2 Proteomics

Proteomics allows the characterization of proteins and the role they play in biological processes as alterations in proteins, which hints at involvement in the development of disease (Bhargava et al. 2014). Unlike transcriptomics, where gene expression is studied by measuring transcriptional regulation of genes through messenger levels, proteomics focuses on proteins that take part in the establishment of the function of genes through enzymatic catalysis, molecular signaling, and physical interactions (Yates et al. 2009). Mass spectrometry (MS) is a tool that is widely used in large-scale proteomics. A comprehensive tool, MS has the capability to quantify proteins, as this provides a depiction of the concentrations of proteins. Due to its dependency on concentration, molecules with the highest concentrations in samples are detected over less abundant proteins (Bhargava et al. 2014).

The CF transmembrane conductance regulator (CFTR) gene codes for a protein transmembrane conductance regulator that functions as a chloride channel and is regulated by cyclic adenosine monophosphate (cAMP) in epithelial tissue. Mutations in this gene lead to the development of cystic fibrosis as cAMP-regulated chloride transport function in the lung epithelial cells becomes defective, leading to chronic bacterial infections that incite inflammation, the most common mutation of this gene being ΔF508CFTR. Whether a mutation in CFTR results in the alteration of protein levels in CF airway epithelial secretome in the absence of infection and inflammatory cells has been tested through comparison of CF and non-CF lung epithelial secretions. Proteins that were secreted were identified using the SecretomeP and SignalP databases. From 666 proteins that were identified as well as quantified, 70 were significant, indicating that CF epithelium displays a unique apical secretome without the presence of immune and inflammatory cells. The structural/molecular function of these proteins was primarily innate immunity (24%), protease/antiprotease activity (17%), cytoskeleton structure (14%), extracellular matrix organization (10%), energy metabolism (12%), and ion-dependent activity (10%). Western blot or ELISA were used to validate specific proteins.

ELISA analysis done on the levels of matrix metalloprotease 9 (MMP-9) in apical secretions from life-extended HBE ALI and primary HBE ALI cultures showed a trend of increased MMP-9 in CF secretion in both that were not significant (Peters-Halls et al. 2015).

Due to the inability to predict which individuals are more likely to develop irreversible airflow obstruction, novel markers for COPD as well as a more thorough understanding of the underlying biological mechanisms are required. Proteomic screening of induced sputum from smokers and patients who have been diagnosed with COPD have shown increased levels of bactericidal/permeability-increasing protein fold containing protein B1 (BPIFB1) as compared to nonsmokers. In order to determine how smoking effects BPIFB1, current smokers and ex-smokers were compared. BPIFB1 levels were found to be higher in COPD patients who were current smokers as compared to current smokers without COPD, while there was no difference in the levels of BPIFB1 between ex-smokers with and without COPD (Gao et al. 2015). As well as having higher sputum levels of BPIFB1, there was an association between increased sputum levels and changes in lung function found most apparently with COPD patients who were current smokers. Such information can be used to show that BPIFB1 may take part in the pathogenesis of smoking-related lung diseases. However, further studies are required in order to validate the role of BPIFB1 in the pathophysiology of COPD.

Cigarette smoking is the main risk factor for the development of COPD; however, only 20%–30% of smokers end up developing COPD. Thus this puts into consideration that there could be a specific genetic background that takes part in the pathogenesis of COPD. The family members of patients who develop severe early-onset COPD are considered "susceptible individuals," as they have an increased risk of developing COPD. An assessment was done to determine if there was a difference between susceptible individuals and age-matched "nonsusceptible individuals." Epithelial lining fluid was collected from young susceptible individuals, young nonsusceptible individuals, and old COPD patients who took part in acute smoking experiments. Epithelial lining fluid was also collected from healthy smoking and nonsmoking individuals, but they did not participate in the smoking experiments and were labeled as controls for COPD patients at baseline. Bronchoscopies were performed at 24 hours after smoking as well as 6 weeks later, and epithelial lining fluid was collected using microsampling probes. Peroxiredoxin I, uteroglobin serpinB3, S100A8, S100A9, and aldehyde dehydrogenase 3A1 were chosen for further analysis because they were significantly up- or downregulated in iTRAQ experiments, had a biological function that may take part in the pathogenesis of COPD, or had quantification with two or more statistically significantly different peptides. When comparing the groups at baseline, there was no difference in peroxiredoxin I, uteroglobin, and ALDH3A1 between young susceptible individuals and young nonsusceptible individuals. The levels of serpinB3, S100A9, and S100A8 were higher in patients who were in the young susceptible group. ALDH3A1 and peroxiredoxin I levels were found to be higher in old healthy smokers when compared to old healthy nonsmokers. When comparing before and after acute smoking, there was a decrease in peroxiredoxin I, S100A9, S100A8, and ALDH3A1 levels in young susceptible patients after acute smoke exposure. In young nonsusceptible individuals, all of the proteins were downregulated. Peroxiredoxin I, serpinB3, and ALDH3A1 were upregulated in old COPD patients, while uteroglobin was downregulated after acute smoke exposure (Franciosi et al. 2014). Due to serpinB3 and uteroglobin showing decreased levels strictly in young nonsusceptible individuals, these two proteins may play an important role in the beginning development of COPD (Table 5.1). The study also supports the use of younger individuals in order to understand what contributes and how it contributes to the beginning development of COPD. Although the study was based on family history, which could have been a weakness, this is not the first time that family history has been used and was able to provide clues for the genetic component of the disease (Franciosi et al. 2014).

The use of sputum can provide information about the presence of inflammatory cells and mediators within the airways, as it is considered to represent bronchial lining fluid. This information can be used for phenotypic characterization of patients who are diagnosed with chronic respiratory diseases. There is difficulty with use of sputum, as there is much effort needed to obtain healthy control samples; in addition, the presence of highly charged mucins within the sputum makes it difficult to separate sputum proteins using techniques such as two-dimensional gel electrophoresis (Pelaia et al. 2014). Saliva and nasal lavage fluid samples can also be obtained noninvasively but are more closely related to the upper airways; thus they are mainly used for investigation of upper respiratory diseases such as allergic rhinitis. The least commonly used samples are lung and bronchial tissue samples, as they are obtained during surgical procedures, making this method invasive (O'Neil et al).

Table 5.1 Proteins Identified in the Study by Franciosi et al. (2014)

Protein	Description	Accession Number
S100A8	Plays a role in antimicrobial activity as well as pro-inflammatory mediators in acute and chronic inflammation	P05109
S100A9	Also plays a role in antimicrobial activity as well as pro-inflammatory mediators in acute and chronic inflammation	P06702
Uteroglobin	Has immunosuppressive and antitumor qualities, but may take part in reducing airway inflammation and providing protection from oxidative stress	P11684
Peroxiredoxins	Controls the response oxidants and has an anti-inflammatory role as well	Q06830
Aldehyde dehydrogenase 3A1	Involved in the detoxification of carcinogenic aldehydes that are associated with smoking	P30838
SerpinB3	Inhibits several types of proteases. Also plays a role in modulating inflammation, fibrosis, and apoptosis	P29508

Hypersensitivity pneumonitis is an inflammation of the lung alveoli caused by exposure to airborne substances such as bacteria and fungi. However, very few people who are exposed to these airborne substances are actually diagnosed with hypersensitivity pneumonitis, which goes to suggest that genetic factors and exposure patterns are required in order for exposure to noninfectious microbial particles to cause hypersensitivity pneumonitis. Although damp building–related illnesses are less established as an illness compared to hypersensitivity pneumonitis, dampness in buildings can still be a risk factor in the development of adverse health effects. Yet there is difficulty in diagnosing damp building–related illnesses and assessing effects due to exposure from noninfectious microbial particles that do not meet the criteria for hypersensitivity pneumonitis. To discover diagnostic markers for pathologic conditions due to exposure to noninfectious microbial particles as well as to examine if there is a relationship between hypersensitivity pneumonitis, agricultural NIMP exposures, and damp building–related illnesses in terms of proteomics, bronchoalveolar lavage fluid was collected. Unlike the noninvasive collection of sputum, bronchoalveolar lavage fluid is collected thorough a more invasive procedure (Pelaia et al. 2014). 2D gel analysis and immunoblot validation studies have shown that there is a difference in protein expression between damp building–related illnesses and hypersensitivity pneumonitis/agricultural NIMP exposure, even though both are due to exposure of noninfectious microbial particles, but protein expression showed that there is a close association between hypersensitivity pneumonitis and agricultural NIMP exposures. Semenogelin and histone 4 were found to be possible diagnostic markers for differential diagnosis between damp building–related illnesses and hypersensitivity pneumonitis-like conditions (Teirilä et al. 2014). Although semenogelins are proteins that take part in the formation of sperm coagulum, they have also been found in the lungs and small-cell lung carcinoma. DeCyder analysis showed that it was upregulated in all of the studied disease patient groups and immunoblot validation confirmed that semenoglobin levels were also increased in agricultural NIMP exposure, hypersensitivity pneumonitis, and sarcoidosis patients when compared to the healthy controls. There was no difference in semenoglobin levels between the damp building–related illnesses group and the healthy controls. Histone variants H2B and H4 were found to be upregulated in all experimental groups, but were slightly less in the damp building–related illnesses group. Increased expression of histone component H4 in bronchoalveolar lavage fluid was associated with AME, HP, and SARC patient samples. H2B, another histone variant, also had increased expression in plasma samples of HP and SARC patients, while H4 could not be detected from plasma. Two-dimensional gel electrophoresis is not without its limitations. Like MS, high-abundant proteins are detected over less abundant proteins, which leads to a less comprehensive proteomic profile. The difficulty in reproducing experiments and protein identification limits its use in large-scale proteomics analysis (Gharib et al. 2011).

5.3 Metabolomics

Metabolomics, the field of study that analyzes molecules or metabolites present within an organism, allows a snapshot reading of gene function, enzyme activity, and physiological landscape. As for previous omics studies, metabolomics is not limited to just one method in order to assess endogenous metabolites within a biologic system. Metabolic finger- or footprinting, target isotope-based analysis or targeted metabolomics, and metabolic targeted profiling are all different methods utilized in metabolomics (Serkova et al.). Lipids, carbohydrates, peptides, and proteins that have different molecular size and charge, whether they are of exogenous or endogenous origin, are metabolites that can be detected (Muhlebach and Sha 2015). Metabolites have the possibility to be good biomarkers due to being easily detectable with analytical methods (Quinn et al. 2016). The metabolome interacts with the transcriptome, genome, or proteome, and any changes that occur within those "-omes" is believed to be reflected in the metabolome, as this then leads to changes in metabolite concentrations in biological fluids (Stringer et al. 2016). Its close relationship with other -omes demonstrates that metabolomics is important for connecting systems biology (Wishart 2014). Use of metabolomics, also known as *metabonomics*, allows detection of changes that result from biological or environmental events over short periods, which proves to be useful in monitoring disease progression or drug response and to be predictive of disease severity, as most acute illnesses are due to disruption in biochemical homeostasis (Stringer et al. 2016). These changes that are linked to biological events can provide information about the pathogenesis of disease with use of the bioinformatics models. Thus any information collected through metabolomics must be linked to biochemical causes and physiological consequences (Wishart 2014).

With metabolomic evaluation of cystic fibrosis airway secretions, biomarkers could be found with the identification of metabolites and metabolic pathways that take part in neutrophilic inflammation, a hallmark of cystic fibrosis. Cellular metabolism can be altered by neutrophilic inflammation, and studies suggest that cystic fibrosis is associated with changes, patterns, and concentrations of metabolites in airway secretions (Esther et al. 2015). MS-based metabolomics was done on bronchoalveolar lavage fluid samples, and targeted MS methods were used in order to identify as well as quantify metabolites related to neutrophilic inflammation. MS determines the composition of a particle based on the mass-to-charge ratio in charged particles. Although its analysis requires more work, it has a higher sensitivity for metabolite detection as compared to nuclear magnetic resonance (NMR) spectroscopy, as well as specificity in metabolite identification at low concentrations. This is especially useful when bronchoalveolar lavage fluid is used, because it contains low levels of metabolites. With the use of positive-mode MS metabolomics discovery profiling, 338 of the 7,791 individual peaks that were detected were associated with neutrophilic inflammation and identified as potential biomarkers. From the metabolites detected, the majority were related to pathways that take part in the metabolism of purines, polyamines, proteins, and nicotinamide. Metabolite identification was done using online resources such as the Human Metabolite Database and comparing with published literature (Esther et al. 2015).

Metabolomics has been applies to urine samples in order to characterize asthma phenotypes and identify metabolites. Urine samples obtained from 41 atopic asthmatic children and 12 healthy controls were profiled using liquid chromatography–mass spectrometry (LC-MS) (Mattarucchi et al. 2011). LC-MS is widely used due to its ability to detect a broad range of different classes of metabolites because it is sensitive to nanomolar concentrations and has good coverage of mass. Its disadvantages, however, are that there is no standardized metabolite library and that it has high variability (Stringer et al). With the use of urine, unlike other biological samples, it does not require the removal of macromolecules. Prior to the use of LC-MS, samples had to be ionized in order for metabolites to be detected, with electrospray ionization being the most common technique (Stringer et al). Coupled with LC-MS, a quadrupole–time-of-flight (Q-TOF) analyzer was used (Figures 5.1 and 5.2).

Untargeted metabolic profiles were studied by multivariate analysis. In multivariate analysis, all metabolites in the data are analyzed simultaneously in one analysis and metabolic variations are detected through dimension reductions (Muhlebach and Sha 2015). A reduction was found in the excretion of urocanic acid and methyl-imidazoleacetic acid contents. Methyl-imidazoleacetic acid is a specific marker of histamine metabolism and urocanic acid is an intermediate produced by histidase in the catabolism of histidine. The reduction of urocanic acid in urine may indicate that it can affect the resolution of the

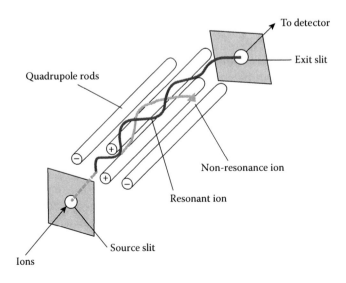

Figure 5.1 *Quadrupole mass analyzer.*

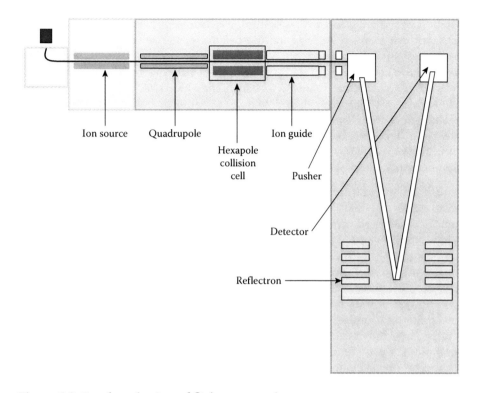

Figure 5.2 Quadrupole–time-of-flight mass analyzer.

inflammation process of asthma. Through this study, metabolic profiles from urine may be able to characterize asthma, and urine may be used as a target for metabolic studies for pulmonary disorders, in contrast to it being used only for systemic disorders.

Serum has also been used to identify the underlying mechanism of asthma as well as potential biomarkers. Serum samples were collected from 39 asthma patients and 17 healthy controls. NMR analysis, using H-NMR spectroscopy more specifically, was then done on these samples. NMR spectroscopy allows the identification of different nuclei based on their resonant frequency when molecules are placed in a magnetic field. Advantages of the use of H-NMR are that it has unbiased metabolite detection, is quantitative, and the experiment and results can be reproduced. "Binning" was done in order to reduce the effect of shifting peaks. In binning, NMR spectra are divided into "bins" that are of equal chemical shift intervals (Stringer et al.). The use of binning in this study did prove to be a bit difficult when assigning metabolites using targeted profiling, because the resolution of the spectra from the integration process was reduced. The metabolites that were detected in the sera of asthmatic patients were involved in hypermethylation and immune reaction, as well as response to hypoxia. From the 10 metabolites that were identified, 5 were related to the enhancement of the methyl transfer pathway (Jung et al. 2013). These five metabolites include formate, choline, methionine, O-phosphocholine, and methanol. An increase in arginine methylation was previously described as a key process in asthma; therefore it is possible that increased methylation takes part in the pathogenesis of asthma. Sera from patients with asthma who had lower $FEV_1\%$ predicted values also had higher levels of VLDL/LDL products. Also shown with the correlation with $FEV_1\%$ predicted values was that the breakdown of these lipids under insufficient glucose conditions can lead to an increase in levels of acetone in patients who have severe asthma (Jung et al. 2013). Therefore, H-NMR-based metabolite profiling of serum may be useful in understanding the pathogenesis of asthma.

Platelet activating factor as well as other inflammatory lipids have been identified as possible biomarkers for COPD. Sputum samples were collected from 11 patients in order to assess the effect of exacerbations on the sputum metabolome. In order to do that, liquid chromatography–tandem mass spectrometry (LC-MS/MS) was used and data were analyzed with MS/MS molecular networking and multivariate statistics. From the two sputum sample sets that were collected, 4,639 unique MS/MS spectra were detected. From the 4,639 unique MS/MS spectra detected, 556 unique metabolites were found in exacerbations samples, 132 metabolites in Tr samples, 781 metabolites in Pt samples, and 100 metabolites in St samples. Across all clinical states, 1,222 metabolites were common. Experiments that use iTRAQ typically use MS/MS spectra in order to infer peptide levels (Yates et al. 2009). Bray–Curtis distance matrix was calculated on the metabolite abundance matrix for each set separately, as LC-MS/MS batch effects did not allow the similarity of each metabolome to be compared across two data sets. Comparison could only have been done within each dataset. From the 556 unique metabolites that were found in exacerbation samples, platelet-activating factor and a related molecule PC were significantly elevated across patient cohort. This implies that lipid remodeling may occur during exacerbation. Platelet-activating factor was previously reported to be at increased levels in exacerbations of inflammatory lung diseases such as asthma. Due to platelet-activating factor having the ability to activate neutrophils, changes in levels of platelet-activating factor can be used to monitor increased neutrophilic inflammation as well as possible onsets of exacerbations (Quinn et al. 2016).

5.4 Breathomics

Breathomics is the noninvasive metabolomics study of exhaled air, where the main aim is to find patterns of volatile organic compounds that are related to metabolic processes that occur within the human body (Smolinska et al. 2014). Exhaled breath has shown to contain hundreds of volatile organic compounds that can be analyzed by high-throughput assessment (Fens et al. 2011). However, exhaled breath volatile organic compounds do not just represent metabolism in the lungs. The collection of exhaled breath is noninvasive, as the subject has a nose-clip applied and breathes quietly through a mouthpiece for 10 minutes. The mouthpiece has a salivary trap and single-way valve attached to it; this diverts the airflow through a Teflon or polypropylene tube that is contained inside a cooling container. The exhaled air is converted from droplets to exhaled-breath condensate (Konstantinidi et al. 2015). Albeit confusing, the terms *exogenous* and *endogenous* have sometimes been used in order to describe the origins of volatile organic compounds. Exogenous volatile organic compounds come from the environment, mainly through inhalation, ingestion of food or drink, and drugs. Endogenous volatile organic compounds reflect metabolites as they arise from processes that occur within the body, and they vary based on the airway compartment that is under study (Bos et al. 2016). There are considerations that should be taken into account when dealing with both breath sampling and analysis (Table 5.2). For example, in analytical methodology, there are methods based on mass spectrometry and electronic noses. For pathophysiological research, methods based on mass spectrometry are done to detect as well as identify volatile organic compounds, especially when the volatile organic compounds of interest have yet to be known. Electronic noses, or eNose, are usually less specific and based on cross-reactive, nonspecific sensors. Sensor properties are changed to respond to patterns of volatile organic compound mixtures, which then produces a quantitative signal change based on pattern recognition algorithms (Bos et al. 2016).

Metabolomic profiling of exhaled breath condensate was shown to have the ability to distinguish different biochemical–metabolic profiles of children with asthma, as well as to differentiate children who had severe asthma from those who had nonsevere asthma and from healthy controls. The study subjects that were recruited were 42 atopic asthmatic children; 31 of the children

Table 5.2 Description of EBC Collection Devices

EBC Collection Device	Description
EcoScreen 2	Allows fractionated collection of EBC from varying parts of the bronchial tree. EBC is collected in two disposable polyethylene bags, which allows the disposal of dead space condensate, which has no biomarkers with clinical relevance. Device is not portable.
TurboDECCS	Consists of a Turbo Unit that is portable and a DECCS collection system that is disposable. The DECCS is equipped with a mouthpiece, a one-way valve, a tube, and a collection cell that is put in an electrical cooling system.
RTube	A portable device that can be used by subjects at home without supervision. The large Tee section made from polypropylene separates saliva from the exhaled breath. The one-way valve is made from silicon and a PP collection tube that has a cooling sleeve placed around it.
ANACON	A device that can be attached to the expiratory branch of a ventilator circuit via two adaptors and two elastomeric connectors. The exhaled air goes through the condensation tubes that pass through the body of the condenser. Condensation temperature can be monitored through the thermometer.

Source: Konstantinidi, E.M., et al., *Scientific World J.*, 2015, 1–25, 2015. With permission.

had nonsevere asthma, 11 children had severe asthma, and 15 children were healthy with no history of respiratory diseases. LC-MS was used in the analysis of metabolites in the exhaled breath condensate samples and bidirectional–orthogonal projections to latent structures–discriminant analysis (O2PLS-DA) was used in order to differentiate between the groups of children. O2PLS-DA is a classification technique that creates classification models in which the information that is produced is summarized in a few predictive scores that are a result of a combination of measured variables (Carraro et al. 2012). Variable 225, a compound that is chemically related to retinoic acid, and variable 127, a compound that is chemically related to deoxyadenosine, were shown to be variables characteristic of severe asthma. Variable 412 was found to characterize the healthy controls and nonsevere asthmatic patients but was lacking in the severe asthma group. This variable was found to be ercalcitriol, which is the active metabolite of vitamin D2. Data in this study showed that unlike lung function and FE_{NO}, metabolomic analysis was able to differentiate between nonsevere and healthy children as well as between severe and nonsevere asthmatic patients (Carraro et al. 2012).

Assessment of inflammatory subtype in mild and moderate COPD by exhaled breath metabolomics was studied. Exhaled breath was collected from 32 patients who had mild to moderately severe COPD by having the patients breathe normally for 5 minutes, with the nose clipped, through a mouthpiece that was connected to a three-way nonrebreathing valve, an inspiratory VOC filter, and an expiratory silica reservoir (Fens et al. 2011). Breath analysis was done using gas chromatography–mass spectrometry (GC-MS). GC-MS is the most commonly used analytical method in order to trace gases within complex mixtures (Smolinska et al. 2014). GC-MS has the advantage of being highly sensitive as well specific when used to separate and detect volatile metabolites. However, this technique is used for thermally stable volatile compounds that have low polarity, as well as those where derivatization can be done. This allows compounds to become less polar and more stable (Stringer et al. 2016). Electronic nose was also used to examine the relationship of exhaled molecular profile, as it has previously been able to differentiate well-defined COPD from asthma. Measurements were performed twice due to deviant sensor deflections and the first analysis done for every measurement was excluded from the analysis. From the exhaled breath samples from the study, 26 volatile organic compounds were found to be correlated to markers of airway inflammation. Also found to be associated with markers of inflammatory cell activation were exhaled compounds. These compounds were eosinophil cationic protein (ECP) for eosinophils and myeloperoxidase (MPO) for neutrophils. From the compounds found, 18 were significantly correlated with ECP and 4 with MPO for patients with GOLD Stage I. GOLD Stage II had nine different compounds correlated with ECP, while one identical compound was found compared with GOLD Stage I. GOLD Stage II also had one different compound that correlated with MPO, and one identical compound was found compared with GOLD Stage I. This study suggests that exhaled breath profiling using the quantitative GC-MS method has the ability to identify the type and activation of inflammation, whether it is eosinophilic or neutrophilic. However, multicompound breath profiling using eNose has more appropriate use for detecting the activation of inflammatory cells.

5.5 Lipidomics

Recently, it has been shown that changes in lipid contents within the airway epithelium may play an important role in chronic airway diseases such as asthma, cystic fibrosis, and COPD. The purpose of lipidomics is to characterize the full lipid complement that is produced by cells, organisms, or tissues. The surfactant that covers the epithelium towards the air spaces is a mixture of approximately 80%–90% lipids and surfactant-specific proteins (Table 5.3). The role of pulmonary surfactant is to lower surface tension as well as stop the occurrence of end-expiratory collapse of the alveoli. The importance of pulmonary surfactant is stressed, as the continued synthesis and secretion of surfactant is important for the maintenance of lung function (Dushianthan et al. 2014). If surface tension is not lowered by the surfactant, high surface tension leads to pulmonary edema, where intra-alveolar fluid continues to accumulate and cause impairment of gas exchange and lung mechanical disturbances (Agassandian and Mallampalli 2013). However, the composition and function can be affected by the occurrence of respiratory diseases. Primary surfactant deficiency in the lungs of preterm infants is known to be the major cause of neonatal respiratory syndrome; secondary surfactant deficiency takes part in the pathology of respiratory diseases of the mature lung such as acute lung injury (ALI)/acute respiratory distress syndrome (ARDS), asthma, COPD, and cystic fibrosis (Dushianthan et al. 2014). To help recognize the individual molecules that vary in molecular lipid structure, lipidomics constantly uses MS (Schwudke et al. 2011). LC-MS–based methods are used due to the fact that lipid extracts contain high amounts of impurities; thus they cannot be analyzed by shotgun lipidomics because of ion suppression effects (Zehethofer et al. 2015).

Table 5.3 The Components of Pulmonary Surfactants as well as the Amount of Each Found in Pulmonary Surfactant

Pulmonary Surfactant Component	% Composition
Dipalmitoylphosphatidylcholine	50
Unsaturated phosphatidylcholine	21
Proteins (SP-A, SP-B, SP-C, SP-D)	10
Phosphatidylglycerol (PC) and phosphatidylinositol	9
Phosphatidylserine, phosphatidylethanolamine, and sphingomyelin	6
Other lipids	4

Source: Agassandian, M., Mallampalli, R.K., Biochim. Biophys. Acta, 1831.3, 612–625, 2013. With permission.

5.5.1 Phosphatidylcholine

Phosphatidylcholine (PC) is the major surfactant phospholipid, comprising 80% of surfactant lipids, where PC16:0/16:0 is the principal PC among several species. This PC is thought to take part in surface reduction at the air–liquid interface. In patients who have respiratory failure that is secondary to ARDS, the pulmonary surfactant complex shows a change in composition as well as lack of adequate surface activity. These changes may then cause severe hypoxemia, poor lung compliance, and lung atelectasis, all of which are characteristic of ARDS. In a study to characterize surfactant PC kinetics in patients with ARDS, patients and controls had an intravenous infusion of *methyl*-D9 choline chloride, as *methyl*-D9 choline chloride has been used to quantify surfactant PC flux via the CDP–choline pathway. Bronchoalveolar lavage fluid was then obtained with the use of a fiber-optic bronchoscope. There was a significant reduction in the total bronchoalveolar lavage fluid PC isolated in patients with ARDS as compared to healthy controls. Bronchoalveolar lavage fluid fractional PC16:0/16:0 absolute concentrations were also found to be lower in patients. Low concentrations of total PC and fractional PC16:0/16:0 may be attributed to reduced synthesis, increased breakdown, or dilution by pulmonary edema (Dushianthan et al. 2014).

As part of a study to determine sensitive biomarkers in peripheral blood for the identification of interstitial lung abnormalities, PC was found to be both a sensitive and reliable biomarker. A metabolomics-based LC-Q-TOF-MS technique was used to show serum metabolic characteristics. Metabolic changes were seen in subjects who were initially healthy and were identified with interstitial lung abnormalities a year later, and the results confirmed the metabolites that took part in the progression from healthy to development of interstitial lung abnormalities. When compared to the initial stage when the subjects were healthy, nine metabolites were identified in the outcome stage when they developed interstitial lung abnormalities. PC, phosphatidic acid, phosphatidylethanolamine, and betaine aldehyde were all found to be upregulated. The upregulation of PC may be associated with epithelial injury in interstitial lung abnormalities (Tan et al. 2016).

5.5.2 Phosphatidylglycerol

Phosphatidylglycerol is the second most abundant surfactant phospholipid and is involved in absorbing and spreading surfactant over the epithelial surface after surfactant films are compressed. The concentration of phosphatidylglycerol is much higher in the lungs when compared to other mammalian tissue (Agassandian and Mallampalli). Bronchoalveolar lavage samples were collected from ARDS patients in order to assess elevation of secretory phospholipases A_2, which hydrolyzes phospholipids in cell membranes and extracellular structures such as pulmonary surfactant, in human lungs during ARDS and whether the levels of secretory phospholipases A_2 are associated with surfactant injury. In ARDS, the alveolar inflammation leads to changes in the biophysical and biochemical properties of pulmonary surfactant, which takes part in how severe the disease becomes. Secretory phospholipase A_2 enzymatic activities were increased when compared to healthy controls. Although PC was found to be the most abundant in terms of the composition of surfactant phospholipids when comparing ARDS patient to healthy controls, there was a decrease in phosphatidylglycerol in the ARDS samples. The decrease of phosphatidylglycerol may take part in the mechanism for surfactant injury in ALI/ARDS (Long et al. 2012).

Lipidomic profiling has been done to see if it could identify certain forms of interstitial lung disease in children with surfactant alterations. Many chronic childhood interstitial lung diseases directly affect different components of pulmonary surfactant, which includes genetically caused deficiency in ABCA3, a lipid transporter. Phosphatidylglycerol was found to be low in the interstitial lung disease group and characteristic changes were seen in species 35:1 and 36:1 in interstitial lung disease related to growth abnormalities as well. Patients who had ABCA3-deficiency from two interstitial lung disease–causing mutations had decreases in phosphatidylglycerols PG 32:1, PG 36:1, PG 36:4, PG 38:4, and PG 38:5 (Griese et al. 2015).

5.5.3 Sphingolipids

Sphingolipids play an important role in signaling molecules and components of other membranes and extracellular fluid, whether it is in normal functioning or pathological settings that involved inflammation. Sphingolipids and altered sphingolipid metabolism have demonstrated to be potential key contributors to the pathogenesis of asthma. The most studied sphingolipids, ceramides and sphingosine-1-phosphate, also play an important role as signaling molecules. Ceramide is a substrate for the production of complex sphingolipids, while sphingosine-1-phosphate acts as both an intracellular second messenger and extracellular ligand for S1P1–S1P5, specific G protein–coupled receptors. Sphingosine-1-phosphate levels are increased in bronchoalveolar lavage from patients with asthma as compared to control subjects. In exhaled breath collections, ceramide levels were increased in very ill patients with asthma. In patients with emphysema, lung ceramide levels were also found to be increased when compared to control subjects without emphysema. Alterations in sphingolipid homeostasis may possibly link ORMDL3 to asthma (Ono et al. 2015). This suggests that smoking and COPD cause impairment in the regulation of sphingolipid metabolism. In a study by Bowler et al. (2015), 26 sphingolipids were identified as significantly associated with emphysema, and 11 sphingolipids were associated with severe COPD exacerbations. Trihexosylceramides had the strongest association with COPD exacerbations; however, this is a lipid class with unknown effects on the lung. MS showed that emphysema was inversely associated with 10 sphingomyelins and that low baseline plasma of sphingomyelin was associated with worse COPD, defined as lower FEV$_1$. Ceramides, gangliosides, and monohexosylceramides, specifically, showed an inverse correlation with emphysema. This may be due to an increase in activity of sphingomyelinase and recycling (from gangliosides) pathways, which is then followed by ceramide consumption/degradation. This study was the largest, as 250 subjects took part, and is the study that combined targeted and nontargeted metabolomics study of plasma sphingolipid (Bowler et al. 2015).

References

Agassandian, M., and R.K. Mallampalli. Surfactant phospholipid metabolism. *Biochimica Et Biophysica Acta (BBA)—Molecular and Cell Biology of Lipids* 1831.3 (2013): 612–25.

Bhargava, M. et al. Application of clinical proteomics in acute respiratory distress syndrome. *Clinical and Translational Medicine* 3 (2014): 34.

Bos, L.D., P.J. Sterk, and S.J. Fowler. Breathomics in the setting of asthma and chronic obstructive pulmonary disease. *Journal of Allergy and Clinical Immunology* 138.4 (2016): 970–6.

Bourdon-Lacombe, J.A. et al. Technical guide for applications of gene expression profiling in human health risk assessment of environmental chemicals. *Regulatory Toxicology and Pharmacology* 72.2 (2015): 292–309.

Bowler, R.P. et al. Plasma sphingolipids associated with chronic obstructive pulmonary disease phenotypes. *American Journal of Respiratory and Critical Care Medicine* 191.3 (2015): 275–84.

Carraro, S. et al. Asthma severity in childhood and metabolomic profiling of breath condensate. *Allergy* 68.1 (2012): 110–17.

Dushianthan, A. et al. Phospholipid composition and kinetics in different endobronchial fractions from healthy volunteers. *BMC Pulmonary Medicine* 14 (2014): 10.

Esther, C.R. et al. Metabolomic evaluation of neutrophilic airway inflammation in cystic fibrosis. *Chest* 148.2 (2015): 507–15.

Fens, N. et al. Exhaled air molecular profiling in relation to inflammatory subtype and activity in COPD. *European Respiratory Journal* 38.6 (2011a): 1301–309.

Fens, N. et al. Breathomics as a diagnostic tool for pulmonary embolism. *Journal of thrombosis and haemostasis* 8.12 (2011b): 2831–3.

Franciosi, L. et al. Susceptibility to COPD: Differential proteomic profiling after acute smoking. Ed. Chris Bullen. *PLoS One* 9.7 (2014): e102037.

Gao, J. et al. Elevated sputum BPIFB1 levels in smokers with chronic obstructive pulmonary disease: A longitudinal study. *American Journal of Physiology—Lung Cellular and Molecular Physiology* 309.1 (2015): L17–26.

Gharib, S.A. et al. Induced sputum proteome in health and asthma. *The Journal of Allergy and Clinical Immunology* 128.6 (2011): 1176–1184.

Griese, M. et al. Surfactant lipidomics in healthy children and childhood interstitial lung disease. Ed. Nades Palaniyar. *PLoS One* 10.2 (2015): e0117985.

Hilzendeger, C. et al. Reduced sputum expression of interferon-stimulated genes in severe COPD. *International Journal of Chronic Obstructive Pulmonary Disease* 11 (2016): 1485–94.

Jung, J. et al. Serum metabolomics reveals pathways and biomarkers associated with asthma pathogenesis. *Clinical & Experimental Allergy Clin Exp Allergy* 43.4 (2013): 425–33.

Kim, W.J. et al. Comprehensive analysis of transcriptome sequencing data in the lung tissues of COPD subjects. *International Journal of Genomics* 2015 (2015): 206937.

Konstantinidi, E.M. et al. Exhaled breath condensate: Technical and diagnostic aspects. *The Scientific World Journal* 2015 (2015): 1–25.

Labib, S. et al. Nano-risk science: Application of toxicogenomics in an adverse outcome pathway framework for risk assessment of multi-walled carbon nanotubes. *Particle and Fibre Toxicology* 13 (2015): 15.

Li, H. et al. TLR4 overexpression inhibits endothelial PAS domain-containing protein 1 expression in the lower respiratory tract of patients with chronic COPD. *Cellular Physiology and Biochemistry* 39.2 (2016): 685–92.

Long, D.L. et al. Secretory phospholipase A2-mediated depletion of phosphatidylglycerol in early acute respiratory distress syndrome. *The American Journal of the Medical Sciences* 343.6 (2012): 446–51.

Mattarucchi, E., E. Baraldi, and C. Guillou. Metabolomics applied to urine samples in childhood asthma: Differentiation between asthma phenotypes and identification of relevant metabolites. *Biomedical Chromatography* 26.1 (2011): 89–94.

Muhlebach, M.S., and W. Sha. Lessons learned from metabolomics in cystic fibrosis. *Molecular and Cellular Pediatrics* 2.1 (2015): 9.

Nikota, J. et al. Meta-analysis of transcriptomic responses as a means to identify pulmonary disease outcomes for engineered nanomaterials. *Particle and Fibre Toxicology* 13 (2015): 25.

Ono, J.G., T.S. Worgall, and S. Worgall. Airway reactivity and sphingolipids—Implications for childhood asthma. *Molecular and Cellular Pediatrics* 2.1 (2015): 13.

Pathak, R.R., and V. Davé. Integrating omics technologies to study pulmonary physiology and pathology at the systems level. *Cellular Physiology and Biochemistry* 33.5 (2014): 1239–60.

Pelaia, G. et al. Application of proteomics and peptidomics to COPD. *BioMed Research International* 2014 (2014): 764581.

Peters-Hall, J.R. et al. Quantitative proteomics reveals an altered cystic fibrosis in vitro bronchial epithelial secretome. *American Journal of Respiratory Cell and Molecular Biology* 53.1 (2015): 22–32.

Quinn, R.A. et al. Metabolomics of pulmonary exacerbations reveals the personalized nature of cystic fibrosis disease. *PeerJ* 4 (2016): e2174.

Schwudke, D. et al. Shotgun lipidomics on high resolution mass spectrometers. *Cold Spring Harbor Perspectives in Biology* 3.9 (2011): a004614.

Smolinska, A. et al. Current breathomics—A review on data pre-processing techniques and machine learning in metabolomics breath analysis. *Journal of Breath Research* 8.2 (2014): 027105.

Stringer, K.A. et al. Metabolomics and its application to acute lung diseases. *Frontiers in Immunology* 7 (2016): 44.

Tan, Y. et al. Potential metabolic biomarkers to identify interstitial lung abnormalities. *International Journal of Molecular Sciences* 17.7 (2016): 1148.

Teirilä, L. et al. Proteomic changes of alveolar lining fluid in illnesses associated with exposure to inhaled non-infectious microbial particles. *PLoS One* 9.7 (2014): e102624.

Wishart, D.S. Advances in metabolite identification. *Bioanalysis* 3.15 (2011): 1769–782.

Yates, J.R., C.I. Ruse, and A. Nakorchevsky. Proteomics by mass spectrometry: Approaches, advances, and applications. *Annual Review of Biomedical Engineering* 11.1 (2009): 49–79.

Yi, Z. et al. Altered microRNA signatures in sputum of patients with active pulmonary tuberculosis. *PLoS One* 7.8 (2012): e43184.

Yick, C. et al. Transcriptome sequencing (RNA-Seq) of human endobronchial biopsies: Asthma versus controls. *European Respiratory Journal* 42.3 (2013): 662–70.

Zehethofer, N. et al. Lipid analysis of airway epithelial cells for studying respiratory diseases. *Chromatographia* 78.5–6 (2015): 403–413.

6

Proteomics as a Comprehensive Molecular Means to Understand Dietary Health Effects

Jayvadan Patel and Anita Patel
Sankalchand Patel University
Visnagar, Gujarat, India

Contents

6.1 A new view of proteins: Historical perspective 135
6.2 What is a proteome and what does proteomics do? 136
6.3 Proteomics technology 138
    6.3.1 Protein identification 138
    6.3.2 Protein quantification 140
    6.3.3 Data processing 143
6.4 Perspectives for proteomics in nutrition 145
6.5 Proteomics in nutritional intervention 145
6.6 Application of proteomics in nutritional interventions 146
6.7 Conclusion 150
References 152

6.1 A new view of proteins: Historical perspective

The neologism *proteome* or *proteomics* was first introduced in 1995 (Wilkins et al. 1995). Proteome analysis is an effort to describe the molecular basis of pathophysiological processes. A proteome is like a snapshot of a physiological state. Life is the translation of the static genome into highly dynamic proteomes. If these single snapshots were mounted together to make a movie, it would describe the dynamics of a living cell. Proteome analysis supplements gene sequence data with protein information about where, in what ratio, and also in which situation proteins are expressed.

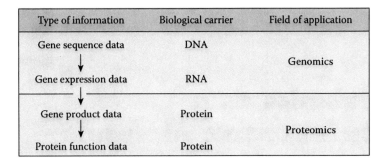

Figure 6.1 *Genomics and proteomics are synergetic.*

The word *proteome* was designed to represent the protein complement of a genome. The challenging fields of proteins and genomics are surprisingly diverse and in addition they are fundamentally interlinked—at this juncture, single compounds exhibiting enormously different properties and requiring labor-intensive studies, in attendance with a full set of information by means of high-throughput techniques has been gaining enormous attention. Figure 6.1 illustrates the synergism of proteomics and genomics.

The historical perspective of proteome analysis comes from protein characterization methods (Dove 1999; Page et al. 1999; Persidis 1998; Wilkins et al. 1997). Over the years a powerful set of protein analytical tools was developed. Moreover, techniques became available that could separate out thousands of proteins in single run, as well as identify proteins with small amounts. The requirements for the study of biologically pertinent questions has been satisfied. Concurrently, the "one gene—one protein" system of belief was no longer accepted. The straightforward view of protein biosynthesis in a chromosomal DNA sequence translating into an analogous RNA sequence that serves as a blueprint for the ribosome to manufacture an amino acid sequence and the resulting protein developing a three-dimensional structure to play a particular role at a particular place in an organism was obsolete. In addition, molecular biology has taught us that a gene can undergo different splicing and that post-translational modifications can result in several active forms of a protein. Sequence information in DNA is not sufficient to describe life. In the life sciences, proteins are the virtual actors.

6.2 What is a proteome and what does proteomics do?

A proteome specifies the quantitative protein expression profile of a cell, an organism, or a tissue under accurately defined conditions. The human genome consists of about 22,000 genes and this gene inventory is applied for a cell-type-specific expression of a set of 10,000 genes. One gene will result in multiple protein products: on average 1.3 proteins per gene in *Escherichia coli*, three proteins per gene in *Saccharomyces cerevisiae*, and maybe more than 10 proteins per gene in humans if one also considers body fluids (Hochstrasser 1997). Therefore, a proteome consists of about 100,000 proteins. These simple numbers demonstrate the enormous variability in the composition of a proteome and the ability to form an infinite number of phenotypes. Slight modifications in the expression parameters, due, for example, to stress or drug effects, will change the protein pattern as well as cause the absence or presence of a protein or gradual variations in abundances. Proteomics analyzes and contrasts protein expression profiles and links the observed protein pattern changes to the causal effects. The key steps in proteomics are the rational design of a proteome project, the quantitative determination of expressed protein patterns by biochemical characterization techniques, and data interpretation and data mining by bioinformatics.

The association between diet and chronic disease has long been documented through epidemiological studies. Modern molecular nutrition focuses on health promotion, disease risk reduction, along with performance enhancement through diet plus lifestyle considerations (Kussmann and Blum 2007; Ronteltap et al. 2008). Innovative genomic, proteomic, and metabolomic techniques are now enabling us to find out more about the basis of these associations through examination of the functional interactions of food with the genome at the molecular, cellular, and systemic levels (Corthésy-Theulaz et al. 2005; Kato 2008; Mariman 2006). Whilst traditional nutrition research has dealt with nourishing populations by providing nutrients, at the present time it focuses on improving the health of individuals through diet. Current nutritional research focuses on health promotion and disease risk reduction and on performance improvement (Trujillo et al. 2006).

Food components interact with our body at the system, organ, cellular, and molecular levels. These nutritional components come in complex mixtures, where not only the presence and concentrations of a single compound but also interactions between numerous compounds decide ingredient bioefficacy and bioavailability (Kussmann et al. 2007).

Recent nutritional research focuses on promoting health, preventing or delaying the onset of disease, and optimizing performance (Kussmann et al. 2006). Deciphering the molecular interplay between food and health requires holistic approaches, for the reason that nutritional improvement of certain health aspects must not be compromised by deterioration of others (Kussmann and Fay 2008).

Proteomics is a central platform in nutrigenomics that describes how our genome expresses itself in response to diet (Ordovas and Corella 2004). Nutrigenetics deals with our genetic predisposition and susceptibility to diet (Kaput 2008) and helps stratify subject cohorts and discern responders from nonresponders (Fay and German 2008). Epigenetics represents DNA sequence–unrelated biochemical modifications of DNA itself and DNA-binding proteins and emerges to provide a format for lifelong or even transgenerational imprinting of metabolism (Gallou-Kabani et al. 2007; Junien et al. 2005). Proteomics in nutrition can identify and quantify bioactive proteins and peptides and address issues of nutritional bioefficacy (Kussmann and Affolter 2006; Kussmann et al. 2005).

The interplay among nutrition along with health has been famous for centuries: the Greek doctor Hippocrates (fourth century BC) can be seen as the father of "functional food," for the reason that he recommended food as medicine and vice versa. Another example is the evidence of traditional Chinese medicine: Sun Simiao, a famous doctor of the Tang dynasty (seventh century AD), affirmed that, "When a person is sick, the doctor should first regulate the patient's diet and lifestyle."

At the present time, dietary research translates this (to a certain extent empirical) knowledge to evidence-based molecular science, as food components interrelate with our body at the system, organ, cellular, and molecular levels (Kussmann and Daniel 2008). Modern nutritional and health research mainly focuses on promoting health, delaying or else preventing the onset of disease, and optimizing performance (Kussmann and Daniel 2008).

Dietary components come in complex mixtures, in which not only the presence and concentrations of a single compound but also interactions of various compounds affect food compound bioefficacy and bioavailability (Kussmann et al. 2007). Thus the need becomes apparent for developing as well as applying comprehensive analytical methods to reveal bioactive ingredients and also their action (Kussmann et al. 2008).

Proteomics is a fundamental platform for elucidating these molecular actions in nutrition, where it can identify as well as quantify bioactive proteins and peptides and address questions of nutritional bioefficacy (Kussmann and Affolter 2006). In this chapter, we focus on these latter aspects and update the reader on technological developments and the most important applications: we also sum up mass spectrometry (MS)-rooted proteomic techniques for protein identification along with quantification and selection of nutritional intervention and bioefficacy studies assessed by proteomics.

In almost all biological processes, proteins are the key actors in the human body—they are the "molecular robots," so as to do all the work. Therefore, since we want to gain a more comprehensive understanding of this mechanism and additionally build up the notion of nutritional systems biology, proteomics is at the center of this concerted action.

6.3 Proteomics technology

6.3.1 Protein identification

A few proteomic studies, be they in a nutritional or other framework, begin with a protein study of what can be "seen" in a given sample and condition. Identifying proteins at a large scale and with high throughput requires MS. Figure 6.2 outlines proteomic workflows for the "discovery mode."

Proteins and peptides can be identified by mass spectrometer by determining their correct masses and information generated on the amino

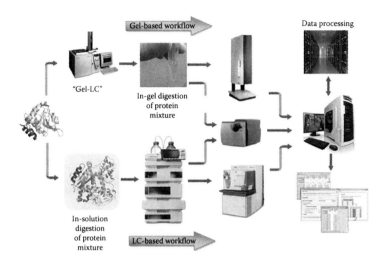

Figure 6.2 *Discovery workflow in mass spectrometry–based proteomics. Gel-LC, gel-LC-based separation; LC, liquid chromatography.*

acid sequences. Nowadays, the main ionization methods deployed are electrospray (Fenn 2003) and matrix-assisted laser desorption (Tanaka 2003), which can put large, delicate biomolecules such as proteins and peptides quietly as well as rapidly into the gas phase and then ionize them while preserving their integrity. These sources of ions appear in a variety of combinations with different mass analyzers that separate the ions by mass over charge. Ion traps, triple quadrupole (triple-Q), time-of-flight (ToF) tubes, Orbitrap, and Fourier-transform ion cyclotron resonance (FT-ICR) cells are the most widely used analyzers in proteomics, with their definite advantages, such as high sensitivity and multiple-stage disintegration for ion traps, high selectivity for triple-Q analyzers, high sensitivity and speed for ToF instruments, and very high resolution and mass accuracy for FT-ICR and Orbitrap analyzers.

Orbitrap (Makarov et al. 2006) and FT-ICR instruments are recent top-end proteomic machines (Nielsen et al. 2005) that rely on frequency readout of oscillating ions rather than ToF or analysis based on scanning. The dynamic range of protein concentrations (e.g., estimated at 10^{12} in human blood) (Jacobs et al. 2005) is the most important analytical challenge, rather than mass accuracy, mass resolution, or absolute sensitivity. Recent MS-based proteomic platforms can carry a dynamic range of protein concentration of 10^4. By depletion of the most abundant proteins, the remaining, as such inaccessible, low-abundant proteome has to be tackled (e.g., commercially available multiple affinity removal system, which particularly removes the top 7 or even 14 plasma proteins) (Gong et al. 2006) or by selective improvement of low-abundant proteins (e.g., by the titanium dioxide techniques for phosphoproteins or immobilized metal affinity chromatography [Thingholm et al. 2009], lectins [Mechref et al. 2008], or the cell surface capture technique for glycoproteins [Wollscheid et al. 2009]). All these enrichment resins, biochemical depletion and columns have matured a great deal and now come in vigorous arrangements.

Subsequent to depletion and/or enrichment, typically further preseparation measurements are taken at the protein–peptide level, anchored in two-dimensional gels, on liquid chromatography (LC), or on hybrid approaches (Gel-LC). Figure 6.2 summarizes these proteomic workflows.

Physically preserving the protein context and generating real protein images is the advantage of gel-based protein separation methods. Nevertheless, they have limited dynamic range, prejudice to the more simply soluble proteins, in addition to a low degree of automation with, in consequence, low throughput. Differential imaging gel electrophoresis is the most sophisticated method for 2D protein separation (Sellers et al. 2007), which depends on multiplexed staining and co-processing of single control plus a maximum of two case samples. Protein spots have then detected, excised, absorbed with trypsin, and moreover amended to LC-MS/MS.

Corresponding to the gels and taking into consideration an increasing demand for speed and throughput, (multi)dimensional LC setups have been coupled online to MS analysis, with straightforward reversed-phase columns in addition to combined strong cation exchange–reversed phase systems being the most commonly applied. The terms *MudPIT* (multidimensional protein identification technology) or *shotgun* proteomics run under these workflows (Swanson and Washburn 2005). One major difference compared with gel approaches is that the protein context is physically given up by upstream tryptic digestion of the protein mixture and subsequent separation and analysis at the peptide level. Reconstruction of the protein context is done *in silico* by reassigning the peptide identification to the same parent protein molecule.

By means of enrichment and/or depletion, gel- and/or LC-based additional preseparation and electrospray ionization–Q/Q-ToF/ion traps/FT-ICR or matrix-assisted laser desorption ionization–ToF/ToF (offline workflow)–based MS, influential platforms exist for quick and complete assessment of proteomes from body fluids, tissues, cells, or organelles.

6.3.2 Protein quantification

Subsequent to a protein review, the first and foremost question asked in proteomic studies comparing manifold conditions is: Which proteins are differentially expressed? Today's means for protein quantification are gel- or MS-based (Moresco et al. 2008).

As mentioned under protein identification, quantification of the gold standard for 2D-rooted proteomics is done by differential imaging gel electrophoresis, that is, by differential staining of the separated protein spots and image analysis.

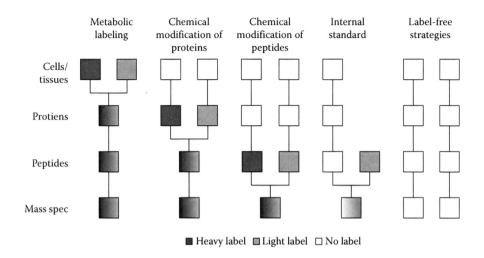

Figure 6.3 *Strategies for relative and absolute protein quantification in mass spectrometry–based proteomics.*

Figure 6.3 summarizes the principal strategies and steps for gel-free global protein quantification, that is, steady isotope entrenched or label-free, metabolic or chemical labeling, and providing relative or absolute quantitative information.

In contrast with discrepancy imaging gel electrophoresis and compatible with online shotgun LC-MS/MS workflows, stable isotopes can be introduced into the circumstances in question, meaning that reagents tagging amino acid side chains at a protein/peptide level are able to introduce a discrepancy isotopic signature so that the conditions can be quantitatively compared at the MS level; for example, the "control" sample can be labeled with the "light," as it is the unlabeled form of the reagent, while the "case" sample can be derivatized with the "heavy" version (e.g., ^{13}C, ^{2}H, or ^{15}N label). These tagging techniques can be implemented at the protein level, for example, aniline-benzoic acid labeling (AniBAL) (Panchaud et al. 2008a), or the peptide level, for example, isotope coded affinity tag (ICAT) (Gygi et al. 1999), tandem mass tag (TMT) (Thompson et al. 2003), and isobaric tag for relative and absolute quantitation (iTRAQ) (Ross et al. 2004), and then can be introduced chemically into the sample (e.g., AniBAL, ICAT, TMT, iTRAQ) otherwise metabolically by feeding cells or even small animals like mices/rats with stable isotopically labeled vital amino acids in cell culture (SILAC) (de Godoy et al. 2006). The quantification readout can be obtained at the MS (AniBAL, ICAT and SILAC) or MS/MS (TMT, iTRAQ) level.

Even though, on the one hand, to maximize co-processing of case(s) and control(s) and minimize bias, it is preferable to introduce a label as upstream as possible in the workflow (e.g., achieved in the cases of the metabolic

SILAC and the chemical AniBAL methods), it is, alternatively, beneficial to not label at all to maximize sample integrity and compare samples directly as they are. Therefore, "label-free" approaches (Figure 6.3) have been developed that deploy spectral counting of peptide coursework for semi-quantitative analysis or compare the peak intensities of the very same peptide by overlaying LC-MS runs of case and control samples (Mueller et al. 2008; Wong et al. 2008).

All previously described methodologies provide information on relative changes in protein abundance. It is advantageous, particularly in nutrition, to generate information on total amounts of proteins present in a given sample. In the context of bioavailability and bioefficacy studies, the bases of proven ingredient bioavailability as well as bioefficacy are complete values of its amounts in the original food matrix and in the pertinent body fluids or tissues. For that reason, proteins and peptides must be completely quantified from the ingredient and biomarker points of view. It is possible to get complete quantitative information by spiking defined amounts of stable isotope-labeled peptides or otherwise entire proteins into the sample of interest and comparing the corresponding mass signals of the sample peptides with those of these internal standards (Brun et al. 2009). The targeted, multiplexed peptide-level version of such an approach is called *AQUA* (absolute quantification) (Gerber et al. 2003); the protein-level alternative is described as *QConCat* (artificial, expressed proteins consist of stable isotope-coded peptides representing the proteins to be quantified and co-processed by the sample) (Pratt et al. 2006) or *PSAQ* (protein standard absolute quantification, that is, spiking the labeled protein of interest and co-processing with the sample) (Dupuis et al. 2008). The approach applied at a proteomic scale by determination as well as synthesis of labeled unique peptide identifiers for almost all proteins to be analyzed is called *proteotypic peptides* (Mallick et al. 2007). The labeled proteotypic peptide standard and its unlabeled, usual counterpart are characteristically monitored, identified, and quantified by a targeted MS/MS acquisition mode, which is known as *selected* or *multiple-reaction monitoring* (Figure 6.4) (Lange et al. 2008; Yocum and Chinnaiyan 2009): quantitative analysis of selected ion transitions explicit for all peptides enables, for example, validation of clinical biomarkers in plasma (Schiess et al. 2009).

Independent of variations of the similar quantification principle, these methods can be understood as highly sensitive methods that are multiplexed MS-based enzyme-linked immune-sorbent "assays" and also do not depend on three-dimensional structure-based recognition of protein epitopes. The Human Proteome Detection and Quantification Project (Anderson et al. 2009) has been recently proposed as an initiative, based on this approach, for development of a complete suite of assays, for example, two peptides from the protein product of about 20,500 human genes, enabling quick and methodical verification of candidate biomarkers and laying a quantitative basis for

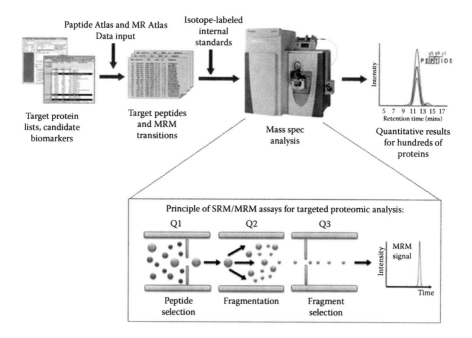

Figure 6.4 *Targeted workflow in mass spectrometry–based proteomics with relative and absolute quantification options. MRM, multiple-reaction monitoring; Q, quadrupole; SRM, selected-reaction monitoring.*

complete human proteome studies. These types of assays could provide an outstanding toolset for future dietary studies for better understanding and correlating the effects of diet as well as food compounds on protein expression plus regulation in humans.

6.3.3 Data processing

In addition to wet laboratory equipment, to generate large proteomic datasets, it takes complicated software to obtain, store, retrieve, process, validate, and interpret these data and ultimately convert them into helpful biological information.

To utilize simply the mass information of a peptide as a sole signature would be the most excellent case scenario in terms of identification. Such approaches were described by Zubarev et al. (1996) and later on by Conrads et al. (2000) as the *accurate mass tag* approach. In this technique, identification depends upon the peptide mass, and for that high-resolution instruments are needed for providing subpart-per-million (0.1 ppm) mass accuracy. However, in spite of such correctness, high levels of confidence in protein identifications can be achieved merely in small eukaryotic systems, like yeast.

Proteins can be identified with good throughput (Pappin 1997) and high sensitivity (Schuerenberg et al. 2000) derived from the set of measured proteolytic peptide masses; this process is called *peptide mass fingerprinting*. Using the similar enzyme cleavage sites, the experimental mass profile is harmonized beside those generated *in silico* from the protein sequences in the database. Consistent with the number of peptide masses matching their succession within a certain mass error tolerance, the proteins are afterward ranked.

On the contrary, MS/MS provides access to sequence data, which enables more confident peptide identifications. A precursor ion with a known mass is selected from the previous MS scan and then isolated for supplementary collision to create daughter ions with sole signature in an MS/MS experiment. This process is described as *peptide mass sequencing*, as it is opposite to peptide mass fingerprinting. Three different approaches have been used for identification of proteins using MS/MS data: (1) peptide sequence tagging (Mann and Wilm 1994), (2) the cross-correlation method (Eng et al. 1994), and (3) probability-based matching (Perkins et al. 1999).

Although peptide and protein identification and database search programs such as Mascot (Perkins et al. 1999) and Sequest (Eng et al. 1994) are well established. Moreover, new software infrastructure for data processing and validation have been built, for example SBEAMS architecture (http://www.sbeams.org), housing the Trans-Proteomic Pipeline and microarray modules, which cover gene and protein expressions. In the Trans-Proteomic Pipeline, the PeptideProphet (Keller et al. 2002) and ProteinProphet (Nesvizhskii et al. 2003) modules are based on a vigorous and precise statistical model for assessment of peptide identification validity made by MS/MS plus database search. The idea behind such resources is to provide the information to researchers for assessment of the quality of the data in a dataset-dependent manner and to control the exchange among false positives (specificity) as well as false negatives (sensitivity) (Urfer et al. 2006). A second strategy for elucidation of the false-positive/false-negative tradeoff depends on a database search using a target-decoy database (Elias and Gygi 2007): first, an appropriate "target" protein sequence database is generated and then a "decoy" database is created, preserving the general composition of the target database while minimizing the number of peptide sequences in common. The search is done next to the target and the composite database. Assuming that no correct peptides are found in the target and decoy entities and those incorrect assignments as of target or decoy sequences are uniformly expected, one can estimate the total number of false positives.

Except for the advancement in proteomics data processing, software platforms enabling cross-correlation with other omics' sources (e.g., SBEAMS, Rosetta Elucidator, Genedata Expressionist, etc.) and supporting pathway understanding (e.g., Ingenuity Pathway Analysis, BioBase Explain module, AffyAnnotator [Staab et al. 2007]) are maturing speedily.

6.4 Perspectives for proteomics in nutrition

With the understanding of disease prevention and health maintenance through adapted nutrition beginning to emerge, the most important challenges for proteomics in nutrition and health still lie ahead, a few of which are relevant to omics disciplines in general and some of which are specific for omics-driven discoveries in the food context: (1) the rate-limiting step is no longer data generation—filtering these data for significant (i.e., high-quality signal-to-noise, solid statistics) and pertinent information (i.e., important for nutrition) is not an easy task; (2) the incorporation of gene plus protein expression profiles with metabolic fingerprints have to advance; we may choose pertinent subsets of information to be merged, for example phenotype-characteristic metabolite profiles with related enzymes and transporter proteins and their corresponding transcripts; (3) *health* and *comfort* are less well defined than disease; (4) in nutrition, proteomics has to disclose many weak signals rather than a few abundant signals to detect early deviations from usual metabolism; (5) from the food context point of view, health cannot be uncoupled from pleasure, that is, food preference and nutritional health are interconnected (Kussmann and Affolter 2006).

Proteomics has evolved as an analogue to genomics, on or after recognizing all proteins present in a given sample at a given time to a global molecular analysis platform that addresses practical aspects of biological systems (Wilkins et al. 1996). Quite the opposite of the genome, the proteome is highly energetic and constantly changing in response to the environment of a cell or an organism. Comparing such variations in the proteome enables the discovery of key proteins and the identification of modulated pathways involved, as in definite nutrition-related processes.

More than the last two decades, proteomics has developed into an established skill for biomarker finding, (Lescuyer et al. 2007; Schrattenholz and Groebe 2007), clinical applications (Mischak et al. 2007), disease profiling along with diagnostics (Marko-Varga et al. 2005), the study of protein interactions (Gingras et al. 2007), and the study of the dynamics of signaling pathways (Scholten et al. 2006). Nutritional proteomics is an emerging field where these technologies are applied to dietary research. It holds vast promise for (a) profiling and characterizing dietary and body proteins, digestion, and absorption, (b) identifying biomarkers of nutritional status and health/disease conditions, and (c) understanding the functions of nutrients and other nutritional factors in growth and reproduction, as well as health (Wang et al. 2006).

6.5 Proteomics in nutritional intervention

Proteomics in nutritional science has the potential to deliver biomarkers for nutritional intervention and individual disposition, assess nutritional status at the molecular level, and discover bioactive food peptides and proteins

(Fuchs et al. 2005a). There have been several papers published summarizing nutritional proteomic applications such as nutritional intervention (Kussmann et al. 2007), elucidation of immune-related gut disorders (Kussmann and Blum 2007), description of functional ingredients such as probiotics or milk and soy proteins (Kussmann et al. 2005), or the study of anxious energy metabolism like in diabetes and obesity (Kussmann and Affolter 2008).

6.6 Application of proteomics in nutritional interventions

Soy isoflavones as well as soybean proteins present in soy-based diets have been shown to promote a cardioprotective effect. Fuchs et al. (2005b) studied the effect of soy isoflavones, through genistein, which is the most plentiful compound, with regard to the protective activity against atherosclerosis. They demonstrated that genistein at low and high concentrations reversed the stressor-induced diminishing of anti-atherogenic proteins. They furthermore identified biomarkers in peripheral blood mononuclear cells (PBMCs) (Fuchs et al. 2007) that reacted to a nutritional intervention with isoflavone-enriched soy extract in postmenopausal women. Approximately 29 proteins were acknowledged that showed appreciably altered expression in PBMCs, including a variety of proteins concerned in anti-inflammatory response, as a result signifying that soy isoflavones increase anti-inflammatory activity in PBMCs. Very recently, Astle et al. (2007) reviewed proteomic and metabolomic responses to nutritional factors (i.e., soy isoflavones, carotenoids, polyphenolic substances) with supplements and moreover concluded that powerful proteomic tools such as top-down MS as well as protein microarrays will seriously contribute to the characterization of subtle proteome changes resulting from the inconsistency in consuming nutritional factors and supplements.

Proteomic investigation of the enteric nervous system (ENS) shows that the nervous system of the gastrointestinal tract (Hansen 2003) has the prospective to deliver insights into gut functionality. It is, for example, recognized that early life events (for instance, neonatal maternal separation) incline adults to develop visceral pain and enhanced colonic motility in response to acute stress. In order to better understand the molecular basis for these functional gut disorders induced by environmental stress, Marvin-Guy et al. (2005) established a proteomic catalogue of the rat intestine.

Barcelo-Batllori et al. (2002) investigated the implications of cytokine-induced proteins in human intestinal epithelial cells (hIECs), which are correlated with inflammatory bowel syndrome (IBS) (Wood et al. 1999). The inspiration behind this study was that cytokine-regulated proteins present in intestinal epithelial cells (IECs) had been associated with the pathogenesis of inflammatory bowel disease (Hansen 2003).

Hang et al. (2009) studied, by a gel-based approach, the molecular mechanism of necrotizing enterocolitis, a serious gastrointestinal inflammatory disease, which frequently takes place in preterm neonates who do not adapt to enteral nutrition. The functional task of the differentially articulated proteins revealed that important cellular functions, such as protein processing, heat shock response, as well as nitrogen, purine, and energy metabolism, were involved in the early progression of necrotizing enterocolitis.

Nutritional components seem to be significant determinants of cancer risk and tumor behavior. To understand the connection between nutritional interventions, proteome changes, and cancer (Milner 2006), functional proteomic studies will be vital. Dietary modifications and interventions have the potential to considerably lower cancer risk and its associated complications, and validated biomarkers will be invaluable tools for this research (Davis and Milner 2007). Four studies have employed proteomics, either as such or else collective with gene expression analysis, to address biomarkers for protection against cancer.

Breikers et al. (2006) recognized 30 proteins differentially expressed in the colonic mucosa of healthy mice upon increased vegetable intake. In one study six proteins identified with changed expression levels could be brought into the context of a protective role in colorectal cancer. In another study, integrated DNA microarrays with proteomics were used to investigate the effects of nutrients by means of recommended anticolorectal cancer properties and to develop a colon epithelial cell line–based screening assay intended for such nutrients (Stierum et al. 2001). The effects of sodium butyrate on growth inhibition of human HT-29 cancer cells *in vitro* were assessed by Tan et al. (2002) using a 2DE-MS-based proteomic strategy. Butyrate treatment changed the expression of a variety of proteins, particularly those of the ubiquitin–proteasome pathway, a result suggesting that proteolysis could be a significant mechanism by which butyrate regulates key proteins in the control of cell cycle, apoptosis, and differentiation.

Combining gene and protein expression profiling in colonic cancer cells, Herzog et al. (2004) identified the flavonoid flavone, present in various fruits and vegetables, as a potent apoptosis inducer in human cancer cells. Flavones display a broad spectrum of effects on gene and protein expression that correlated to apoptosis induction and cellular metabolism. The effect of the flavonoid quercetin on normal and malignant prostate cells was evaluated by Aalinkeel et al. (2008) and identified the possible target of quercetin action. Their results confirmed that quercetin treatment of prostate cancer cells resulted in decreased cell proliferation as well as viability. By downregulating the levels of heat shock protein-90, quercetin encouraged cancer cell apoptosis but put forth no scientific effect on normal prostate epithelial cells (Aalinkeel et al. 2008).

Zhang et al. (2008) studied altered protein expression levels of fructose-induced fatty liver in the hamsters. High fructose consumption is linked through the development of fatty liver in addition to dyslipidemia. Matrix-assisted laser desorption ionization–MS-based proteomic analysis of the hamster's liver tissue revealed a number of proteins whose expression levels were altered by more than double. The recognized proteins were grouped into categories such as fatty acid metabolism, triacylglycerol and cholesterol metabolism, enzymes in fructose catabolism, molecular chaperones, and proteins with housekeeping functions.

Not only the presence but also the absence of a particular nutrient can have a marked effect on an organism. The consequences of nutrient deficiency were studied by tom Dieck et al. (2005) by force-feeding rats with a zinc-deficient diet and analyzing the lipidome, hepatic transcriptome, and proteome. The major metabolic pathways of hepatic glucose and lipid metabolism and their changes with zinc deficiency were identified through this mutual omics analysis, which caused liver lipid accumulation and hepatic inflammation. In the same context, Fong et al. (2005) showed that alleviation of zinc deficiency by zinc supplementation resulted in an 80% reduction of COX-2 mRNA, a prime enzyme involved in inflammation.

Generally, samples of body fluids are relatively easy to process for proteomic analysis, for the reason that, unlike complex solid tissues, the separation of cellular fractions is usually not necessary. In a rat model to investigate the effect of cobalamin deficiency on the proteome of cerebrospinal fluid, Gianazza et al. (2003) used 2D gel electrophoresis. In totally gastrectomized animals there was an increase in total protein in cerebrospinal fluid, which reached a peak 4 months following surgery. A cobalamin-deficient state was maintained in rats by dietary depletion, and a comparable peak occurred 6 months subsequent to introduction of the diet. The 4-month peak in protein concentration was associated by means of a specific raise in alpha-1 antitrypsin and the *de novo* appearance of thiostatin and haptoglobin-b, but all these changes were corrected with supplementation with cobalamin.

More recently, Linke et al. (2004) described the application of proteomics to plasma samples as of rats with conflicting retinol status. Plasma samples were analyzed directly using SELDITOF MS, and prefractionation of the samples done by anion-exchange chromatography, using 96-well filter plates, was shown to markedly increase the total number of peptides and proteins detectable by this method. Three proteins with molecular mass between 10,000 and 20,000 were shown to be present at reduced concentration in the plasma of retinol-deficient rats, and the authors concluded that their approach provided a hopeful means of detecting changes in nutritional status at the level of whole-body.

Park et al. (2004) recently described the use of proteomic techniques to explore the impact of atherogenic diets on hepatic protein expression in C3H/HeJ mice (C3H, atherosclerosis-resistant strain) and C57BL/6J mice (B6, atherosclerosis-susceptible strain). Both strains were fed atherogenic diets and each showed a different pattern of both plasma lipids and intracellular lipid droplets. Proteomic analysis of liver from the two strains revealed a complex response. Overall, a total of 30 hepatic proteins were significantly changed by exposure to the diets, and, of these, 14 including carbonic anhydrase III, senescence marker protein 30, and Se-binding protein 2 were differentially changed in B6 mice only. The remaining 16 proteins, including the proteins glutathione S-transferase, chaperonin, and apo E, were altered in both strains. Another 28 proteins were differentially expressed in the livers of both C3H and B6 mice, despite diet feeding condition. The authors concluded that the proteomic approach had revealed obvious differences in expression of both lipid metabolism-related proteins and oxidative stress proteins in both strains in response to the atherogenic diets, and that these differences could account for their differing susceptibility to atherogenesis.

Food deficiency results in metabolic, functional, and structural changes in the small intestine. As a result, it influences gut mucosal integrity, mucin synthesis, epithelial cell proliferation, and other processes (Lenaerts et al. 2006). A comparative proteomics study in mice identified intestinal proteins whose expression was changed under different starvation conditions. The results of this study provide novel insights into the intestinal starvation response and may contribute to providing better nutritional support during conditions characterized by malnutrition.

Proteomic analysis of depleted human serum samples from a dietary intervention study with supplemented vegetables (broccoli) provided biomarkers for evaluating dietary exposure (Mitchell et al. 2005). MALDI-TOF analysis allowed the identification of the B-chain of α2-HS-glycoprotein (fetuin), a serum protein previously found to show a discrepancy with diet and to be involved in insulin resistance and immune function.

Food components may not only change gene and protein expression but also target post-translational modifications (Davis and Milner 2004). Diet-induced protein modifications can ideally be assessed by proteomic techniques. For instance, the protein phosphorylation position of the protein ERK is altered after exposure to diallyl disulfide, a compound present in processed garlic, which results in cell cycle arrest (Knowles and Milner 2003). Another example is the modification of thiol groups in the cytoplasmic protein Keap1, which results in alteration of the protein redox status, affecting its binding to the protein Nrf2, which acts as a transcriptional regulator (Dinkova-Kostova et al. 2002).

Briefly, nutritional proteomics is an emerging field of proteomics and its victory will depend on many factors. First, technology platforms will profit from further improvements including advanced protein/peptide separation techniques, more sensitive and specific mass analysis methods, and better depletion and enrichment methods. Second, bioinformatics tools to assess data quality and to convert data into interpretable information are proceeding quickly. New systems will be able to support the reconstruction of pathways in addition to regulatory networks even in the presence of fragmentary data (Staab et al. 2007), as a result helping to integrate incomplete omics data sets. Third, intelligent focusing on proteome subsets (at the level of cell organelles, along with protein subclasses, or else the mass spectral level, that is, proteotypic peptides and multiple-reaction monitoring) will offer deeper insights into molecular networks. Fourth, addressing protein turnover at the proteomic scale, that is, interpretation of protein abundance changes as a result of protein synthesis and degradation (Doherty and Beynon 2006) will add value to dietary intervention studies performed with stable-isotope-labeled amino acids, peptides, and proteins. In addition, such data should facilitate an enhanced correlation between transcript, protein, and metabolite data, as an increased protein synthesis rate is more consistent in the biological context than just the change at the transcript level. Finally, nutritional changes in humans signify somewhat subtle interventions, resulting in many small rather than a few large molecular changes, rendering data interpretation challenging. As a result, improved definition of human cohorts undergoing nutritional interventions all the way through appropriate genotyping can be predicted to deliver clearer readouts from omics applications.

6.7 Conclusion

Nutrition is a young field of proteomics compared with clinical (Mueller et al. 2008) and medical (Brun et al. 2009) applications. The success of proteomics in nutrition and health will rely on a number of factors. As such, the proteomic technologic platforms, independent of their application, will benefit from further superior protein/peptide separation techniques, better depletion and enrichment methods, and more sensitive as well as specific mass analysis techniques.

Bioinformatics is the second area of platform-related improvements. For assessment data quality and conversion of data into interpretable information, the tools used are improving quickly (Panchaud et al. 2008b). Current gaps in omics datasets and hidden regulation motifs upstream of the observed gene product regulation may be elucidated by means of interpretation tools that are able to reconstruct pathways and regulatory networks even in the presence of fragmentary data (Staab et al. 2007). If these network-reconstructing and motif-elucidating tools prove to be successful, they may also shed a different light on the terms reproducibility and comparability of "omic" studies: rather than searching for the same transcripts/proteins/metabolites found regulated between related studies, one may focus on the common motifs behind these—often at first glance divergent—datasets to find congruence between them.

The third area of development for proteomic methods concerns the analytical approach. Intellectual focusing on proteome subsets, be it at the level of cell organelles, protein subclasses (Bantscheff et al. 2007; Mancone et al. 2007), or the mass spectral level (targeted proteomics with proteotypic peptides) (Mallick et al. 2007), or else selected-reaction monitoring (Anderson and Hunter 2006), will yield less comprehensive proteomes but provide deeper insights into molecular networks.

Despite this predictable advancement within proteomics, the technology will largely profit from its cross-correlation with gene expression analysis at the mRNA level along with metabolite profiling. In the search of the causality and "wiring" between these three observational levels, one has to be conscious of the fact that the interrelated timing of gene and protein expression as well as metabolite generation remains implicit (Nicholson et al. 2002). One possible solution to this is addressing protein revenue at a proteomic scale, that is to say, rather than taking proteomic snapshots, interpreting protein abundance changes because of the interplay among changing protein synthesis and degradation (Doherty and Beynon 2006). Proteome turnover information will add value to dietary intervention studies performed with stable isotope- labeled amino acids and peptides, as well as proteins.

What takes proteomics in nutritional and food research beyond the pure technologic advances is that human genetic heterogeneity comes into play. Genetic susceptibility might predispose an individual to a diet-induced disease in addition to this as well relates to biomarker profiles in individuals (Chen et al. 2007; Siffert 2005). This can be additional illustrated by a nutritionally pertinent example: Siffert (2005) and Holtmann et al. (2004) identified and characterized metabolically applicable single nucleotide polymorphisms in G-proteins, the latter representing a significant "funnel" of cellular signaling. These types of polymorphisms predispose individuals of different ethnicity to a higher risk of developing atherosclerosis, hypertension, metabolic syndrome, or functional dyspepsia (Holtmann et al. 2004; Siffert 2005).

Epigenetic regulation such as DNA methylation (gene silencing) and histone acetylation (chromatin structure) must preferably be included in dietary systems biology, because these mechanisms strongly influence gene transcription and expression. Extraordinarily, MS-based proteomic methods have started to contribute in this regard: Beck et al. (2006) presented a quantitative analysis of human histone post-translational modifications, whereas Bonenfant et al. (2006) focused on the histone codes of H2A and H2B variants.

In humans, dietary changes represent rather subtle interferences, frequently resulting in several small rather than a few large molecular changes, making data interpretation most complicated. Enhanced definition of human cohorts undergoing dietary interventions through proper geno- and phenotyping may be capable of and expected to transport clearer readouts from omics applications. As nutritional science develops into a holistic molecular science by means of systems biology character, all intervention studies, including those that use proteomic approaches, should be rooted in standardized diets, ingredients, and stratified cohorts and ideally follow the double-blinded, placebo-controlled crossover design.

Proteomics will carry on to play a key role in systems biology, because it can not only identify and quantify the "molecular robots" that do all the work in biological systems but also map the networks of their physical interactions between each other and with nutrients, drugs, and other small molecules.

An imposing example of such thematic network organization was given by Bantscheff et al. (2007), who revealed the mechanisms of action of clinical kinase inhibitors through MS profiling of small-molecule interactions with hundreds of endogenously expressed protein kinases.

References

Aalinkeel R, Bindukumar B, Reynolds JL, Sykes DE, Mahajan SD, Chadha KC, Schwartz SA. The dietary bioflavonoid, quercetin, selectively induces apoptosis of prostate cancer cells by down-regulating the expression of heat shock protein 90. *Prostate.* 2008; 68: 1773–89.

Anderson L, Hunter CL. Quantitative mass spectrometric multiple reaction monitoring assays for major plasma proteins. *Mol Cell Proteomics.* 2006; 5: 573–88.

Anderson NL, Anderson NG, Pearson TW, Borchers CH, Paulovich AG, Patterson SD, Gillette M, Aebersold R, Carr SA. A human proteome detection and quantitation project. *Mol Cell Proteomics.* 2009; 8: 883–6.

Astle J, Ferguson JT, German JB, Harrigan GG, Kelleher NL, Kodadek T, Parks BA, et al. Characterization of proteomic and metabolomic responses to dietary factors and supplements. *J Nutr.* 2007; 137(12): 2787–93.

Bantscheff M, Eberhard D, Abraham Y, Bastuck S, Boesche M, Hobson S, Mathieson T, et al. Quantitative chemical proteomics reveals mechanisms of action of clinical ABL kinase inhibitors. *Nat Biotechnol.* 2007; 25: 1035–44.

Barcelo-Batllori S, Andre M, Servis C, Levy N, Takikawa O, Michetti P, Reymond M, Felley-Bosco E. Proteomic analysis of cytokine induced proteins in human intestinal epithelial cells: Implications for inflammatory bowel diseases. *Proteomics.* 2002; 2: 551–60.

Beck HC, Nielsen EC, Matthiesen R, Jensen LH, Sehested M, Finn P, Grauslund M, Hansen AM, Jensen ON. Quantitative proteomic analysis of post-translational modifications of human histones. *Mol Cell Proteomics.* 2006; 5: 1314–25.

Bonenfant D, Coulot M, Towbin H, Schindler P, van Oostrum J. Characterization of histone H2A and H2B variants and their post-translational modifications by mass spectrometry. *Mol Cell Proteomics.* 2006; 5: 541–52.

Breikers G, van Breda SG, Bouwman FG, van Herwijnen MH, Renes J, Mariman EC, Kleinjans JC, van Delft JH. Potential protein markers for nutritional health effects on colorectal cancer in the mouse as revealed by proteomics analysis. *Proteomics.* 2006; 6: 2844–52.

Brun V, Masselon C, Garin J, Dupuis A. Isotope dilution strategies for absolute quantitative proteomics. *J Proteomics.* 2009; 72: 740–9. doi: 10.1016/j.jprot.2009.03.007.

Chen Y, Rollins J, Paigen B, Wang X. Genetic and genomic insights into the molecular basis of atherosclerosis. *Cell Metab.* 2007; 6: 164–79.

Conrads TP, Anderson GA, Veenstra TD, Pasa Tolic L, Smith RD. Utility of accurate mass tags for proteome-wide protein identification. *Anal Chem.* 2000; 72: 3349–54.

Corthésy-Theulaz I, den Dunnen JT, Ferré P, Geurts JM, Müller M, van Belzen N, van Ommen B. Nutrigenomics: The impact of biomics technology on nutrition research. *Ann Nutr Metab.* 2005; 49: 355–65.

Davis CD, Milner J. Frontiers in nutrigenomics, proteomics, metabolomics and cancer prevention. *Mutat Res.* 2004; 551: 51–64.

Davis CD, Milner JA. Biomarkers for diet and cancer prevention research: Potentials and challenges. *Acta Pharmacol Sin.* 2007; 28: 1262–73.

de Godoy LM, Olsen JV, de Souza GA, Li G, Mortensen P, Mann M. Status of complete proteome analysis by mass spectrometry: SILAC labeled yeast as a model system. *Genome Biol.* 2006; 7: R50.

Dinkova-Kostova AT, Holtzclaw WD, Cole RN, Itoh K, Wakabayashi N, Katoh Y, Yamamoto M, Talalay P. Direct evidence that sulfhydryl groups of Keap1 are the sensors regulating induction of phase 2 enzymes that protect against carcinogens and oxidants. *Proc Natl Acad Sci U S A.* 2002; 99: 11908–13.

Doherty MK, Beynon RJ. Protein turnover on the scale of the proteome. *Expert Rev Proteomics.* 2006; 3: 97–110.

Dove A. Proteomics: Translating genomics into products? *Nat Biotechnol.* 1999; 17: 233–36.

Dupuis A, Hennekinne JA, Garin J, Brun V. Protein standard absolute quantification (PSAQ) for improved investigation of staphylococcal food poisoning outbreaks. *Proteomics.* 2008; 8: 4633–6.

Elias JE, Gygi SP. Target-decoy search strategy for increased confidence in large-scale protein identifications by mass spectrometry. *Nat Methods.* 2007; 4: 207–14.

Eng JK, McCormack AL, Yates JR. An approach to correlate tandem mass spectral data of peptides with amino acid sequences in a protein database. *J Am Soc Mass Spectrom.* 1994; 5: 976–89.

Fay LB, German JB. Personalizing foods: Is genotype necessary? *Curr Opin Biotechnol.* 2008; 19: 121–8.

Fenn JB. Electrospray wings for molecular elephants (Nobel lecture). *Angew Chem Int Ed Engl.* 2003; 42: 3871–94.

Fong LY, Zhang L, Jiang Y, Farber JL. Dietary zinc modulation of COX-2 expression and lingual and esophageal carcinogenesis in rats. *J Natl Cancer Inst.* 2005; 97: 40–50.

Fuchs D, Pascual-Teresa S, Rimbach G, Virgili F, Ambra R, Turner R, Daniel H, Wenzel U. Proteome analysis for identification of target proteins of genistein in primary human endothelial cells stressed with oxidized LDL or homocysteine. *Eur J Nutr.* 2005b; 44: 95–104.

Fuchs D, Vafeiadou K, Hall WL, Daniel H, Williams CM, Schroot JH, Wenzel U. Proteomic biomarkers of peripheral blood mononuclear cells obtained from postmenopausal women undergoing an intervention with soy isoflavones. *Am J Clin Nutr.* 2007; 86: 1369–75.

Fuchs D, Winkelmann I, Johnson IT, Mariman E, Wenzel U, Daniel H. Proteomics in nutrition research: Principles, technologies and applications. *Br J Nutr.* 2005a; 94: 302–14.

Gallou-Kabani C, Vige A, Gross MS, Junien C. Nutri-epigenomics: Lifelong remodelling of our epigenomes by nutritional and metabolic factors and beyond. *Clin Chem Lab Med.* 2007; 45: 321–7.

Gerber SA, Rush J, Stemman O, Kirschner MW, Gygi SP. Absolute quantification of proteins and phosphoproteins from cell lysates by tandem MS. *Proc Natl Acad Sci USA.* 2003; 100: 6940–5.

Gianazza E, Veber D, Eberini I, Buccellato FR, Mutti E, Sironi L, Scalabrino G. Cobalamin (vitamin B12)-deficiency-induced changes in the proteome of rat cerebrospinal fluid. *Biochem J.* 2003; 374: 239–46.

Gingras AC, Gstaiger M, Raught B, Aebersold R. Analysis of protein complexes using mass spectrometry. *Nat Rev Mol Cell Biol.* 2007; 8: 645–54.

Gong Y, Li X, Yang B, Ying W, Li D, Zhang Y, Dai S, Cai Y, Wang J, He F, Qian X. Different immuno affinity fractionation strategies to characterize the human plasma proteome. *J Proteome Res.* 2006; 5: 1379–87.

Gygi SP, Rist B, Gerber SA, Turecek F, Gelb MH, Aebersold R. Quantitative analysis of complex protein mixtures using isotope-coded affinity tags. *Nat Biotechnol.* 1999; 17: 994–9.

Hang P, Sangild PT, Sit WH, Ngai HH, Xu R, Siggers JL, Wan JM. Temporal proteomic analysis of intestine developing necrotizing enterocolitis following enteral formula feeding to preterm pigs. *J Proteome Res.* 2009; 8: 72–81.

Hansen MB. The enteric nervous system I: Organisation and classification. *Pharmacol Toxicol.* 2003; 92: 105–13.

Herzog A, Kindermann B, Doring F, Daniel H, Wenzel U. Pleiotropic molecular effects of the npro-apoptotic dietary constituent flavone in human colon cancer cells identified by protein and mRNA expression profiling. *Proteomics.* 2004; 4: 2455–64.

Hochstrasser DF. Clinical and biomedical applications of proteomics. In Wilkins MR, Williams KL, Appel RD, Hochstrasser DF, editors. *Proteome Research: New Frontiers in Functional Genomics.* Springer, Heidelberg; 1997. p. 211.

Holtmann G, Siffert W, Haag S, Mueller N, Langkafel M, Senf W, Zotz R, Talley NJ. G-protein beta 3 subunit 825 CC genotype is associated with unexplained (functional) dyspepsia. *Gastroenterology.* 2004; 126: 971–9.

Jacobs JM, Adkins JN, Qian WJ, Liu T, Shen Y, Camp DG, Smith RD. Utilizing human blood plasma for proteomic biomarker discovery. *J Proteome Res.* 2005; 4: 1073–85.

Junien C, Gallou-Kabani C, Vige A, Gross MS. Nutritional epigenomics: Consequences of unbalanced diets on epigenetic processes of programming during lifespan and between generations. *Ann Endocrinol.* 2005; 66(pt 3): 2S19–28.

Kaput J. Nutrigenomics research for personalized nutrition and medicine. *Curr Opin Biotechnol.* 2008; 19: 110–20.

Kato H. Nutrigenomics: The cutting edge and Asian perspectives. *Asia Pac J Clin Nutr.* 2008; 17 Suppl 1: 12–15.

Keller A, Nesvizhskii AI, Kolker E, Aebersold R. Empirical statistical model to estimate the accuracy of peptide identifications made by MS/MS and database search. *Anal Chem.* 2002; 74: 5383–92.

Knowles LM, Milner JA. Diallyl disulfide induces ERK phosphorylation and alters gene expression profiles in human colon tumor cells. *J Nutr.* 2003; 133: 2901–6.

Kussmann M, Affolter M. Proteomic methods in nutrition. *Curr Opin Clin Nutr Metab Care.* 2006; 9: 575–83.

Kussmann M, Affolter M. Proteomics and metabonomics routes towards obesity. In Sorensen CK, editor. *Obesity-Genomics and Postgenomics.* Informa Health Care Inc., New York; 2008. p. 527–35.

Kussmann M, Affolter M. Proteomics at the center of nutrigenomics: Comprehensive molecular understanding of dietary health effects. *Nutrition.* 2009; 25: 1085–93. doi: 10.1016/j.nut.2009.05.022.

Kussmann M, Affolter M, Fay LB. Proteomics in nutrition and health. *Comb Chem High Throughput Screen.* 2005; 8: 679–96.

Kussmann M, Affolter M, Nagy K, Holst B, Fay LB. Mass spectrometry in nutrition: Understanding dietary health effects at the molecular level. *Mass Spectrom Rev.* 2007; 26: 727–50.

Kussmann M, Blum S. OMICS-derived targets for inflammatory gut disorders: Opportunities for the development of nutrition related biomarkers. *Endocr Metab Immune Disord Drug Targets.* 2007; 7: 271–87.

Kussmann M, Daniel H. Editorial overview. *Curr Opin Biotechnol.* 2008; 19: 63–5.

Kussmann M, Fay LB. Nutrigenomics and personalized nutrition: Science and concept. *Pers Med.* 2008; 5: 447–55.

Kussmann M, Raymond F, Affolter M. OMICS-driven biomarker discovery in nutrition and health. *J Biotechnol.* 2006; 124: 758–87.

Kussmann M, Rezzi S, Daniel H. Profiling techniques in nutrition and health research. *Curr Opin Biotechnol.* 2008; 19: 83–99.

Lange V, Picotti P, Domon B, Aebersold R. Selected reaction monitoring for quantitative proteomics: A tutorial. *Mol Syst Biol.* 2008; 4: 222.

Lenaerts K, Sokolovic M, Bouwman FG, Lamers WH, Mariman EC, Renes J. Starvation induces phase-specific changes in the proteome of mouse small intestine. *J Proteome Res.* 2006; 5: 2113–22.

Lescuyer P, Hochstrasser D, Rabilloud T. How shall we use the proteomics toolbox for biomarker discovery? *J Proteome Res.* 2007; 6: 3371–76.

Linke T, Ross AC, Harrison EH. Profiling of rat plasma by surface-enhanced laser desorption/ionization time-of-flight mass spectrometry, a novel tool for biomarker discovery in nutrition research. *J Chromatogr A.* 2004; 1043: 65–71.

Makarov A, Denisov E, Kholomeev A, Balschun W, Lange O, Strupat K, Horning S. Performance evaluation of a hybrid linear ion trap/orbitrap mass spectrometer. *Anal Chem.* 2006; 78: 2113–20.

Mallick P, Schirle M, Chen SS, Flory MR, Lee H, Martin D, Ranish J, et al. Computational prediction of proteotypic peptides for quantitative proteomics. *Nat Biotechnol.* 2007; 25: 125–31.

Mancone C, Amicone L, Fimia GM, Bravo E, Piacentini M, Tripodi M, Alonzi T. Proteomic analysis of human very low-density lipoprotein by two-dimensional gel electrophoresis and MALDI-TOF/TOF. *Proteomics.* 2007; 7: 143–54.

Mann M, Wilm M. Error-tolerant identification of peptides in sequence databases by peptide sequence tags. *Anal Chem.* 1994; 33: 4390–9.

Mariman EC. Nutrigenomics and nutrigenetics: The 'omics' revolution in nutritional science. *Biotechnol Appl Biochem.* 2006; 44: 119–28.

Marko-Varga G, Lindberg H, Lofdahl CG, Jonsson P, Hansson L, Dahlback M, Lindquist E, Johansson L, Foster M, Fehniger TE. Discovery of biomarker candidates within disease by protein profiling: Principles and concepts. *J Proteome Res.* 2005; 4: 1200–12.

Marvin-Guy L, Lopes LV, Affolter M, Courtet-Compondu MC, Wagniere S, Bergonzelli GE, Fay LB, Kussmann M. Proteomics of the rat gut: Analysis of the myenteric plexus-longitudinal muscle preparation. *Proteomics.* 2005; 5: 2561–69.

Mechref Y, Madera M, Novotny MV. Glycoprotein enrichment through lectin affinity techniques. *Methods Mol Biol.* 2008; 424: 373–96.

Milner JA. Diet and cancer: Facts and controversies. *Nutr Cancer.* 2006; 56: 216–24.

Mischak H, Apweiler R, Banks RE, Conaway M, Coon J, Dominiczak A, Ehrich JHH, Fliser D, Girolami M, Hermjakob H, et al. Clinical proteomics: A need to define the field and to begin to set adequate standards. *Proteomics Clin Appl.* 2007; 1: 148–56.

Mitchell BL, Yasui Y, Lampe JW, Gafken PR, Lampe PD. Evaluation of matrix-assisted laser desorption/ionization-time of flight mass spectrometry proteomic profiling: Identification of alpha 2-HS glycoprotein B-chain as a biomarker of diet. *Proteomics.* 2005; 5: 2238–46.

Moresco JJ, Dong MQ, Yates JR III. Quantitative mass spectrometry as a tool for nutritional proteomics. *Am J Clin Nutr.* 2008; 88: 597–604.

Mueller LN, Brusniak MY, Mani DR, Aebersold R. An assessment of software solutions for the analysis of mass spectrometry based quantitative proteomics data. *J Proteome Res.* 2008; 7: 51–61.

Nesvizhskii AI, Keller A, Kolker E, Aebersold R. A statistical model for identifying proteins by tandem mass spectrometry. *Anal Chem.* 2003; 75: 4646–58.

Nicholson JK, Connelly J, Lindon JC, Holmes E. Metabonomics: A platform for studying drug toxicity and gene function. *Nat Rev Drug Discov.* 2002; 1: 153–61.

Nielsen ML, Savitski MM, Zubarev RA. Improving protein identification using complementary fragmentation techniques in Fourier trans-form mass spectrometry. *Mol Cell Proteomics.* 2005; 4: 835–45.

Ordovas JM, Corella D. Nutritional genomics. *Ann Rev Genomics Hum Genet.* 2004; 5: 71–118.

Page MJ, Amess B, Rohlff C, Stubberfield C, Parekh R. Proteomics: A major new technology for the drug discovery process. *Drug Discovery Today.* 1999; 4: 55–62.

Panchaud A, Affolter M, Moreillon P, Kussmann M. Experimental and computational approaches to quantitative proteomics: Status quo and outlook. *J Proteomics.* 2008b; 71: 19–33.

Panchaud A, Hansson J, Affolter M, Bel RR, Piu S, Moreillon P, Kussmann M. ANIBAL, stable isotope-based quantitative proteomics by aniline and benzoic acid labeling of amino and carboxylic groups. *Mol Cell Proteomics.* 2008a; 7: 800–12.

Pappin DJ. Peptide mass fingerprinting using MALDI-TOF mass spectrometry. *Methods Mol Biol.* 1997; 64: 165–73.

Park JY, Seong JK, Paik YK. Proteomic analysis of diet-induced hypercholesterolemic mice. *Proteomics.* 2004; 4: 514–23.

Perkins DN, Pappin DJ, Creasy DM, Cottrell JS. Probability-based protein identification by searching sequence databases using mass spectrometry data. *Electrophoresis.* 1999; 20: 3551–67.

Persidis A. Proteomics. *Nat Biotechnol.* 1998; 16: 393–94.

Pratt JM, Simpson DM, Doherty MK, Rivers J, Gaskell SJ, Beynon RJ. Multiplexed absolute quantification for proteomics using concatenated signature peptides encoded by QconCAT genes. *Nat Protoc.* 2006; 1: 1029–43.

Ronteltap A, van Trijp JC, Renes RJ. Consumer acceptance of nutrigenomics-based personalised nutrition. *Br J Nutr.* 2008; 15: 1–13.

Ross PL, Huang YN, Marchese JN, Williamson B, Parker K, Hattan S, Khainovski N, et al. Multiplexed protein quantitation in Saccharomyces cerevisiae using amine-reactive isobaric tagging reagents. *Mol Cell Proteomics.* 2004; 3: 1154–69.

Schiess R, Wollscheid B, Aebersold R. Targeted proteomic strategy for clinical biomarker discovery. *Mol Oncol.* 2009; 3: 33–44.

Scholten A, Poh MK, van Veen TA, van Breukelen B, Vos MA, Heck AJ. Analysis of the cGMP/cAMP interactome using a chemical proteomics approach in mammalian heart tissue validates sphingosine kinase type 1-interacting protein as a genuine and highly abundant AKAP. *J Proteome Res.* 2006; 5: 1435–47.

Schrattenholz A, Groebe K. What does it need to be a biomarker? Relationships between resolution, differential quantification and statistical validation of protein surrogate biomarkers. *Electrophoresis.* 2007; 28: 1970–79.

Schuerenberg M, Luebbert C, Eickhoff H, Kalkum M, Lehrach H, Nordhoff E. Prestructured MALDI-MS sample supports. *Anal Chem.* 2000; 72: 3436–42.

Sellers KF, Miecznikowski J, Viswanathan S, Minden JS, Eddy WF. Lights, camera, action! Systematic variation in 2-D difference gel electrophoresis images. *Electrophoresis.* 2007; 28: 3324–32.

Siffert W. G protein polymorphisms in hypertension, atherosclerosis, and diabetes. *Ann Rev Med.* 2005; 56: 17–28.

Staab CA, Ceder R, Jagerbrink T, Nilsson JA, Roberg K, Jornvall H, Höög JO, Grafström RC. Bioinformatics processing of protein and transcript profiles of normal and transformed cell lines indicates functional impairment of transcriptional regulators in buccal carcinoma. *J Proteome Res.* 2007; 6: 3705–17.

Stierum R, Burgemeister R, van Helvoort A, Peijnenburg A, Schutze K, Seidelin M, Vang O, van Ommen B. Functional food ingredients against colorectal cancer. An example project integrating functional genomics, nutrition and health. *Nutr Metab Cardiovasc Dis.* 2001; 11 Suppl 4: 94–98.

Swanson SK, Washburn MP. The continuing evolution of shotgun proteomics. *Drug Discov Today.* 2005; 10: 719–25.

Tan S, Seow TK, Liang RC, Koh S, Lee CP, Chung MC, Hooi SC. Proteome analysis of butyrate-treated human colon cancer cells (HT-29). *Int J Cancer.* 2002; 98: 523–31.

Tanaka K. The origin of macromolecule ionization by laser irradiation (Nobel lecture). *Angew Chem Int Ed Engl.* 2003; 42: 3860–70.

Thingholm TE, Jensen ON, Larsen MR. Analytical strategies for phosphoproteomics. *Proteomics.* 2009; 9: 1451–68.

Thompson A, Schafer J, Kuhn K, Kienle S, Schwarz J, Schmidt G, Neumann T, Hamon C. Tandem mass tags: A novel quantification strategy for comparative analysis of complex protein mixtures by MS/MS. *Anal Chem.* 2003; 75: 1895–904.

tom Dieck H, Doring F, Fuchs D, Roth HP, Daniel H. Transcriptome and proteome analysis identifies the pathways that increase hepatic lipid accumulation in zinc-deficient rats. *J Nutr.* 2005; 135: 199–205.

Trujillo E, Davis C, Milner J. Nutrigenomics, proteomics, metabolomics, and the practice of dietetics. *J Am Diet Assoc.* 2006; 106: 403–13.

Urfer W, Grzegorczyk M, Jung K. Statistics for proteomics: A review of tools for analyzing experimental data. *Proteomics.* 2006; 6: 48–55.

Wang J, Li D, Dangott LJ, Wu G. Proteomics and its role in nutrition research. *J Nutr.* 2006; 136: 1759–62.

Wilkins MR, Sanchez JC, Gooley AA, Appel RD, Humphrey-Smith I, Hochstrasser DF, Williams KL. Progress with proteome projects: Why all proteins expressed by a genome should be identified and how to do it. *Biotechnol Gene Eng Rev.* 1995; 13: 19–50.

Wilkins MR, Williams KL, Appel RD, Hochstrasser D. *Proteome Research: New Frontiers in Functional Genomics.* Springer-Verlag Berlin, Heidelberg; 1997.

Wilkins MS, Sanchez JC, Gooley AA, Appel RD, Humphery-Smith I, Hochstrasser DF, Williams KL. Progress with proteome projects: Why all proteins expressed by a genome should be identified and how to do it. *Biotechnol Genet Eng Rev.* 1996; 13: 19–50.

Wollscheid B, Bausch-Fluck D, Henderson C, O'Brien R, Bibel M, Schiess R, Aebersold R, Watts JD. Mass-spectrometric identification and relative quantification of N-linked cell surface glycoproteins. *Nat Biotechnol.* 2009; 27: 378–86.

Wong JW, Sullivan MJ, Cagney G. Computational methods for the comparative quantification of proteins in label-free LCn-MS experiments. *Brief Bioinform.* 2008; 9: 156–65.

Wood J, Alpers D, Andrews P. Fundamentals of neurogastroenterology. *Gut.* 1999; 45 Suppl 2: II6–II16.

Yocum AK, Chinnaiyan AM. Current affairs in quantitative targeted proteomics: Multiple reaction monitoring–mass spectrometry. *Brief Funct Genomic Proteomic.* 2009; 8: 145–57.

Zhang L, Perdomo G, Kim DH, Qu S, Ringquist S, Trucco M, Dong HH. Proteomic analysis of fructose-induced fatty liver in hamsters. *Metabolism.* 2008; 57: 1115–24.

Zubarev RA, Hakansson P, Sundqvist B. Accuracy requirements for peptide characterization by monoisotopic molecular mass measurements. *Anal Chem.* 1996; 68: 4060–3.

7

Application of Nutritional Metabolomics for Better Health and Healthcare

Avipsha Sarkar and Shampa Sen
VIT University
Vellore, India

Yashwant V. Pathak
University of South Florida
Tampa, Florida

Contents

7.1 Introduction	160
7.1.1 Metabolomics	160
7.1.1.1 Targeted metabolomics	160
7.1.1.2 Untargeted metabolomics	160
7.1.2 Pharmacogenomics to nutrigenomics	161
7.1.3 Personalized medicine includes personalized nutrition	161
7.2 Metabolomics in nutrition and toxicology	161
7.3 Metabolomics in medicine	162
7.4 Conceptual developments	162
7.5 Diet and gene expression	162
7.6 Risks of nutrigenomics and nutrigenetics	163
7.7 Practice of dietetics	163
7.8 Interindividual response to nutrients	164
7.9 Nutritional epigenetics	164
7.10 Microbiome-related metabolome	164
7.11 Future of nutrigenomics	165
7.12 Conclusion	165
References	166

7.1 Introduction

Nutrition is a very well-established foundation of health. The observed data account for the information that a low-nutritional diet, though defined rudimentarily, is the cause of disorders such as diabetes, metabolic imbalances, obesity, infectious and inflammatory diseases, hypertension, and osteoporosis [1].

A vast array of food chemicals can be metabolized by the human body. The way in which the metabolism of a human body reacts or responses to type as well as concentration variations of food chemicals provide a hint to perceive how health is affected by a diet. The mutual communication between genetic mechanisms and these dietary chemicals has a strong participation in managing health issues and inhibiting chronic disorders that are diet influenced [2].

7.1.1 Metabolomics

The complete testing and observation of metabolites in microbes, plants, and animals is known as metabolomics [3–5]. This so-called metabolome provides a better picture of the entire procedure of metabolism along with the fingerprint in the molecular level. Consequently, such a categorization acts as a biomarker and depicts the biological condition of any being [3,4]. Grouping or sorting between normal and diseased or test and control can be done by comparing the metabolome reports [3–5]. Metabolomic studies also help to supervise the outcome of various nutritional as well as pharmacological intrusions. Such a supervision is done by monitoring the phenotypic manipulations in the metabolome of test and unhealthy subjects toward healthier metabolome [3].

7.1.1.1 Targeted metabolomics

Under targeted metabolomics, certain definite metabolic procedures, for example, amino acids or fatty acids or other plant-derived chemicals related to particular metabolites, are analyzed [6–12]. This approach in almost all cases is influenced by hypothesis. Initially, there is a question that needs to be solved according to which the metabolites to be analyzed are chosen and they are completely quantified using certain analytical techniques. Targeted metabolomics thus provides an opportunity to emancipate information about various nutritional components with respect to their turnover, metabolism, concentration, or bioavailability.

7.1.1.2 Untargeted metabolomics

Under this category, all metabolites present in a biological being are screened. This is done for the metabolite profile comparison between samples. The ultimate goal of this procedure is almost similar to that of targeted approach. This helps to categorize the phenotype of a person in terms of their metabolism, to conclude the result of various nutritional intrusions, and also to determine the components present in food. The initial step in a traditional method is to extract the metabolites present in the samples, which is then isolated by techniques including gas and liquid chromatography or by mass spectrometer [13,14].

7.1.2 Pharmacogenomics to nutrigenomics

Explorations in the concepts of pharmacogenomics have highly emphasized the mutual interactions between the genotype and the environment. This recent advancement has helped to understand that a particular drug's efficiency as well as the extent of side effects varies with the variation in the genotype of humans. To enhance the safety issues of the drug along with its toxicity and efficiency, the clinical trials integrate genotyping in the process. Improved drugs are being produced that has smaller amount of side effects by the companies with the help of the relationship between genotype and phenotype. The part of the population that do not respond are identified, and novel drugs are being produced using compounds that were once considered to be very toxic to humans [2].

7.1.3 Personalized medicine includes personalized nutrition

The idea of "personalised" drugs has gained entry into the playing pitch of nutrition. Due to advancements in this area, the fact that both macro- and micronutrients play an important role in altering the genetic mechanisms like gene expression as well as the structure of DNA is now accepted. These alterations in turn change the beginning and progression of the disease. The metabolism, excretion, and incorporation of nutrients can also be manipulated by the genetic distinction of the individual [2].

7.2 Metabolomics in nutrition and toxicology

Nutrition can help inhibit as well as can be the reason for a particular disease. When the metabolomic is traced, certain compounds are disclosed by the diet intake report, for example, normal uptake of meat has been correlated with higher amounts of two compounds: 1-methylhistidine and anserine [3]. Red meat intake has been associated with the compound O-acetylcarnitine, and high amounts of phenylacetylglutamine are linked to the intake of vegetables [4]. Recent explorations have suggested that the concentration of chains of saturated fatty acids comprising glycerophosphatidylcholine is inversely linked to the ingestion of polyunsaturated fatty acids in adult men [5]. The epidemiological explorations can be perked up using metabolomics to calculate food occurrence surveys [3]. Deficit in certain nutrients can be detected using metabolomics. An individual's metabolomic summary at the baseline when studied with respect to choline (decrease and increase) was able to forecast whether the person will have liver dysfunction or not due to low intake of choline [6].

7.3 Metabolomics in medicine

Conventional definition of health is the deficit of any observable disorder. A disease is categorized as possessing a single origin and thus having one target of diagnosis. Since the complete mechanistic properties of most of the disorders are not known, cardiovascular disorders (CVDs) provide a prosperous area of explorations. Certain compounds present in the diet can either cause or inhibit CVD. Report suggests that the level of atherogenicity among hamsters that are hyperlipidemic are positively associated with the quantity of milk fat present in one's diet [7]. Esters present in plant sterols contain stearate that according to studies have lowered the low-density lipoprotein (LDL) present in cholesterol among humans [8]. There has been a huge difference in the metabolome of the hypercholesteremic pig's plasma with a special mention to betaine concentration due to intake of whole-grain rye diets when compared with wheat diets (nonwhole grain) [9]. The effect of diet on CVDs is the recent area of interest. Metabolomics tend to present hints of disease outcomes sooner by making available a clearer image of disease progression. In humans, this has provided new biomarkers for better diagnosis and treatment of acute myocardial ischemia [10]. The metabolites present in the plasma of normal human beings had specific differences from that of an individual having coronary syndrome and also those having unwavering atherosclerosis [11].

7.4 Conceptual developments

The change or shift to targeted metabolic explorations that unfolds the personal dietary needs from biochemical ones that gives the averages of the population is due to improvement in the concepts. The concepts are:

1. The collective exposures of an individual throughout have been integrated into health models. These are known as exposomes [12].
2. The replacement of dietary guidance to inhibit disorders with diet that is planned to provide optimal well-being that is known as predictive health [13].
3. The concept of using more than one interacting networks known as individual complexity [14].

7.5 Diet and gene expression

Though the degree of understanding of nutrigenomics is still very basic, it can be very clearly observed that the genomic reaction of a person completely synced to his dietary conditions. Other than humans, insects also react to the qualitative as well as quantitative intake of nutrients with the help of their biochemical and behavioural mechanistic properties [15]. At the molecular stage, these reactions are easily and clearly detectable. The insect *Locusta migratoria* experiences a low expression of the gene responsible for proliferation of nuclear antigen due to change in the ratio of protein and carbohydrate [16]. According to Zinke et al., when *Drosophlia melanogaster* was made to starve and also fed with high sugar, it induces the expression of certain genes [17].

7.6 Risks of nutrigenomics and nutrigenetics

Different methods can be utilised to understand both nutrigenetics and nutrigenomics. Ronteltap et al. [18] in 2007 reported that some scientists makes the study of interacting genes with nutrition narrow, whereas the rest along with the interactions also explores the applications of nutrigenetics in both inhibition and promotion of the disease [18]. The difference between the two is often unclear due to several contradictory definitions. Both nutrigenomics and nutrigenetics have gained interest for their prospective applications that benefits human health. Research in this field predicts the inhibition of dreadful diseases like diabetes a well as cancer with the help of personalized nutritional involvement. These include modified dietary components that are specific toward an individual's genetic properties, which enhance the health of the consumers [18,19]. The development in this field is challenged by socioethical contemplations, which in turn questions the probable achievability.

7.7 Practice of dietetics

The mechanistic epigenetic as well as genetic properties can be changed by a number of nutritional compounds, which in turn control the health. In addition to the indispensible dietary nutrients such as zinc, folate, calcium, vitamin C, selenium, and vitamin E, some bioactive compounds as well as the nonessential dietary nutrients also manipulate health notably. Figure 7.1 discusses about the nonessential nutrients that are known to affect health.

Nutrient group	Example
Bacteriochemicals	Butyrate and aspartame along with other components produced from fermentation of gastrointestinal flora
Phytochemicals	Indoles, carotenoids, isothiocyanates, floavonoids
Fungochemicals	Schizophyllan, beta-glucans lentinan

Figure 7.1 *Some nonessential nutrients and bioactive components that can alter genetic and epigenetic events.*

Application of Nutritional Metabolomics for Better Health and Healthcare   163

Several cellular mechanisms that are related to inhibition of the disease and maintaining health can be altered by both essential and nonessential dietary compounds. The mechanisms include balance of the hormones, apotosis, metabolism of the carcinogen, angiogenesis, and control of the cell cycle [20].

7.8 Interindividual response to nutrients

Almost all the genes consist of small variations after each 1,500 bases in their sequence among every person [21]. The efficiency of the protein and its interaction capability with its substrates as well as other proteins are affected by the polymorphisms. Motulsky in 1999 reported that the prediction of certain diseases used these gene polymorphisms as tools to screen and identify certain risks. Alzheimer's and cholesterol homeostasis could be predicted by using the gene polymorphisms of the E4 allele present on the APOE gene [22 and 34].

Some situations can depend entirely on single-nucleotide polymorphisms (SNPs), but the phenotype is majorly affected by a number of genes along with behavioural and surrounding environmental aspects. The introduction of changeability can be done successfully on SNPs or differences present on a single base in the DNA. Such locations that amount to three million have been recognised by scientists [23]. Polymorphic markers have become very useful for exploring any genetic mechanisms. SNPs are being used as markers since these are the most frequent type of sequence deviation in DNA.

7.9 Nutritional epigenetics

The activation of genes and other epigenetic proceedings can be altered by bioactive compounds. A number of enzymatic proteins such as histone-modifying enzymes, DNA methyltransferases, chromatin remodelling factors, and methyl cytosine guanine dinucleotide–binding proteins along with the molecular complexes are required for the epigenetic mechanisms [24]. Immediate development of tumor and DNA hypomethylation in rats were seen after administering them with methionine along with choline-deficit diet continuously [25].

7.10 Microbiome-related metabolome

It has been found out that the mammalian metabolome includes a huge input from the enteric microbiome leading to advancements in research. The mutual communication between the metabolism of a mouse with its gut microbial population was done by Martin et al. [26] utilising a top-down procedure of metabolomics. The top-down technique does not concentrate only on a targeted group but studies all the chemicals produced. When comparisons were done between a germ-free set of mice populated by human microflora to a traditional set of mice, it showed a simple linked network of metabolome. This network was observed to directly affect the capability of the host in terms of lipid metabolism. It was finally declared that at the level of organization, the microbiome present can manipulate the storage and absorption capabilities along with the energy that is harvested from nutrition. Early nutritional links with the host's immune system and the microbiota present are explored extensively as the association is thought to cause obesity and other chronic disorders [27,28]. Reports suggested that the metabolites consisting of indole that has been taken from tryptophan-like indoxyl sulphate are produced by certain bacteria [29]. According to the results, there is a noteworthy relationship existing between the metabolism of mammals and bacteria at the point where certain pathways are associated with a disease.

7.11 Future of nutrigenomics

Various techniques have been applied in genomic studies like metabolomics as well as transcriptomics or proteomics to produce information that is complimentary to each other, and each of these techniques stand at a different position in terms of their current development. The main target of nutritional biology is the complete phenotypic description of a complex biologically active system like a human being. The target can be achieved by utilising the above-mentioned methods [30,31,32]. Research does not depend on a single technique to answer all the questions and, therefore, a researcher should be absolutely lucid about what the study aims and its potential restrictions. The human hepatic system is very complex that requires a complete proteome as well as transcriptome study. The limitation is that there is no availability of hepatic tissue section readily. To the contrary, the analysis of metabolite plasma that acts as a marker would be a more viable option to detect any dysfunction of liver.

The technique of metabolomics [32–37]. is still in its developmental stage, where the number of metabolites located endogenously are still unknown and also the exact number of metabolites taken from food cannot be calculated from the human plasma or urine. Quite a lot of barriers should be conquered by the researchers that include the complete revival of metabolites that are present in tissue sections and other body fluids. The scientists should also build a large thorough database having complete information about the metabolome that is important nutritionally. The data mining requires modernized techniques and novel softwares to provide the required information from the huge data produced by the complete metabolomic study. Though the techniques are quite modern, the current softwares pose restrictions in the extraction of data. These restrictions are being looked after by a few groups of scientists since metabolomics have a high prospective in dietary applications [37,38].

7.12 Conclusion

A comment stated by Peter Medawar said that expectations regarding the future are built by wiser group of the population, whereas the foolish ones only craft predictions [39]. This was perceived as a clever advice by all the molecular nutritionists. The studies related to nutrigenomics as well as nutrigenetics are expected to detect as well as validate the SNPs and the genes that can be manipulated by nutrients thereby inhibiting any disease progression and hence maintaining health. These studies will incorporate a huge set of novel data as well as new food components thereby promoting the initialization of guidelines based on diet. The ultimate goal of nutritional science is to manage health issues and also inhibit the progression of disease which has gained high acceleration recently due to improved techniques of computational biology with a helping hand from molecular biology. Inspite of everything, the proper deciphering of scientific and therapeutic advice still depends on the researchers along with the physicians. The obstinacy of medicine based on evidence is thought to play a crucial function in the proliferation of nutrigenetic proposal. The society of health care with such nutrigenetic studies provides a prospect for dietitians to define their position in a novel way. Along with their redefined position that can be termed as "nutrigenetic counselors," they are endowed with responsibilities and innovative training.

The complete knowledge of nutrigenomics has the potential to increase business load among the various industries dealing with food since "mass-marketing" shifts to "mass-customization." At the end, there still remains a dilemma among the people whether or not to accept nutrigenetic procedures. This dilemma arises due to a debate regarding bioethical issues in terms of worldwide and personal equity in health. To overcome this, the provision of guidelines with respect to nutrigenetics should be highly encouraged [40,41].

References

1. German JB, Roberts MA, Watkins SM. Genomics and metabolomics as markers for the interaction of diet and health: Lessons from lipids. *J Nutr* 2003; 133: 2078S–83S.
2. *The NCMHD Centre for Excellence for Nutritional Genomics.*
3. Nicholson JK, Holmes E, Kinross JM, Darzi AW, Takats Z, Lindon JC. Metabolic phenotyping in clinical and surgical environments. *Nature* 2012; 491: 384–392.
4. Patti GJ, Yanes O, Siuzdak G. Innovation: Metabolomics: The apogee of the omics trilogy. *Nat Rev Mol Cell Biol* 2012; 13: 263–269.
5. Fiehn O. Metabolomics—The link between genotypes and phenotypes. *Plant Mol Biol* 2002; 48: 155–171.
6. Nicolaou A, Masoodi M, Mir A. Lipidomic analysis of prostanoids by liquid chromatography-electrospray tandem mass spectrometry. *Methods Mol Biol* 2009; 579: 271–286.
7. Lundstrom SL, Saluja R, Adner M, Haeggstrom JZ, Nilsson G, Wheelock CE. Lipid mediator metabolic profiling demonstrates differences in eicosanoid patterns in two phenotypically distinct mast cell populations. *J Lipid Res* 2013; 54: 116–126.
8. Giordano G, Di Gangi IM, Gucciardi A, Naturale M. Quantification of underivatised amino acids on dry blood spot, plasma, and urine by HPLC-ESI-MS/MS. *Methods Mol Biol* 2012; 828: 219–242.
9. Gucciardi A, Pirillo P, Di Gangi IM, Naturale M, Giordano G. A rapid UPLC-MS/MS method for simultaneous separation of 48 acylcarnitines in dried blood spots and plasma useful as a second-tier test for expanded newborn screening. *Anal Bioanal Chem* 2012; 404: 741–751.

10. Serhan CN, Samuelsson B. Lipoxins: A new series of eicosanoids (biosynthesis, stereochemistry, and biological activities). *Adv Exp Med Biol* 1988; 229: 1–14.
11. Cortina MS, Bazan HE. Docosahexaenoic acid, protectins and dry eye. *Curr Opin Clin Nutr Metab Care* 2011; 14: 132–137.
12. Vrhovsek U, Masuero D, Gasperotti M, Franceschi P, Caputi L, Viola R, et al. A versatile targeted metabolomics method for the rapid quantification of multiple classes of phenolics in fruits and beverages. *J Agric Food Chem* 2012; 60: 8831–8840.
13. Rainville PD, Stumpf CL, Shockcor JP, Plumb RS, Nicholson JK. Novel application of reversed-phase UPLC-oaTOF-MS for lipid analysis in complex biological mixtures: A new tool for lipidomics. *J Proteome Res* 2007; 6: 552–558.
14. Castro-Perez JM, Kamphorst J, DeGroot J, Lafeber F, Goshawk J, Yu K, et al. Comprehensive LC-MS E lipidomic analysis using a shotgun approach and its application to biomarker detection and identification in osteoarthritis patients. *J Proteome Res* 2010; 9: 2377–2389.
15. Dragsted LO. Biomarkers of meat intake and the application of nutrigenomics. *Meat Sci* 2010; 84: 301–307.
16. O'Sullivan A, Gibney MJ, Brennan L. Dietary intake patterns are reflected in metabolomic profiles: Potential role in dietary assessment studies. *Am J Clin Nutr* 2011; 93: 314–321.
17. Altmaier E, Kastenmuller G, Romisch-Margl W, Thorand B, Weinberger KM, Illig T, et al. Questionnaire-based self-reported nutrition habits associate with serum metabolism as revealed by quantitative targeted metabolomics. *Eur J Epidemiol* 2010; 26(2): 145–156.
18. Sha W, da Costa KA, Fischer LM, Milburn MV, Lawton KA, Berger A, et al. Metabolomic profiling can predict which humans will develop liver dysfunction when deprived of dietary choline. *FASEB J* 2010; 24: 2962–2975.
19. Martin JC, Canlet C, Delplanque B, Agnani G, Lairon D, Gottardi G, et al. 1H NMR metabonomics can differentiate the early atherogenic effect of dairy products in hyperlipidemic hamsters. *Atherosclerosis* 2009; 206: 127–133.
20. Carr T, Krogstrand K, Schlegel V, Fernandez M. Stearate-enriched plant sterol esters lower serum LDL cholesterol concentration in normo- and hypercholesterolemic adults. *J Nutr* 2009; 139: 1445–1450.
21. Bertram HC, Malmendal A, Nielsen NC, Straadt IK, Larsen T, Knudsen KE, et al. NMR-based metabonomics reveals that plasma betaine increases upon intake of high-fiber rye buns in hypercholesterolemic pigs. *Mol Nutr Food Res* 2009; 53: 1055–1062.
22. Sabatine MS, Liu E, Morrow DA, Heller E, McCarroll R, Wiegand R, et al. Metabolomic identification of novel biomarkers of myocardial ischemia. *Circulation* 2005; 112: 3868–3875.
23. Vallejo M, García A, Tuñón J, García-Martínez D, Angulo S, Martin-Ventura JL, et al. Plasma fingerprinting with GC-MS in acute coronary syndrome. *Anal Bioanal Chem* 2009; 394: 1517–1524.
24. Wild CP. Complementing the genome with an "exposome": The outstanding challenge of environmental exposure measurement in molecular epidemiology. *Cancer Epidemiol Biomarkers Prev* 2005; 14: 1847–1850.
25. Markley JL, Anderson ME, Cui Q, Eghbalnia HR, Lewis IA, Hegeman AD, et al. New bioinformatics resources for metabolomics. *Pac Symp Biocomput* 2007; 12: 157–168.
26. Draper J, Enot DP, Parker D, Beckmann M, Snowdon S, Lin W, et al. Metabolite signal identification in accurate mass metabolomics data with MZedDB, an interactive m/z annotation tool utilising predicted ionisation behaviour 'rules'. *BMC Bioinformatics* 2009; 10: 227.
27. Chown SL, Nicholson SW. *Insect Physiological Ecology: Mechanisms and Patterns.* Oxford University Press, Oxford; 2004, pp. 14–48.
28. Zudaire E, Simpson SJ, Illa I, Montuenga LM. Dietary influences over proliferating cell nuclear antigen expression in the locust midgut. *J Exp Biol* 2004; 205: 2255–2265.

29. Zinke I, Schutz S, Kattzenberger D, Bauer M, Panratz MJ. Nutrient control of gene expression in *Drosophila:* Microarray analysis of starvation and sugar-dependent response. *EMBO J* 2002; 21: 6162–6173.
30. Ronteltap A, van Trijp H, Renes RJ. Expert views on critical success and failure factors for nutrigenomics. *Trends Food Sci Technol* 2007; 18: 189–200. doi:10.1016/j.tifs.2006.12.007.
31. Godard B, Hurlimann T. Nutrigenomics for global health: Ethical challenges for underserved populations. *CPPM* 2009; 7: 205–214.
32. Davis CD, Uthus EO. DNA methylation, cancer susceptibility, and nutrient interactions. *Exp Biol Med (Maywood)* 2004; 229: 988–995.
33. Livingston RJ, von Niederhausern A, Jegga AG, Crawford DC, Carlson CS, Rieder MJ, et al. Pattern of sequence variation across 213 environmental response genes. *Genome Res* 2004; 14: 1821–1831.
34. Motulsky AG. If I had a gene test, what would I have and who would I tell? *The Lancet* 1999; 354(suppl 1): SI35–SI37.
35. Jiang R, Duan J, Windemuth A, Stephens JC, Judson R, Xu C. Genome-wide evaluation of the public SNP databases. *Pharmacogenomics* 2003; 4: 779–789.
36. Ross SA. Diet and DNA methylation interactions in cancer prevention. *Ann N Y Acad Sci* 2003; 983: 197–207.
37. Poirier LA. The role of methionine in carcinogenesis in vivo. *Adv Exp Med Biol* 1986; 206: 269–282.
38. Martin FP, Dumas ME, Wang Y, Legido-Quigley C, Yap IK, Tang H, et al. A top-down systems biology view of microbiome mammalian metabolic interactions in a mouse model. *Mol Syst Biol.* 2007; 3: 112.
39. Campbell P. Tales of the expected. *Nature* 1999; 402(suppl): C7–C9.
40. Editorial. Defining a new bioethic. *Nat Genet* 2001; 28: 297–298.
41. Singer P. *University of Toronto Program in Applied Ethics and Biotechnology.* Canadian Program in Genomics and Global Health; 2001. Available at: www.utoronto.ca/jcb.

8

Facts and Controversies Based on Diet, Genomics, and Cancer

Roland Cadet, Charles Preuss, and Yashwant V. Pathak
University of South Florida
Tampa, Florida

Contents

8.1 Introduction 170
8.2 Diet and cancer facts and controversies 171
    8.2.1 Cancer causes and controversies: Understanding risk reduction and prevention 171
    8.2.2 Toxicological aspects of saccharin 173
    8.2.3 Nutrients 174
    8.2.4 New insights into the health effects of dietary saturated and omega-6 and omega-3 polyunsaturated fatty acids 175
    8.2.5 Dietary fats and health: Dietary recommendations in the context of scientific evidence 177
    8.2.6 Fruit and vegetable consumption in adolescence and early adulthood and risk of breast cancer: Population-based cohort study 178
8.3 Genomics/cancer 178
    8.3.1 Current concepts of pheochromocytoma 178
    8.3.2 Genomics and health in the developing world 179
    8.3.3 Mitochondria organelle transplantation: A potential cellular biotherapy for cancer 181
    8.3.4 A specific mesothelial signature marks the heterogeneity of mesenchymal stem cells from high-grade serous ovarian cancer 182
    8.3.5 Network-based proteomic approaches reveal the neurodegenerative, neuroprotective, and pain-related mechanisms involved after retrograde axonal damage 183
    8.3.6 Combining clinicopathological and molecular pathway signatures for improving clinical decisions through an understanding of CRC biology 184

8.4 Diet/genomics/cancer..185

    8.4.1 Impact of genetic and epigenetic variations within the fatty acid desaturase cluster on the composition and metabolism of PUFAs in PCa 185

    8.4.2 Meta-analysis of genome-wide association study of homeostasis model assessment beta cell function and insulin resistance in East Asian population and the European results...186

    8.4.3 Plasma 25-hydroxyvitamin D3 is associated with decreased risk of postmenopausal breast cancer in whites: A nested case-control study in a multiethnic cohort study 187

8.5 Conclusion 188

References...189

8.1 Introduction

Cancer, the uncontrolled growth and spread of abnormal cells, is the second leading cause of death in the United States, after heart or cardiovascular disease. According to the American Cancer Society in *Cancer Facts and Figures 2016*, cancer accounts for one of every four deaths in the United States, and 595,690 Americans are expected to die of cancer in 2016. Although the number of expected deaths from cancer seems high for this year, the report revealed that cancer deaths and cancer prevalence have been reduced considerably since 1991. This decrease resulted from the intensive cancer prevention effort in the US population and new effective treatments that were discovered. For example, the intensive prevention program against cigarette smoking and unhealthy diet contributed a lot to reducing cancer in United States (American Cancer Society 2016).

According to the same report from the American Cancer Society, the risk of developing cancer is 42% (one in two) in men and 38% (one in three) in women. Cigarette smoking, eating unhealthy food, and physical inactivity are the most common risk factors associated with cancer. As a result, unhealthy behaviors increase cancer risks. As cigarette smoking has decreased over the last two decades, unhealthy diet has remained one important risk factor for cancer to be controlled. Junk and fast food continue to dominate the food culture in the United States. Fast food restaurants and supermarkets are growing considerably in United States. Still, vegetable and organic products remain expensive and less available in many US supermarkets. Consequently, the US government must continue the effort to promote "Healthy Plate" among the US population to reduce the cancer rate. Public or government action must be taken to reduce the consumption of unhealthy foods that remain one important risk factor of many types of cancer (American Cancer Society 2016).

Food is an important cultural indicator in American society. Regulation of diet to combat cancer and whether food causes cancer has been a source of many

170   Nutrigenomics and Nutraceuticals

disputes and controversies among scientists, researchers, businesspeople, and politicians. It is very important to be informed about the last statistics and controversies surrounding diet and cancer. Prevention, action, and treatment cannot be improved without a good understanding of the information about diet and cancer.

In recent years, researchers and scientists have discovered that most cancers are also a result of gene mutations. Genetics and the human genome are involved in many types of cancer. This fact has led researchers to study the human genome and gene-associated cancer. They believe that a comprehensive analysis of the human genome and the mutated genes involved in cancer could help them to find a better cure or treatment for cancer. As a result, a new discipline called *genomics* was introduced in the study and treatment of cancer. More importantly, the introduction of genomics to cancer treatment has allowed researchers to combine the molecular specificity of a drug with the genetic and pathophysiologic specificity of a drug target to provide more and more selective therapies (Golan 2012).

Cancer is the second leading cause of death after heart disease in the United States. There has been a great deal of research about cancer treatment and many cancer prevention programs throughout the country and worldwide. After the decrease in cigarette smoking, diet constitutes an important cancer risk factor to be controlled. In addition, gene mutations are involved in most cancers, so scientists developed a new discipline called *genomics* for the study and treatment of cancer. In their cancer studies, scientists sought to support their hypotheses regarding cancer study and treatment. As a result, many controversies and disputes among cancer specialists emerged. Today, the need for constant review on diet, genomics, and cancer has become important for better decision-making and better therapy options. In this paper, a review of different facts and controversies based on diet, genomics, and cancer will be developed.

8.2 Diet and cancer facts and controversies

8.2.1 Cancer causes and controversies: Understanding risk reduction and prevention

In his book *Cancer Causes and Controversies: Understanding Risk Reduction and Prevention*, Bernard Kwabi-Addo, the author, recaps how cancer was an old incurable disease discovered in the United States a long time ago. Most of the different types of cancer that were diagnosed were caused by the environment, people's lifestyles, or DNA modification. During the early and mid-twentieth century, cancer cases were high. CRC, stomach cancer, prostate cancer (PCa), and breast cancer were increasing. However, when authorities started to prevent cancer by educating the population, bringing refrigeration to store food to the population, and improving the living conditions of the population, the US cancer rate declined. In recent years, there have been far fewer people living with cancer or dying from cancer despite the fact that most cancer has no cure. Why? The author believes that the authorities and many organizations helped the population to make healthier lifestyle choices such as eating well, exercising, and not smoking or drinking alcohol excessively. A healthier diet has been linked to cancer reduction in the United States. In addition, the population was warned to avoid occupational exposure to toxins and infection. In term of prevention, the US authorities and many organizations have educated the population and encourage the population to do screenings for early diagnostic. Most often, the authorities and organizations did prevention without a deep action. As a result, the author wanted to put emphasis on the understanding of risk and prevention for a better cure for cancer. US authorities and organizations need to examine and understand the different screening techniques, dietary supplements, and potentially toxic environmental exposures.

Among the most common types of cancer, bladder cancer was first associated with industrial environments, according to Kwabi-Addo. A long time ago, in 1885, Dr. Ludwig Rhen, a German surgeon, discovered that some workers were being exposed to a dangerous dye that contained the cancerous constituents alpha- and beta-naphthylamine. Bladder cancer is mainly due to workplace environment. According to the National Cancer Institute, about 70,530 cases of bladder cancer were diagnosed in the United States in 2010. Men are two to three times more vulnerable to bladder cancer compared to women. Smokers are also two to three times more subject to bladder cancer than nonsmokers. Like most cancer, the risk of bladder increases with age. If a person is old and is exposed to risk factors, he or she has a better chance of getting bladder cancer (Kwabbi-Addo et al. 2011).

Patients diagnosed with bladder cancer often see blood in the urine, and sometimes they cannot urinate even though they feel the urge. If the bladder cancer persists, they may experience abdominal pain and aches in their bones. These symptoms are not sure, but they can be an indicator to see a urologist for diagnostic and treatment. In addition, smoking, occupational exposure, and environment are the most common risk factors associated with bladder cancer. First, according to studies, current and former smokers are at great risk of bladder cancer, even though former smokers showed a 30%–40% reduction in bladder cancer risk after 1 year. Second, there are many carcinogenic or toxic compounds that workers are exposed to in industry. For example, the aromatic amines that are used in many dyes and pigments for plastics, paints, textiles, hair dyes, drugs, and pesticides increase the risk of bladder cancer among industrial workers. In consequence, printers, autoworkers, dry cleaners, metal workers, textile workers, dental technicians, leather workers, truck drivers, hairstylists, and barbers are all exposed to bladder cancer risks. Third, the authors stated that all things that are natural are safe to consume. For example, in Taiwan, people are at risk of bladder cancer because researchers found that the groundwater contained arsenic. Even though it has not been confirmed, some studies have pointed out that nitrogen-based fertilizers and pesticides in Spain and the United States often contaminate well water with nitrates, increasing the risk of bladder cancer. Fourth, some parasites may be involved in bladder cancer risks in developing countries. For example, a parasite called *Schistosomiasis haematobium* located in Egypt's Nile River valley and other parts of Africa is primarily responsible for some bladder cancer cases. Finally, there may be a genetic risk factor for bladder cancer, but it is uncommon. Generally, bladder cancer is due to occupational exposure and tobacco (Kwabbi-Addo et al. 2011).

According to many studies, bladder cancer can be prevented and reduced. First, fruits and vegetables are largely recommended to reduce bladder cancer risks. Green and yellow varieties of fruits and vegetables have the most protective effect against bladder cancer. Second, nonsmokers who eat well also have less risk of having bladder cancer. Third, people who eat high levels of saturated fats multiply their risks of having bladder cancer. Fourth, many studies have suggested that drinking a lot of water could possibly reduce the risk of bladder cancer. These studies believed that water has the power to dilute carcinogens found in the body and excrete them through urine. However, other studies have minimized the fact that drinking a lot of water can reduce bladder cancer, making this fact controversial. More studies must be done to confirm the evidence that drinking a lot of water can reduce or eliminate bladder cancer risks. Finally, scientists discovered that people in Asia have the fewest bladder cancer cases in the world. They discovered that the green tea contains polyphenols that interfere with many processes that can damage DNA and induce cancer (Kwabbi-Addo et al. 2011).

8.2.2 Toxicological aspects of saccharin

Saccharin is a chemical food additive recognized for its sweetness. For this reason, researchers believed that saccharin could replace the sugar or glucose that human consumed. Saccharin could be used as an excellent sugar replacement for diabetics. However, after its discovery in 1879, researchers found that saccharin could cause bladder cancer in rats that consumed too much saccharin. After that discovery, the use of saccharin in humans became controversial. Many researchers continued to study the carcinogenicity of saccharin. While some researchers remained skeptical, many others were persuaded that these results concerned only rats or animals, and they let people or industries continue to use low doses of saccharin in human consumption (Singh 2013).

In 1958, saccharin was classified as "generally recognized as safe." However, this status did not remove the doubts about saccharin use in humans. Again in 1970, researchers discovered a positive association between saccharin and bladder cancer in two generations of bioassays in rats. After that, the controversy flared up again. In 1973, Hick's research paper titled, "Impurities in Saccharin and Bladder Cancer," confirmed these doubts (Singh 2013).

The 1970s and 1980s was a period of great controversy about the carcinogenicity of saccharin. In England, in 1975, Armstrong and Doll conducted a study on bladder cancer mortality in diabetics who consumed saccharin. They analyzed the death certificates of 18,377 diabetic patients who died from bladder cancer. Despite the diabetics consuming more saccharin than the nondiabetics, the researchers found no relation between diabetes of long duration and increased bladder cancer risk (Singh 2013).

In 1977, after Culliton's article titled, "Cancer Society Take Pro-Saccharin Stand," the controversy flared up again. Then, in 1978, researchers started to study saccharin again and publish research papers on saccharin carcinogenicity. For example, in 1979, Cohen revealed that saccharin was a potent agent of short latent bladder cancer in male Fischer rats. Then, in 1980, Hooson discovered the carcinogenicity of saccharin and ortho-toluene sulfonamide in rats. However, his study did not find any of the tumor-promoting abilities that Cohen evoked in his research. Nonetheless, he did notice an increase in proliferative lesions in rat urinary bladders. Then, in the same year, Schmahl and Habs showed that the application of cyclamate and saccharin during pregnancy does not cause any type of cancer risk in Sprague Dawley rats. Despite the results of these studies, the possible carcinogenicity of saccharin still animated different debates among researchers. Thus, researchers tried to look at the mechanisms of saccharin that cause cancer. Between 1980 and 1993, many studies were conducted on saccharin carcinogenicity. In 1991, Okamura demonstrated that sodium saccharin was not related to bladder cancer in male rats fed an AIN-76A diet. Then, Chappel reviewed his study in 1992. He discovered that saccharin did not cause bladder cancer in humans. Finally, in 2000, as a result of the lack of evidence in previous research, the US National Toxicology Program removed saccharin from its list of carcinogens and the International Agency for Research on Cancer changed the saccharin rating from Group 2B (possibly carcinogenic to humans) to Group 3 (not classifiable as to the carcinogenicity to humans). Now, saccharin can be used as an additive in the food industry (Singh 2013).

8.2.3 Nutrients

Humans need nutrients such as carbohydrates, protein, and lipids to survive. These nutrients are so essential that everyone is aware of their benefits. However, excess of these nutrients can cause serious problems to the human body. Some types of cancer, from colorectal to breast cancer, may develop. In this article, the author put emphasis on the association between carbohydrates and breast cancer. Excessive consumption of starch, a carbohydrate, could provoke breast cancer. There are very few research papers and studies about this association. The few that are available never put in evidence the relative association between breast cancer risk and carbohydrates (Ronco 2012).

In many countries like Italy and the United States, the consumption of starch is high among the population. The vast majority of foods contain a high percentage of starch. For example, in Italy, the major foods consumed by the population are white bread and pasta that are rich in starch. According to one study in Italy, the researchers were the first to reveal an association between starch consumption and breast cancer. The results were significant but they remain small (40%) to predict that consumption of starch is related to breast cancer risk. The researchers deduced that the metabolic link between high-glycemic foods, insulin peaks, inflammation, and the development of cancers should be taken into account for verification of the association of starch with breast cancer risk. After the negative result from the previous study, other researchers studied Asian-Americans whose diet consisted of low-starch intake and high intake of legumes. They discovered that this diet contributed to a reduced breast cancer risk. The Asian Americans who consumed more legumes than starch presented no association between starch association and breast cancer risk (Ronco 2012).

According to many studies, dietary fiber is always viewed as a good component of food. It helps people digest their food and it prevents many types of cancer. Hypothetically, dietary fiber has a good virtue into people's food consumption. Many cohort studies showed a protective association of dietary fiber against breast cancer risk. For example, consumption of high fiber bread significantly decreased breast cancer incidence in Sweden (odds ratio [OR] = 0.75, 95% CI 0.57–0.98). In another study in England premenopausal women, not postmenopausal women, also presented a significant inverse relationship between total fiber intake and risk of breast cancer (OR = 0.48, 95% CI 0.24–0.96). In other parts of the world, in a rural Chinese population who consumed 70–80 g/day of fiber, compared to the lower fiber intake in Western countries (5–20g/day), researchers also found a reduced association between dietary fiber consumption and breast cancer risk (Ronco 2012).

According to many studies presented in this article, there is no significant relationship between carbohydrate or starch intake and breast cancer risk. The epidemiologic associations between fiber and the risk of breast cancer are probaby due to the presence of bioactive components of fiber-rich foods such as carotenoids, isoflavones, or lignans (Ronco 2012).

8.2.4 New insights into the health effects of dietary saturated and omega-6 and omega-3 polyunsaturated fatty acids

A long time ago, fats were recognized as a risk factor for cardiovascular diseases and cancer, especially breast cancer. There are two main types of fats that often capture the attention of scientists and dieticians. The first type is saturated fats, which contain no double bonds. These fats are usually considered bad fats, since they increase cardiovascular risks in humans. The second type is polyunsaturated fats, which contain one or more double bonds in their structure. Polyunsaturated fats are usually viewed as good fats, since they show reduced cardiovascular and cancer risks in humans (De Lorgeril et al. 2012).

Among polyunsaturated fats, omega-3 fatty acids and omega-6 fatty acids, found especially in marine plant and animals, became a type of polyunsaturated fat available for human consumption. The Mediterranean diet is a good example of the complex combination of saturated fats, omega-6 and omega-3 unsaturated fats, and conjugated and nonconjugated animal or industrial trans-fatty acids. This complex combination of fats in the Mediterranean diet makes the epidemiological data difficult to interpret and it explains the controversy about dietary fats and cardiovascular disease risks. In this article, the author tries to analyze the complexity of dietary fats in the Mediterranean diet in order to provide new insights concerning the effects of dietary fats on cardiovascular disease complications and mortality (De Lorgeril et al. 2012).

Recent studies have come up with a new concept called *preconditioning* to approach the association between dietary fats and cardiovascular diseases. By definition, preconditioning is the ability of the myocardium to withstand an ischemia–reperfusion injury. This has become a major concept in cardiology. However, drug makers have failed to identify pharmacological methods capable of inducing chronic preconditioning. As a result, according to clinical and experimental data, researchers revealed that lifestyle, including moderate alcohol drinking and physical exercise, is the potent preconditioner (De Lorgeril et al. 2012).

In many animal studies, researchers found that omega-6 polyunsaturated fatty acids (PUFAs) could cause mammary tumors. Omega-6 PUFAs, common in Western foods, undergo oxidative metabolization through the lipoxygenase and cyclooxygenase pathways to exert their carcinogenic effect. Dietary linoleic acid becomes arachidonic acid through this transformation. This oxidation of omega-6 showed that omega-6 fatty acids are linked to breast cancer risk. The researchers found that 5-lipoxygenase, which is a genetic predisposition related to omega-6 fatty acid metabolism, determined the breast cancer risk. The other factors that might influence breast cancer risk are the obesity profile and the amount of omega-3 and omega-6 fatty acids that people consume (De Lorgeril et al. 2012).

In sum, in this article, the author demonstrated the potential confusion about the effects of dietary fats on cardiovascular diseases and breast cancer. The complex mixture of saturated and polyunsaturated omega-3 and omega-6 fatty acids refined the theories regarding the positive association between dietary fats and cardiovascular disease and breast cancer. However, these studies have allowed a better approach to the use of dietary fats. Like in Mediterranean cultures, people should consume small amounts of saturated fats, moderate amounts of omega-6 PUFAs, and more omega-3 PUFAs to reduce the risk of cardiovascular disease and breast cancer (De Lorgeril et al. 2012).

8.2.5 Dietary fats and health: Dietary recommendations in the context of scientific evidence

According to early studies, saturated fats are associated with cardiovascular disease. They increase the LDL cholesterol serum in the body. Lawrence (2013) suggests that all coronary artery diseases or cardiovascular diseases are associated with dietary saturated fats. Other risk factors could come into play and cause cardiovascular disease and death. The author mentioned that saturated fatty acids (SFAs) found in dairy products and coconut oil can ameliorate health. For this reason, the author called for a rational reevaluation of existing dietary recommendations that separate dietary SFAs that lack a mechanism for adverse health effects (Lawrence 2013).

High levels of LDL cholesterol serum from saturated fats have always been tied to cardiovascular diseases. However, later on, researchers found that high levels of HDL cholesterol in the blood could also induce cardiovascular disease risks. As a result, many researchers started to study the mechanisms by which dietary fats and specific types of fatty acids regulate cholesterol and lipoprotein serum. In the 1990s, they discovered a family of proteins known as *sterol regulatory element binding proteins* (SREBPs). These proteins travel to the nucleus via cholesterol-depleted cells to modify the transcription of several genes involved in lipid metabolism. When intracellular cholesterol levels are low, SREBP-1 promotes the expression of genes for synthesis of cholesterol and LDL receptors that remove cholesterol from circulation. When intracellular cholesterol is high, SREBP-1 is not activated by protease cleavage, and the genes for cholesterol production and LDL receptors are downregulated. Moreover, SREBP-1 also activates promoters for genes involved in fatty acids synthesis and lipid storage. As a result, when PUFAs are present, one can notice decreased expression of SREBPs and enzymes for cholesterol synthesis, and the serum cholesterol pool decreases (Lawrence 2013).

Dairy fat and coconut contain short-chain SFAs that can influence gene expression via interactions with G-protein-coupled receptor, linked to hormonal responses such as insulin and leptin. Attempts to correlate saturated fats with disease are complicated by human food preferences that favor both fats and sugar. Sugars in food undergo oxidation with fructose, and they get oxidized many times faster than glucose. The main products from sugar oxidation are glyoxal, methylglyoxal, and formaldehyde. According to many clinical studies, fewer events are observed when polyunsaturated oils replace saturated fats. However, a recent meta-analysis showed that interventions using mixed omega-3 and omega-6 PUFAs resulted in a 22% decrease in coronary artery disease events. Then, the interventions that used omega-6 PUFAs with no omega-3 fatty acids showed 16% more cardiovascular events. However, more studies are required to confirm the significance of these interventions (Lawrence 2013).

Finally, many diseases such as cancer, atherosclerosis, type 2 diabetes, and endothelial dysfunction seem to be related to the oxidation of PUFAs.

Thus, SFAs may not be responsible for many of the adverse health effects. Instead, oxidation of PUFAs in those foods may be the cause of any associations that may be found. As a result, the dietary recommendations to restrict saturated fats in the diet should be revised to reflect the differences in handling before consumption (Lawrence 2013).

8.2.6 Fruit and vegetable consumption in adolescence and early adulthood and risk of breast cancer: Population-based cohort study

In this article, the researchers evaluated the association between fruit and vegetable intake during adolescence and early adulthood and risk of breast cancer. They designed a prospective cohort study and they invited health professionals in the United States. This cohort study included 90,476 premenopausal women aged 27–44 from the Nurses' Health Study II who completed a questionnaire on diet in 1991. The cohort also contained 44,223 women who completed a questionnaire about their diet during adolescence in 1998 (Farvid et al. 2016).

The researchers noted 3,235 cases of invasive breast cancer during follow-up in 2013. Among these cases, 1,347 cases were women who had completed a questionnaire about their diet during adolescence (ages 13–18). Thus, total fruit consumption during adolescence was associated with lower risk of breast cancer. However, the association of fruit intake during adolescence was independent of adult fruit intake. Thus, the researchers confirmed that they observed no association between breast cancer risk and total fruit intake in early adulthood and total vegetable intake in either adolescence or early adulthood. Only higher early adulthood intake of fruits and vegetable rich in alpha carotene was capable of reducing premenopausal breast cancer. For example, individuals who consumed a great quantity of apples, bananas, and grapes during adolescence and oranges and kale during early adulthood showed a significantly reduced risk of breast cancer. However, fruit juice intake in adolescence or early adulthood was related to breast cancer risk (Farvid et al. 2016).

In this study, the author confirmed the existence of an association between higher fruit intake and lower risk of breast cancer. Thus, food choices during adolescence have a great impact on breast cancer risk (Farvid et al. 2016).

8.3 Genomics/cancer

8.3.1 Current concepts of pheochromocytoma

Pheochromocytoma (PCC) is a rare neuroendocrine tumor initiated from the adrenal medulla or from chromaffin cells in sympathetic ganglia. This disease is more common in women in their forties and fifties. In the United States, the incidence rate is 2–8 cases per million per year. The only treatment is

178 Nutrigenomics and Nutraceuticals

surgical resection, which carries a high risk of hypertensive crises. One in ten patients has malignant PCC; in one of ten cases the tumor is bilateral. Inheritance genetic and surgical management is one of the controversies with PCC (Conzo 2014).

PCC is a hereditary disease. The most common hereditary causes of PCC include multiple endocrine neoplasia type 2A and 2B (MEN2A/2B), von Hippel–Lindau syndrome, neurofibromatosis type 1, and familial PCC/paraganglioma syndromes. MEN2A is characterized by a lifelong risk of developing medullary thyroid carcinoma (MTC), which occurred in 95% of patients. PCC is associated with MEN2A and MEN2B but rarely with familial MTC (Conzo 2014).

MEN2 is an autosomal dominant inherited syndrome. Its occurrence is estimated at 1 in 35,000 persons. Twenty years ago, germline mutations of the rearranged during transfection (RET) proto-oncogene were responsible for the disease. RET activation leads to stimulation of multiple downstream pathways, including mitogen-activated protein kinase B, signal transducer and activator of transcription 3, and proto-oncogene tyrosine-protein kinase B, which all promote cell growth, proliferation, survival, and differentiation. MEN2-associated mutations are located in Exons 10, 11, or 13–16 of the gene (Conzo 2014).

PCC occurs in up to 50% of individuals with MEN2A and MEN2B that bear mutation of codon 634 (MEN2A) and codon (MEN2B) respectively. PCC is often associated with high risk of mutations for MTC; thus its presence may imply a more aggressive thyroid tumor. PCC developed after the identification of MTC constitutes the initial manifestation of the syndrome (Conzo 2014).

Less than 3% of sporadic PCC occurs before the age of 50 years. These cases are due to germline mutations of the RET proto-oncogene. In order to detect MEN2-associated PCC, researchers must use routine biochemical screening or screen for symptoms such as hypertension, palpitations, headache, tachycardia, or sweating. The typical age of onset is the third decade of life, 10–20 years earlier than the typical age of sporadic PCC development. As the treatment of PCC rise controversies among scientists, the American Thyroid Association has published management guidelines for initial diagnosis, therapeutic intervention, and long-term follow-up based on the patient's genotype and the current understanding of the natural history of the disease associated with each RET mutation (Conzo 2014).

8.3.2 Genomics and health in the developing world

All inherited disorders derive from a genetic abnormality present in the DNA of cells such as germ cells. These abnormalities from the germ cells can be transmitted. However, genetic abnormalities in somatic cells cannot be transmitted. Genetic abnormalities in somatic cells can occur anytime from the conception stage to late adult life. Consequently, somatic cell disorder results in cancer, where the malignancy is often the consequence of mutations in the gene that control cellular growth. There are many types of these genes and they are called *oncogenes*. Thus, all human cancer results from mutations in the nuclear DNA of somatic cells (Kumar et al. 2012).

Interaction of mutations within these genes and with other genomic polymorphisms such as single-nucleotide polymorphisms (SNPs) is probably important in general acute medical conditions including trauma. However, the role of SNPs in modulating complex medical disorders (diabetes mellitus, coronary heart disease, hypertension, and various forms of cancer) is unclear. As a result, the complexity of interaction of SNPs with other genetic traits and loci is probably important in the prognosis of these disorders, specifically the outcome of therapeutic interventions (Kumar et al. 2012).

Various cancers and degenerative diseases occur with increasing frequency in old age. However, this disease may also present in childhood leukemia at a younger age. The molecular mechanisms of these diseases are not clear. However, they probably include defects in the DNA repair mechanism, accelerated apoptosis, deregulation of imprinted genomic regions, and *de novo* chromosome rearrangement involving specific genomic regions (Kumar et al. 2012).

Epigenetic changes can play an important role in the development of human cancer. For example, a high percentage of patients with sporadic CRC have microsatellite instability. They also show methylation and silencing of the gene encoding MLH1. As a result, epigenetic changes lead to instability (Kumar et al. 2012).

Promoter of associated methylation of MLH1 is found in the tumor and normal somatic tissues, including spermatozoa. These germline epimutations lead individuals carrying abnormal methylation patterns to develop various cancers. Often, a disruption of pathways that lead to cancer occurs. This disruption is often caused by the *de novo* methylation of the relevant gene's promoter. For the silencing of the tumor suppressor genes, epigenetic silencing is recognized as the third pathway satisfying Knudson's two-hit hypothesis (Kumar et al. 2012).

Generally, human leukemia is a result of chromosomal rearrangement. In acute promyelocytic leukemia, the oncogenic fusion protein PML-RAR-alpha causes repression of genes that are essential for the differentiation of hematopoietic cells. In the same manner, the AML-ETO fusion recruits the repressive N-COR-Sin3-HDAC1 complex and inhibits myeloid development in acute myeloid leukemia. Among the other complex genomic arrangements that result in cancer and modification of therapeutic response, mutations in the genes for ATPase complex are an example. These mutations usually cause a poorer prognosis in patients with non-small-cell lung cancer (Kumar et al. 2012).

8.3.3 Mitochondria organelle transplantation: A potential cellular biotherapy for cancer

Mitochondria is an active organelle cell that has many functions: energy conservation in the form of ATP, regulation of membrane potential, signaling through reactive oxygen species, calcium signaling, apoptosis and autophagy, cellular metabolism, iron metabolism and heme synthesis, and steroid synthesis. Beginning in 1930, Otto Warburg argued that mitochondrial dysfunction caused many human diseases such as metabolic, aging, cardiovascular, and neurodegenerative diseases. Dysfunction of the mitochondria leads to many consequences. Mitochondria process control is very important for determination of the lifespan of eukaryotic cells and mitochondrial disorders (Elliott et al. 2015).

After the work of Otto Warburg, Thomas Seyfried wrote a great book titled *Cancer as a Metabolic Disease.* In his book, he wanted to explain why only the body cells capable of increasing glycolysis during respiratory damage can promote tumorigenesis. However, cells not capable of inducing glycolysis in response to respiratory damage will die because of the lack of energy (Elliott et al. 2015).

Later on, many other mitochondrial studies were published. One of the best was a research paper published by Fogg, Lanning, and MacKeigan. This paper was entitled "Mitochondria in Cancer: At the Crossroads of Life and Death." In this work, the authors discussed the mitochondrial processes that play an important role in tumor initiation and progression. Despite the controversy, retrograde response is an epigenetic system responsible for nuclear genomic stability. However, a persistent retrograde response will cause respiratory damage that leads to genomic instability. This instability will result in the Warburg effect, genomic instability, and tumorigenesis (Elliott et al. 2015).

In his theory, Warburg presented respiratory insufficiency as the cause of the origin of cancer. In contrast, Seyfried claimed that genome instability is related to mitochondrial dysfunction through retrograde signaling. As a result, cancer with defective mitochondria can be prevented if the defective mitochondria are replaced by normal mitochondria (Elliott et al. 2015).

Nuclear cytoplasm transfer studies are very important to confirm the hypothesis that normal mitochondria can really suppress cancer and tumor. The mitochondria from human skin fibroblasts are a good illustration. Fibroblast mitochondria were stained, isolated, and co-cultured with cancer cells. After the mitochondria entered the cells easily, the researchers noticed no increase in drug sensitivity and no inhibition of proliferation. This discovery made clear that mitochondrial activities are highly tissue specific. Consequently, a reversal of glycolysis, decreased expression of glucose transporter III (Glut III), and the promotion of apoptosis present a novel strategy to overcome drug resistance in cancer cells (Elliott et al. 2015).

According to this article, the introduction of normal isolated mitochondria in cancer cells inhibits proliferation and increases drug sensitivity. Thus, the mitochondrion is a powerful biologic intracellular organelle for cell-based therapy such as cancer therapy (Elliott et al. 2015).

8.3.4 A specific mesothelial signature marks the heterogeneity of mesenchymal stem cells from high-grade serous ovarian cancer

Mesenchymal stem/stromal cells (MSCs) are present in almost all types of tissue. They have a wide range of functions in the human body such as tissue regeneration, wound repair, and maintenance of tissue homeostasis. They are also heterogeneous, so they can support the widely diversified parenchymal cells and tissue organization. In addition, mesenchymal interactions with epithelial parenchyma are very important for organogenesis. Thus, they play a critical role in cancer progression by providing more scaffolding/structural elements in the tumor microenvironment. In the dynamic homeostasis ecosystem of cancer, the secretome of the MSCs produces many bioactive molecules that have both immunomodulatory and general trophic functions such as angiogenesis/vasculogenesis regulators that can respond to local inflammation. As a result, the exploration of the presence of MCSs in human tumors, their functions, and their prognostic significance has become an area of investigation for researchers and scientists (Verardo et al. 2014).

For the study of MSCs, human samples were collected according to the Declaration of Helsinki. Normal MSCs were isolated from adult human tissues such as bone marrow, heart, and adipose tissues. High-grade serous ovarian cancer (HG-SOC) MSCs were isolated from primary HG-SOC. All of these samples were cultured under normal conditions. Then, the cultured N-MSCs and HG-SOC-MSCs were subjected to flow cytometry and immunofluorescence, cell proliferation assays, multilineage differentiation, high-resolution genotyping analysis, FANTOM 5 data matrix and sample ontology, cluster analysis, differential expression analysis, annotation of functional analysis, real-time quantitative PCR, and survival analysis, respectively (Verardo et al. 2014).

After the researchers isolated and characterized the MSCs from HG-SOC-MSCs, they compared them with the primary cells and tissues of the FAMTOM5 project by applying deepCAGE technology. As a result, the researchers discovered that the MSCs derived from HG-SOC compared with similarly derived normal tissue MSCs, possessed a specific tissue that showed a relationship with mesothelial-derived cells. There was a correlation between HG-SOC-MSC gene expression signature and the clinical outcome in the specific tumor (Verardo et al. 2014).

8.3.5 Network-based proteomic approaches reveal the neurodegenerative, neuroprotective, and pain-related mechanisms involved after retrograde axonal damage

This article is about to establish network-based proteomic approaches to reveal the neurodegenerative processes after retrograde axonal damage. Neuronal dysfunction and synaptic disconnection always follow neurodegenerative processes. What are axonal injuries? They are generally described as a permanent loss of vital neuronal functions, which appears with a retrograde process of neuronal atrophy or death. Axonal injuries usually occur in neurodegenerative diseases or after acute peripheral nerve disease or trauma. For example, traumatic axotomy or mechanical traction (avulsion) of the nerves can result from traffic accidents or work and sports activities, or as a consequence of obstetric complications. These lesions or injuries are difficult to reconstitute with surgery because the proximal nerve stump is absent (Casas et al. 2015).

In order to study this phenomenon, researchers acquired female Sprague-Dawley rats aged 12 weeks. These rats were kept under standard conditions of light and temperature and given food and water. The researchers performed surgical procedures such as extra-vertebral nerve root avulsion of the L4–L5 roots under anesthesia with a ketamine/xylazine cocktail. Then, the researchers snap-froze the anesthetized groups of rats in liquid nitrogen. Their tissues were homogenized in a lysis buffer (Casas et al. 2015).

For the proteomic analysis, the researchers analyzed the samples using an LTQ-OrbitrapVelos mass spectrometer coupled to a ProxeonEasyLC. They loaded the peptide mixtures directly into the analytical column and separated them by reversed-phase chromatography on a 15-centimeter column with an inner diameter of 100 micrometers, packed with 5-micrometer C18 particles. The researchers acquired all data with Xcalibur software v2.1. They used the Proteome Discover software suite and the Mascot search engine for peptide identification and quantification. They analyzed the data against the SwissProt Rat database containing the most common contaminants (Casas et al. 2015).

After the previous procedures, the researchers begin to make protein–protein interaction (PPI) networks. This interaction network helped the researchers to notice the presence of apoptotic, necrotic death-associated pathways such as anoikis, nucleolar stress, and mitochondrial dysfunction in the described neurodegenerative processes. For the protein interaction data, the researchers collected all the available PPIs from an integrated database that contains data from nine major public PPI databases: Intact, MINT, DIP, MatrixDB, InnateDB, BIOGRID, BIND, MPIDB, and HPRD. Then, the researchers collected all the experimentally verified direct interactions. They added only those described as binary according to the associated detection methods. This binary interactome generated a second interactome by collecting all experimentally interactions using the "spoke expanded" model that transforms protein complexes into binary interactions (Casas et al. 2015).

These interactomes allowed the construction of two types of networks: first-degree networks and second-degree networks. The first-degree networks consisted of adding the direct interactors of the motive seeds. The second-degree networks consisted of adding an extra level of interactors to the first-degree networks. Each interaction was observed based on the size and type of the experiment, as well as the number of publications supporting the interaction, to build high-confidence networks (Casas et al. 2015).

In order to determine whether a predefined list of genes shows significant differences between two biological phenotypes, the researchers conducted a gene set enrichment analysis (GSEA). They performed the GSEA using the lists of biological process–associated genes and the set of PPI networks. The GSEA required first ranking genes according to their association with a given phenotype. Then, the researchers determined whether the genes included in the signature presented positive or negative enrichment values. The estimated log2 fold changes from the proteomic analysis was used to measure the association with each model. The size of the gene set being tested, the p-value, and the estimated false discovery rate constituted the output of the GSEA. Finally, the researchers made a data validation by using immunohistochemistry and Western blot. This study is very important because it allows the presentation of a network-based proteome, which can be relevant for trauma therapy (Casas et al. 2015).

8.3.6 Combining clinicopathological and molecular pathway signatures for improving clinical decisions through an understanding of CRC biology

CRC is a worldwide cancer. Over 1 million patients are affected every year. Surgery is the best therapy method to treat patients with localized disease. Sometimes, physicians use adjuvant chemotherapy in their attempts to prevent future relapse. However, not all CRC patients can be treated with this chemotherapy. Thus, physicians must be very careful in identifying patients for chemotherapy, because the current available clinical and pathological information is insufficient (Mehta 2013).

In order to better predict CRC progression, researchers combined RNA abundance signatures from tumors with the clinical data from patients and made laboratory-defined mutagens using microarray data from HT-29 CRC cells. These cells were treated with the following:

1. siRNAs that knock down the levels of specific transcripts
2. Conditions that modify proliferation and differentiation
3. Chemotherapeutic drugs

From the results of the experiment, the researchers observed that combined clinicopathological and molecular pathway signatures can cluster CRC patients into groups significantly associated with survival outcomes. In addition, the use of putative classifiers that used these pathways signatures was a good method to predict CRC patient disease-free survival. However, none of the assessed classifiers could predict disease-free survival effectively for stage II CRC patients (Mehta 2013).

To conclude, the researchers found that the molecular pathway information inferred from tumor genomics, especially when combined with clinicopathological information, can provide a great deal of information about the individual tumor and predict clinical outcomes for some patients. They deduced that the molecular pathway-based signatures could provide a promising method to understand the biology of individual tumors and personalize patient care, for example, predicting CRC outcome in the clinic (Mehta 2013).

8.4 Diet/genomics/cancer

8.4.1 Impact of genetic and epigenetic variations within the fatty acid desaturase cluster on the composition and metabolism of PUFAs in PCa

This article is about the *in vitro* and experimental animal that was set to show that high levels of omega-6 PUFAs and high ratio of omega-6 to omega-3 PUFAs are strongly associated with the development and progression of PCa. This discovery caused much controversy among scientists. When the researchers looked into epidemiological studies in humans, they found that the association between PUFAs and PCa was inconsistent. Thus, they deduced that the genetic and epigenetic variations within the FADS were responsible for these PUFA and PCa associations (Cui et al. 2016).

For this study, the author began to test the relationship of the genotype of an SNP, rs174537, the methylation of a CpG site, cg2738632 with PUFA composition, and markers of PUFA biosynthesis in PCa tissue. For the study method, the author selected 60 PCa specimens from patients undergoing radical prostatectomy. These specimens were genotyped, pyrosequenced, and quantitated for fatty acids (Cui et al. 2016).

As a result, the researcher found many long chains of PUFAs such as arachidonic acid in these specimens. These arachidonic acids in the specimens accounted for 15.8% of the total fatty acids. The researcher also found a positive association between the G allele at rs174537 with the concentrations of arachidonic and adrenic acid and ratios of products to precursor within the omega-6 PUFA pathway. Thus homozygous G individuals exhibited higher values as compared to specimens from heterozygous individuals and homozygous T individuals. Finally, the researchers found out that the methylation status of cg27386326 is inversely correlated with tissue concentrations of long-chain PUFA (LC-PUFA) biosynthesis (Cui et al. 2016).

According to this study, the data reveal that genetic and epigenetic variations within the fatty acid desaturase (FADS) cluster are highly related to LC-PUFA concentrations and LC-PUFA biosynthetic capacity in PCa tissue. Thus, gene–PUFA interactions can play a vital role in PCa risk and severity (Cui et al. 2016).

8.4.2 Meta-analysis of genome-wide association study of homeostasis model assessment beta cell function and insulin resistance in East Asian population and the European results

In recent years, many Asian countries have undergone rapid economic development and urbanization. Many Western food industries like McDonald's and Burger King have expanded into those Asian countries. Their presence has really changed the diet of these Asian populations, whose food culture previously involved eating fresh fruit, vegetables, and legumes. This change in diet led to an increase in the risk of type 2 diabetes in these Asians. In this chapter, the author discovered that Asians develop diabetes at younger ages and at lower degrees of obesity in comparison with Western populations. Genetic and environmental factors have a considerable effect on the diabetes incidence rate. As a result, the author felt that it was urgent to understand the genetic differences between Asian and Western populations (Hong et al. 2014).

Beta cell function and insulin resistance play a key role in type 2 diabetes. For this reason, the researchers used the homeostasis model assessment (HOMA) to evaluate the maintenance of glucose levels and insulin resistance. HOMA-B was used to measure beta cell function and HOMA-IR was used for insulin resistance (Hong et al. 2014).

Because few replication studies confirmed the association with HOMA-%B or HOMA-IR, the researchers, in this study preferred examine the results of the Meta-Analyses of Glucose- and Insulin-Related Traits Consortium (MAGIC) for HOMAs in East Asians, specifically in two Korean community-based cohorts (Hong et al. 2014).

The two population-based cohorts chosen—Ansung and Ansan—were part of the Korean Genome and Epidemiology Study (KoGES). This study was approved by the Institutional Review Board of the Korea National Institute of Health, and these two populations lived in Ansung and Ansan, near Seoul. However, for the triage, the researchers did include people with genotype accuracies below 98%, and high missing genotype call rates (less than or equal to 4%), high heterozygosity (>30%), or inconsistency in sex. Then, the researchers collected 8,842 samples from the selected group (Hong et al. 2014).

186   Nutrigenomics and Nutraceuticals

Then, the researchers began to conduct laboratory analysis and establish inclusion criteria. For example, the researchers applied the hexokinase method on an ADIVA 1650 Auto Analyzer to determine plasma glucose concentrations. Then, they started the HOMA calculation by using the following formulas: HOMA1-IR = (FSI × FSG)/22.5 and HOMA1-%B = (20 × FSI)/(FSG-4.5). The HOMA2 model was calculated using a program that is available at http://www.OCDEM.ox.ac.uk (Hong et al. 2014).

In addition, the researchers used genotyped SNPs from the Affymetrix 5.0 SNP array and imputed SNPs to examine the MAGIC SNPs in the two Korean cohorts. Then, the researchers performed a statistical analysis where the effect of a genotype was analyzed by linear regression. The calculations of effect size (beta), standard error, HOMA1-%B, HOMA1-IR, HOMA2-%B, and HOMA2-IR values were also performed. The researchers used PLINK for all statistical tests (Hong et al. 2014).

In the study, the researchers identified that the effects of SNPs from 16 loci were associated with HOMAs. They also confirmed five loci (MTNR1B, DGKB, GCK, GLIS3, and FDS1) that were significantly replicated for HOMA-%B. In conclusion, the findings of this study increased the understanding of glucose homeostasis in humans. Thus, this study revealed new pathways for diabetes therapy (Hong et al. 2014).

8.4.3 Plasma 25-hydroxyvitamin D3 is associated with decreased risk of postmenopausal breast cancer in whites: A nested case-control study in a multiethnic cohort study

In this article, the researchers studied the possible correlation between plasma 25-hydroxyvitamin D3 and breast cancer risk. In contrast to previous preliminary studies where the results were null, for this study the researchers took into account a variety of factors such as ultraviolet radiation exposure, skin sensitivity to sun exposure, and diet. Also, the researchers decided to focus on circulating 25-hydroxyvitamin D as the most reliable indicator of vitamin D even they differ between race/ethnic groups with varying diets and ability to synthesize vitamin D in the skin (Kim et al. 2014).

There are many forms of vitamin D. However the two major forms are vitamin D3 (cholecalciferol) and vitamin D2 (ergocalciferol). Vitamin D3 is synthesized mostly from the irradiation of 7-hydrocholesterol on the skin and only a few foods (fortified products, supplements) naturally contain vitamin D3. Consequently, the body has a lower concentration of vitamin D3 in the body (Kim et al. 2014).

To implement the study, the researchers conducted a nested case-control study within a multiethnic cohort in Hawaii and Los Angeles to test the association between plasma levels of 25-hydroxyvitamin D2 [25(OH)D2] and 25-hydroxyvitamin D3 [25-(OH)D3] and breast cancer risk. More than 215,000 adults from five race/ethnic groups (white, African-American, native Hawaiian, Japanese, Latino) established in Los Angeles and Hawaii between 1993 and 1996 were selected. The plasma levels of 25(OH)D2 and 25(OH)D3 were analyzed by isotope dilution liquid chromatography–Orbitrap mass spectrometry. Then, the researchers validated the assay by the Vitamin D External Quality Assessment Scheme (DEQAS) and National Institute of Standards and Technology quality assurance programs. In addition, the researchers performed sensitivity analyses for 25(OH)D3 and 25(OH)D among whites only by excluding women within 6 months, 2, 3, and 4 years from the date of blood draw. Then, they implemented a two-segmented piecewise-linear logistic regression for each race/ethnic group to find the change-point in the ORs to identify the threshold effect of 25(OH)D3 and 25(OH)D on breast cancer risk (Kim et al. 2014).

From this study, researchers confirmed the potential beneficial effect of vitamin D against breast cancer and other malignancies. For example, the researchers observed that white women whose circulating 25(OH)D3 and 25(OH)D exceeded that of women in other race/ethnic groups had a lower risk of postmenopausal breast cancer. The reason for this inverse association is the high levels of circulating vitamin D3 produced among whites living in Los Angeles and Hawaii, who are exposed to ambient levels of ultraviolet radiation. Consequently, the researchers concluded that only a minimum threshold of vitamin D exposure from both sun and diet is required to reduce breast cancer risk among postmenopausal white women (Kim et al. 2014).

8.5 Conclusion

Cancer is one of the chronic diseases that continue to affect the US population. Although the cancer rate has been decreasing significantly since 1991, it is still expected that 595,690 Americans will die from cancer in 2016. In order to fight cancer, researchers and health professionals have conducted many research studies and prevention programs to inform and educate the US population and around the world. However, different studies show contrasting results. For example, one study may promote polyunsaturated fats while others advance the benefits of some saturated fats against cancer (CRC, breast cancer). Thus, the main studies concerning diet, genetic, or mutated genes and cancer must be reevaluated to reduce the cancer rate.

American culture is also characterized by food. Fast foods restaurants such as McDonald's, Burger King, Kentucky Fried Chicken, and Pizza Hut occupy an important place in the US economy and American society. The menus of these fast food restaurants contain a lot of fat. In addition, menu items usually consist of processed food rich in chemical preservatives or additives. For these reasons, researchers have conducted many research studies that can inform and help health professionals to implement prevention programs against cancer, to promote healthy diets rich in fruit and vegetable, and to encourage physical activity and smoking cessation.

Mutated genes and genetics can be also a risk factor for cancer. In recent years, this discovery has led to the creation of a new discipline called *genomics*, which is a comprehensive analysis of the human genome and mutated genes to find a better cure and treatment for cancer. Diet, genomics, and cancer are important factors that must be taken into account to treat or reduce cancer.

In my opinion, this research was a great opportunity to expand my knowledge about the associations between diet, genomics, and cancer. Now, I am aware of some of the major controversies related to cancer, diet, and genomics. This research will further motivate me to participate in cancer prevention.

References

American Cancer Society. (2016). *Cancer Facts and Figures 2016.* American Cancer Society, Atlanta, GA.

Casas, C. et al. (2015). Network based proteomic approaches reveal the neurodegenerative, neuroprotective, and pain-related mechanisms involved after retrograde axonal damage. *Scientific Reports* 5, 9185.

Conzo, G. et al. (2014). Current concepts of pheochromocytoma. *International Journal of Surgery* 12, 469–474.

Cui, T. et al. (2016). Impact of genetic and epigenetic variations within the FADS cluster on the composition and metabolism of polyunsaturated fatty acids in prostate cancer. *Prostate* 76, 1182–1191.

De Lorgeril, M. et al. (2012). New insights into the health effects of dietary saturated and omega-6 and omega-3 polyunsaturated fatty acids. *BMC Medicine* 10, 50.

Elliott, R. et al. (2015). Mitochondria organelle transplantation: A potential cellular biotherapy for cancer. *Journal of Surgery* S(2):9, 6–9.

Farvid, M. et al. (2016). Fruit and vegetable consumption in adolescence and early adulthood and risk of breast cancer: Population based cohort study. *BMJ: British medical journal* 353, i2343.

Golan, D. (2012). *Principles of Pharmacology: The Pathophysiology Basis of Drug Therapy.* Philadelphia, PA: Lippincott Williams & Wilkins.

Hong, K. et al. (2014). Meta-analysis of genome wide association study of homeostasis model assessment beta cell function and insulin resistance in East Asian population and the European Results. *Molecular Genetic Genomics* 289, 1247–1255.

Kim, Y. et al. (2014). Plasma 25-hydroxyvitamin D3 is associated with decreased risk of postmenopausal breast cancer in whites: A nested case-control study in the multiethnic cohort study. *BMC Cancer* 14, 29.

Kumar, D. et al. (2012). *Genomics and Health in the Developing World.* Oxford University Press, Oxford.

Kwabbi-Addo, B. et al. (2011). *Cancer Causes and Controversies: Understanding Risk Reduction and Prevention.* ABC-CLIO, Santa Barbara, CA.

Lawrence, G. D. (2013). Dietary fats and health: Dietary recommendations in the context of scientific evidence. *Advances in Nutrition: An International Review Journal* 4, 294–302.

Mehta, S. (2013). Combining clinicopathological and molecular pathway signatures for improving clinical decisions through an understanding of colorectal cancer biology. *Doctoral Dissertation*, Auckland University.

Ronco, A. D. (2012). Nutrients. *Nutritional Epidemiology of Breast Cancer* 119, 35–51.

Singh, Z. (2013). Toxicological aspects of saccharin. *Food Biology* 2, 4–7.

Verardo, R. et al. (2014). Specific mesothelial signature marks the heterogeneity of mesenchymal stem cells from high-grade serous ovarian cancer. *Stem Cells* 32, 2998–3011.

9

Chronic Degenerative Diseases in Adults and Their Correlation with Childhood Feeding and Genomic Composition

Adnan Ali and Yashwant V. Pathak
University of South Florida
Tampa, Florida

Contents

9.1 Introduction 191
9.2 Common and rare variants and their roles in chronic
debilitating disease 192
    9.2.1 Alzheimer's disease 193
    9.2.2 Type 2 diabetes 196
9.3 Conclusion 197
References 197

9.1 Introduction

Chronic degenerative diseases impose a heavy toll on modern human society. Consisting of diseases that manifest themselves in a chronic manner and impose degenerative cell changes, this definition encompasses many of the chronic diseases that have a disproportionate impact on quality of life, such as AD, diabetes mellitus, and macular degeneration. The etiology of these chronic degenerative diseases, although some are less well understood than others, often involve disparate factors such as genetics, nutrition, and other sociobehavioral choices. It's been known for over two dozen years that nutritional behavior plays a large role in not only the general health of individuals, but also the likelihood that an individual will develop chronic degenerative diseases (Campbell and Chen 1994; Eaton et al. 1988). However, these diseases often have a key genetic component as well, and numerous genome-wide association studies (GWAS) and other genetic-related studies (such as linkage studies) have been conducted to root out the genetic components of chronic disease. In some cases, this has been spectacularly successful, such as the identification of repetitive CAG repeats in the key gene huntingtin (*HTT*) as the dominant factor in Huntington's disease pathogenesis. In some other cases, even after population-level GWAS, there is still ongoing debate about the effect of genetics on certain conditions, such as diabetes mellitus or AD. One might in fact ask, why isn't genetics able to give us more information regarding chronic disease etiologies? This question touches on a key debate regarding how genetic variation actually impacts chronic disease risk. Here, we will briefly introduce several competing models as to how genetic variants impact disease risk.

9.2 Common and rare variants and their roles in chronic debilitating disease

Through the transformative power of GWAS, genetics have begun to unravel the immense complexity hidden in the human genome. In an average human, there are over 20 million base pairs of DNA that differ relative to an arbitrary reference (Auton et al. 2015). With thousands of potential diseases and disorders that can harm human health, it is perhaps self-evident that many of these polymorphisms contribute to disease risk. Geneticists have debated over several competing models of how exactly genetic polymorphisms cause disease. This debate is also tightly intertwined with the debate regarding the missing heritability problem, which is discussed in-depth in Chapter 1 of this review. If the reader is unfamiliar with the material, we suggest revisiting the material in Chapter 1 or utilizing a reference text (Hartl et al. 1997). In short, the *common-disease–common-variant hypothesis*—the earliest model of how genetics impacts disease risk—suggests that several common variants (defined as those variants with frequency ≥0.5% in the population) contribute a significant proportion of the variance in the heritability of common diseases (Gibson 2012; Zuk et al. 2014). However, as more GWAS datasets have become available, this hypothesis has quickly been refuted as a result of the "missing heritability" problem (Gibson 2012). Soon, other competing hypotheses were proposed regarding the missing variants. The *infinitesimal model* suggests that hundreds or even thousands of loci contribute minimally to the overall phenotype and that the common variants we are able to detect only constitute a small percentage of the total phenotypic heritability explainable by genotype alone. Only with GWAS of ever-increasing sample size are we able to capture the effects of these marginally impactful variants; however, in the worst case, these sample sizes could be even larger than the available human population (Gibson 2012). The *rare allele hypothesis* suggests that extremely rare alleles—those with minor allele frequencies of <1%—have major effect sizes. However, the expressivity—the severity of the disease or phenotype—is heavily modulated by the environment. Instead of thinking of alleles as imparting disease, it is perhaps better to think of alleles as imparting risk for a particular disease or phenotype. Under this interpretation, a complex disease such schizophrenia can be

192   Nutrigenomics and Nutraceuticals

explained by the fact that multiple different loci each impart some risk, and nearly every adult is a carrier for some of these risk alleles. Only in individuals with some sufficient number of these risk alleles—and with the correct environmental factors—will present with schizophrenia. Evidence from GWAS experiments surrounding schizophrenia suggests over 100 different loci might be implicated in the manifestation of the disease (Ripke et al. 2014). There is still ongoing theoretical debate about the problem of missing heritability and the factors that contribute to missing heritability. Recent works suggest that better designed GWAS—known as *rare-variant association studies*—and better analytical methods are able to better identify the effects of rare alleles (Zuk et al. 2012, 2014). Another major model, the *broad sense heritability model*, suggests that the additive effect of alleles is insufficient to explain the observed missing heritability in many diseases and phenotypic traits. Instead, the model proposes that missing genotype-by-genotype interactions, also known as *epistasis*, and genotype-by-environment interactions (potentially mediated by epigenetic mechanisms) provide a significant part of the missing heritability. It is likely that some combination of the broad sense heritability model and the rare allele hypothesis can make up the heritability gap that current GWAS experiments observe.

These models offer a lens into the mechanistic basis of how chronic disease develops. Through the rare allele model, a simple interpretation is that one's genotype confers some level of risk to an individual, and one's environment and actions—for example, the patterns of childhood feeding—might will turn that risk into a reality. The infinitesimal hypothesis suggests that for some disorders, we might require decades of development in genomics and GWAS experiments before we can hope to understand the potential causes of certain chronic diseases. Although a victor has not yet been selected from these competing models for explaining the missing heritability gap, we have provided a detailed discussion of these models in order to illustrate the pitfalls of pinpointing the root cause of chronic disease to either genetics or the environment. It is still an extremely active research area in human genetics, and developments in this field will dramatically influence the way we understand and treat chronic diseases in the future. Here, we recap the current stage of knowledge of how genetic and environmental factors impact a number of chronic diseases, with a focus on childhood diet and feeding. The label *degenerative chronic disease* is a wide label that covers a variety of diseases that afflict millions of individuals around the world. By concentrating on AD, we hope to illustrate not only how the link between childhood diet (an environmental factor) and genomics factors into disease pathogenesis but hopefully also the enormous potential of nutrigenomics in understanding disease pathogenesis.

9.2.1 Alzheimer's disease

AD is the poster child of debilitating chronic degenerative diseases (Reitz and Mayeux 2014). It costs developed countries more than $602 billion a year, and with rates of diagnosis increasing over the past two decades poses a significant financial and social burden for developed countries (Huang and Mucke 2012). Characterized by worsening neurodegeneration and loss of brain mass, AD initially presents with memory loss and personality changes. Evidence suggests that the synapses and dendrites that enable neuronal connections are particularly at risk, and their loss may contribute more than the loss of neurons (Palop et al. 2006). Several heritable mutations have been shown to have a causal influence on the development of AD. These mutations are concentrated in three genes: amyloid precursor protein (APP), presenilin-1, and presenilin-2. APP is intricately linked to deposits of amyloid plaques, made up of fibroid amyloid-β, which is often observed in radiological imaging of AD patients. Patients with Down's syndrome, whose extra copy of Chromosome 21 confers an additional copy of APP, tend to develop early-onset dementia and AD-like symptoms (Huang and Mucke 2012). Thus, these mutations cause autosomal dominant AD and contribute to roughly 1% of the incidence of AD in the population (Huang and Mucke 2012). However, the preponderance of AD present in the population is characterized as late onset and is regarded as a multifactorial disorder with a strong genetic disposition (Van Cauwenberghe et al. 2016).

This fact has driven geneticists to undertake a series of GWAS experiments in order to determine the underlying cause of AD. Recent estimates place the overall heritability of AD at over 80% (Lambert et al. 2013). A number of risk alleles can be found in the apolipoprotein E4 locus. This gene has been consistently one of the top variants found in GWAS experiments on AD, and it was implicated as early as 1997 in various studies as a strong risk factor (Farrer et al. 1997).

The APOE gene contains three major allelic variants, known as ε2, ε3, and ε4, at a single gene locus that produces three different isoforms of APOE: ApoE2, ApoE3, and ApoE4 (Van Cauwenberghe et al. 2016). An example of an allele that confers risk, the APOE ε4 allele is carried by 40%–65% of AD patients, whereas only 20%–25% of the general population has the APOE ε4 allele (Harold et al. 2009). The APOE ε4 allele is estimated to account for 27.3% of the 80% heritability of AD (Lambert et al. 2013). Surprisingly, another allele, the ε2 allele, seems to confer protective power and reduce the risk of AD in carriers (Van Cauwenberghe et al. 2016). In the last decade, with almost exponential increases in the power of GWAS experiments, several more loci associated with immune function, such as several HLA genes, and a number of other proteins involved in endosomal cycling, lipid and cholesterol metabolism, and inflammatory response have been significantly implicated as harboring potential risk alleles for AD (Van Cauwenberghe et al. 2016). The variety of disparate systems that these risk genes influence again supports the hypothesis that late-onset AD has a multifactorial basis.

Could one of these factors be nutritional? All isoforms of APOE are significantly involved in lipid metabolism and cholesterol control. Indeed, there has been a high correlation observed between high cholesterol levels and AD risk (Luchsinger and Mayeux 2004). It might appear that the dual roles of APOE might confound any link between diet and AD; however, additional studies have confirmed that there is a significant correlation between cholesterol and AD risk, regardless of APOE ε4 status (Morris et al. 2003). Indeed, several epidemiological studies have implicated diet as a significant factor associated with AD risk. One such study, which evaluated dietary transitions and their impact on AD rates, saw a significant correlation between total energy and animal fat consumption and AD (Grant 2014). Another meta-analysis of dietary trends and AD prevalence concluded that advanced glycation end products (ADEs). Consumption of ADEs has been significantly linked to not only AD but also inflammation and oxidative stress, both of which have also been implicated in the pathogenesis of AD (Luchsinger and Mayeux 2004; Uribarri et al. 2010). Oxidative stress, in particular, has been repeatedly linked with neuronal damage and AD risk. This is due to the fact that reactive oxygen species can cause significant neuronal damage (Luchsinger and Mayeux 2004). Moreover, this is supported by the positive correlation between intake of dietary antioxidants and slower mental decline in older adults (Morris et al. 2002). A number of other studies have shown that alcohol consumption might play a role in AD risk (Luchsinger and Mayeux 2004). However, one must take this evidence with caution, as there is significant uncertainty over the latency period of AD and when disease progression actually starts. This uncertainty could impact any retrospective correlational study between dietary factors and AD risk.

This uncertainty over the initialization of AD progression has driven researchers to explore the role of APOE in childhood. Several studies have shown that APOE, especially the ε4 allele, has a significant role in mental development. In a recent study of 1,187 children ages 4–20, researchers found that the ε4 allele impacted brain development relative to children with ε2 or ε3 alleles (Chang et al. 2016). The hippocampus, which is disproportionately impacted by AD, showed the greatest difference in structural integrity. This experiment not only confirmed the correlation between APOE allele status and brain morphology but also showed that this correlation begins in childhood (Hostage et al. 2013). Due to the key role of APOE in diet, AD risk, and neurological development, one can reasonably speculate that childhood diet may play a role in AD risk. However, as with so many genetic and environmental effects, teasing out the specific effects and the mechanistic basis that certain pleiotropic genes might play is difficult, if not impossible, with the current state of genomics. Indeed, as discussed earlier, most of the fundamental models regarding the effects of alleles on phenotypes typically only account for the additive effects of each variant. More complex models that factor in the potential pleiotropic effects of risk alleles are needed to elucidate the proper balance between environmental effects and genetic effects in complex, multifactorial diseases. Furthermore, epigenetic changes must also be considered when attempting to understand these diseases. Recent evidence utilizing epigenomic profiling has shown that AD might also have an immunological basis (Gjoneska et al. 2015).

Nutrigenomics offers an attractive role in delineating between the genetic, environmental, and the gene–environment interactions that play a role in causing chronic degenerative diseases. With the advent of CRISPR-based genome editing techniques and a variety of other methods to modify the genetics of both model organisms and cell lines, scientists have vastly increased their power to dissect the mechanistic interactions between disease variants and their role in diet. Through such dissection, a better understanding of genetic–environmental interactions can be gained. Armed with this knowledge, we can, for example, better dissect the interplay between childhood diet, APOE ε4 allele status, and AD progression and pathogenesis.

9.2.2 Type 2 diabetes

T2D is also a chronic degenerative disease with complex underpinnings. Affecting more than 370 million people around the world, this degenerative disease involves the body's development of insulin resistance and pancreatic β-cell dysfunction. Both play a key role in the feedback loop that controls blood glucose levels, and a debate is still ongoing regarding which component contributes more to T2D development (Kahn et al. 2014). Indeed, even the main feedback loop in controlling insulin still has yet to be finely mapped to individual genes. Due to the complex nature of the disease, several GWAS have been attempted to dissect the disease. A recent meta-analysis found that over a dozen different genetic loci are associated with T2D development, with each loci potentially housing hundreds of risk SNPs in linkage disequilibrium with each other (Billings and Florez 2010). The majority of these are associated with insulin resistance, with only two, the *FTO* and *PPARG* loci, associated with β-cell function (Billings and Florez 2010). However, the effect sizes of these (mostly rare) variants are much smaller relative to the impact of the APOE ε4 allele, further confusing scientists as to the true cause of diabetes (Hakonarson and Grant 2011).

The link between childhood diet and T2D development has been virtually established as scientific fact. The observation that 75% of new childhood obesity cases are also from chronically obese children suggests that childhood diet plays a critical part in T2D development (D'Adamo and Caprio 2011). A number of epidemiological studies have conclusively shown that childhood diet is significantly linked with both obesity and T2D (Steyn et al. 2004). This link is genetic, with common variants in the *FTO* locus being significantly correlated with both increased weight and over a 1.67-fold increased risk for obesity (Frayling et al. 2007). Obesity itself has a heavy genetic component, with numerous genes implicated in T2D also significantly associated with BMI (Walley 2006). This "pleiotropy" clearly has implications for dissecting the mechanistic basis of T2D, as several risk alleles may play both causal and confounding roles at the same time. Moreover, similar to AD, the genetic, environmental, and gene–environment effects have not yet been clearly elucidated in T2D.

Nutrigenomics might prove to be a valuable solution to unraveling this complex problem. As evidenced by recent CRISPR-enabled dissections of the *FTO* locus, scientists finally have the capacity to establish causality—both at the level of contributing to diet and to T2D—for individual alleles (Claussnitzer et al. 2015). As noted in Chapter 1, approaches such as the one employed by Claussnitzer et al.—when merged with nutrigenomics—have the potential to transform our understanding of nutrition, chronic degenerative diseases, and disease genomics. Combined with detailed models of development offered by pluripotent stem cells, these technologies enable scientists to study the development of heritable diseases *in vitro* (Teo et al. 2015). By combining epigenomics, GWAS experimental results, and careful genetic editing, in-depth dissections and teasing apart the nutritional and disease impacts of genetic variants can finally begin.

9.3 Conclusion

Returning to our original discussion on the various models for explaining missing heritability, we see that different diseases may have significantly different genetic architectures. With APOE, we see that a common variant (the ε4 allele) can have significant impact on the risk status of an individual. This is also the case with the IL23R loci in Crohn's disease. However, in T2D, although there have been common variants identified, the majority of variants tend to have minimal effect (Sanghera and Blackett 2012). These differences illustrate the potentially dramatic differences in the complex genetic architecture of these diseases. One must take a balanced view of how rare alleles, common alleles, and other genetic interactions (e.g., pleiotropy) might play in the etiology of complex degenerative diseases. Combined with the almost infinite space of potential diets and environmental exposures, it seems almost impossible for scientists to solve all potential combinations of the genetic, environmental, and gene–environment interactions that lead to complex chronic degenerative diseases. Through epidemiological studies and GWAS experiments, we can gain insights into the correlations between various factors and the disease of interest; however, true scientific understanding can only come from careful genetic manipulations and thoughtful experiments that prove a mechanistic link. With complex genetic and epigenetic interactions, and with an immense space of nutritional and dietary practices, associating chronic disease with a factor such as childhood feeding is a complex task. Fortunately, the postgenomics era has progressed to a point where such associations can not only be made statistically but also linked mechanistically. With a greater number of studies in these areas, we can hopefully identify more promising drug targets or dietary/lifestyle patterns that can serve as a point of therapeutic intervention.

References

Auton, A., Abecasis, G. R., Altshuler, D. M., Durbin, R. M., Abecasis, G. R., Bentley, D. R., et al. (2015). A global reference for human genetic variation. *Nature, 526*(7571), 68–74. http://doi.org/10.1038/nature15393

Billings, L. K., & Florez, J. C. (2010). The genetics of type 2 diabetes: What have we learned from GWAS? *Annals of the New York Academy of Sciences, 1212*(1), 59–77. http://doi.org/10.1111/j.1749-6632.2010.05838.x

Campbell, T. C., & Chen, J. S. (1994). Diet and chronic degenerative diseases—Perspectives from China. *American Journal of Clinical Nutrition, 59*(Suppl) 553S–1161S.

Chang, L., Douet, V., Bloss, C., Lee, K., Pritchett, A., Jernigan, T. L., et al. (2016). Gray matter maturation and cognition in children with different APOE ε genotypes. *Neurology, 87*(6), 585–594. http://doi.org/10.1212/WNL.0000000000002939

Claussnitzer, M., Dankel, S. N., Kim, K.-H., Quon, G., Meuleman, W., Haugen, C., et al. (2015). FTO obesity variant circuitry and adipocyte browning in humans. *The New England Journal of Medicine, 373*(10), 895–907. http://doi.org/10.1056/NEJMoa1502214

D'Adamo, E., & Caprio, S. (2011). Type 2 diabetes in youth: Epidemiology and pathophysiology. *Diabetes Care, 34*(Suppl 2), S161–S165. http://doi.org/10.2337/dc11-s212

Eaton, S. B., Konner, M., & Shostak, M. (1988). Stone agers in the fast lane: Chronic degenerative diseases in evolutionary perspective. *American Journal of Medicine, 84*(4), 739–749. http://doi.org/10.1016/0002-9343(88)90113-1

Farrer, L. A., Cupples, L. A., Haines, J. L., Hyman, B., Kukull, W. A., Mayeux, R., et al. (1997). Effects of age, sex, and ethnicity on the association between apolipoprotein E genotype and Alzheimer disease. A meta-analysis. APOE and Alzheimer Disease Meta Analysis Consortium. *JAMA, 278*(16), 1349–1356. Retrieved from http://www.ncbi.nlm.nih.gov/pubmed/9343467

Frayling, T. M., Timpson, N. J., Weedon, M. N., Zeggini, E., Freathy, R. M., Lindgren, C. M., et al. (2007). A common variant in the FTO gene is associated with body mass index and predisposes to childhood and adult obesity. *Science, 316*(5826), 889–894. http://doi.org/10.1126/science.1141634

Gibson, G. (2012). Rare and common variants: Twenty arguments. *Nature Reviews Genetics, 13*(2), 135–145. http://doi.org/10.1038/nrg3118

Gjoneska, E., Pfenning, A. R., Mathys, H., Quon, G., Kundaje, A., Tsai, L.-H., et al. (2015). Conserved epigenomic signals in mice and humans reveal immune basis of Alzheimer's disease. *Nature, 518*(7539), 365–369. http://doi.org/10.1038/nature14252

Grant, W. B. (2014). Trends in diet and Alzheimer's disease during the nutrition transition in Japan and developing countries. *Journal of Alzheimer's Disease : JAD, 38*(3), 611–20. http://doi.org/10.3233/JAD-130719

Hakonarson, H., & Grant, S. F. A. (2011). Genome-wide association studies (GWAS): Impact on elucidating the aetiology of diabetes. *Diabetes/Metabolism Research and Reviews, 27*(7), 685–696. http://doi.org/10.1002/dmrr.1221

Harold, D., Abraham, R., Hollingworth, P., Sims, R., Gerrish, A., Hamshere, M. L., et al. (2009). Genome-wide association study identifies variants at CLU and PICALM associated with Alzheimer's disease. *Nature Genetics, 41*(10), 1088–1093. http://doi.org/10.1038/ng.440

Hartl, D. L., Clark, A. G., & Clark, A. G. (1997). *Principles of Population Genetics* (Vol. 116). Sinauer associates, Sunderland.

Hostage, C. A., Roy Choudhury, K., Doraiswamy, P. M., & Petrella, J. R. (2013). Dissecting the gene dose-effects of the APOE ε4 and ε2 alleles on hippocampal volumes in aging and Alzheimer's disease. *PLoS One, 8*(2), e54483. http://doi.org/10.1371/journal.pone.0054483

Huang, Y., & Mucke, L. (2012). Alzheimer mechanisms and therapeutic strategies. *Cell, 148*(6), 1204–1222. http://doi.org/10.1016/j.cell.2012.02.040

Kahn, S. E., Cooper, M. E., & Del Prato, S. (2014). Pathophysiology and treatment of type 2 diabetes: Perspectives on the past, present, and future. *The Lancet, 383*(9922), 1068–1083. http://doi.org/10.1016/S0140-6736(13)62154-6

Lambert, J.-C., Ibrahim-Verbaas, C. A., Harold, D., Naj, A. C., Sims, R., Bellenguez, C., et al. (2013). Meta-analysis of 74,046 individuals identifies 11 new susceptibility loci for Alzheimer's disease. *Nature Genetics, 45*(12), 1452–1458. http://doi.org/10.1038/ng.2802

Luchsinger, J. A, & Mayeux, R. (2004). Dietary factors and Alzheimer's disease. *The Lancet Neurology, 3*, 579–587. http://doi.org/10.1016/S1474-4422(04)00878-6

Morris, M. C., Evans, D. A., Bienias, J. L., Tangney, C. C., & Wilson, R. S. (2002). Vitamin E and cognitive decline in older persons. *Archives of Neurology, 59*(7), 1125–32.

Morris, M. C., Evans, D. A., Bienias, J. L., Tangney, C. C., Bennett, D. A., Aggarwal, N., et al. (2003). Dietary fats and the risk of incident Alzheimer disease. *Archives of Neurology, 60*(2), 194–200.

Palop, J. J., Chin, J., & Mucke, L. (2006). A network dysfunction perspective on neurodegenerative diseases. *Nature, 443*(7113), 768–73. http://doi.org/10.1038/nature05289

Reitz, C., & Mayeux, R. (2014). Alzheimer disease: Epidemiology, diagnostic criteria, risk factors and biomarkers. *Biochemical Pharmacology, 88*(4), 640–51. http://doi.org/10.1016/j.bcp.2013.12.024

Ripke, S., Neale, B. M., Corvin, A., Walters, J. T. R., Farh, K.-H., Holmans, P. A., et al. (2014). Biological insights from 108 schizophrenia-associated genetic loci. *Nature, 511*(7510), 421–427. http://doi.org/10.1038/nature13595

Sanghera, D. K., & Blackett, P. R., (2012). Type 2 diabetes genetics: Beyond GWAS. *Journal of Diabetes & Metabolism, 3*(5). http://doi.org/10.4172/2155-6156.1000198

Steyn, N., Mann, J., Bennett, P., Temple, N., Zimmet, P., Tuomilehto, J., et al. (2004). Diet, nutrition and the prevention of type 2 diabetes. *Public Health Nutrition, 7*(1A), 147–165. http://doi.org/10.1079/PHN2003586

Teo, A. K. K., Gupta, M. K., Doria, A., & Kulkarni, R. N. (2015). Dissecting diabetes/metabolic disease mechanisms using pluripotent stem cells and genome editing tools. *Molecular Metabolism, 4*(9), 593–604. http://doi.org/10.1016/j.molmet.2015.06.006

Uribarri, J., Woodruff, S., Goodman, S., Cai, W., Chen, X., Pyzik, R., et al. (2010). Advanced glycation end products in foods and a practical guide to their reduction in the diet. *Journal of the American Dietetic Association, 110*(6), 911–916.e12. http://doi.org/10.1016/j.jada.2010.03.018

Van Cauwenberghe, C., Van Broeckhoven, C., & Sleegers, K. (2016). The genetic landscape of Alzheimer disease: Clinical implications and perspectives. *Genetics in Medicine : Officiassl Journal of the American College of Medical Genetics, 18*(5), 421–430. http://doi.org/10.1038/gim.2015.117

Walley, A. J. (2006). Genetics of obesity and the prediction of risk for health. *Human Molecular Genetics, 15*(Review Issue 2), R124–R130. http://doi.org/10.1093/hmg/ddl215

Zuk, O., Hechter, E., Sunyaev, S. R., & Lander, E. S. (2012). The mystery of missing heritability: Genetic interactions create phantom heritability. *Proceedings of the National Academy of Sciences of the United States of America, 109*(4), 1193–1198. http://doi.org/10.1073/pnas.1119675109

Zuk, O., Schaffner, S. F., Samocha, K., Do, R., Hechter, E., Kathiresan, S., et al. (2014). Searching for missing heritability: Designing rare variant association studies. *Proceedings of the National Academy of Sciences of the United States of America, 111*(4), E455–E464. http://doi.org/10.1073/pnas.1322563111

10

Biology and Optimal Health

Amanda Lasher and Yashwant V. Pathak
University of South Florida
Tampa, Florida

Contents

10.1   Introduction 201
10.2   Theme 1: Two perspectives on systems biology in medicine 203
      10.2.1   The narrow perspective 204
      10.2.2   The broad perspective..205
10.3   Theme 2: The top-down and bottom-up approaches to
      systems biology...206
      10.3.1   The top-down approach...207
      10.3.2   The bottom-up approach...208
10.4   Theme 3: Applying systems biology to medicine..............................208
      10.4.1   Using systems biology to understand disease and
               health problems..209
      10.4.2   Using systems biology to develop drugs and vaccines..........210
10.5   Conclusion...211
References...212

10.1 Introduction

Over the past few decades, scientists and researchers have continuously expanded the field of biology in order to gain more knowledge on essential biological elements such as environmental sustainability and population health. With consistent improvements in methods and research come more opportunities and new discoveries. For instance, advances in chemical engineering have sparked ideas to design methods to convert reusable biomass into valuable fuel sources. At the same time, geneticists have been able to recognize the value of reverse genetics for use in vaccinations.[3] Researchers around the globe are constantly looking to make a difference and take their discoveries to greater depths.

One of the most impressive fields in the scientific community is that of biomedical research. These researchers aim to design products and methods for use in a variety of health-related practices such as pharmaceutical companies and patient care facilities. In order to be successful, these researchers need to have a strong foundation of knowledge pertaining to biology's essential goal: understanding how organisms work. This knowledge places biomedical scientists and engineers at the forefront of advancing the field of medicine. With the help of advancements and new technology, geneticists, chemists, and other researchers have inadvertently propagated a new approach to studying the world around us. This new and upcoming field is known as *systems biology*.

The study of systems biology provides a strong foundation of knowledge with regard to the behavior and function of all organisms. The understanding of organisms at the system level is garnered by observing individual aspects of organisms from the cellular to the ecological level. These aspects can be thoroughly analyzed as separate pieces in order to gain further insight into the dynamics and functionality of the whole. The use of the systemic approach in biology has sculpted new ideas and methods for researchers. The realization that the integration of molecular events with higher level events produces an efficient way of studying has changed the field of biology immensely.[4] Consistent advancements in technology make it possible for modern scientists to design innovative ways to study organisms at the system level.

Although systems biology may sound eccentric, there are some methods biologists use to generalize the subject. The top-down method and bottom-up method are two approaches that can accomplish this. While the top-down method begins by focusing on observing a broad range of systems and later delving deeper into more narrow systems, the bottom-up method does just the opposite. Studying using these methods is mostly accomplished using methods such as quantitative measurements, systematic measurement technologies, and mathematical and computational models.[5] Both methods have their own unique outcomes; however, they still provide further insight to organisms at the system level and produce intricate and reliable data needed to further prepare improvements for disease prevention and better health care. Using either the top-down or bottom-up method helps researchers by organizing ideas and data in such a way that they can be compared to one another more easily. In order to be successful in using one of these approaches, researchers must first decide which approach would be best to use. This determination depends on a few key factors such as how much information has already been gathered about the subject.

Understanding organisms at the system level also helps progress advancements within the scientific community. For instance, by developing a strong understanding of the metabolic system, researchers have the capacity to design vaccines capable of producing the antibodies needed in order to prevent humans from a particular disease.[6] Also, comprehension as to how one specialized system may influence another is advantageous when it comes to developing tools and methods to prevent disease.

The aim of this article is to discuss how systems biology can be used when studying broad and narrow subjects, examine the top-down and bottom-up methods used in systems biology, as well as expand on how the study can further be used to understand diseases and health conditions with hopes of developing drugs and vaccinations for patients.

10.2 Theme 1: Two perspectives on systems biology in medicine

Over the past several decades, biologists and other scientists have continuously gathered information in order to understand everything there is to know about how cells function.[7] Being the smallest functional units in living organisms, cells were difficult to study before some of the major advancements in technology emerged. For example, the invention of the microscope catapulted the desire for scientists to study cellular properties.[8] Thanks to this essential tool, scientists were given the capability to observe the structure of various types of cells in organisms. By having the ability to closely observe cells, they were able to make valuable hypotheses such as how humans emerged and how various species relate to one another. At the same time, the expanding array of cellular detail sparked the development of new methods of researching these tiny units. A popular method used to research the function of cells includes growing a selected type of cell in a petri dish containing materials that allow cells to replicate and survive *in vitro*.[9] This method allows researchers to study living cells and helps them analyze cellular activity outside the organism. Today, upgrades in methods and technology allow cell biologists to create 2D or 3D representations of cells for use in the development of medicine and research.[10]

With technology becoming more and more advanced and new methods being practiced, the scientific field is progressively expanding. As more discoveries are made, more possibilities arise within the field. This growth has and will continue to initiate more specified substudies within the field of science. Biological researchers, for instance, have divided amongst themselves in order to study particular aspects of ourselves as well as the world we live in. Today, the field of biology branches into almost a hundred different specified areas of study. Among them is an up-and-coming approach to biology, namely, systems biology.

Systems biology focuses on studying the interactions of specific components in a system. These systems could range from broad systems such as ecological systems to smaller, narrower systems such as those at the cellular level within the human body.[4] The systemic approach helps researchers develop a more generalized manner of studying ourselves and the world we live in.

Driven by the curiosity of scientists, it has the potential to be applied to a wide array of research studies.[7] This expanding field is steadily providing essential tools that give researchers and healthcare professionals the capacity to describe, model, and visualize the various aspects of systems at all biological levels.[3]

Unlike other branches of biology, systems biology integrates numerous other fields of biology in order to understand different aspects of our world. For instance, a study performed by a team of immunologists, pharmacologists, and systems biologists was conducted in order to assess the vaccine-induced immunity in humans. This study used the systemic approach to produce models and computational analysis that helped to accurately produce data that supported the initial hypothesis.[11]

Furthermore, the systematic approach to studying biology has become increasingly popular with the help of advancements in technology and medicine. Over the past few decades, steady advancements in scientific technology have produced devices and computers with more powerful processing capabilities.[12] Advanced technology makes it possible to visualize pieces of our world that we never thought existed. Thanks to continual advancements in research-based technology, scientists have made astonishing realizations pertaining to the diversification of species and the function and structure of microbacteria.[13] Through this developing research and technology, the field of systems biology has aided in the improvement of medicine and vaccinations.

In pharmacological studies, researchers can use this approach to develop alternate drug therapies for patients as well as manufacture vaccinations. For instance, by sustaining a strong understanding of the dynamics and structure of the major organ systems in our bodies, pharmacologists can use the systemic approach to biology when developing medications for patients. This study also makes it possible for them to design medications that best fit the needs of patients with specific health-related issues.

10.2.1 The narrow perspective

When researchers use the systemic approach in application to medicine, one of the two perspectives that can be used is the narrow perspective. In the medical field, this perspective focuses on the microscopic networks and cellular processes of the human body. This method is utilized when doctors and researchers are presented with a difficulty of some sort and must use theoretical knowledge in order to determine a solution.[14] In other words, given the cause of the health condition of a patient, doctors and researchers are able to use the systemic approach in order to develop a solution for the patient. This is made possible by focusing on the minute systems of our bodies. For example, if a patient were previously diagnosed with a malignant tumor within the abdomen, a doctor could use background knowledge of how cancerous tumors impact the body. Using this knowledge, the doctor could use a method, such as chemotherapy, to provide a solution for the patient.

This perspective is advantageous in conjugation with developing vaccines to prevent prevalent diseases in the overall population. For instance, the systemic approach and decades of research has embellished our understanding of how the HIV/AIDS virus thrives and hides in an infected person (Simon). Over the past few decades, researchers around the globe have dedicated themselves to designing a vaccine to prevent the spread of this fatal virus. Geneticists, micro-biologists, and system biologists have discovered how the HIV/AIDS virus replicates and manipulates the genetic sequences with those infected. So far, some biomedical researchers have shown success in using a vaccine that induces a strong T-cell-mediated immune response.[15] These studies remain at the forefront of developing a vaccine for the HIV/AIDS virus, thanks to the use of systemic approaches to biology. Further advancements in methods and technology are expected to help to progressively develop a vaccine for use by the general public.

Furthermore, a narrow perspective to systems biology makes designing prescription drugs for patients possible. In the global population today, some of the leading health concerns are high blood pressure, diabetes, and obesity.[16] By studying some of the major organ systems of the human body at the microscopic level, biomedical researchers can target specific components within the metabolic system of the body in order to treat patients with these health issues. For patients suffering from an abnormally high amount of glucose in their blood stream (i.e., type 2 diabetes), medical professionals can provide prescriptions that reduce the release of glucose from the liver as well as increase the patients' sensitivity to insulin.[2] This is only one example of how using the narrow perspective of systems biology is shaping the lives of patients and providing the population with prescriptions needed to live a long and healthy life.

10.2.2 The broad perspective

Unlike the narrow perspective of systems biology in medicine, the broad perspective uses an influx of information in order to determine the specific cause of a medical concern. While the narrow perspective is often used when the cause of a medical concern is already known, the broad perspective is used when the underlying cause of a health concern is unknown. This perspective is more commonly practiced in the medical field, due to the fact that health risks usually presented to doctors are more common than not. When treating patients, doctors often proceed by treating the patients depending on the specific symptoms he or she may be presenting. So, when a patient presents a doctor with various symptoms of an illness, the doctor can use this perspective to eliminate potential causes of the illness.

When using this perspective in the medical field, it can also be used to determine the underlying cause of an illness. A macroscopic way of diagnosing a patient can easily be associated with environmental factors that influence the health of patients. In order to diagnose the cause of an illness, doctors can examine potential causes by examining the environment in which a patient may live. For instance, a doctor can accurately diagnose a patient by investigating if the patient has recently moved to a location with a very different environment, that is, from a suburban area to a rural area. According to an observational study conducted in 2007, an industrial environment with a high population of people has proven to have an astonishingly negative effect on the overall health of the population.[17] By living in these areas, people are significantly more likely to be exposed to surroundings that are considered unsanitary. These surroundings can house various forms of bacteria, including super bugs such as MRSA. By using a broad perspective when analyzing patients, medical professionals can determine potential causes of illnesses in patients.

10.3 Theme 2: The top-down and bottom-up approaches to systems biology

When a scientist or researcher studies something, whether it may be the anatomy of a plant, the solar system, or the deepest parts of the ocean, he or she must always develop some sort of method or approach. These are crucial to successfully understanding the subject and help researchers to be able to accurately analyze their observations and data collected. In systems biology, there are two common approaches researchers use to study the world around us. These approaches are known as the *top-down* and *bottom-up approaches*.

Regardless of the subject, researchers need to be able to organize information gained by performing research in order to progressively study a subject. When it comes to research, specific methods and approaches can be designed for specific subjects. In genomics, computer software systems are used to track samples and data, search results, and modify data. These systems have an efficient impact on the way laboratories function by organizing data in such a way that it is easily accessible as well as performing tasks that would otherwise be time-consuming to the researcher.[18] Without any sort of method to research, data could easily be misinterpreted or lost. This would not only be time-inefficient, but it would also hinder the progress of the study.

The top-down and bottom-up approaches to studying organisms at the system level are strictly opposite. As mentioned previously, the top-down approach begins by first observing and analyzing an organism as one entire unit and then continues to break down the organism into smaller segments. On the other hand, the bottom-up approach does just the opposite. This approach aims to understand individual segments of the organism and further build on the understanding of these small segments to later understand the entire unit.

10.3.1 The top-down approach

One of the most common approaches to systems biology is the top-down approach. By definition, this approach uses background knowledge of the subject to develop more specified concepts pertaining to the subject.[2] The approach begins with one general goal in mind, such as finding the cause of cancer, and is further utilized by developing theories related to that goal. This helps researchers identify desired properties and establish a certain algorithm for a set of goals in order to be able to define the system being studied.[19] In order to accomplish the overall goal of a study, macroscopic properties must first be analyzed and understood. Figure 10.1 displays the method behead using the top-down approach. By understanding the macroscopic elements first, researchers can develop a model network that resembles how the properties and subproperties function together. For instance, when a biologist examines the anatomy of a human, they may first begin by observing some of the major organs such as the brain, heart, and lungs. By understanding these components, the biologist can use this information in order to further examine more microscopic elements of the body, which can be used to understand how the circulatory, nervous, and respiratory systems all function together to make for a healthy individual.

This approach is especially useful in the medical field because it provides doctors with the ability to make accurate diagnoses for patients using observational techniques. For instance, by observing the symptoms of a patient, a doctor can use background knowledge to theorize about the diagnosis

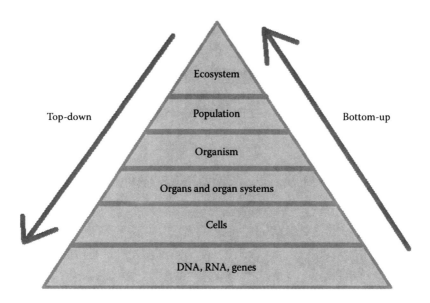

Figure 10.1 A way in which two of the most common approaches to system biology are studied.

of the patient. With theories in mind, the doctor can utilize the top-down approach to run the necessary tests in order to rule out possible causes for the symptoms of the patient.

10.3.2 The bottom-up approach

While the top-down approach begins by looking at a broad range of systems and further analyzes the smaller networks within them, the bottom-up approach does just the opposite. This approach begins by unravelling the more biologically complex foundation of a subject and progressively develops concepts that bring forth a broad understanding of the subject as a whole. This is achieved with the help of the latest advances in technology, experimental design, and theoretical modeling.[20] The ultimate goal of this approach is to incorporate various pathway models into a model for the entire system level.[7] This approach has proven to be effective in a diversity of branches in the scientific field such as genetics, cell biology, and ecology.

In the medical field, the bottom-up approach focuses on using fine elements in order to develop solutions for patients. These elements include, but are not limited to, neurological, hematological, and metabolic aspects of patients. By examining these elements in patients, doctors can assess potential causes for medical altercations. In turn, this would help to produce a plausible solution. A team of researchers at the University of Sydney applied the bottom-up approach in order to formulate nanoparticles by building the particles from drug molecules in a solution.[21] Nanoparticle-encapsulated drugs are currently being studied in order to determine potential solutions to common medical conditions. The use of nanoparticles in pharmacological research is just one example in which this approach can be applied to medical research. An alternate example of using the bottom-up approach would be in the hospital setting. When assisting patients, doctors commonly inquire about past medical conditions of close relatives of patients. By evaluating the health of close relatives, doctors can assess and determine if a condition is hereditary. With this information in mind, a plausible solution can be attained by building onto the theoretical knowledge gained.

10.4 Theme 3: Applying systems biology to medicine

Understanding organisms at the systemic level is fundamental for understanding how diseases pervade human bodies, how vaccines are developed, and how to actively improve the health of the general population. So far, the use of this approach in medicine has paved new ways of understanding the dynamics and structure of the human body in ways that have proven vital to revolutionary drug discoveries. For instance, the systemic approach in medicine has been particularly motivational when it comes to studying the metabolic processes involved in the breakdown of drugs in the body. One researcher,

Marcel de Groot, demonstrated the importance of this approach when observing enzymes of the cytochrome P450 superfamily. According to this researcher, the enzyme is responsible for approximately 90% of the metabolism of all drugs. By actively studying this family of enzymes, researchers can use 3D modeling techniques to help guide the development of new medicinal drugs.[22] This is only one example of the many ways scientists can apply systems biology when designing medicinal drugs.

Furthermore, the use of systems biology in the field of medicine helps scientists and medical professionals understand the behavior and foundation of various diseases. Understanding how diseases thrive within a living host as well as how they are contracted influences the development of preventive health care. Without knowledge on how a certain disease functions, making a vaccine to prevent the disease is virtually impossible. Systems biology allows these researchers to study diseases inside and out in order to prevent the spread of diseases as well as eliminate them. The approach sparks the development of an essential part of modern medicine: vaccines and medicinal drugs.

10.4.1 Using systems biology to understand disease and health problems

There are many methods and techniques available for researchers to use when studying diseases and health conditions. Systems biology greatly influences these procedures by providing modular networks that can be studied from the larger components and then delving into the smaller ones or vice versa. The systemic approach allows researchers and medical professionals to be able to fully perceive the various systems of the human body as well as understand how these systems contribute to one another. With this proficiency, diseases and health problems implementing the population can be more efficiently understood.

In modern medical technology, geneticists and microbiologists are capable of using methods involving genetic testing to understand genetic mutations and anomalies that could be pathogenic. Genetic testing offers insight into the nature of certain diseases and health conditions by analyzing a small sample of a patient's DNA, RNA, chromosomes, metabolites, or the like.[23] With this sample, researchers can visualize the chemical makeup of a patient's genes and look for deletions or mutations that may cause phenotypical health conditions. This innovative way of understanding the health of patients applies the bottom-up systematic approach to biology by analyzing the microscopic systems and building upon these findings. By doing so, researchers can determine the root cause of diseases and health conditions. This could potentially lead to the development of preventative medical treatment or even a cure.

Systems biology is also applied to understanding health conditions and diseases in hospitals and patient care facilities on a regular basis. Instances of the application occur when doctors inquire about the medical history of a patient's family.

By using this technique to determine if a condition is hereditary, a systemic approach is being applied. Determining the inheritance of a disease or condition can lay a foundation for which doctors can determine a cause. For instance, a model known as a *pedigree* that presents the inheritance of a condition can be developed using a family tree. This inheritance model can help medical professionals and geneticists visualize if the condition is sex-linked or autosomal, as well as determine the likelihood of it being passed to offspring. Researchers at the Wuhan University of Science and Technology collected data from a family of nine individuals, three generations in all, and used this data to produce a pedigree. This pedigree served as a foundation for which the researchers could examine the inheritance of a blood-clotting disorder within this specific bloodline. With information from studies such as this one provided by geneticists, microbiologists can produce theories and ideas regarding how the condition can be genetically altered or edited. With the help of new technology, genes that code for a health condition can be snipped or altered in such a way that it is no longer expressed when passed to offspring. Another team of researchers from the National Institute of Allergy and Infectious Diseases examined the use of gene editing in hopes of acquiring a cure for HIV/AIDS. The study used the Cas9/guide RNA system to inactivate the viral genome in an infected person. The study proved to be promising in developing a cure for this tenacious disease. Using techniques and models such as these, researchers and medical professionals can use the information obtained to advance medical research and possible work on the development of a cure.

10.4.2 Using systems biology to develop drugs and vaccines

Medicinal drugs and vaccines play a pivotal role when it comes to providing optimum health for the overall population. Without therapeutic techniques, diseases would be practically unavoidable and minor health problems would be devastating. Since the early years of the twentieth century, medicinal drugs have provided a longer lifespan for the public and improved the quality of life of patients.[24]

As time goes on, bacteria and viruses are slowly and steadily adapting to drug therapies aimed to eliminate them from living hosts. These new, and stronger, strains of disease-causing agents are now easier to contract and harder to avoid. Using systems biology, medical professionals can collaborate with cell biologists and other researchers in order to develop vaccines capable of preventing new strains of diseases. By studying the structure and dynamics of viral beings as well as the capabilities of the human immune system, researchers have the capacity to develop vaccines that target specific viruses. For instance, in 2009 a virus containing a unique combination of gene segments from both North American and Eurasian swine lineage began to circulate in humans.[25] This virus, H1N1 influenza (swine flu), emerged undetected and proved to be resistant to modern vaccinations for swine flu. By closely analyzing the classical form of swine flu, researchers were able to accumulate data and information pertaining to the function of this new strain in order to develop a vaccine. With the help of modern technology, researchers were soon able to use functional assays to determine that the strain was sensitive to the antiviral drugs oseltamivir and zanamivir.[26] Using this information, researchers were able to compound a vaccine that successfully prevents the contraction of this new form of swine flu. Within a few years, the vaccine was available for public use and successfully reduced the number of people infected with H1N1 influenza by approximately 60%.[27]

When it comes to bacterial infections, treatment can be challenging, as there are many different infectious bacteria in the environment and many different symptoms that can be expressed. When a person is infected by bacteria, improper hygiene and misuse of antibiotics can make infectious bacteria more resistant to therapies. These "superbugs" can lay dormant in settings with a high population of people such as gyms, hospitals, and schools. They can be easily contracted and can cause moderate to severe infections in hosts. In order to eliminate the bacteria from an infected person, scientists and medical professionals use research techniques that incorporate things such as bacteriophages and gel electrophoresis.[28] By evaluating the use of binary fission in the bacteria and understanding the cellular properties of humans, researchers can develop antibiotics aimed to disintegrate the cell wall of infected cells, eventually causing cellular death. The bacterial response to antibiotic treatment is highly complex and is ultimately based on subcellular pathways, such as genetic and biochemical pathways. The role of systems biology in drug discovery lies within these early developmental stages. These stages of the developmental process are essential because they compile information and observational data on the major biological processes and apply them to developing drugs for medicinal purposes.

10.5 Conclusion

In conclusion, systems biology is continuously expanding within the field of science. It harnesses the ability to bring various divisions of science together in order to generate new discoveries and further explore things we have already learned. This approach pushes scientists and researchers to a new level of understanding, allowing for new methods and techniques for use in research. Medical professionals are steadily teaming up with microbiologists, geneticists, pharmacologists, and many more in an effort to provide optimal health care for the overall population.

Using one of the major approaches in systems biology, namely the top-down or bottom-up approaches, researchers and medical professionals can observe various aspects of our world and further understand the systematic functions between them. This allows for a stronger foundation of knowledge pertaining to the subject at hand, which can further be applied to advances in medicine.

Biology and Optimal Health   211

For instance, microbiologists are able to merge information pertaining to the function and dynamics of viruses and bacteria with geneticists in order to develop vaccines and medicinal drugs. By bringing researchers of various fields together, systems biology is at the forefront of progressing advancements within the field of medicine. The approach organizes information and data collected, which helps researchers understand the functions and dynamics of various diseases. By doing so, the production of vaccinations for the public's use is made possible. This greatly reduces the number of infected individuals within our population.

Overall, the field of systems biology is boundless. It has and will continue to expand our knowledge of everything this world has to offer. With its efforts, advancements in the field of medicine will continue to evolve for the better by providing an understanding of our own complex systems. Researchers and medical professionals around the globe are incorporating theories and data in order to better the health of patients. With the help of improvements in technology, the study of systems biology is expected to lengthen the average lifespan by providing new methods for the treatment of patients. For instance, some researchers today are developing alternative treatments for patients with cancer. Using prostate cancer as a model, researchers at the Massachusetts Institute of Technology have developed a method for treating patients using docetaxel-encapsulated nanoparticles. When tested *in vivo*, an astonishing 100% of the animals survived the 109-day study (Farokhzad). Promising research such as this can provide cancer patients with treatments that have fewer side effects and health risks. Systems biology will continue to influence medical research in ways that will improve medicine and health care.

References

1. Kitano, H. (2002). Systems biology: A brief overview. *Science, 295*(5560), 1662–1664. doi:10.1126/science.1069492.
2. Khan, S. (2016). *Bottom-up vs. Top-down Processing.* Retrieved August 3, 2016, from https://www.khanacademy.org/science/health-and-medicine/nervous-system-and-sensory-infor/sensory-perception-2014-03-27T18:45:20.451Z/v/bottom-up-versus-top-down-processing
3. Blaney, J. E., Durbin, A. P., Murphy, B. R., & Whitehead, S. S. (2006). Development of a live attenuated dengue virus vaccine using reverse genetics. *Viral Immunology, 19*(1), 10–32. doi:10.1089/vim.2006.19.10
4. Bard, J. (2013). Systems biology—The broader perspective. *Cells, 2*(2), 414–431. doi:10.3390/cells2020414.
5. Welcome to the Department of Systems Biology @HMS. *Systems Biology—Harvard Medical School.* Harvard Medical School Department of Systems Biology, 2010. Web. 24 July 2016.
6. Buonaguro, L., & Pulendran, B. (2010). Immunogenomics and systems biology of vaccines. *Immunological Reviews, 239*(1), 197–208. doi:10.1111/j.1600-065x.2010.00971.x.
7. Bruggeman, F. J., & Westerhoff, H. V. (2007). The nature of systems biology. *Trends in Microbiology, 15*(1), 45–50. doi:10.1016/j.tim.2006.11.003.

8. Frost, W. N., Wang, J., & Brandon, C. J. (2007). A stereo-compound hybrid microscope for combined intracellular and optical recording of invertebrate neural network activity. *Journal of Neuroscience Methods, 162*(1–2), 148–154. doi:10.1016/j.jneumeth.2007.01.003.
9. Mohanty, B. K., & Kushner, S. R. (2006). The majority of *Escherichia coli* mRNAs undergo post-transcriptional modification in exponentially growing cells. *Nucleic Acids Research, 34*(19), 5695–5704. doi:10.1093/nar/gkl684.
10. Xu, F., Wu, J., Wang, S., Durmus, N. G., Gurkan, U. A., & Demirci, U. (2011). Microengineering methods for cell-based microarrays and high-throughput drug-screening applications. *Biofabrication, 3*(3), 034101. doi:10.1088/1758-5082/3/3/034101.
11. Li, S., Rouphael, N., Duraisingham, S., Romero-Steiner, S., Presnell, S., Davis, C., et al. (2013). Molecular signatures of antibody responses derived from a systems biology study of five human vaccines. *Nature Immunology, 15*(2), 195–204. doi:10.1038/ni.2789.
12. Lu, W., & Lieber, C. M. (2007). Nanoelectronics from the bottom up. *Nature Materials, 6*(11), 841–850. doi:10.1038/nmat2028.
13. Scher, J. U., & Abramson, S. B. (2011). The microbiome and rheumatoid arthritis. *Nature Reviews Rheumatology, 7*, 569–578. doi:10.1038/nrrheum.2011.121.
14. Klipp, E., Herwig, R., Kowald, A., Wierling, C., & Lehrach, H. (2005). *Systems Biology in Practice: Conceptions, Implementation, and Application*. Berlin, Germany: Wiley-VCH Verlag GmbH.
15. Johnston, M. I., & Fauci, A. S. (2007). An HIV vaccine—Evolving concepts. *New England Journal of Medicine, 356*(20), 2073–2081. doi:10.1056/nejmra066267.
16. World Health Organization. (2009). *Global Health Risks: Mortality and Burden of Disease Attributable to Selected Major Risks*. Geneva: World Health Organization.
17. Rao, M., Prasad, S., Adshead, F., & Tissera, H. (2007). The built environment and health. *The Lancet, 370*(9593), 1111–1113. doi:10.1016/S0140-6736(07)61260-4.
18. Truong, C. V., Groeneveld, L. F., Morgenstern, B., & Groeneveld, E. (2011). MolabIS—An integrated information system for storing and managing molecular genetics data. *BMC Bioinformatics, 12*(1), 425–440. doi:10.1186/1471-2105-12-425.
19. Haken, H. (2004). *Synergetic Computers and Cognition: A Top-Down Approach to Neural Nets* (2nd ed., Vol. 50). Springer-Verlag, Berlin, Heidelberg.
20. Bausch, A. R., & Kroy, K. (2006). A bottom-up approach to cell mechanics. *Nature Physics, 2*(4), 231–238. doi:10.1038/nphys260.
21. Chan, H., & Kwok, P. C. (2011). Production methods for nanodrug particles using the bottom-up approach. *Nanodrug Particles and Nanoformulations for Drug Delivery, 63*(6), 406–416. doi:10.1016/j.addr.2011.03.011.
22. Groot, M. J. (2006, July). Designing better drugs: Predicting cytochrome P450 metabolism. *Drug Discovery Today, 11*(13–14), 601–606. doi:10.1016/j.drudis.2006.05.001.
23. Burke, W. (2002). Genomic medicine: Genetic testing. *New England Journal of Medicine, 347*(23), 1867–1875. Retrieved August 30, 2016.
24. The History of Prescription Drugs. (2012). Retrieved August 20, 2016, from http://www.goodmedicinebadbehavior.org/explore/history_of_prescription_drugs.html.
25. Garten, R. J., Davis, C. T., Russell, C. A., Shu, B., Lindstrom, S., Balish, A., et al. (2009). Antigenic and genetic characteristics of swine-origin 2009 A (H1N1) influenza viruses circulating in humans. *Science, 325*(5937), 197–201. doi:10.1126/science.1176225.
26. Dawood, F. S., Iuliano, A. D., Reed, C., Meltzer, M. I., Shay, D. K., Cheng, P., et al. (2012). Estimated global mortality associated with the first 12 months of 2009 pandemic influenza A H1N1 virus circulation: A modelling study. *The Lancet Infectious Diseases, 12*(9), 687–695. doi:10.1016/s1473-3099(12)70121-4.
27. Vaccine Effectiveness—How Well Does the Flu Vaccine Work? (2016). Retrieved August 25, 2016, from http://www.cdc.gov/flu/about/qa/vaccineeffect.htm.
28. Singh, A., Goering, R. V., Simjee, S., Foley, S. L., & Zervos, M. J. (2006). Application of molecular techniques to the study of hospital infection. *Clinical Microbiology Reviews, 19*(3), 512–530. doi:10.1128/cmr.00025-05.

29. Alon, U. (2006). *An Introduction to Systems Biology: Design Principles of Biological Circuits.* Boca Raton, FL: Chapman & Hall/CRC.

30. Belda-Lois, J., Horno, S. M., Bermejo-Bosch, I., Moreno, J. C., Pons, J. L., Farina, D., et al. (2011). Rehabilitation of gait after stroke: A review towards a top-down approach. *Journal of NeuroEngineering and Rehabilitation, 8*(1), 66. doi:10.1186/1743-0003-8-66.

31. Berg, J. M., Tymoczko, J. L., Gatto, G. J., Jr., & Stryer, L. (2015). *Biochemistry* (8th ed.). W. H. Freeman, New York.

32. Bleakley, H. (2007). Disease and development: Evidence from hookworm eradication in the American South. *The Quarterly Journal of Economics, 122*(1), 73–117. doi:10.1162/qjec.121.1.73.

33. Borenstein, E., & Ullman, S. (2008). Combined top-down/bottom-up segmentation. *IEEE Transactions on Pattern Analysis and Machine Intelligence, 30*(12), 2109–2125. doi:10.1109/tpami.2007.70840.

34. Cooper, G. M., & Hausman, R. E. (2013). *The Cell: A Molecular Approach* (6th ed.). Sunderland, MA: Sinauer Associates.

35. Daszak, P., Zambrana-Torrelio, C., Bogich, T. L., Fernandez, M., Epstein, J. H., Murray, K. A., et al. (2012). Interdisciplinary approaches to understanding disease emergence: The past, present, and future drivers of Nipah virus emergence. *Proceedings of the National Academy of Sciences, 110*(Suppl 1), 3681–3688. doi:10.1073/pnas.1201243109.

36. Farokhzad, O. C., Cheng, J., Teply, B. A., Sherifi, I., Jon, S., Kantoff, P. W., et al. (2006). Targeted nanoparticle-aptamer bioconjugates for cancer chemotherapy in vivo. *Proceedings of the National Academy of Sciences, 103*(16), 6315–6320. doi:10.1073/pnas.0601755103.

37. Feng, K., Chapagain, A., Suh, S., Pfister, S., & Hubacek, K. (2011). Comparison of bottom-up and top-down approaches to calculating the water footprints of nations. *Economic Systems Research, 23*(4), 371–385. doi:10.1080/09535314.2011.638276.

38. Fraser, E. D., Dougill, A. J., Mabee, W. E., Reed, M., & Mcalpine, P. (2006). Bottom up and top down: Analysis of participatory processes for sustainability indicator identification as a pathway to community empowerment and sustainable environmental management. *Journal of Environmental Management, 78*(2), 114–127. doi:10.1016/j.jenvman.2005.04.009.

39. Goodwin, R., Haque, S., Neto, F., & Myers, L. B. (2009). Initial psychological responses to Influenza A, H1N1 ("Swine flu"). *BMC Infectious Diseases, 9*(1), 166. doi:10.1186/1471-2334-9-166.

40. Guido, N. J., Wang, X., Adalsteinsson, D., Mcmillen, D., Hasty, J., Cantor, C. R., et al. (2006). A bottom-up approach to gene regulation. *Nature: International Weekly Journal of Science, 439*(7078), 856–860. doi:10.1038/nature04473.

41. Holmes, E., Wilson, I. D., & Nicholson, J. K. (2008). Metabolic phenotyping in health and disease. *Cell, 134*(5), 714–717. doi:10.1016/j.cell.2008.08.026.

42. Kahn, S. E., Haffner, S. M., Heise, M. A., Herman, W. H., Holman, R. R., Jones, N. P., et al. (2006). Glycemic durability of rosiglitazone, metformin, or glyburide monotherapy. *New England Journal of Medicine, 355*(23), 2427–2443. doi:10.1056/nejmoa066224.

43. Karp, G., & Geer, P. V. (2013). *Cell and Molecular Biology: Concepts and Experiments* (7th ed., Vol. 1). Hoboken, NJ: John Wiley.

44. Kemp, P. (2006, September). History of regenerative medicine: Looking backwards to move forwards. *Regenerative Medicine, 1*(5), 653–669. doi:10.2217/17460751.1.5.653.

45. Lipinski, C. A., Lombardo, F., Dominy, B. W., & Feeney, P. J. (2012). Experimental and computational approaches to estimate solubility and permeability in drug discovery and development settings. *Advanced Drug Delivery Reviews, 64*, 4–17. doi:10.1016/j.addr.2012.09.019.

46. Murphy, F. A. (1995). *Virus Taxonomy: Classification and Nomenclature of Viruses* (Vol. 6). Wien: Springer-Verlag.

47. Nicholson, J. K. (2006). Global systems biology, personalized medicine and molecular epidemiology. *Molecular Systems Biology, 2*, 52. doi:10.1038/msb4100095.

48. Simon, V., Ho, D. D., & Abdool Karim, Q. (2006, August 5–11). HIV/AIDS epidemiology, pathogenesis, prevention, and treatment. *The Lancet, 368*(9534), 489–504.
49. Slonczewski, J., & Foster, J. W. (2009). *Microbiology: An Evolving Science.* New York: W.W. Norton &. Co.
50. Taylor, A. G., Goehler, L. E., Galper, D. I., Innes, K. E., & Bourguignon, C. (2010). Top-down and bottom-up mechanisms in mind-body medicine: Development of an integrative framework for psychophysiological research. *EXPLORE: The Journal of Science and Healing, 6*(1), 29–41. doi:10.1016/j.explore.2009.10.004.
51. Wang, Z., Zhao, Z., Xu, K., Sun, G., Song, L., Yin, H., et al. (2015). Hereditary protein S deficiency leads to ischemic stroke. *Molecular Medicine Reports, 12*, 3279–3284. doi:10.3892/mmr.2015.3793.

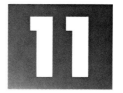

The Role of Pro-Inflammatory Factors and Metabolic Stress in Disease

Christopher T. Kaul, Aditya Grover, and Yashwant V. Pathak
University of South Florida
Tampa, Florida

Contents

11.1 Introduction	217
11.2 Intestinal regulation and dysregulation	218
11.3 Chronic inflammatory state and its effects on aging and the cardiovascular and pulmonary systems	220
11.4 Diabetes	220
11.5 Inflammation and diabetes	221
11.6 Diabetic nephropathy	222
11.7 Diabetic neuropathy	223
11.8 Conclusion	223
References	224

11.1 Introduction

The human body is an incredible biochemical laboratory that runs with the continuous goal of achieving homeostasis in response to external and internal stimuli. Homeostasis is a series of mechanical, chemical, and biological reactions within the body that one undergoes in order to maintain an internal environment that is suitable for survival. A simple example that is often used to describe the phenomenon is sweating when the body becomes too hot in order to bring down temperature. Without this, the body would become too hot, proteins would begin to denature, and widespread damage would ensue. In many cases, metabolic abnormalities and disease processes are in fact the human body's failing attempts or inability to regulate its internal environment. Therefore, the pathology of many diseases is the inability to achieve this homeostasis. This chapter will highlight the various ways that the body's normal regulatory functions are in some way damaged or affected within specific disease processes. In order to accomplish this, one must understand the role of pro-inflammatory cells, as well as immunological cells that play a role in specific disease processes. With this knowledge one can then begin to understand the impact of various anti-inflammatory medications, specific therapies, and the potential within nutrigenomics that is discussed in different parts of this book.

11.2 Intestinal regulation and dysregulation

In all regions of the body there are regulatory cells and molecules that work together in a symphony of reactions to maintain normal bodily functions. Within the intestinal tract, the pulmonary system of the body is a flurry of such reactions, working continuously to maintain homeostasis. The gut has a unique epithelium that constantly undergoes regeneration and growth in an ongoing battle to selectively uptake nutrients for survival [1]. The internal environment of the gut also is home to 10–100 trillion different microbes that make up what is known as the *microbiome* [2]. In order to understand the ways in which the body regulates itself, one must understand the barrier functions, autography, and cytokines of the gut.

The interstitial immunity of the gut starts with the functions of the mucosal barrier [1]. The intestinal mucosal surface is comprised of a physical outer barrier of intestinal epithelial cells joined by tight junctions and arranged into pore-like crypts, and in the small intestine protruding villi, protected by a layer of protective mucus that harbors a variety of secreted factors [1]. Underneath this layer are interstitial stem cells that continuously divide in order to maintain this border [1]. These cells then go on to form the various epithelial monolayer of the gut, including absorptive enterocytes, hormone-secreting enteroendocrine cells, mucin-producing goblet cells, and antimicrobial peptide-producing Paneth cells [1]. Connecting these cells are a series of tight junctions composed of adhesive molecules that prevent unregulated passage of biotic and abiotic material into the body. As a result, the sterile environment within the body is physically separated from the heavily populated microbiome of the intestines.

There is also a series of immunological regulatory molecules known as *cytokines* that play major roles in regulating the microbiome. Paneth cells have been shown to play a major role in regulating the immune response to microbes within the gut [3]. These cells are rich in granules that contain α-defensins, lysozyme, lipopolysaccharide-binding protein, and RegIII-γ. These encompass a large amount of the antimicrobial regulators to inhibit growth of the foreign cells that would otherwise run unchecked in the gut, leading to a variety of diseases. These granules are released in response to cytokines such as TNF-α, IL1-β, and IL-6, as well as intrinsic components of potentially invading microbes [1,3]. Mucosal immunoglobulin, IgA, is also secreted by B-cells in order to defend against such microbes [1]. These pro-inflammatory molecules

218   Nutrigenomics and Nutraceuticals

are usually held in check by other cytokines, such as IL-10 and IL-22, which downregulate the immune response [1].

Autophagy is another important factor within immune regulation within the gut. Autophagy in the gut is a process in which specific white blood cells, known as *phagocytes*, consume cellular material in order to maintain homeostasis by recycling cellular debris for nutrients, attacking pathogenic microbes and playing a role in programmed cell death [1]. Macrophages and dendritic cells, the phagocytes within the gut, play a major role in the immune response to foreign material by consuming material that would otherwise cause harm to the body [1]. These cells also upregulate pro-inflammatory cytokines and chemokines such as IFN-γ, TNF-α, IL-1α, IL-2, and IL-6 and are normally downregulated by IL-4, IL-10, and IL-13 [1].

Dysregulation of pro-inflammatory molecules and cells can lead to various disease processes as well. One dysregulation of this intestinal border of note is irritable bowel disease (IBD). IBD is a chronic relapsing-remitting disease where the tight junctions and cellular lining of the gut are not properly maintained, leading to a failure of homeostasis [1]. As a result, the intestinal contents have an increased ability to interact with the normally sterile environment of the gut. This disease is characterized by unregulated pro-inflammatory processes within intestinal mucosa leading to diarrhea, often associated with blood [4]. Unopposed IL-6 within the gut is often implicated as one of the prevalent overactive pro-inflammatory cytokines, which leads to a breakdown in the tight junctions of the mucosa [1]. Invasion of microbes past the mucosal barrier can then ensue.

IBD is often treated with corticosteroids, which are designed to downregulate the immune response. These treatments also have major side effects on the body, including osteoporosis, hypertension, diabetes, weight gain, infections the body would normally be able to fight off, and Cushing syndrome. These treatments often require high dosages for long periods of time during flare-ups, further increasing the likelihood of side effects. As a result, they are not an ideal treatment. One of the proposed adjunctive therapies for IBD is omega-3 fatty acid [5]. Omega-3 is a popular anti-inflammatory fatty acid found in high concentrations in fish oils. Omega-3 has been shown to decrease the synthesis of inflammatory markers such as TNF-α, IL-6, IL-1β, and prostaglandin E2 and expression of TLR4 and NF-κB [5]. Therefore, omega-3 has been researched as a potential treatment for IBD. Unfortunately, the data gathered from this research is conflicted. Although studies have shown a decrease in symptoms of IBD, other studies have shown that the efficacy of omega-3 is highly dependent on the specific origin of the omega-3 fatty acid (native within fish versus synthetic), genetic variations of individuals being treated, as well as the methodology of the studies [5]. As a result, further research is needed to elucidate the exact extent to which omega-3 fatty acids can be used as a therapy for IBD [5].

11.3 Chronic inflammatory state and its effects on aging and the cardiovascular and pulmonary systems

Aging is a process still under research. One of the leading theories is that the aging process is highly connected to telomere reduction. Telomeres are non-transcribable regions of DNA located at the ends of chromosomes. As cells divide, a small amount of these telomeres are depleted, leading to DNA damage and eventual programmed cell death. However, with increased chronic inflammation, this process is accelerated. A chronic inflammatory state is also highly connected with cancer [6]. Cancer is a disease where, through a variety of mechanisms, unregulated cell growth occurs, leading to growth of tumors. Normally a single cell has a limited number of times it can divide, but in the case of cancer, cellular growth can continue indefinitely due to activation of a particular gene that transcribes telomerase. Telomerase is an enzyme that when activated allows for the prolongation of telomeres, therefore bypassing the normal innate limit a cell can divide. Smoking tobacco is one particular way in which the body can achieve a pro-inflammatory state, leading to increased cellular aging and predisposing individuals to cancer [6].

There are multiple ways in which a pro-inflammatory state can lead to an increase in cellular aging. For instance, activation of the NF-κB pathway is one of the key players in a chronic inflammatory state leading to aging. NF-κB is responsible for increased transcription of a variety of genes that lead to the production of pro-inflammatory molecules such as TNF-α, interleukins, AMs, and COX [6].

The effects of chronic low-grade inflammation is also the key mediator in cardiovascular diseases, such as coronary artery disease. At sites of injury, inflammatory cells and local cells alike release inflammatory markers that increase oxidative stress, damaging tissue and leading to atherosclerosis of vessels. This atherosclerosis can then evolve into a plaque, predisposing an individual to myocardial infarctions and emboli. Under normal situations, after tissue injury there is acute inflammation and resolution of the inflammation upon healing, mediated through specialized pro-resolving mediators (SPMs) [7]. These SPMs are free polyunsaturated fatty acids that are released from membrane phospholipids, which include arachidonic acid and various omega-3 fatty acids [7]. Their release provides an anti-inflammatory effect that locally blunts the innate immune system and promotes cellular restoration [7]. As a result, this diminishes cytokine release, leukocyte–endothelium interaction, and reactive oxygen species production, while at the same time increasing nitrous oxide production and prostacyclin release [7].

11.4 Diabetes

Diabetes is a chronic medical condition that currently affects around 300 million individuals around the world and is estimated to effect around 600 million in the next 20 years, with the greatest increase occurring in developing nations [8]. Diabetes results in a hyperglycemic state with serious long-term complications including nephropathy, neuropathy, and retinopathy, among others. The decrease in insulin secretion by pancreatic islet β-cells is thought to be one of the main pathogenic factors behind the disease process; however, evidence has shown that chronic inflammation due to obesity and resident tissue macrophages play an important role in pancreatic β-cell dysfunction characteristic of diabetic pathogenesis [9].

11.5 Inflammation and diabetes

Although there are multiple environmental and genetic factors that contribute to the development of diabetes, obesity is one of the largest contributors to development of the condition, with almost 80% of diabetic patients being overweight or obese [9]. Adipose tissue secretes a number of compounds apart from fatty acids, such as polypeptides, including hormones, cytokines, and chemokines, with varied effects on systemic inflammation and insulin resistance [10]. Insulin sensitivity is increased through secreted adipokines such as leptin and adiponectin, while other compounds such as resistin and retinol-binding protein 4 promote insulin resistance [10].

Further, the accumulation of adipose tissue in obese individuals serves not only the function of storage of excess calories and energy sources but also plays a reported role in chronic inflammation. Adipose tissue has been found to be closely associated with bone marrow–derived macrophages and lymphocytes and the density of inflammatory cells in adipose tissue is directly correlated to the magnitude of obesity [10,11]. The activation of these resident macrophages leads to the further activation of an increased number of macrophages in a self-propagating manner, which leads to the development of a chronic inflammatory state [10]. These inflammatory mediators lead to the development of an insulin-resistant state in multiple tissue types, including liver and skeletal muscle cells, which leads to the release of pro-inflammatory factors from these tissues, thereby further propagating the release of inflammatory factors from adipose tissue. For example, TNFα, IL-6, and IL-1β released from adipose tissue macrophages lead to the activation of serine kinases such as JNK and IKKβ in insulin-targeted cells, leading to insulin resistance through the phosphorylation of insulin resistance substrate proteins and receptors; furthermore, JNK and IKKβ lead to the upregulation of AP1 and NF-κB, which upregulate inflammatory mediators [10,12–14]. Indeed, cell and mouse models in which JNK and IKKβ are knocked out do not show insulin resistance through the above mentioned pathway [10,15,16].

It is hypothesized that the resident adipose tissue macrophages induce liver and skeletal muscle insulin resistance through inflammatory mediators. These act on liver Kupffer cells, resident bone-derived macrophages, to release local inflammatory mediators that induce insulin resistance in a paracrine fashion [10]. Indeed, knockout models that decrease the pro-inflammatory activity of Kupffer cells do not exhibit an insulin-resistant state [10,17]. Furthermore, Kupffer cells have been shown to be upregulated and highly activated in rat models fed a high-fat diet, leading to nonalcoholic steatohepatitis [18]. M1 macrophages in skeletal muscle adipose tissue may also function in a similar fashion, that is, adipose-derived inflammatory mediator–induced inflammatory mediator release, which acts in a paracrine fashion to induce insulin resistance in these tissues [10,19]. Free fatty acids have also been shown to induce macrophage cell–derived inflammation in fatty tissue through the increased expression of TNFα, IL-6, IL-1β, and MCP-1; furthermore, these inflammatory mediators have been shown to increase insulin resistance in L6 myoblasts [9,20,21]. These molecules may further activate resident skeletal muscle macrophages to increase inflammatory mediator release in a synergistic fashion to propagate the inflammatory reaction in high-fat exposure, thereby leading to insulin resistance [7,22].

IL-1β also plays a role in pancreatic islet β-cell inflammation through the induction of a local inflammatory response, which leads to the infiltration of macrophages in islet cell tissue. This leads to the release of local inflammatory mediators, which act in a paracrine fashion to induce the further migration of macrophages, eventually leading to fibrosis, apoptosis, and decreased insulin secretion [10,23]. Indeed, Ehses et al. have shown an increase in CD68+ inflammatory cells in diabetic patients [24].

11.6 Diabetic nephropathy

Diabetes-induced nephropathy has been shown to be caused by a hyperglycemic state as well as inflammatory responses that lead to proteinuria, glomerular hypertrophy, and fibrosis [25,26]. These processes are largely mediated through the function of renal macrophages recruited through a pro-inflammatory state. Human renal tissue samples from diabetic patients show an increased level of macrophages and activated T lymphocytes in the glomeruli and interstitium, which may cause an inflammatory state leading to glomerular immune complex deposition and eventual tissue fibrosis [27–29]. Indeed, the degree of fibrosis from human renal biopsies was found to be directly correlated to the amount of tissue macrophages and was also found to be highly correlated to signs of nephropathy, namely increased serum creatinine and proteinuria [30,31].

A number of pro-inflammatory mediators have been documented in diabetic renal tissue. Among these, the effects of IL-1 and TNFα have been studied and reported. IL-1 has been shown to alter the interaction of mesangial cells with podocytes to favor a pro-hyperplastic state by affecting the dynamics of the extracellular matrix apart from upregulating mesangial cell proliferation rate and adhesion molecule expression on endothelial cells and vascular smooth muscle cells [32]. TNFα has been shown to alter glomerular capillary permeability and the balance of vasodilatory and vasoconstrictive effects through the actions of reactive oxygen species, which are also a marker of inflammation [33].

11.7 Diabetic neuropathy

Diabetic neuropathy is characterized by axonal atrophy and demyelination, which may lead to the development of gangrenous foot ulcers and possible nontraumatic limb amputation [33]. Although a hyperglycemic state plays a role in the development of neuropathy, inflammation has also been suggested to be involved in the pathogenesis of diabetic neuropathy.

IL-1, IL-6, and IL-17 have been shown to be induced in peripheral neurons through persistent hyperglycemic state leading to neuropathic pain. Hyperglycemia leads to the glycosylation of neuron myelin, which induces an inflammatory response through the activity of macrophages and lymphocytes due to altered self-antigenicity. These inflammatory cells secrete local mediators, which leads to the recruitment of an increased number of inflammatory cells; these secrete cytokines, which further damage neuronal tissue [34,35]. One such molecule is TNFα, increased serum levels of which are directly correlated with the level of pain experienced and reported by diabetic patients [36]. Indeed, anti-TNFα antibody medication, such as infliximab, has been shown to decrease the level of pain reported in diabetic patients and TNFα knockout diabetic animal models exhibited lower incidences of neuropathy [37].

11.8 Conclusion

All in all, the body is constantly evaluating its current state in order to produce the appropriate response for that moment in time. These collective actions are in response to disease and external stimuli. They elicit metabolic consequences that if left unchecked could lead to disastrous long-term effects. These effects can lead to wide-ranging problems, from atherosclerosis to long-term inflammation, all of which lead to complex disease states. There are normal physiological responses to try and curb these responses, but when those mechanisms are broken or underutilized, homeostasis cannot be achieved properly. In the cases of IBD and cardiovascular disease, the body fails to diminish the inflammatory response. In diabetes, the body cannot control blood sugar levels due to desensitization, leading to widespread damage. The metabolic state of disease is an ongoing topic of research that continues to uncover new and exciting discoveries that can lead to improved treatments in the future.

References

1. Elshaer D, Begun J. 2016. The role of barrier function, autophagy, and cytokines in maintaining intestinal homeostasis. *Semin Cell Devel Biol.* 2017;61:51–59.
2. Turnbaugh PJ, Ley RE, Hamady M, Fraser-Liggett CM, Knight R, Gordon JI. The human microbiome project. *Nature* 2007;449:804–810.
3. Bevins CL, Salzman NH. Paneth cells, antimicrobial peptides and maintenance of intestinal homeostasis. *Nat Rev Microbiol.* 2011;9(5):356–368.
4. Silverberg MS, Satsangi J, Ahmad T, Arnott ID, Bernstein CN, Brant SR, et al. Toward an integrated clinical, molecular and serological classification of inflammatory bowel disease: Report of a Working Party of the 2005 Montreal World Congress of Gastroenterology. *Can J Gastroenterol.* 2005;19 Suppl A:5A.
5. Barbalho SM, Goulart Rde A, Quesada K, Bechara MD, de Carvalho Ade C. Inflammatory bowel disease: Can omega-3 fatty acids really help? *Ann Gastroenterol.* 2016;29(1):37–43.
6. Zhang J, Rane G, Dai X, Shanmugam MK, Arfuso F, Samy RP, et al. Ageing and the telomere connection: An intimate relationship with inflammation. *Ageing Res Rev.* 2016; 25:55–69.
7. Deeb RS, Hajjar DP. Repair mechanisms in oxidant-driven chronic inflammatory disease. *Am J Pathol.* 2016;186(7):1736–1749.
8. Guariguata L, Whiting DR, Hambleton I, Beagley J, Linnenkamp U, Shaw JE. Global estimates of diabetes prevalence for 2013 and projections for 2035. *Diabetes Res Clin Pract.* 2014;103(2):137–149.
9. Meshkani R, Vakili S. Tissue resident macrophages: Key players in the pathogenesis of type 2 diabetes and its complications. *Clin Chim Acta.* 2016;462:77–89. doi: 10.1016/j.cca.2016.08.015
10. Olefsky JM, Glass CK. Macrophages, inflammation, and insulin resistance. *Annu Rev Physiol.* 2010;72:219–246.
11. Weisberg SP, Hunter D, Huber R, Lemieux J, Slaymaker S, Vaddi K, et al. CCR2 modulates inflammatory and metabolic effects of high-fat feeding. *J Clin Investig.* 2006;116:115–124.
12. Bandyopadhyay GK, Yu JG, Ofrecio J, Olefsky JM. Increased p85/55/50 expression and decreased phosphotidylinositol 3-kinase activity in insulin-resistant human skeletal muscle. *Diabetes* 2005;54:2351–2359.
13. Itani SI, Ruderman NB, Schmieder F, Boden G. Lipid-induced insulin resistance in human muscle is associated with changes in diacylglycerol, protein kinase C, and Iκß-α. *Diabetes* 2002;51:2005–2011.
14. Nguyen MT, Favelyukis S, Nguyen AK, Reichart D, Scott PA, Jean A, et al. A subpopulation of macrophages infiltrates hypertrophic adipose tissue and is activated by free fatty acids via Toll-like receptors 2 and 4 and JNK-dependent pathways. *J Biol Chem.* 2007;282:35279–35292.
15. Hirosumi J, Tuncman G, Chang L, Gorgun CZ, Uysal KT, Maeda K, et al. A central role for JNK in obesity and insulin resistance. *Nature* 2002;420:333–336.
16. Solinas G, Vilcu C, Neels JG, Bandyopadhyay GK, Luo JL, Naugler W, et al. JNK1 in hematopoietically derived cells contributes to diet-induced inflammation and insulin resistance without affecting obesity. *Cell Metab.* 2007;6:386–397.
17. Schenk S, Saberi M, Olefsky JM. Insulin sensitivity: Modulation by nutrients and inflammation. *J Clin Investig.* 2008;118:2992–3002.
18. Su GL. Lipopolysaccharides in liver injury: Molecular mechanisms of Kupffer cell ctivation. *Am J Physiol Gastrointest Liver Physiol.* 2002;283(2):G256–G265.
19. Patsouris D, Li PP, Thapar D, Chapman J, Olefsky JM, Neels JG. Ablation of CD11c-positive cells normalizes insulin sensitivity in obese insulin resistant animals. *Cell Metab.* 2008;8:301–309.

20. Varma V, Yao-Borengasser A, Rasouli N, Nolen GT, Phanavanh B, Starks T, et al. Muscle inflammatory response and insulin resistance: Synergistic interaction between macrophages and fatty acids leads to impaired insulin action. *Am J Physiol Endocrinol Metab.* 2009;296(6):E1300–E1310.
21. Samokhvalov V, Bilan PJ, Schertzer JD, Antonescu CN, Klip A. Palmitate-and lipopolysaccharide-activated macrophages evoke contrasting insulin responses in muscle cells. *Am J Physiol Endocrinol Metab.* 2009;296(1):E37–E46.
22. Pillon NJ, Arane K, Bilan PJ, Chiu TT, Klip A. Muscle cells challenged with saturated fatty acids mount an autonomous inflammatory response that activates macrophages. *Cell Commun Signal.* 2012;10(1):30.
23. Abdulreda MH, Berggren PO. Islet inflammation in plain sight. *Diabetes Obes Metab.* 2013;15(s3):105–116.
24. Ehses JA, Perren A, Eppler E, Ribaux P, Pospisilik JA, Maor-Cahn R, et al. Increased number of islet-associated macrophages in type 2 diabetes. *Diabetes* 2007;56(9):2356–2370.
25. Sun Y-M, Su Y, Li J, Wang L-F. Recent advances in understanding the biochemical and molecular mechanism of diabetic nephropathy. *Biochem Biophys Res Commun.* 2013;433(4):359–361.
26. Lim AK, Tesch GH. Inflammation in diabetic nephropathy. *Mediat Inflamm.* 2012;2012:146154.
27. Hickey FB, Martin F. Diabetic kidney disease and immune modulation. *Curr Opin Pharmacol.* 2013;13(4):602–612.
28. Sassy-Prigent C, Heudes D, Mandet C, Bélair M-F, Michel O, Perdereau B. Early glomerular macrophage recruitment in streptozotocin-induced diabetic rats. *Diabetes* 2000;49(3):466–475.
29. Chow F, Ozols E, Nikolic-Paterson DJ, Atkins RC, Tesch GH. Macrophages in mouse type 2 diabetic nephropathy: Correlation with diabetic state and progressive renal injury. *Kidney Int.* 2004;65(1):116–128.
30. Furuta T, Saito T, Ootaka T, Soma J, Obara K, Abe K, et al. The role of macrophages in diabetic glomerulosclerosis. *Am J Kidney Dis.* 1993;21(5):480–485.
31. Nguyen D, Ping F, Mu W, Hill P, Atkins RC, Chadban SJ. Macrophage accumulation in human progressive diabetic nephropathy. *Nephrology* 2006;11(3):226–231.
32. Dalla Vestra M, Mussap M, Gallina P, Bruseghin M, Cernigoi AM, Saller A, et al. Acute-phase markers of inflammation and glomerular structure in patients with type 2 diabetes. *J Am Soc Nephrol.* 2005;16(3 Suppl. 1):S78–S82.
33. McCarthy ET, Sharma R, Sharma M, Li J-Z, Ge X-L, Dileepan KN, et al. TNF-alpha increases albumin permeability of isolated rat glomeruli through the generation of superoxide. *J Am Soc Nephrol.* 1998;9(3):433–438.
34. Sandireddy R, Yerra VG, Areti A, Komirishetty P, Kumar A. Neuroinflammation and oxidative stress in diabetic neuropathy: Futuristic strategies based on these targets. *Int J Endocrinol.* 2014;2014: 674987.
35. King R. The role of glycation in the pathogenesis of diabetic polyneuropathy. *Mol Pathol.* 2001;54(6):400.
36. Purwata TE. High TNF-alpha plasma levels and macrophages iNOS and TNF-alpha expression as risk factors for painful diabetic neuropathy. *J Pain Res.* 2011;4:169.
37. Yamakawa I, Kojima H, Terashima T, Katagi M, Oi J, Urabe H, et al. Inactivation of TNF-α ameliorates diabetic neuropathy in mice. *Am J Physiol Endocrinol Metab.* 2011;301(5):E844–E852.

12

The Influence of Dietary Components on Gene Expression

Hamid Zand, Katayoun Pourvali, Azam Shakeri, and Asieh Mansour
Shahid Beheshti University of Medical Sciences
Tehran, Iran

Contents

Overview	228
12.1 Epigenetic control of gene expression	229
12.1.1 Introduction	229
12.1.1.1 DNA methylation	230
12.1.1.2 Histone modifications and chromatin structure	231
12.1.1.3 Micro RNAs	232
12.1.2 Effect of dietary components on epigenetics	233
12.1.2.1 Energy, carbohydrates, and lipids	233
12.1.2.2 Protein and amino acid content of diet	237
12.1.2.3 The role of bioactive food components in regulation of epigenetics	238
12.1.2.4 Nutritional regulation of miRNAs	242
12.1.2.5 Prenatal nutrition status and epigenetic	243
12.2 Transcriptional control of gene expression	247
12.2.1 Introduction	247
12.2.2 Transcription factors	249
12.2.3 Nuclear receptor superfamily	250
12.2.3.1 RAR/RXR nuclear receptor	252
12.2.3.2 Vitamin D nuclear receptor	253
12.2.3.3 PPARs	253
12.3 Translational control of protein synthesis	255
12.3.1 Introduction	255
12.3.2 The role of energy and amino acids in protein synthesis	257
References	258

Overview

Diet and food played important roles in traditional medicine. Our ancestors believed that most diseases were caused by bad diet. This historical perspective continued until the recent era. Anthelme Brillat-Savarin in 1826 wrote: "Tell me what you eat and I will tell you what you are." The meaning of this quote in language of modern science is that the human diet affects phenotype [1]. Recent advances in the field of genetic and molecular biology indicate that the phenotypes of an organism are related to their genetic background and environmental factors. *Nutrigenomics* explains the effect of dietary components on gene expression patterns, whereas *nutrigenetics* is defined as the effects of genetic variations on the response of an organism to diet [2].

In multicellular organisms, different cell types have distinct gene expression patterns, which are highly affected by physiological, environmental, and pathological factors. Some genes are expressed in almost all circumstances and in all cells, including those that encode cytoskeleton proteins, essential metabolic pathways, and transcription- or translation-related proteins. These are called *housekeeping genes*. They are often expressed constitutively without any specific regulation. There are some other genes that encode specific proteins for specialized cell types. These genes determine cell identity and are under tight regulation during differentiation. As opposed to housekeeping genes, some genes are induced when needed. The expression of these genes depends on changes in stimuli, for example, cell environment. Among the environmental factors, dietary components have a more important impact on gene expression programs [3].

Eukaryotic gene expression occurs at several levels through more complex and precise temporal and spatial regulation. The gene expression might be regulated at DNA methylation and chromatin structure, gene transcription, nuclear RNA export, post-transcriptional regulation of mRNA stability, translation, and post-translational modification levels. There is strong evidence showing the effect of dietary components and nutrients on almost all levels of gene regulation [3].

Energy content and some nutrients exert their effects on gene expression through covalent modification of DNA and histones. This level of eukaryotic gene expression is called *epigenetics* [4]. Some nutrients directly act on gene expression through activation of specific ligand-dependent transcription factors (TFs) such as vitamin D and retinoic acid, which exert their effects through some nuclear receptors and alteration of their responsive gene expression [5,6].

Dietary nutrients also affect signaling pathways. Some phytochemical compounds inhibit the NF-κB pro-inflammatory pathway, possibly through inhibition of the canonical NF-κB signaling pathway [7].

Also indirectly, dietary components could act on gene expression by affecting metabolic pathways [8,9]. Energy acts on all levels of gene expression from chromatin structure to mRNA translation and post-translation. Caloric restriction diets cause inhibition of cellular anabolic pathways, induce energy-producing catabolic pathways through energy-sensing proteins, and thus reprogram gene expression, which leads to a decrease in age-related diseases and increases longevity in different species from yeasts to mice (Guarente). It has been suggested that high calorie diets increase a common fuel-sensing pathway: hexosamine synthesis and its product, N-acetylglucosamine (GlcNAc). O-linked N-acetylglucosamine (O-GlcNAc) of key proteins and enzymes alters their function; for example O-GlcNAcylation of insulin-signaling protein decreases insulin post-receptor action and promotes insulin resistance. Also, histones modification by O-GlcNAcylation changes chromatin structure and gene expression [10].

There is a tight link between metabolism and inflammation and immune system response. Inflammation-induced insulin resistance is the evolutionary preference to change glucose flux from insulin target tissues to the immune system. Several lines of studies have also shown that high-fat (HF) diets promote insulin resistance through toll-like receptors 2 and 4 and activation of NF-κB canonical pathway. Subsequently, NF-κB induces proinflammatory genes including TNFα, interleukin 1, and interleukin 6. It was shown recently that p53 is activated in the insulin target tissues of obese subjects, which inhibits insulin post-receptor signaling in those tissues [11,12].

This chapter will focus on recent findings on mechanisms by which dietary components act on regulation of gene expression and investigate new opportunities to apply this knowledge to human health and diseases.

12.1 Epigenetic control of gene expression

12.1.1 Introduction

The term *epigenetics* refers to modifications on DNA or histones that alter gene expression without changing DNA sequences. These modifications are heritable by daughter cells in dividing cells but not germ cells, whereas genetic traits are inherited by germ cells. The most important epigenetic alterations are DNA methylation, histone modifications (histone codes), and micro RNAs (miRNAs). Epigenetic variations may explain some aspects of human complex phenotypes more convincingly than genetic variations. There is increasing interest in this field of molecular biology in order to resolve some important mysterious questions in human health and disease [13].

Epigenetic modifications create a link between environmental alterations and gene expression. Epigenetic marks are created by enzymes called *writers* that catalyze covalent modification on DNA or histones, recognized by effector proteins, known as *readers*, that have specific domains for specific marks on histones or nucleotides, and erased by enzymes generally called *erasers* that remove the covalent modifications. When the results of the Human Genome Project were released in 2001, scientists found that there was no proportionality between the number of human genes and complex phenotypes. Since epigenetic changes are reversible, nutritional and pharmaceutical means may prevent or promote these alterations and provide revolutionary effects on human health [14].

12.1.1.1 DNA methylation

Methylation of DNA is the most important investigated epigenetic mechanism in eukaryotes that represses gene transcription. DNA methylation occurs by addition of a methyl (CH_3) group to the fifth carbon of the cytosine ring, resulting in 5-methylcytosine (5-mC). Methylation often occurs on the cytosines in CpG sites, where a cytosine nucleotide and a guanidine nucleotide are located next to each other. Approximately 1.5% of the human genome is 5-mC, mostly found in CpG sites. Some genes contain a cluster of CpG sites in their regulatory elements, called *CpG islands*. Approximately 70% of genes have CpG islands in their promoters, including housekeeping and tissue-specific genes. Most CpG islands containing genes are not methylated. Non-CpG methylation in somatic cells is rare, whereas embryonic stem cells contain a considerable amount of 5-mC in non-CpG sites [15].

During the first stages of fertilization, the pronucleus genome of the sperm and ovule undergo DNA demethylation. Following developmental stages, *de novo* DNA methylation occurs according to the development program. Differentiation of cells from embryonic stem cells to somatic cells requires methylation of genes that are involved in maintenance of stemness. These methylation patterns should be stable in terminally differentiated somatic cells to prevent conversion of the cell to a different cell type [16].

DNA methylation is catalyzed by DNA methyltransferases (DNMTs) and requires S-adenosyl methionine as the methyl donor. There are three major DNMTs in mammalians: DNMT1, DNMT3a, and DNMT3b. DNMT1 is responsible for methylation of a new strand of hemi-methylated DNA during DNA replication and maintenance of methylation pattern. Several lines of evidence have shown that DNMT1 is also involved in *de novo* methylation of DNA. *De novo* DNA methylation by DNMT3a and DNMT3b do not require hemi-methylated DNA. These DNMTs have major roles in early development so loss of their genes in mice can be lethal. Although tissue-specific DNA methylation patterns are established from early embryonic stages to terminally differentiated states, they can be modified by environmental factors [17].

To ensure well-tuned regulation of gene expression, demethylation of DNA has equal importance. DNA demethylation is accomplished in both passive and active manners. Passive DNA demethylation is performed in the absence of methylation of a new replicated strand during replication. In spite of well-characterized DNMTs in DNA methylation, the mechanism of active demethylation of DNA remained enigmatic until recently. New findings showed that the ten-eleven translocation (TET) family of enzymes can catalyze oxidation of 5-mC to 5-hydroxymethylcytosine (5-hmC) requiring O_2, vitamin C, alpha-ketoglutarate, and iron (He, Yu-Fei). Although some studies have suggested that 5-hmC may be a new epigenetic mark, independent of its role in demethylation mechanism, others believe that the mechanisms for active DNA demethylation by TETs are further oxidation of 5-hmC to 5-formylcytosine and 5-carboxylcytosine (5-cmC). Then, 5-hmC is deaminated to 5-hydroxymethyluracil. Subsequently, both 5-cmC and 5-hydroxymethyluracil are repaired by thymine-DNA glycosylase and base excision repair system [18].

12.1.1.2 Histone modifications and chromatin structure

The total length of human DNA in each cell is approximately 2 meters. This length is placed in the cellular nucleus with a diameter of approximately 6 micrometers. In eukaryotic cells it is packed into the nucleus as chromatin structure. Nucleosome, the basic unit of chromatin, consists of 146 base pairs wrapped around a histone octamer. One pair of each histone core (H2A, H2B, H3, and H4) makes a histone octamer. The linker DNA between nucleosomes can be further packed through formation of a coil from nucleosomes and H1 histone. Further condensation is achieved by other proteins, including nuclear scaffolding proteins. Chromatin is folded and tightly coiled to reach maximum condensation in metaphasic chromosomes. Condensed chromatin structure is called *heterochromatin* and is transcriptionally inactive, whereas euchromatin is less condensed and transcriptionally active [19].

Chromatin structure dynamically changes during developmental stages and in response to environmental alterations. Histone tails extend from the histone octamer. Chemical modification of histone tails by histone writers regulates interaction of DNA and histones. The list of covalent modifications of histones is expanding fast and many may not have a clear regulatory role in chromatin structure and gene expression. The most investigated posttranslational modifications of histones are acetylation/deacetylation of lysine or arginine residues, methylation and demethylation of lysine residues, phosphorylation and dephosphorylation of serine or threonine residues, and ubiquitination of lysine residues [20].

Histone acetyltransferases (HATs) catalyze the addition of acetyl group mainly to lysines of histone tails. Negatively charged acetyl groups neutralize positively charged histones and reduce their interaction with the DNA. Acetylation of lysine 9 and 14 in the tail of histone H3 by HAT enzymes is generally associated with transcriptional permission. Histone deacetylases (HDACs) remove acetyl moiety from lysines and reverse histone acetylation function [21]. Conversely, histone methylation by histone methyltransferases stabilizes positively charged histones and chromatin structure. Methylation of lysine 27 in histone H3 (H3K27) has an essential role in tissue development via transcriptional repression. Trimethylation of H3K27 is accomplished by catalytic subunit (enhancer of zeste homolog 2, or EZH2) of a polycomb repressive complex 2 (PRC2) [22]. The trimethylated H3K27 is recognized by a subunit of another polycomb protein complex (PRC1), which then monoubiquitinates H2A on K119 and leads to chromatin stabilization and gene silencing. Histone demethylases also remove a methyl group from the lysine of histones [23].

A large number of cellular proteins in eukaryotes are modified on serine and threonine residues by the O-GlcNAc. O-GlcNAc transferase enzyme (OGT) adds the sugar and β-N-acetylglucosaminidase (OGA) removes it. GlcNAc is the product of the hexosamine pathway, which uses fructose-6-phosphate, glutamine, acetyl CoA, and UTP to synthesize UDP-GlcNAc, which represents glucose flux into the cell; therefore nutritional status and metabolism are the main factors affecting histone GlcNAcylation. Nonhistone protein O-GlcNAcylation also has major roles in physiologic and pathologic states. Several studies have showed that GlcNAcylation of some TFs promotes nuclear localization [24]. Histone O-GlcNAcylation is a new epigenetic mark that may exhibit strong link between metabolism and gene expression. New findings indicate that TETs directly interact with OGT and promote histone O-GlcNAcylation during gene transcription [25]. OGT also catalyzes O-GlcNAcylation and nuclear export of TET3, therefore downregulating its activation [26]. These results exhibit a correlation between distinct epigenetic mechanisms that regulate gene expression.

Transcription of protein-coded genes requires both covalent modification of histone tails to loosen histones/DNA affinity and chromatin remodeling complexes. These proteins rearrange chromatin structure to expose cis-acting regulatory DNA elements for transcription machinery proteins in an ATP-dependent manner. Several families of chromatin remodeling complexes are found in eukaryotes, including SWItch/sucrose nonfermentable (SWI/SNF) and nucleosome remodeling deacetylase [27].

12.1.1.3 Micro RNAs

miRNAs are a family of short length noncoding RNAs that are transcribed from DNA but not translated into proteins. miRNAs were initially discovered in C elegance in 1993; however, the term *miRNA* was introduced in 2001 by Ruvkun et al. In general, miRNAs regulate gene expression at the posttranscriptional level. It has been suggested that approximately 60% of all human genes are regulated by miRNAs. They bind to the 3′-untranslated regions (3′-UTR) of target mRNAs and repress translation through several mechanisms, including translational repression, mRNA degradation, and deadenylation. They are encoded by independent genes (intergenic) or processed introns (intronic) [28,29].

RNA polymerase II transcribes a large primary transcript (pri-miRNAs). Pri-miRNAs are subjected to nuclear processing before entering the cytoplasm. A complex, called a *microprocessor*, consisting of Drosha (a type of RNase) and DiGeorge syndrome critical region 8/Pasha, processes pri-miRNA to around 70 nucleotides pre-miRNA. Pre-miRNA is exported to the cytoplasm via the nuclear/cytoplasmic shuttling system (exportin 5 and Ran-GTP complex) that is similar to protein nuclear export. In the cytoplasm, additional processing takes place on pre-miRNA by Dicer RNase, producing a double-stranded, 20–25 nucleotide, and two-base 3′ overhang miRNA. Dicer also unwinds double strand. RNA-induced silencing complex (RISC) recruits one-stranded miRNAs and targets mRNAs based on complementation between miRNA sequences and 3′-UTR of specific mRNA. It is evident that any changes in the miRNA expression pattern can be highly relevant to pathologic states [28].

12.1.2 Effect of dietary components on epigenetics
12.1.2.1 Energy, carbohydrates, and lipids

Energy metabolism is the way that fuels convert to cellular current form of energy, ATP. Glucose, fatty acids, and amino acids are the major fuels for eukaryotic cells. Several metabolite ratios represent cell energetic states including AMP:ATP, NAD$^+$:NADH, and Acetyl CoA:CoA. Some nutrients and energy sensors also gauge cellular nutritional status and regulate metabolic pathways accordingly. AMP-activated protein kinase (AMPK) is allosterically activated by elevation of the AMP:ATP ratio. AMPK generally inhibits energy-consuming pathways and promotes energy-producing catabolic pathways. Another master serine/threonine protein kinase that regulates cell growth, cell proliferation, protein synthesis, autophagy, and transcription is also regulated by energy and nutrient availability in addition to oxygen and growth factors [30].

Dietary components may act on epigenetic regulation of gene expression through several pathways, which will be discussed in ensuing sections.

Histone acetylation and deacetylation

Chromatin modification and subsequent transcription regulation requires modifying enzymes that utilize metabolite resources as cofactors. Histone lysine acetylation requires acetyl CoA as the cofactor, located mainly in mitochondria. Availability of acetyl CoA in cytoplasm depends on the activity of two enzymes: ATP-citrate lyase (ACL) and acetyl CoA synthetase. The latter recruits acetate, ATP, and coenzyme A to produce acetyl CoA. It has been proposed that the intracellular level of acetyl CoA is dependent on the energy and nutrient status. The histone acetylation capacity is affected by the cellular acetyl CoA:coenzyme A ratio [31]. In low energy states, the Krebs cycle oxidizes acetyl CoA produced by fuels to generate reducing equivalents. In nutritional repletion states, the intracellular level of acetyl CoA increases dramatically and vice versa. In support of these data, glucose depletion in cell culture globally reduces histone acetylation levels. Also, it has been shown that transcription of the ACL gene is elevated by the calorie content of the diet and insulin. Therefore, it is conceivable to propose that some physiological effect of calorie-restricted diets and nutritional repletion result from histone acetylation and alteration of transcriptional patterns. Imbalance between fuel resources may also change the histone acetylation pattern. A diet with a high carbohydrate-to-fat ratio promotes the acetylation of histone H3 on the transcriptional region and H4 on the promoter region of sucrase-isomaltase in mouse small intestine [32]. In addition, expression of HDACs in the medial hypothalamus of mice was changed in response to either a fasting or a high-fat diet [33]. Dietary fructose also increases acetylation of histone H3 at the glucose transporter 5 (Glut5) promoter [34]. Pancreatic duodenal homeobox 1 (PDX1) transactivates the insulin gene by recruiting p300 histone acetylase in a serum glucose level–dependent manner. PDX1 interacts with HDAC1 and 2 and represses insulin expression at low levels; however, it binds to p300 at high glucose levels and promotes insulin expression [35].

During starvation or in low carbohydrate/HF diets, overload of acetyl CoA in the liver saturates the Krebs cycle, and the additional acetyl CoA enters the ketogenesis pathway to produce ketone bodies. Beta-hydroxybutyrate (β-OHB) and acetoacetate carry energy from the liver to extrahepatic tissues. Intense exercise can also cause elevation of ketone bodies to levels caused by prolonged fasting [36]. In the past two decades, several lines of evidence have revealed that calorie-restricted diets improve longevity and decrease age-related diseases. Recently some pioneering studies revealed that β-OHB exerts longevity-promoting effects through inhibition of HDAC and subsequent chromatin structure regulation and alteration of several gene expressions [37,38].

Histone O-GlcNAcylation

The hexosamine biosynthetic pathway is a nutrient sensor pathway that responds to excess nutrients. A high energy diet can increase the hexosamine biosynthesis pathway. Subsequently, it decreases expression of some nuclear-encoded genes involved in skeletal muscle oxidative phosphorylation via O-GlcNAcylation of nucleo-cytoplasmic proteins [39]. Hyper activation of this pathway in adipocytes disrupts insulin-stimulated AKT activation and glucose uptake [40]. In agouti-related peptide (AgRP) neurons, O-GlcNAc signaling is an important factor for inhibiting thermogenesis to conserve energy during fasting. O-GlcNAcylation of cytoplasmic and nuclear proteins in AgRP neurons increases with fasting and ablation of OGT prevents diet-induced obesity in mice [41].

Some observation revealed that activation of OGA reduces obesity and subsequent insulin resistance through activation of thermogenic signaling in white adipose tissue [42]. Researchers have found that high glucose and insulin cause O-GlcNAcylation of proteins [43]. Some of the scientific evidence indicates that diets high in saturated fat and sugar may be involved in the metabolic syndrome via an O-GlcNAc modification of proteins [44]. It has been indicated that O-GlcNAcylation and acetylation may act as glucose-sensitive histone posttranslational modifications that can contribute to hepatic glucose sensing by targeting the epigenome [45]. An increase in glucose uptake and glycolysis in normal breast cancer cells lead to oncogenic activation, at least in part, through O-GlcNAc modification [46].

Histone methylation

Generally, it has been indicated that high energy conditions promote histone lysine acetylation and low calorie diets cause histone methylation (GUT P). Histone H3 lysine 9 (H3K9) methylation plays an important role in promotion of heterochromatin and transcriptional silencing. The H3K9-specific demethylase, Jhdm2a, has an essential role in expression of metabolic genes including *PPARγ* and *UCP1*. Genetically, loss of function of this enzyme results in obesity and metabolic syndrome in mice [47,48].

In yeast, nutrient depletion causes growth arrest and quiescence; however, nutrient availability causes exit from quiescence by histone modification. During escape from quiescence, histone acetylation responds to metabolic state dramatically, while methylation is interestingly static during the cell cycle [49].

Nicotinamide N-methyltransferase (Nnmt) transfers the methyl group to nicotinamide (vitamin B3) using S-adenosylmethionine (SAM) as the methyl donor. It has been shown that Nnmt expression is increased in the white adipose tissue and liver of obese and diabetic mice. Nnmt inhibition decreases diet-induced obesity by regulation of histone methylation and expression of key enzymes in polyamine biosynthesis pathway [50]. Hyperglycemia is usually associated with microcirculation disorder. It seems that monocyte chemoattractant protein-1 (MCP-1) expression mediates hyperglycemia-induced microcirculation dysfunction. Also, glucose reduces H3K4me2/3 of MCP-1 gene expression and subsequently MCP-1 expression [51].

DNA methylation

It seems that DNA methylation as a profound epigenetic mark should be affected by calorie content of the diet. Research by Bouchard et al. showed that a calorie-restricted diet for weight loss alters the methylation pattern of different genes in adipose tissue [52]. However, most of these studies have investigated the effect of nutritional factors in gestation and subsequent alteration of DNA methylation pattern and future metabolic health of the offspring. Therefore, some differences in susceptibility to metabolic disorders among people could result from different DNA methylation patterns. For instance, response to calorie-restricted diet is variable among different people.

During aging, the DNA methylation pattern is disrupted by global hypomethylation and hypermethylation of many specific genes. Some evidence shows that calorie-restricted diets reverse these aging-induced aberrant DNA methylation patterns by DNA methylation regulation of specific genes. These genes include oncogenes, tumor suppressors, and regulator of metabolic pathways [53]. In a pioneering study, Spanish researchers found that in a low-calorie diet regimen, successful diet responders had lower initial levels of DNA methylation in both TNF-alpha and leptin gene promoters. However, low calorie diet had no significant effect on the DNA methylation pattern of these genes [54].

Adiponectin as the main regulator of energy homeostasis is encountered by change in methylation at promoter. HRAS in the pancreas and cMYC in the liver of old mice are hypomethylated; however, low calorie restriction diet prevent these age-induced epigenetic effects [55,56]. Inhibition of DNMT1 reduces obesity-induced insulin resistance in an adiponectin-dependent manner [57]. In this regard, some researchers have suggested a type of diet called an *epigenetic diet*. The components of this type of diet prevent or restore deleterious epigenetic changes induced by pathological states [58].

Many researchers believe that fructose may play a role in the development of metabolic disorders. An interesting study demonstrated that a fructose diet significantly reduces mRNA levels for peroxisome proliferator-activated receptor alpha (PPARα) and carnitine palmitoyltransferase 1A (CPT1A) in rat liver. This study suggested that fructose-mediated reduced gene expression may be exerted through induction of DNA methylation of related genes [59].

Few studies have evidenced the role of n-3 polyunsaturated fatty acids on regulation of DNA methylation. For instance, eicosapentaenoic acid (EPA) demethylates a single CpG of CCAAT/enhancer-binding protein delta in leukemia cells [60]. Moreover, Kulkarni et al. observed that docosahexaenoic acid (DHA) acts on placental global DNA methylation patterns in Wistar rats [61].

Histone modification and energy sensors

One of the main sensors and master regulators of energy homeostasis is AMPK. This serine/threonine protein kinase exerts a regulatory effect through alteration of AMPK-dependent genes expression by direct association with chromatin and phosphorylation of histone H2B at serine 36. Phosphorylation of H2B by AMPK takes place both in promoters and in transcribed regions of AMPK-dependent genes [62]. Another potential mechanism by which AMPK regulates gene expression is direct phosphorylation of HADC5 at serine 259 and 498. AMPK-dependent HADC5 phosphorylation and inhibition increases GLUT4 gene expression (McGee SL2008). In addition, exercise activates AMPK and calmodulin-dependent protein kinase II (CaMKII), an upstream activator of AMPK, in muscle tissues. These effects are associated with increased acetylation of H3K36 via regulation of HDACs [63]. The energy-sensing pathway also has crosstalk in epigenetic regulation of gene expression. Furthermore, activation of AMPK decreases histone H2B O-GlcNAcylation via phosphorylation of OGT. This inhibits the OGT–chromatin association. OGT also O-GlcNAcylates AMPK and upregulates AMPK activity in a positive feedback manner [64].

Sirtuins are a class III protein deacetylase family whose activity is dependent on intracellular NAD^+ levels. Cellular energy status may directly affect chromatin structure and gene expression through sirtuins and the $NAD^+/NADH$ ratio [65]. Some sirtuins have only deacetylase activity, including SIRT1, 2, and 3, while others act as ADP-ribosyl transferase, for example, SIRT6. In addition to cellular energy, several lines of evidence now propose that some naturally occurring small molecules may also activate SIRT1 allosterically. Resveratrol is at the top of the sirtuin activator list; however, the search for selective and more potent activators is actively underway. The precursors of NAD^+ such as nicotinamide may also mimic the intrinsic pathway of sirtuin activation [66].

12.1.2.2 Protein and amino acid content of diet

Prenatally induced effects aside, it seems that the epigenetic landscape of body cells is influenced by the protein and amino acid content of the diet. However, studies on this effect after development are scarce, specifically in humans.

The one-carbon metabolism pathway consists of the vitamins folic acid, B12, B6, and B2 in its coenzyme form, as well as seine, glycine, and threonine amino acids. In addition to dietary methyl donors such as choline, catabolism of serine and threonine provides a one-carbon source. Tetrahydrofolate, as the active form of folate, and vitamin B12 transfer one-carbon groups to *de novo* purine synthesis pathways. Moreover, methyl-tetrahydrofolate and vitamin B12, as coenzyme, converts homocysteine to methionine, which can then be further converted to SAM as the main methyl donor in the methylation reaction including histones and DNA methylation [67].

Dietary protein restriction attenuates tumor growth in human xenograft models of prostate and breast cancer through reduction of the histone methyltransferase EZH2 and the associated histone mark H3K27me3 [68]. Diets containing low lysine globally decrease chromatin protein in comparison to normal diets [69]. Amino acid deprivation of mammalian cells alters the gene-associated chromatin structure of asparagine synthetase and activating TF 3 [70].

Folate and methyl-group deficiency may influence susceptibility to several cancers (e.g., colon, stomach, uterine, cervix, prostate, thyroid, and breast) in humans (ROSS [71]). It was shown that a methyl-deficient diet caused significant decreases in repressive histone modifications (dimethyl-H3K9) within the H19 promoter, as well as Igf2 P2 and P3 promoters in C57BL/6 mice. DNA methylation in these loci was not changed. These observations suggest that chromatin modifications are more susceptible to methyl-deficient diets than DNA methylation at this locus [72].

It is hypothesized that dietary methionine may affect the SAM–SAH ratio and DNA methylation pattern. Some researchers propose that schizophrenia has an epigenetic basis and supplementation with methionine promotes schizophrenic behavior by regulation of DNA methylation at some genes [73]. Locasale and colleagues recently showed that modulation of dietary methionine and methionine availability may directly influence histone methylation and gene expression in the liver [74]. Intercellular s-adenosylhomocysteine inhibits DNMTs; therefore, methionine supplementation alters the DNA methylation pattern. In another study, Devlin et al. observed that supplementation of wild-type and heterozygous methylenetetrahydrofolate reductase knockout mice with methionine had no significant effect on global DNA methylation [75]. Methionine supplementation also induces DNA damage in the peripheral blood of mice.

In contrast, a low methionine diet decreases basal DNA damage in liver of mice [76]. Methionine-restricted diet improved lifespan in many species including Caenorhabditis elegance and rodents. Methionine restriction reverses the adverse effects of aging on metabolic pathways. Methionine-limited diet improves metabolism and increases longevity, perhaps in part through epigenetic regulation [77]. The mechanism underlying the longevity induced by methionine restriction is not fully understood; however, epigenetic alteration, specifically the alteration in DNA methylation patterns, may be involved as an underlying mechanism [78].

12.1.2.3 The role of bioactive food components in regulation of epigenetics

Bioactive compounds are non-nutrient components of foods that have biological effects on organisms through several molecular mechanisms. It is accepted that these naturally occurring botanicals have numerous health benefits. Phytochemicals are the most abundant food-derived bioactive compounds, including flavonoids, phenolic acids, and lignans. They are classified into subgroups, according to their chemical structure: flavanones, flavones, flavonols, flavan-3-ols, anthocyanins, and isoflavones. Moreover, the antioxidant, anti-inflammatory, and chemopreventive effect of phytochemicals is exerted via modulation of the epigenetic landscape [79]. It is worth noting that most studies have investigated the anticarcinogenic effect of polyphenols. In this part, some of these compounds would be reviewed.

Curcumin

Curcumin is a polyphenol derived from turmeric and to a lesser extent ginger. Several molecular pathways are affected by curcumin, including apoptosis, cell cycle, survival, and inflammation. A study using colorectal cancer cell lines showed that curcumin modulates demethylation of a subset of partially methylated genes. Other research data indicate that curcumin inhibits DNA DNMT1, with the EC_{50} = 30 nM. These data suggest that curcumin is a potent hypomethylation factor [80]. Curcumin-modulated DNA methylation is accompanied by corresponding alterations in gene expression, both up- and downregulation of genes in various colorectal cell lines [81]. In addition, CpG demethylation of the Neurog1 gene and its subsequent expression by curcumin is observed in human prostate LNCaP cells. The Neurog1 gene is highly methylated and suggested as a cancer methylation marker [82].

HATs are another epigenetic target of curcumin. It has been shown that curcumin induces hypoacetylation through downregulation of HAT [83]. It inhibits CBP/p300 acetyltransferase activity in MCF7 cell lines [84]. However, in contrast to those studies, various studies have suggested that curcumin is an HDAC inhibitor, too [85]. In this manner, some studies also revealed that HDAC 1, 3, and 8 protein levels were significantly lowered by curcumin. Attenuation of HDACs by curcumin results in increased histone H4 acetylation [86].

The chemopreventive effects of curcumin have been also linked to its effect on histone methylation regulation. EZH2 is upregulated in some human cancers with poor prognosis, such as breast cancer [87]. It has been shown that EZH2 is downregulated by curcumin in the MDA-MB-435 breast cancer cell line through stimulation of three major members of the mitogen-activated protein kinase (MAPK) pathway: c-Jun NH2-terminal kinase, extracellular signal-regulated kinase, and p38 kinase [88]. A novel analogue of curcumin, difluorinated curcumin, reduces EZH2 and prevents cell growth in the human pancreatic cancer cell lines AsPC-1 and MiaPaCa-2 [89]. In conclusion, it seems that curcumin is more effective at regulation of histone acetylation than histone methylation [90].

Epigallocatechin gallate

Epigallocatechin gallate (EGCG) is the most abundant polyphenolic catechin in green tea. Green tea is a popular beverage in East Asia and the world. Numerous health benefits and therapeutic effects of green tea have been noted in traditional Chinese medicine.

Hypomethylation of tumor suppressor genes is a common effect of green tea polyphenols [91]. Hypermethylation and silencing of the glutathione-S-transferase *pi* (GSTP1) gene promoter is a hallmark of prostate cancer. Green tea polyphenols restore GSTP1 expression by DNMT1 inhibition in human prostate cancer LNCaP cells [92]. Moreover, some studies have shown that EGCG demethylates and re-expresses genes involved in antitumor signaling by inactivation of enzymes involved in DNA methylation [93–96]. EGCG inhibits expression of the oncogenic gene hTERT (the catalytic subunit of telomerase) by modulation of chromatin structure and DNA methylation in (ER)-positive MCF-7 and ER-negative MDA-MB-231 cells [97]. However, EGCG does not promote global hypomethylation of the genome similar to that seen in cancer cells.

It has been reported that EGCG can inhibit HDACs and relax the chromatin structure at some gene promoters. In 2010, Li and colleagues found that EGCG can reactivate ERα expression through chromatin remodeling of its promoter by altering histone acetylation and methylation in MDA-MB-231 breast cancer cells [98]. EGCG may promote proteasomal degradation of class I HDACs in human prostate cancer cells, too [99].

Modulation of polycomb proteins is another epigenetic chemopreventive mechanism in regulation of gene expression that has been reported by some studies [100–102]. Deb et al. reported that EGCG reduces H3K27me3 at the promoter of some genes such as metalloproteinases and TIMP-3, by proteasomal degradation of PcG proteins including EZH2, EED, SUZ12, and BMI-1 in breast cancer cells [94].

Genistein

Genistein is an isoflavone with phytoestrogenic properties. Similar to other isoflavones such as daidzein, genistein is found abundantly in a number of plants including soybeans, fava beans, lupin, and kudzu. A large number of studies have demonstrated that genistein has numerous biological activities including estrogenic, antioxidative, anticarcinogenic, and antiatherosclerosis properties [103]. It has been suggested that genistein exerts its biological effect through nuclear receptors, regulation of several tyrosine kinases, or inhibition of DNMTs. Fang et al. observed that genistein is a more potent DNMT inhibitor than other isoflavones and reactivates the p16INK4a, RARbeta, and MGMT genes in the esophageal squamous carcinoma cells KYSE 510 and the prostate cancer cells LNCaP and PC3 [104]. In a recent study, genistein directly interacted with the catalytic domain of DNMT1 and had no significant effect on DNMT3A and DNMT3B. Moreover, genistein reduces DNA methylation in the promoter of some tumor suppressor genes in MCF-7 and MDA-MB-231 human breast cancer cells [105]. Furthermore, intake of genistein by rats alters DNA methylation of CpG islands at promoter of GLUT4 [106].

Genistein also modifies gene expression by influencing histone modification and chromatin remodeling. The acetylation of estrogen receptor-alpha via modulation of HAT activity is reported as the mechanism by which genistein and daidzein regulate gene expression [107,108]. It activates PTEN, p53, and FOXO3a gene expression by altering chromatin structure at their promoters via modulating histone H3-lysine 9 (H3K9) methylation and deacetylation in prostate cancer cells [109]. Genistein induces histone H3K9 acetylation and increases expression of HAT1 in several prostate cancer cell lines, including ARCaP-E/ARCaP-M [110]. It also promotes histone H3 acetylation of the antagonist Dickkopf 1 (DKK1) promoter region in the SW480 and HCT15 human colon cancer cell lines [111]. Genistein induces the expression of activating transcription factor 3 (ATF3) by decreasing phosphorylation of histone H3 serine 10 (H3S10p) at both the promoter and coding regions of ATF3 and increasing methylation of histone H3 lysine 36 (H3K36me3) at the coding region and dimethylated histone H3 lysine 4 (H3K4me2) at the promoter region [112].

This isoflavone increases trimethylation of H3K9 and decreases dimethylation of H3K4 at the hTERT promoter, therefore repressing hTERT expression in MCF10AT and MCF-7 breast cancer cells [113].

Resveratrol

Resveratrol is a stilbenoid, a type of polyphenol, and a phytoalexin. Several plants produce it in response to stress, injury, fungal infection, and radiation. It is found in the skin of red grapes, peanuts, and some berries. There are numerous studies showing that resveratrol has biological effects including antioxidant, anticarcinogenic, anti-atherosclerotic, and anti-aging properties. A recent paper by Qin et al. reported that resveratrol reduces DNMT1 and 3b expression *in vitro* and promotes hypomethylation of RASSF-1a tumor suppressor in women with high breast cancer risk [114]. It was shown in another study that 3-month treatment of diabetic rats with resveratrol reduces methylation of the IL-1β, IL-6, TNF-α, and IFN-γ genes concomitant with a decrease in their gene expression. In contrast, simultaneously resveratrol decreased methylation of the anti-inflammatory cytokine IL-10 in those rats [115].

It has been observed that resveratrol deacetylates the surviving gene promoter through SIRT1 activation and in turn reduces its expression in mouse BRCA1 mutant cell lines [116]. Resveratrol treatment also increases peroxisome proliferator-activated receptor gamma coactivator 1-alpha (PGC-1α) mediated by SIRT1 activation [117]. Docking studies indicated that resveratrol may inhibit the activity of different human HDAC enzymes. It inhibits inhibition of HDACs and subsequently the histone hyperacetylation of HepG2 hepatocellular carcinoma cells [118].

According to a new study, resveratrol (50 mg/L in drinking water) prevented deoxycorticosterone acetate-induced hypertension through alteration of the H3K27me3 epigenetic mark in the aorta and renal artery sections, suggesting that resveratrol might improve hypertension by changing the epigenetic landscape of genes in vessels [119].

Sulforaphane

Sulforaphane is an organosulfur compound belonging to the isothiocyanate group. It is found abundantly in cruciferous vegetables, including broccoli, brussels sprouts, and cabbage. It has been proposed that sulforaphane has antioxidative, anticancer, and antineurodegenerative effects and stimulates phase 2 detoxifying enzymes. Sulforaphane treatment decreased DNMT expression in normal prostate epithelial cells (PrEC), as well as androgen-sensitive (LnCAP) and androgen-insensitive (PC3) prostate cancer cells [120]. DNMTs were decreased in sulforaphane-treated breast cancer cells and in turn repressed hTERT by hypomethylation [121]. Sulforaphane may decrease the risk of some type of cancers such as breast, bladder, and prostate cancer. It was found that sulforaphane at physiologically relevant concentration decreases hypomethylation of PTEN and RARbeta2 promoters with concomitant increase in their gene expression [122].

Dietary sulforaphane is known as HDAC inhibitor, according to several studies. It increases histone acetylation globally and locally in p21 and bax promoters in *Apc*min mice [123,124]. Also, it increases the activity of a β-catenin-responsive reporter in a dose-dependent manner, without changing HDAC or β-catenin protein levels. Sulforaphane causes an increase in acetylation of histones bound to the p21Cip1/Waf1 promoter [125]. Recent experiments indicated that dietary sulforaphane prevents HDAC activity in B16 melanoma cells and subsequently promotes apoptosis [126]. In a randomized controlled trial, a group of women with abnormal mammograms received a placebo or a sulforaphane analog supplement. After 8 weeks, HDAC activity was measured in peripheral blood mononuclear (PBMC) cells. Supplementation caused a significant decrease in PBMC HDAC activity in PBMC [127].

12.1.2.4 Nutritional regulation of miRNAs

It has been indicated that miRNAs have pivotal roles in the post-transcriptional regulation of biological processes. They are found in biological fluids, such as serum, urine, saliva, and cerebrospinal fluid [128]. The circulating levels of some miRNAs, including miR-142-3p, miR-140-5p, miR-222, miR-15a, miR-520c-3p, miR-423-5p, and miR-130b, is altered in severe obesity. Bariatric surgery and subsequent weight loss causes those mRNA to change in an opposite manner [129]. It was found that several miRNAs in circulation are associated with body weight and body mass index and can be potentially used as biomarkers for weight management programs [130]. Recently, researchers showed that an increase in circulating miR-122 is associated with obesity and insulin resistance in young adults, confirming the role of miRNAs in obesity and insulin resistance [131].

It has been suggested that the biological effect of some dietary phytochemicals is mediated by alteration of the miRNAs profile. Curcumin reduces expression of Notch-1 specific microRNAs, miR-21, and miR-34a, and increases let-7a miRNA concomitant with inhibition of cell growth and induction of apoptosis in esophageal cancer cell lines [132]. Moreover, curcumin inhibits proliferation of BxPC-3 and MIAPaCa-2 cells through upregulation of let-7a miRNA and downregulation of Ras signaling [133]. It may also prevent Bcl-2 activation and promote apoptosis through upregulation of mir-15 [134].

Green tea catechins and EGCG also upregulate let-7a and miR-16 miRNAs and concomitantly decrease Ras and cMYC signaling in some cell types [135]. Green tea catechins also target C-myc and the oncogenic miRNA LIN-28 to inhibit growth of human lung cancer cells [136]. Genistein decreases cell growth of prostate cancer PC3 cells through upregulation of miR-1296. Inhibition of miR-1296 upregulates MCM2 mRNA and expression of related protein [137]. In another study, genistein caused a decrease in miR-21 expression in A-498 cells and consistent reduction in p21, p38MAPK, and cyclin E2 [138]. Moreover, genistein significantly inhibits melanoma cell growth in a time- and dose-dependent manner. In agreement, the levels of miR-27a and its target gene ZBTB10 decreased according to genistein concentrations [139]. Upregulation of miR-34a prevents pancreatic cancer cell growth and promotes apoptosis. Incubation of these cells with genistein results in the upregulation of miR-34a and subsequent downregulation of Notch-1 signaling [140]. Genistein suppresses NF-κB through upregulation of miRNA-29b and subsequent proliferation in human multiple myeloma cells [141].

There are examples in which grape polyphenol and resveratrol also modulate miRNA expression profiles in experimental models. AKT activation in PC-3M-MM2 cells was decreased by resveratrol via inhibiting the AKT/miRNA-21 pathway [142]. Resveratrol modulated the expression pattern of miR-20b in an ischemia/reperfusion model in rats. Downregulation of miR-109 is also related to the potent anti-angiogenic action of resveratrol [143]. It has been shown that the anti-inflammatory action of resveratrol depends on reduction of miR-21, miR-181b, miR-663, miR-30c2, miR-155, and miR-34a and their pro-inflammatory target genes, including CL3, IL-1β, and TNF-α [144]. Tumor-suppressive miRNAs including miR-125b-5p, miR-200c-3p, miR-409-3p, miR-122-5p, and miR-542-3p were modulated by resveratrol in breast cancer cells. Alteration of their target genes promotes apoptosis in those cells [145].

It was proposed that sulforaphane has chemopreventive activity against tumor initiation and carcinogenesis. Sulforaphane inhibits the epithelial-to-mesenchymal transition (EMT) in human bladder cancer cell lines through miR-200c-induced suppression of ZEB1 and E-cadherin [146]. Treatment of oral squamous carcinoma cells by sulforaphane caused a reduction of stemness properties including ALDH1 activity and CD44 positivity of cells. These results suggest that sulforaphane may prevent the cancer stemness and tumor-initiating processes [147]. The anti-inflammatory effect of sulforaphane against amyloid-β peptide also mediates the attenuation of miRNA-146a expression, which is usually upregulated in the temporal cortex and hippocampus of Alzheimer's patients [148].

12.1.2.5 Prenatal nutrition status and epigenetic

Recently, a growing body of information has accumulated to suggest that the *in utero* environment including nutritional status and diet composition impacts fetal metabolism and has a potential influence on gene expression, changing the risk of offspring developing subsequent chronic disease susceptibility through epigenetic modifications. Epigenetic dysregulation is reported in individuals following periconceptional and prenatal exposure to famine [149,150], for example, methylation changes in insulin-like growth factor 2 (IGF2) [150]. Here in this section, we examine the influences of maternal intake of protein, fat, and carbohydrate and also some micronutrients that may influence the health of offspring through epigenetic alteration.

12.1.2.5.1 Protein

There is growing evidence, predominantly in rodents, that early life protein restriction can cause deficits in metabolic pathways in offspring. For example, it has been reported that the male offspring of rat dams fed on a protein-restricted diet had early growth restriction and higher susceptibility to developing diabetes in old age [151]. Also, a very recent data by Han et al. showed that elevated abdominal fat content and glucose dysregulation in female (but not male) offspring of mice following a protein-restricted diet in gestation and lactation may result from high expression levels of neuropeptide Y (NPY) and its Y2 receptor in the visceral fat [152].

Diet low in protein during gestation is associated with reduction in methylation status of the PPARα promoter in the liver of offspring in their adult life [153–155]. Lillycrop et al. [155,156] has reported hypomethylation of the glucocorticoid receptor (GR) promoter in the liver of offspring following a protein-restricted diet. Another study suggested significantly increased GLUT4 gene expression in the skeletal muscle of female offspring of rats fed on a protein-restricted diet during pregnancy through epigenetic changes in the chromatin structure [157]. Moreover, PPARγ coactivator-1α (PGC-1α) is related to insulin resistance. PGC-1α mRNA expression has been found to be reduced in the skeletal muscle in the offspring of rats, following a gestational protein-restricted diet. This effect was due to increased DNA methylation of PGC-1α promoter [158].

A severe protein-restricted diet (5% protein) in mice altered pancreatic development, impaired its function, and also reduced pancreatic β-cells mass, which affected three generations [159]. The adult offspring of dams who experienced a reduction in protein intake during pregnancy showed minimal hypermethylation at the P2 promoter and reduction of Hnf4a mRNA in islets and so represent one candidate epigenetic mechanism for the development of type 2 diabetes [160]. The regulation of hepatic glucose-6-phosphatase (G6PC) by several epigenetic modifications, including miRNA expression, DNA methylation, and modifications in histones in a sex-specific manner, was reported in the newborn piglets of dams fed a low protein diet during pregnancy [161]. Prenatal exposure to a protein-restricted diet resulted in changes in histone modifications and the alteration of CCAAT/enhancer-binding protein (C/EBPβ) gene expression and phosphoenolpyruvate carboxykinase (PEPCK) transcription with the risk of metabolic syndrome in female rat offspring [162].

Multiple experimental studies aimed at determining the role of a protein-restricted diet on fetal blood pressure. As an example, female Wistar rats exposed to a PR diet (9% casein) throughout pregnancy developed adult systolic blood pressure and endothelial dysfunction compared to the control group (18% casein), which was also transferred to the second generation [163]. Harrison et al. [164] showed that a prenatal PR diet led to hypertension and decreased nephron number in offspring and that this phenotype is transgenerationally passed to the F2 offspring via both parental lines. In addition, expression of angiotensinogen and angiotensin-converting enzyme-1 (ACE-1) are both increased with changes in DNA methylation and miRNA expression in fetal brains born to mice dams fed a PR diet of 50% during pregnancy [165].

Vucetic et al. showed that a maternal low protein diet during gestation could negatively influence the expression of dopamine-related genes in the offspring. These changes could have long-term consequences for the development of ADHD via epigenetic mechanisms [166]. Studies have also shown that restricted prenatal protein consumption led to decreased content of lipids, particularly docosahexaenoic acid (DHA), status in the offspring brain, which may impair brain function [167,168].

As mentioned above, some of the evidence shows that maternal protein deficiency in gestation may cause epigenetic modification to the fetal genome, which may be prevented or negated by supplementation with specific nutrients such as folic acid [169–171], glycine [172], and taurine [173] throughout gestation. For instance, in mice, Mortensen et al. showed dysregulation of mitochondrial genes mainly in the liver and muscle by protein restriction during pregnancy. They also examined the effect of oral administration of taurine with low protein diet. In this study, gene expression patterns in both the liver and skeletal muscle were normalized, and also mitochondrial gene expression in offspring was rescued. Although the exact mechanism was unclear, the authors hypothesized that regulating gene expression possibly by an epigenetic mechanism led to this result [173].

Much of the work previously undertaken on epigenetic regulation by maternal dietary protein has focused on assessment of protein restriction, with little effort to demonstrate that high protein could affect offspring phenotype. However, it seems that both low and high maternal protein intakes are responsible for altered epigenetic marks and gene expression [174]. In a follow-up study of 34 men and women born during 1967–1968, whose mothers ate an unbalanced diet (rich in protein and low in carbohydrate) in pregnancy, Drake et al. reported that changes in GR promoter methylation was linked with elevated risk of high blood pressure and adiposity later in life [175].

12.1.2.5.2 Fat

Maternal HF diet is associated with higher fat mass and lower size of liver in offspring [176]. Moreover, maternal obesity impairs fetal bone formation through homeodomain-containing factor A10 (HoxA10) promoter hypermethylation, leading to downregulation of gene expression when challenged with HF diet [177]. Despite minimal weight gain, similar results were also reported by Liang et al. [178], who found impairment of the osteogenic pathway among fetuses of HF diet users during pregnancy. The HF exposure led to increased body length and reduced insulin sensitivity in both genders of F1 and F2 generations [179]. However, only F3 females, but not males, displayed increased body length [180]. Epigenetic factors (decreased methylation at the GH secretagogue receptor [GHSR] promoter) affecting the GH-IGF signaling cascade may cause an increase in body length that was inherited into the second generation [179].

It has been reported that consumption of a HF diet during pregnancy resulted in steatohepatitis in adult offspring (BRUCE KD). Kelsall et al. observed that hypermethylation of CpG-394 in the fatty acid desaturase (FADS2) gene with increased maternal fat intake induced dysregulation in gene expression of desaturase (FADS1 and FADS2) in offspring aorta, in a dose-dependent manner [181]. Recently Hoile et al. showed that both the amount and also the type of maternal fat intake (for example, consumption of fish oil more than butter) induces methylation of four CpG dinucleotides in the FADS2 promoter in offspring liver during their adulthood [182]. In mice, a maternal HF diet has been shown to reduce adiponectin levels by modification of H3K9 in the adiponectin promoter and to increase leptin levels by methylation of H4K20 in the leptin promoter. These changes were accompanied by enhancement of leptin and suppression of adiponectin gene expression in adipose tissues, which might cause metabolic syndrome [183]. Furthermore, male and female offspring exposed to a HF diet *in utero* had a higher risk for obesity in later life, via altered epigenomic modifications of the thyroid axis [184].

12.1.2.5.3 Carbohydrate

Carbohydrate intake during gestation can also affect the metabolic fate of the offspring. In adulthood, offspring who were exposed to a sucrose-rich diet in uterus had higher adiposity and more extensive increases in triglyceride liver content than those who were exposed to a standard diet [185]. Moreover, increased capacity to store excess triglyceride in the liver and adipose tissue in rat offspring with a HF diet has been suggested [186,187]. Furthermore, increased adiponectin levels and insulin sensitivity of skeletal muscle has been reported for individuals exposed to high sucrose *in utero* [185]. Maternal fructose (10%) intake contributed toward metabolic syndrome progression in adult male offspring, but not female, which was accompanied by hyperleptinemia [188]. Additionally, maternal consumption of high fructose can change the offspring's epigenetic marks in the kidney and alter the expression of genes related to blood pressure [189].

12.1.2.5.4 Micronutrients

High levels of maternal folate and low B12 status have been associated with higher insulin resistance in offspring. In the same study, high maternal circulating folate levels correlated with higher adiposity in 6-year-old offspring [190]. Maternal vitamin B12 restriction reduced the percent of lean body mass (LBM) and fat-free mass (FFM) in Wistar rats, probably by increasing oxidative stress and altering epigenetics in the offspring [191]. Interestingly, the risk of developing obesity was protected against in mice offspring exposed to hypermethylating dietary supplement (with folic acid, betaine, vitamin B12, and choline) *in utero*, despite a genetic tendency toward gaining weight [192]. Furthermore, maternal folic acid administration was found to counteract altered mRNA expression of genes involved in lipid metabolism induced by IUGR in the early development of piglets [193]. Choline deficiency in pregnant rats induced IGF2 gene hypermethylation in the offspring by hypomethylation of CpGs in the DNMTs (Dnmt1) gene regulatory region [194]. Very importantly, a maternal diet low in choline diminished *in utero* methylation of fetal DNA at the CpG islands of the genes that control cell cycling, affecting the memory performance of the offspring [195]. Thus, data suggest changes in fetal brain structure and performance may occur in response to a maternal diet rich in choline by altering epigenetic marks [196].

Moreover, for the first time Dolinoy et al. [197] showed that *in utero* genistein intake resulted in hypermethylation at CpG sites in the promoter region of agouti viable yellow (Avy) IAP, which persisted into adulthood and protected against obesity by decreasing expression of ectopic Agouti.

In 2004 Venu et al. showed that, in rodents, consistent with maternal vitamin restriction, *in utero* restriction of minerals (50%) is important in programming body adiposity in offspring [198]. Later they provided evidence that even a single maternal mineral restriction such as magnesium or zinc could have long-term effects on offspring, alter the body composition (increasing the percentage of body fat and decreasing FFM), and impair glucose-induced insulin release [199–201]. Moreover, they found that maternal chromium restriction also increased adiposity in rat offspring [202].

12.2 Transcriptional control of gene expression

12.2.1 Introduction

Eukaryotic gene expression regulation occurs at several levels. Gene transcription is the most important and widely used strategy used by some nutrients to control gene expression control. Transcription is the molecular process by which transcriptional units (genes), as template, are utilized by transcription machinery to make a copy of RNA. This process is fully controlled by tight regulatory pathways. It has been estimated that human cells contain some 21,000 genes. Some of these genes are required by all cells and in all circumstances. These are called *housekeeping genes*, and the genes of master enzymes in metabolic pathways, genes of cytoskeleton, and RNA polymerases belong to this group. Some are expressed as cells differentiated to specific cells. Another group are those whose products require to respond environmental alterations and stimulations. The principle of transcription in eukaryotes is similar to that in simple prokaryotes; however, the whole process is more complex. Unlike prokaryotes, which contain one RNA polymerase, eukaryotes have three distinct RNA polymerases. RNA polymerases I and III are involved in synthesis of ribosomal RNAs and transfer RNAs. RNA polymerase II transcribes all genes to mRNAs, which are committed to translate to proteins [3].

Transcription consists of three steps: initiation, elongation, and termination. The main step in regulation of gene transcription is initiation. Eukaryotic protein-coding genes contain coding sequences called *exons* and spacer sequences called *introns*. There are also regulatory regions in upstream flanking of genes. Promoter regions are elements located near the transcription initiation sites and contain the RNA polymerase II binding site and TATA box in some genes. Some eukaryotic genes have an initiator element instead of a TATA box. In addition to RNA polymerase II, several general TFs bind to the promoter. Eukaryotic promoters are more complex and longer than the ones in prokaryotes. Enhancers and silencers are other cis-acting elements on DNA that are located thousands of base pairs away from their related genes [203].

In prokaryotes, RNA polymerase binds to the gene promoter by itself; however, in eukaryotes several TFs are required to initiate transcription. They bind to promoter and RNA polymerases to form initiation complex in the right manner. About 10%–15% of mammalian genes have TATA boxes in the core promoter. Transcription factor IID (TFIID) contains a TATA box binding subunit called *TBP*. Several more general TFs such as TFIIA, B, E, and F and also RNA polymerase enzyme are recruited around the promoter in a stepwise manner. TFIIH unzips double-stranded DNA for accessibility of RNA polymerase to the noncoding DNA strand (DNA template). Kinase activity of TFIIH promotes phosphorylation of RNA polymerase at the C-terminal domain (CTD) to move it away from the initiation site. RNA polymerization along the template DNA strand in the 3′ to 5′ direction using nucleotide triphosphates continues until the end of the transcription unit. RNA copied from the DNA template is similar to nontemplate strand, except thymine-containing nucleotides, which are replaced by uracil.

During elongation, it is necessary to relax the structure of chromatin by moving histones away from DNA. RNA polymerases recruit histone-modifying proteins such as HDACs to overcome DNA restricted by nucleosomes. Some elongation factors (EFs) help transcription machinery to stimulate transcription elongation. These factors associate to RNA polymerase after initiation to prevent RNA polymerase dissociation before it completes the program. The protein-coding genes that are transcribed by RNA polymerase II do not contain any conserved site for termination, unlike ribosomal rRNA genes transcribed by RNA polymerase I. The transcript is cleaved from transcription machinery before finishing the transcription by RNA polymerase II. Termination is linked with the 3′-end polyadenylation process of the pre-mRNA. The two ends of mRNA are modified at the end of transcription [203].

Two proteins, cleavage and polyadenylation specificity factor (CPSF) and cleavage stimulation factor (CSF), recognize the polyA signal and cleave the pre-mRNA. Polyadenylation and cleavage take place 10–30 nucleotides downstream from the conserved sequence, AAUAAA, and almost 30 nucleotides upstream from the GU-rich sequence. The AAUAAA hexanucleotide is identified by CPSF. PolyA polymerase (PAP), as a member of cleavage and polyadenylation complex, helps to cleave transcript and adds almost 200 adenine nucleotide to the 3′-end. Polyadenylation of the 3′-end is a signal for export to cytoplasm, protects pre-mRNA from nuclease degradation, and is involved in initiation of ribosomal translation. When the RNA polymerase creates 25 nucleotide segments from the new RNA, its 5′-end is modified by 5′ cap. The pre-mRNA 5′-end is also capped with 7-methylguanosine prior to completing transcription. Adding a 7-methylguanosine moiety by 5′ to 5′ bond is important for linking small subunits of ribosome and formation of the initiation complex in the translation step.

Pre-mRNA in eukaryotes contains interstitial sequences, introns, between protein-coding sequences. These spacer sequences should be removed and protein-coding segments joined together before nuclear export of mRNA for the protein synthesis step in cytoplasm. The RNA splicing process in most mammalian genes occurs in different ways; therefore it produces several forms of mRNA with one gene origin. A free 2′-hydroxyl (OH) group from a specific adenine in the 3′-end of intron attacks the 5′ nucleotide in splice site, binds to it, and produces a free 3′-hydroxyl at the end of the exon. The free 3′-OH attacks the first nucleotide at the next exon, binds to it, and releases intron to form a lariat shape [3,203].

Recognition of these nucleotides in the splicing processes and catalysis of the splicing reaction are performed by several ribonucleoprotein structures called *small nuclear ribonucleoprotein* (snRNP), which consist of small nuclear RNAs (snRNAs) and about seven protein polypeptides. U1 snRNP binds to 5′ splicing sites and U2 snRNP specifies adenine nucleotide in the 3′ region of intron. snRNPs U4, 5, and 6 catalyze nucleophilic reactions, remove intron, and ligate two exons. mRNA combines with several proteins and forms a ribonucleoprotein called *mRNP*. These proteins include cap-binding protein complex (CBC), poly (A)-binding protein (PAB), and mRNA export complex TREX, which itself consists of several subunits [203,204].

Mature mRNA nuclear export to cytoplasm differs from proteins, tRNAs, and miRNAs. A heterodimer protein consisting of Nxf1-Nxt1 binds to the new mRNP via a subunit of TREX, ALY. Then, ALY is removed and the Nxf1-Nxt1 heterodimer facilitates the binding of mRNP to nucleoporins and helps cytoplasmic export [205].

12.2.2 Transcription factors

Unlike general TFs, which are recruited by transcription machinery assembly at promoters, specialized TFs bind to a specific sequence of DNA far from the promoter. They activate or suppress expression of their target genes through binding to specific elements on DNA and recruitment of several coregulators. Like other DNA-binding proteins, some motifs are responsible for direct binding to DNA, including helix-turn-helix domain, zinc finger domain, leucine zipper, and helix-loop-helix DNA-binding domain (DBD). Many genes have cis-regulatory elements upstream, downstream, or within introns that are called *enhancers*. They can be located a thousand base pairs away from the transcription site. TFs can bind to enhancers or promoters of their target genes. TF binding to specific elements on DNA causes conformational changes in their three-dimensional structures. When TFs and their related coactivators bind to an enhancer, the DNA is looped. This loop facilitates interaction between the TFs bound to the enhancers and the transcription machinery bound to the promoter to promote gene expression. A mechanism for gene silencing in eukaryotes is considered to prevent gene expression. Some TF repress gene expression through recruitment of corepressors. The availability of coactivators or corepressors determines the fate of gene expression regulation by specific TFs in the nucleus. Coregulator proteins, including coactivators and corepressors, cannot directly bind to DNA. Some of them possess histone-modifying properties. For instance, CBP/p300 proteins as coactivators have HAT effects and facilitate accessibility of TFs to DNA. Some corepressors possess HDAC activity and inhibit accessibility of related TF to DNA. It has been shown that DNMTs also act as corepressors in some TFs [203,206].

12.2.3 Nuclear receptor superfamily

It is well known that some dietary factors like retinoids, vitamin D3, and lipophilic hormones, including steroids, thyroid hormones, and other small lipid-soluble metabolites, do their physiologic actions in regulation of proliferation, development, cell metabolism, and differentiation through control of gene expression. Unlike water-soluble peptide hormones and growth factors, these lipid-soluble molecules can pass through the lipid bilayer membrane of the cell and directly interact with their receptors inside the cell to act as a TF.

The classic model of their action, as first identified for steroid hormones, comprises an allosteric change following the binding of the hormone to its specific receptor, which enables the hormone-receptor complex to bind to specific binding sites on the genome and modulate transcription [207]. Nowadays 48 codes for nuclear receptors have been identified in the human genome; for many of them their ligand has been recognized but some of them have remained orphan receptors with unknown ligands [208].

The characteristic structural features of nuclear receptors are composed of a variable amino-terminal domain that includes several distinct transactivation regions (called *AF1* for activation function 1), a conserved DBD that includes two Zn finger motifs for binding to specific sequences of DNA called *hormone response element* (HRE), a short linker region for nuclear localization called *hinge*, a conserved carboxy-terminal ligand-binding domain (LBD), which is involved in specificity and selectivity of the biologic response following ligand receptor interaction and also imparts to interactions of coregulators and the subfamily of nuclear receptors to form heterodimers. Some of them also have a variable carboxy-terminal end (also called *activation function 2*, AF2) [209].

Some receptors bind to a solitary 6 base pair (bp) motif on DNA as a monomer, but the remaining receptors bind as homodimer or heterodimer to specific sequences on DNA that contains two 6 bp motifs with palindromic, reverse repeats or direct repeats. The consensus nucleotides of these motifs are AGAACA palindromic repeats separated by three nucleotides in steroid hormones except estrogen receptor, and AGGTCA conserved order for the remaining receptors. The arrangement and number of separating nucleotides between repeats are responsible for the specificity and selectivity of receptors. Therefore, direct repeats with 3, 4, and 5 bp distances (i.e., DR3, DR4, DR5) are specifically recognized by vitamin D receptor, thyroid hormone receptor, and retinoic acid receptor, respectively [210].

Based on their style of action, nuclear receptors can be divided into four subtypes. In type I, the receptor is held in the cytoplasm by chaperon proteins including Hsp90 and Hsp56 in the absence of ligand. Following ligand binding, the chaperon is released and homodimerization of the receptor helps the disclosure of nuclear localizing sequence (NLS) and translocation to nucleus. In the nucleus, ligand homodimer receptor complex adjoins to pair inverted repeats on enhancer sequences of the target gene, so association between them and coactivators leads to activation of target genes. Estrogen and androgen receptors are examples of this type [207,208,211].

Type II receptors like thyroid, VDR, PPARs, and retinoic acid receptors are placed in contact with their HRE in the nucleus, regardless of the existence of ligand. They form heterodimers with retinoid X receptor (RXR) and bind to direct repeats or sometimes symmetric repeats of DNA. In the absence of ligand, incorporation with nuclear corepressor complexes such as nuclear receptor corepressor (NCoR) or silencing mediator of retinoid and thyroid receptors (SMRT) and HDACs cause repression of gene expression. Ligand binding induces conformational changes that allow displacement of the corepressor complexes and recruitment of transcriptional coactivators like HATs and chromatin remodeling factors that open up chromatin to facilitate gene expression and exert epigenetic modification supporting gene activation.

Type III receptors are like the type I family, except that HRE arrangement in type 3 receptors consists of direct repeats that homodimers adjoin. In type IV receptors like FXR, receptors bind to one part of HRE pair sequences as a monomer [207,208].

The effects of nuclear receptors on gene expression is mediated through interactions with coregulators like the SWI/SNF chromatin remodeling complex, CBP/p300 (as histone acetyl transferase) and steroid receptor coactivator (SRC)/p160 factors through their LXXLL motifs (*L* indicates leucine and *X* indicates any amino acid) [210,212]. Moreover, the action of nuclear receptors can be modified by post-translational modifications such as phosphorylation, ubiquitination, O-GlcNAcylation, acetylation, and SUMOylation that could impact their affinity for their ligands and thus functions [213]. Nuclear receptors can also affect other TFs like STAT5, OCT2A, etc. So there are surprising complexities for gene expression regulation procedures and crosstalk between nuclear receptors and their ligands [214].

12.2.3.1 RAR/RXR nuclear receptor

Retinoids are vitamin A derivatives that exert their biological actions, including regulating development, cell proliferation, differentiation, immunity, and embryonic organogenesis, through heterodimerization of two nuclear receptors, such as retinoic acid receptors (including RAR α, β, and γ isoforms) and the indiscriminate retinoid X receptors (including RXR α, β, and γ isoforms) [215].

All-trans retinoic acid is the ligand for RARs that, with the involvement of cellular retinoic acid-binding protein 2 (CRABP2), is transported from cytosol to RARs in the nucleus, where it binds to RA response element (RARE) on DNA that is classically (notably there are also DR1 and DR0 for RAR/RXR) composed of 5 bp spaced direct repeat (DR5), which is found in the promoter of some target genes like HOX and HNF. CRABP2 can also be a coactivator agent as chromatin remodeling factor [216]. 9-cis retinoic acid is the ligand for both RXR and RAR [217]. RA can directly activate the transcription of target genes that have RARE such as the Hoxa1 gene, which is a TF that regulates differentiation [218]. Phosphoenolpyruvate carboxykinase (PEPCK), the key enzyme of the fatty acid reesterification pathway, can be induced by RA through interaction with RAR/RXR and the ATP-dependent chromatin remodeling SWI/SNF complex [219].

Some other types of RA targets do not have RARE but are indirectly induced by the TFs that are modulated by RA. FOX03 is a TF that leads to natural regulatory T-cell differentiation, which is critical in immunity regulation. FOX03 activation is induced by RA [220].

Sometimes RA signaling induces transcriptional repression. For example, RA, by preventing attachment of the TF OCT4 to the promoter of its target gene Rex1, which causes maintenance of embryonic stem cell pluripotency, can induce differentiation [221].

Control of duration and magnitude of retinoid mediated transcription involves ubiquitylation of RARs or their coregulators in response to retinoids, which targets them for proteosomal degradation [222].

RA can inhibit adipogenesis indirectly through inducing the TGF-β/smad3 pathway, which can interfere with C/EBPβ DNA binding, which is the master regulator of adipocyte differentiation [223].

12.2.3.2 Vitamin D nuclear receptor

The biologically active form of vitamin D is $1\alpha,25\text{-}(OH)_2D$ (calcitriol), through its nuclear receptor VDR, is involved in regulation of its target genes at the transcriptional level, which controls physiological functions such as calcium and phosphate homeostasis, cell differentiation, immunity, xenobiotic detoxification, and antiproliferative actions in various tissues [5].

VDRE is a DNA sequence of direct repeat of six base pairs with a three-nucleotide spacer upstream of the 5′ end of the vitamin D target genes. The liganded VDR, along with its heterodimeric partner RXR attached to VDRE, recruits coactivators such as vitamin D receptor interacting protein (DRIP)/T3 receptor auxiliary protein (TRAP) multimeric complex and eliminates the transcriptional inhibitory factors to transactivate its target genes [224].

The calcemic roles of vitamin D3 are composed of positive and negative gene regulation. Vitamin D can positively induce the genes of the transient receptor potential vanilloid (TRPV) family that are calcium channels responsible for the influx of calcium into the epithelial cells, calcium binding proteins, calbindins (CaBPs), the plasma membrane calcium ATPase ($PMCA_{1b}$) that regulates calcium extrusion in intestine and Na^+/Ca^{2+} exchanger (NCX1) pomps in the kidney, osteopontine, and BGP (osteocalcin) to control calcium absorption and homeostasis [225].

VDR can directly downregulate transcription of some genes like PTH and CYP27B1 that catalyze 1α-hydroxylation of D3 (feedback loop). These negative VDREs are transcriptionally active, even in the absence of $1\alpha, 25\text{-}(OH)_2D$, and are bound to VDR-interacting repressor, a basic helix-loop-helix TF that recruits CBP/p300 HAT activity upon phosphorylation by protein kinase A. Liganded VDR/RXR results in replacement of the CBP/p300 HAT coactivator by HDACs and NCoR/SMRT corepressors. The WINAC multimeric complex facilitates chromatin remodeling during this replacement process that ultimately causes gene silencing [226].

The noncalcemic role of vitamin D is upregulation of p21 and p27 cyclin-dependent kinase inhibitors, resulting in the dephosphorylation of retinoblastoma protein, which inhibits the transcription of E2F, the necessary TF for cell cycle growth [227]. Vitamin D may also suppress cell growth by altering the signaling pathways of TGFβ, IGF, and Wnt/β-catenin [228]. Moreover, vitamin D increases apoptosis in prostate cancer cell lines through downregulation of the Bcl-2 family of antiapoptotic proteins [229].

12.2.3.3 PPARs

Naturally occurring long-chain fatty acids and their eicosanoid derivatives play critical roles in lipid and carbohydrate metabolism and other different biologic pathways by modulating the expression of their target genes at the transcriptional level through interaction with their nuclear receptor PPARs.

PPARs form a heterodimer with RXR and bind to a specific site composed of a direct repeat of consensus 6 bp sequence spaced by one nucleotide (DR1). The three isoforms of PPARs in mammals—PPARα, PPARβ (also called PPARδ), and PPARγ—have different functions and tissue distributions [230].

12.2.3.3.1 PPARα

PPARα is involved in mitochondrial and peroxisomal β-oxidation, fatty acid binding and uptake, and lipoprotein assembly and transport in tissues with active fatty acid catabolism like liver, heart, kidney, muscle, and brown adipose tissue [231].

The genes regulated by PPARα include apolipoprotein (Apo) genes such as APOA1, APOA2, and APOA5, genes involved in fatty acid oxidation (acyl-CoA oxidase, CPT-I, and CPT-II), those required for the desaturation of fatty acyl CoA (delta-6-desaturase), and genes involved in HDL metabolism (PLTP) and ketone body synthesis (HMGCS2) [232].

PPARα agonists also increase the activity of the sterol regulatory element binding protein 1c (SREBP1c) promoter, which plays a key role in regulation of gene expression of lipogenic enzymes and is essential for the genomic actions of insulin on the metabolism of both carbohydrates and lipids, depending on nutritional status [233].

PPARα reduces gene expression of apolipoprotein CIII, so helps to control hypertriglyceridemia [234]. By downregulation of activator protein 1 and nuclear factor-κB signaling, PPARα exhibits anti-inflammatory effects [235]. Moreover, PPARα inhibits tumor growth and angiogenesis through repressing hypoxia inducible factor 1α in cancer cells [236].

Activation of PPARα by its ligand enhances the expression of some cytochrome p-450 enzymes such as CYP3A4, which is the major detoxifying enzyme [237].

12.2.3.3.2 PPARβ and PPARδ

PPARδ has emerged as a powerful metabolic regulator in diverse tissues including fat, skeletal muscle, and the heart. It enhances fatty acid catabolism and energy uncoupling, resulting in decreased triglyceride stores, improved endurance performance, and enhanced cardiac contractility. PPARδ modulates lipoprotein metabolism to lower triglycerides and robustly raise HDL cholesterol. Additionally, recent studies reveal that PPARδ activation in the liver suppresses hepatic glucose output, contributing to improved glucose homeostasis [238]. PPARδ activation induces genes in fatty acid oxidation, including CPT1, acyl-CoA oxidase (AOX), and long chain acyl-CoA dehydrogenase (LCAD), and in mitochondrial thermogenesis including uncoupling protein 1 (UCP1) and UCP3 [239].

Recently, it has been shown that PPARδ is a target gene for the β-catenin/TCF transcription pathway and, as a consequence, is overexpressed in tumoral intestinal cells from human familial adenomatous polyposis and can be induced by HF diet that leads to stemness [240].

12.2.3.3.3 PPARγ

There are two isoforms of PPARγ in humans—PPARγ1 and PPARγ2, and PPARγ2 is the strongest TF during adipogenesis. PPARγ is expressed in adipose tissue, muscle, gastrointestinal tract, blood cells, macrophages, and liver [241]. The eminent effect of this receptor is regulating fatty acid storage through adipose tissue differentiation and survival and glucose metabolism by improving insulin sensitivity [242]. An unliganded receptor represses gene transcription by stabilizing its interactions with corepressor complexes such as NCoR or SMRT at the promoter region of the target genes. Ligand binding recruits coactivators like SRC, P300/CBP, and HDAC (notably HDAC3), favoring transcription, albeit in some cases this can led to gene repression in a ligand-dependent manner through protein–protein interactions with NF-κB, AP1, Smads, STATs, and NFATs [243].

A functionally special form of PPARγ liganded by TZD, which is susceptible to ligand-dependent SUMOylation at lysine 365, through the recruitment and stabilization of the N-CoR complexes at the NF-κB-responsive promoters of pro-inflammatory genes in inflammatory bowel diseases, inhibits the expression of several inflammatory genes in macrophages [244].

PPAR coactivator-1α (PGC-1α), a potent coactivator of PPARγ, is expressed in brown adipose tissue and induced by adrenergic signals; it enhances mitochondrial thermogenesis and cellular respiration by inducing UCP-1 in accordance with PPARγ [245].

In adenocarcinoma cell lines, PPARγ prevents invasiveness of tumors by inhibiting the TGF-β/Smad3 pathway [246].

Liganded PPARγ induces the expression of genes such as P2 (fatty-acid binding protein), CD36 (receptor for lipoproteins), lipoprotein lipase (hydrolysis of lipoproteins), FATP-1 (fatty acid transporter), glycerol kinase, SREBP-1 and SCD-1 (regulators of sterol and fatty acid synthesis, respectively), adiponectin (insulin sensitizing factor), c-Cbl-associated protein (CAP), which stimulates glucose transport, and PEPCK [242,247].

In vitro studies suggest that PPARγ is the ultimate effector of adipogenesis in a transcriptional cascade that also involves members of the C/EBP transcription factor family [248].

12.3 Translational control of protein synthesis

12.3.1 Introduction

Translation is the process by which codes provided by the genome are converted to functional proteins. This takes place in the cytoplasm and mainly requires messenger RNA (mRNA), transfer RNA (tRNA), and ribosomal RNA (rRNA). mRNA carries the genetic information as three-nucleotide sets called codons. Each codon on mRNA is translated into an amino acid. tRNA specifically binds amino acids at one end and selects them based on its three-nucleotide sequence, called *anticodon*, at the other end. The tRNA binds amino acids with a high energy link made by the catalytic action of the aminoacyl-tRNA synthetase enzyme. Amino acids are bound to the 3′ hydroxyl group of the terminal adenosine. During translation, the tRNA base pairs with the mRNA through its anticodon and delivers the attached amino acid to the polypeptide chain. Any error can lead to addition of an incorrect amino acid. Finally, rRNA forms ribonucleoprotein structure (ribosome) that provide a scaffold to assemble amino acids into a polypeptide chain.

Protein synthesis can be divided into three distinct steps: initiation, elongation, and termination.

In eukaryotes, during the initiation step, the two ribosomal subunits form a complex that can move along the mRNA. Also involved in the process are eukaryotic translation initiation factors (eIFs). By hydrolyzing GTP to GDP, eIFs stabilize the formation of the functional ribosome and act as proofreading switches. The translation moves forward if only the former step has occurred correctly. The tRNA initiator (tRNAiMet) is bound to eIF2, while the 40s subunit is associated with eIF1, 1A, and 3, leading to inhibition of premature binding between small and large ribosomal subunits. mRNA is also activated by the addition of eIF4 at the 5′ end and attaching to the poly(A)-binding protein (PAPB) bound to the mRNA poly(a) tail at the 3′ end. Then, the eIF4 complex binds to the 43s preinitiation complex, formed by the addition of eIF5 to the 40s. This way, the small ribosomal subunit attaches to the mRNA. Recently, it was shown that the 5′ end of mRNA is important in ribosome recruitment and also can affect translation efficiency [249]. The eIF4A, which has helicase activity, unwinds the mRNA and the subunits move from the 5′ to 3′ end, scanning for the start codon. Following recognition of the start codon (most commonly AUG), the 60S subunit binds the preinitiation complex, eIF5B GTP is hydrolyzed to GDP, some eIFs are released, and subsequently the initiation complex is formed. The tRNA$_i$^{Met} is localized in the P site formed in the initiation complex. Two other sites are also found in the initiation complex, the A and E sites. The first aminoacyl-tRNA attaches to the A site. The E site is the exit location for free tRNAs in the elongation step [203].

In the elongation step, the ribosome moves along the mRNA codon by codon and recruits new aminoacyl-tRNAs, forming a peptide bond between the corresponding amino acids, by peptidyl transferase. Similar to initiation, the elongation step requires special proteins called *translation elongation factors*. The first aminoacyl-tRNA along with EF1α-GTP is recruited by ribosome and enters the A site. Simultaneously, the EF1α-GTP is hydrolyzed to GDP. This induces a conformational change in the ribosome and the peptide bond is formed between the new amino acid and the last one—in the case of the first codon, methionine.

256   Nutrigenomics and Nutraceuticals

Hydrolyses of EF2-GTP causes another conformational change that moves the ribosome along the mRNA as one codon and results in translocation of the peptide chain bound aminoacyl-tRNA from the A site to the P site and the unacylated tRNA from the P to E site, where it exits the ribosome in the next cycle. This process repeats until the stop codon is recognized. As the polypeptide chain becomes longer, it leaves through a channel found in the large subunit, opposite the position the tRNAs enter [203].

The final step of protein synthesis, termination, also needs special proteins called *eukaryotic release factors* (eRFs). In eukaryotes, when the ribosome reaches one of the stop codons (UAA, UGA, UAG), eRF1 with a similar shape to tRNAs recognizes and binds to the A site along with the eRF3.GTP, a GTP-binding protein. Hydrolysis of GTP cleaves and releases the completed nascent peptide chain from the tRNA in the P site [250]. Finally, the two ribosomal subunits are separated.

12.3.2 The role of energy and amino acids in protein synthesis

Mammalian target of Rapamycin (mTOR), a 289-kDa serine-threonine kinase, plays an important role in protein translation regulation by energy and nutrients, growth factors, and stress (251–253). The mTOR signaling senses both intracellular and extracellular cues and affects cell metabolism and protein synthesis, among others. mTOR is part of two multiprotein complexes, mTORC1 and mTORC2 [254]. The former is a major regulator of cell metabolism. It controls the translation process and through this specifically facilitates cell growth and proliferation. S6Ks and 4E-BPs, two mTORC1 substrates, regulate translation. When dephosphorylated, 4E-BPs affects translation initiation by preventing assembly of the eIF-4 to the 5′ cap complex and therefore stops cap-dependent mRNA translation. mTORC1 can phosphorylate 4E-BPs and prevents its inhibitory effect [255,256].

The mTORC1 complex also includes regulatory-associated protein of mTOR (RAPTOR) and DEP domain-containing mTOR-interacting protein (DEPTOR), which are negative regulators of mTORC1, and mammalian lethal with SEC13 protein 8 (mLST8; also known as GβL) as a positive regulator [252]. Some signals that affect the mTORC1 activity come via the tuberous sclerosis complex (TSC, comprising TSC1 and TSC2), a GTPase activating protein that hydrolyses RHEB. GTP to GDP (RAS homologue enriched in brain) and thus TSC negatively regulates mTORC1. However, inhibition of TSC results in increase of mTORC1 kinase activity [257,258].

In addition, mTORC1 can be inhibited by the action of AMPK, which in low energy status can phosphorylate RAPTOR and TSC2 [259]. AMPK is a well-known energy sensor inside the cell and affects mTORC1 activity according to the cellular AMP:ATP ratio. Recently, it was shown that inhibiting mTOR by rapamycin administration leads to preservation of neural ATP levels, probably by a decrease in protein synthesis; hence this was proposed as a possible treatment for neurodegeneration caused by defective mitochondria [260].

Unlike energy, amino acids do not signal through TSC-RHEB and the mechanism by which they affect mTORC was obscure for a long time, while amino acids seem to be the most important signal sensed by mTORC1 as they positively regulate it [254]. Leucine is known to activate the mTORC1 signaling pathway and enters the cells in exchange with glutamine via the SLC (solute carrier) family of transporters [261]. Although it is known that leucine, glutamine, and arginine activate mTORC1 [261–263], no clear data are available for other amino acids on how and where they are sensed.

It has been shown that other than RHEB, the four members of the Rag protein family, small guanosine triphosphates (GTPases), can affect mTORC1 in an amino acid–dependent manner [264,265]. In mammalians, amino acid sufficiency leads to enhancement of the active state of these proteins as a complex of the RAGA/RAGB.GTP-RAGC/RAGD.GDP forms. This complex binds RAPTOR and induces mTORC1 relocalization to lysosome, where it interacts with RHEB and hence is activated; however, in amino acid deficiency mTORC1 is distributed across the cytoplasm, physically distant from its activator RHEB [265,266].

mTORC1 activity has been linked to aging and lifespan in several different studies as inhibition of mTORC1 signaling led to longer life in yeast, worms, flies, and rodents [267]. As mentioned above, mTOR activation leads to protein synthesis and proliferation and its inhibition causes autophagy and blocks growth [258]. Most studies leading to longer life have involved protein and/or calorie-restricted diets and seem to be reducing insulin/IGF signaling and activation of AMP kinase. Therefore, it has been suggested that mTORC1 might be involved in the process. In addition, S6Ks and 4E-BPs have been linked to longevity. Loss of S6K and increased 4E-BPs activity has caused longer life in different organisms [267,268].

Use of rapamycin, a pharmacological agent that is a specific inhibitor of mTOR, as an anti-aging drug is very interesting. It has also been shown that with rapamycin administration in mice both mean and maximum life spans were extended. However, due to the side effects, it may not be suggested as an anti-aging treatment in humans and more current studies are being carried out to confirm the safety and effectiveness of this drug [268,269].

It has also been reported that resveratrol, a naturally occurring polyphenol, can slow aging-associated pathologies in animal models [270]. It can improve endothelial function by recoupling eNOS, preventing superoxide formation, and increasing endothelial NO production by inhibition of mTORC1–S6K1 signaling [271].

References

1. Prasad C. Improving mental health through nutrition: The future. *Nutritional Neuroscience.* 2001;4(4):251–72. PubMed PMID: 11842893. Epub 2002/02/15. eng.

2. Trujillo E, Davis C, Milner J. Nutrigenomics, proteomics, metabolomics, and the practice of dietetics. *Journal of the American Dietetic Association.* 2006;106(3):403–13. PubMed PMID: 16503231. Epub 2006/03/01. eng.
3. Alberts B. *Molecular Biology of the Cell with CD.* New York, Garland; 2008.
4. Choi S-W, Friso S. Epigenetics: A new bridge between nutrition and health. *Advances in Nutrition: An International Review Journal.* 2010;1(1):8–16.
5. Haussler MR, Haussler CA, Bartik L, Whitfield GK, Hsieh JC, Slater S, et al. Vitamin D receptor: Molecular signaling and actions of nutritional ligands in disease prevention. *Nutrition Reviews.* 2008;66(10 Suppl 2):S98–112. PubMed PMID: 18844852. Epub 2008/12/05. eng.
6. Haussler MR, Whitfield GK, Kaneko I, Haussler CA, Hsieh D, Hsieh J-C, et al. Molecular mechanisms of vitamin D action. *Calcified Tissue International.* 2013;92(2):77–98.
7. Killeen MJ, Linder M, Pontoniere P, Crea R. NF-κβ signaling and chronic inflammatory diseases: Exploring the potential of natural products to drive new therapeutic opportunities. *Drug Discovery Today.* 2014;19(4):373–8.
8. Wellen KE, Thompson CB. A two-way street: Reciprocal regulation of metabolism and signalling. *Nature Reviews Molecular Cell Biology.* 2012;13(4):270–6.
9. Gut P, Verdin E. The nexus of chromatin regulation and intermediary metabolism. *Nature.* 2013;502(7472):489–98. PubMed PMID: 24153302. Epub 2013/10/25. eng.
10. Ruan H-B, Singh JP, Li M-D, Wu J, Yang X. Cracking the O-GlcNAc code in metabolism. *Trends in Endocrinology & Metabolism.* 2013;24(6):301–9.
11. Minamino T, Orimo M, Shimizu I, Kunieda T, Yokoyama M, Ito T, et al. A crucial role for adipose tissue p53 in the regulation of insulin resistance. *Nature Medicine.* 2009;15(9):1082–7.
12. Homayounfar R, Jeddi-Tehrani M, Cheraghpour M, Ghorbani A, Zand H. Relationship of p53 accumulation in peripheral tissues of high-fat diet-induced obese rats with decrease in metabolic and oncogenic signaling of insulin. *General and Comparative Endocrinology.* 2015;214:134–9.
13. Berger SL, Kouzarides T, Shiekhattar R, Shilatifard A. An operational definition of epigenetics. *Genes & Development.* 2009;23(7):781–3.
14. Qiu J. Epigenetics: Unfinished symphony. *Nature.* 2006;441(7090):143–5.
15. Cedar H, Bergman Y. Linking DNA methylation and histone modification: Patterns and paradigms. *Nature Reviews Genetics.* 2009;10(5):295–304.
16. Wu SC, Zhang Y. Active DNA demethylation: Many roads lead to Rome. *Nature Reviews Molecular Cell Biology.* 2010;11(9):607–20.
17. Okano M, Bell DW, Haber DA, Li E. DNA methyltransferases Dnmt3a and Dnmt3b are essential for *de novo* methylation and mammalian development. *Cell.* 99(3):247–57.
18. Kohli RM, Zhang Y. TET enzymes, TDG and the dynamics of DNA demethylation. *Nature.* 2013;502(7472):472–9.
19. Bannister AJ, Kouzarides T. Regulation of chromatin by histone modifications. *Cell Research.* 2011;21(3):381–95.
20. Karlić R, Chung H-R, Lasserre J, Vlahoviček K, Vingron M. Histone modification levels are predictive for gene expression. *Proceedings of the National Academy of Sciences of the United States of America.* 2010;107(7):2926–31.
21. Wang Z, Zang C, Cui K, Schones DE, Barski A, Peng W, et al. Genome-wide mapping of HATs and HDACs reveals distinct functions in active and inactive genes. *Cell.* 2009;138(5):1019–31.
22. Margueron R, Reinberg D. The Polycomb complex PRC2 and its mark in life. *Nature.* 2011;469(7330):343–9.
23. Greer EL, Shi Y. Histone methylation: A dynamic mark in health, disease and inheritance. *Nature Reviews Genetics.* 2012;13(5):343–57.
24. Karunakaran U, Jeoung NH. O-GlcNAc modification: Friend or foe in diabetic cardiovascular disease. *Korean Diabetes Journal.* 2010;34(4):211–19. PubMed PMID: 20835337. Pubmed Central PMCID: PMC2932889. Epub 2010/09/14. eng.

25. Chen Q, Chen Y, Bian C, Fujiki R, Yu X. TET2 promotes histone O-GlcNAcylation during gene transcription. *Nature.* 2013;493(7433):561–4. PubMed PMID: 23222540. Pubmed Central PMCID: PMC3684361. Epub 2012/12/12. eng.
26. Zhang Q, Liu X, Gao W, Li P, Hou J, Li J, et al. Differential regulation of the ten-eleven translocation (TET) family of dioxygenases by O-linked β-N-acetylglucosamine transferase (OGT). *Journal of Biological Chemistry.* 2014;289(9):5986–96.
27. Witkowski L, Foulkes WD. In brief: Picturing the complex world of chromatin remodelling families. *The Journal of Pathology.* 2015;237(4):403–6.
28. Krol J, Loedige I, Filipowicz W. The widespread regulation of microRNA biogenesis, function and decay. *Nature Reviews Genetics.* 2010;11(9):597–610.
29. Ha M, Kim VN. Regulation of microRNA biogenesis. *Nature Reviews Molecular Cell Biology.* 2014;15(8):509–24.
30. Hardie DG, Schaffer BE, Brunet A. AMPK: An energy-sensing pathway with multiple inputs and outputs. *Trends in Cell Biology.* 2016;26(3):190–201.
31. Wellen KE, Hatzivassiliou G, Sachdeva UM, Bui TV, Cross JR, Thompson CB. ATP-citrate lyase links cellular metabolism to histone acetylation. *Science (New York, NY).* 2009;324(5930):1076–80.
32. Honma K, Mochizuki K, Goda T. Carbohydrate/fat ratio in the diet alters histone acetylation on the sucrase-isomaltase gene and its expression in mouse small intestine. *Biochemical and Biophysical Research Communications.* 2007;357(4):1124–9. PubMed PMID: 17466947. Epub 2007/05/01. eng.
33. Funato H, Oda S, Yokofujita J, Igarashi H, Kuroda M. Fasting and high-fat diet alter histone deacetylase expression in the medial hypothalamus. *PLoS One.* 2011;6(4):e18950. PubMed PMID: 21526203. Pubmed Central PMCID: PMC3078138. Epub 2011/04/29. eng.
34. Suzuki T, Douard V, Mochizuki K, Goda T, Ferraris RP. Diet-induced epigenetic regulation in vivo of the intestinal fructose transporter Glut5 during development of rat small intestine. *The Biochemical Journal.* 2011;435(1):43–53. PubMed PMID: 21222652. Epub 2011/01/13. eng.
35. Mosley AL, Ozcan S. Glucose regulates insulin gene transcription by hyperacetylation of histone h4. *The Journal of Biological Chemistry.* 2003;278(22):19660–6. PubMed PMID: 12665509. Epub 2003/04/01. eng.
36. Newman JC, Verdin E. β-hydroxybutyrate: Much more than a metabolite. *Diabetes Research and Clinical Practice.* 2014;106(2):173–81.
37. Sassone-Corsi P. When metabolism and epigenetics converge. *Science (New York, NY).* 2013;339(6116):148–50.
38. Newman JC, Verdin E. Ketone bodies as signaling metabolites. *Trends in Endocrinology & Metabolism.* 2014;25(1):42–52.
39. Obici S, Wang J, Chowdury R, Feng Z, Siddhanta U, Morgan K, et al. Identification of a biochemical link between energy intake and energy expenditure. *The Journal of Clinical Investigation.* 2002;109(12):1599–605. PubMed PMID: 12070307. Pubmed Central PMCID: PMC151013. Epub 2002/06/19. eng.
40. Wells L, Vosseller K, Hart GW. A role for N-acetylglucosamine as a nutrient sensor and mediator of insulin resistance. *Cellular and Molecular Life Sciences.* 2003;60(2):222–8. PubMed PMID: 12678487. Epub 2003/04/08. eng.
41. Ruan HB, Dietrich MO, Liu ZW, Zimmer MR, Li MD, Singh JP, et al. O-GlcNAc transferase enables AgRP neurons to suppress browning of white fat. *Cell.* 2014;159(2):306–17. PubMed PMID: 25303527. Pubmed Central PMCID: PMC4509746. Epub 2014/10/11. eng.
42. Yang YR, Jang HJ, Choi SS, Lee YH, Lee GH, Seo YK, et al. Obesity resistance and increased energy expenditure by white adipose tissue browning in Oga(+/-) mice. *Diabetologia.* 2015;58(12):2867–76. PubMed PMID: 26342595. Epub 2015/09/08. eng.

43. Walgren JL, Vincent TS, Schey KL, Buse MG. High glucose and insulin promote O-GlcNAc modification of proteins, including alpha-tubulin. *American Journal of Physiology Endocrinology and Metabolism.* 2003;284(2):E424–34. PubMed PMID: 12397027. Epub 2002/10/25. eng.

44. Medford HM, Chatham JC, Marsh SA. Chronic ingestion of a Western diet increases O-linked-beta-N-acetylglucosamine (O-GlcNAc) protein modification in the rat heart. *Life Sciences.* 2012;90(23–24):883–8. PubMed PMID: 22575823. Pubmed Central PMCID: PMC3372663. Epub 2012/05/12. eng.

45. Oosterveer MH, Schoonjans K. Hepatic glucose sensing and integrative pathways in the liver. *Cellular and Molecular Life Sciences.* 2014;71(8):1453–67. PubMed PMID: 24196749. Epub 2013/11/08. eng.

46. Onodera Y, Nam JM, Bissell MJ. Increased sugar uptake promotes oncogenesis via EPAC/RAP1 and O-GlcNAc pathways. *The Journal of clinical investigation.* 2014 Jan;124(1):367–84. PubMed PMID: 24316969. Pubmed Central PMCID: PMC3871217. Epub 2013/12/10. eng.

47. Tateishi K, Okada Y, Kallin EM, Zhang Y. Role of Jhdm2a in regulating metabolic gene expression and obesity resistance. *Nature.* 2009;458(7239):757–61. PubMed PMID: 19194461. Pubmed Central PMCID: PMC4085783. Epub 2009/02/06. eng.

48. Inagaki T, Tachibana M, Magoori K, Kudo H, Tanaka T, Okamura M, et al. Obesity and metabolic syndrome in histone demethylase JHDM2a-deficient mice. *Genes to cells: Devoted to Molecular & Cellular Mechanisms.* 2009;14(8):991–1001. PubMed PMID: 19624751. Epub 2009/07/25. eng.

49. Mews P, Zee BM, Liu S, Donahue G, Garcia BA, Berger SL. Histone methylation has dynamics distinct from those of histone acetylation in cell cycle reentry from quiescence. *Molecular and Cellular Biology.* 2014;34(21):3968–80. PubMed PMID: 25154414. Pubmed Central PMCID: PMC4386454. Epub 2014/08/27. eng.

50. Kraus D, Yang Q, Kong D, Banks AS, Zhang L, Rodgers JT, et al. Nicotinamide N-methyltransferase knockdown protects against diet-induced obesity. *Nature.* 2014;508(7495):258–62. PubMed PMID: 24717514. Pubmed Central PMCID: PMC4107212. Epub 2014/04/11. eng.

51. Han P, Gao D, Zhang W, Liu S, Yang S, Li X. Puerarin suppresses high glucose-induced MCP-1 expression via modulating histone methylation in cultured endothelial cells. *Life Sciences.* 2015;130:103–7. PubMed PMID: 25817234. Epub 2015/03/31. eng.

52. Bouchard L, Rabasa-Lhoret R, Faraj M, Lavoie ME, Mill J, Perusse L, et al. Differential epigenomic and transcriptomic responses in subcutaneous adipose tissue between low and high responders to caloric restriction. *The American Journal of Clinical Nutrition.* 2010;91(2):309–20. PubMed PMID: 19939982. Epub 2009/11/27. eng.

53. Li Y, Daniel M, Tollefsbol TO. Epigenetic regulation of caloric restriction in aging. *BMC Medicine.* 2011;9:98. PubMed PMID: 21867551. Pubmed Central PMCID: PMC3175174. Epub 2011/08/27. eng.

54. Cordero P, Campion J, Milagro FI, Goyenechea E, Steemburgo T, Javierre BM, et al. Leptin and TNF-alpha promoter methylation levels measured by MSP could predict the response to a low-calorie diet. *Journal of Physiology and Biochemistry.* 2011;67(3):463–70. PubMed PMID: 21465273. Epub 2011/04/06. eng.

55. Hass BS, Hart RW, Lu MH, Lyn-Cook BD. Effects of caloric restriction in animals on cellular function, oncogene expression, and DNA methylation *in vitro. Mutation Research.* 1993;295(4–6):281–9. PubMed PMID: 7507563. Epub 1993/12/01. eng.

56. Miyamura Y, Tawa R, Koizumi A, Uehara Y, Kurishita A, Sakurai H, et al. Effects of energy restriction on age-associated changes of DNA methylation in mouse liver. *Mutation Research.* 1993;295(2):63–9. PubMed PMID: 7680421. Epub 1993/03/01. eng.

57. Kim AY, Park YJ, Pan X, Shin KC, Kwak SH, Bassas AF, et al. Obesity-induced DNA hypermethylation of the adiponectin gene mediates insulin resistance. *Nature Communications.* 2015;6:7585. PubMed PMID: 26139044. Pubmed Central PMCID: PMC4506505. Epub 2015/07/04. eng.

58. Meeran SM, Ahmed A, Tollefsbol TO. Epigenetic targets of bioactive dietary components for cancer prevention and therapy. *Clinical Epigenetics.* 2010;1(3–4):101–16. PubMed PMID: 21258631. Pubmed Central PMCID: PMC3024548. Epub 2011/01/25. Eng.

59. Ohashi K, Munetsuna E, Yamada H, Ando Y, Yamazaki M, Taromaru N, et al. High fructose consumption induces DNA methylation at PPARalpha and CPT1A promoter regions in the rat liver. *Biochemical and Biophysical Research Communications.* 2015;468(1–2):185–9. PubMed PMID: 26519879. Epub 2015/11/01. eng.

60. Ceccarelli V, Racanicchi S, Martelli MP, Nocentini G, Fettucciari K, Riccardi C, et al. Eicosapentaenoic acid demethylates a single CpG that mediates expression of tumor suppressor CCAAT/enhancer-binding protein delta in U937 leukemia cells. *The Journal of Biological Chemistry.* 2011;286(31):27092–102. PubMed PMID: 21659508. Pubmed Central PMCID: PMC3149302. Epub 2011/06/11. eng.

61. Kulkarni A, Dangat K, Kale A, Sable P, Chavan-Gautam P, Joshi S. Effects of altered maternal folic acid, vitamin B12 and docosahexaenoic acid on placental global DNA methylation patterns in Wistar rats. *PLoS One.* 2011;6(3):e17706. PubMed PMID: 21423696. Pubmed Central PMCID: PMC3053375. Epub 2011/03/23. eng.

62. Bungard D, Fuerth BJ, Zeng PY, Faubert B, Maas NL, Viollet B, et al. Signaling kinase AMPK activates stress-promoted transcription via histone H2B phosphorylation. *Science (New York, NY).* 2010;329(5996):1201–5. PubMed PMID: 20647423. Pubmed Central PMCID: PMC3922052. Epub 2010/07/22. eng.

63. McGee SL, Fairlie E, Garnham AP, Hargreaves M. Exercise-induced histone modifications in human skeletal muscle. *The Journal of Physiology.* 2009;587 (Pt 24):5951–8. PubMed PMID: 19884317. Pubmed Central PMCID: PMC2808551. Epub 2009/11/04. eng.

64. Xu Q, Yang C, Du Y, Chen Y, Liu H, Deng M, et al. AMPK regulates histone H2B O-GlcNAcylation. *Nucleic Acids Research.* 2014;42(9):5594–604. PubMed PMID: 24692660. Pubmed Central PMCID: PMC4027166. Epub 2014/04/03. eng.

65. Nakagawa T, Guarente L. Sirtuins at a glance. *Journal of Cell Science.* 2011;124(Pt 6):833–8. PubMed PMID: 21378304. Pubmed Central PMCID: PMC3048886. Epub 2011/03/08. eng.

66. Guarente L. Calorie restriction and sirtuins revisited. *Genes & Development.* 2013;27(19):2072–85. PubMed PMID: 24115767. Pubmed Central PMCID: PMC3850092. Epub 2013/10/12. eng.

67. Anderson OS, Sant KE, Dolinoy DC. Nutrition and epigenetics: An interplay of dietary methyl donors, one-carbon metabolism and DNA methylation. *The Journal of Nutritional Biochemistry.* 2012;23(8):853–9.

68. Fontana L, Adelaiye RM, Rastelli AL, Miles KM, Ciamporcero E, Longo VD, et al. Dietary protein restriction inhibits tumor growth in human xenograft models. *Oncotarget.* 2013;4(12):2451–61. PubMed PMID: 24353195. Pubmed Central PMCID: PMC3926840. Epub 2013/12/20. eng.

69. Astrom S, von der Decken A. Lysine deficiency reduces transcription activity and concentration of chromatin proteins reversibly in rat liver. *Acta Physiologica Scandinavica.* 1983;117(4):519–25. PubMed PMID: 6410687. Epub 1983/04/01. eng.

70. Balasubramanian MN, Shan J, Kilberg MS. Dynamic changes in genomic histone association and modification during activation of the ASNS and ATF3 genes by amino acid limitation. *The Biochemical Journal.* 2013;449(1):219–29. PubMed PMID: 22978410. Pubmed Central PMCID: PMC3608204. Epub 2012/09/18. eng.

71. Ross SA. Diet and DNA methylation interactions in cancer prevention. *Annals of the New York Academy of Sciences*. 2003;983:197–207. PubMed PMID: 12724224. Epub 2003/05/02. eng.

72. Dobosy JR, Fu VX, Desotelle JA, Srinivasan R, Kenowski ML, Almassi N, et al. A methyl-deficient diet modifies histone methylation and alters Igf2 and H19 repression in the prostate. *The Prostate*. 2008;68(11):1187–95. PubMed PMID: 18459101. Epub 2008/05/07. eng.

73. Tremolizzo L, Carboni G, Ruzicka W, Mitchell C, Sugaya I, Tueting P, et al. An epigenetic mouse model for molecular and behavioral neuropathologies related to schizophrenia vulnerability. *Proceedings of the National Academy of Sciences of the United States of America*. 2002;99(26):17095–100.

74. Mentch SJ, Mehrmohamadi M, Huang L, Liu X, Gupta D, Mattocks D, et al. Histone methylation dynamics and gene regulation occur through the sensing of one-carbon metabolism. *Cell Metabolism*. 2015;22(5):861–73. PubMed PMID: 26411344. Pubmed Central PMCID: PMC4635069. Epub 2015/09/29. eng.

75. Devlin AM, Arning E, Bottiglieri T, Faraci FM, Rozen R, Lentz SR. Effect of Mthfr genotype on diet-induced hyperhomocysteinemia and vascular function in mice. *Blood*. 2004;103(7):2624–9. PubMed PMID: 14630804. Epub 2003/11/25. eng.

76. Aissa AF, Gomes TD, Almeida MR, Hernandes LC, Darin JD, Bianchi ML, et al. Methionine concentration in the diet has a tissue-specific effect on chromosomal stability in female mice. *Food and Chemical Toxicology: An International Journal Published for the British Industrial Biological Research Association*. 2013;62:456–62. PubMed PMID: 24036140. Epub 2013/09/17. eng.

77. Orgeron ML, Stone KP, Wanders D, Cortez CC, Van NT, Gettys TW. The impact of dietary methionine restriction on biomarkers of metabolic health. *Progress in Molecular Biology and Translational Science*. 2014;121:351–76. PubMed PMID: 24373243. Pubmed Central PMCID: PMC4049285. Epub 2014/01/01. eng.

78. Ables GP, Hens JR, Nichenametla SN. Methionine restriction beyond life-span extension. *Annals of the New York Academy of Sciences*. 2016;1363(1):68–79. PubMed PMID: 26916321. Epub 2016/02/27. eng.

79. Hauser AT, Jung M. Targeting epigenetic mechanisms: Potential of natural products in cancer chemoprevention. *Planta Medica*. 2008;74(13):1593–601. PubMed PMID: 18704881. Epub 2008/08/16. eng.

80. Liu Z, Xie Z, Jones W, Pavlovicz RE, Liu S, Yu J, et al. Curcumin is a potent DNA hypomethylation agent. *Bioorganic & Medicinal Chemistry Letters*. 2009;19(3):706–9. PubMed PMID: 19112019. Epub 2008/12/30. eng.

81. Link A, Balaguer F, Shen Y, Lozano JJ, Leung HC, Boland CR, et al. Curcumin modulates DNA methylation in colorectal cancer cells. *PLoS One*. 2013;8(2): e57709. PubMed PMID: 23460897. Pubmed Central PMCID: PMC3584082. Epub 2013/03/06. eng.

82. Shu L, Khor TO, Lee JH, Boyanapalli SS, Huang Y, Wu TY, et al. Epigenetic CpG demethylation of the promoter and reactivation of the expression of Neurog1 by curcumin in prostate LNCaP cells. *The AAPS Journal*. 2011;13(4): 606–14. PubMed PMID: 21938566. Pubmed Central PMCID: PMC3231852. Epub 2011/09/23. eng.

83. Kang J, Chen J, Shi Y, Jia J, Zhang Y. Curcumin-induced histone hypoacetylation: The role of reactive oxygen species. *Biochemical Pharmacology*. 2005;69(8):1205–13. PubMed PMID: 15794941. Epub 2005/03/30. eng.

84. Collins HM, Abdelghany MK, Messmer M, Yue B, Deeves SE, Kindle KB, et al. Differential effects of garcinol and curcumin on histone and p53 modifications in tumour cells. *BMC Cancer*. 2013;13:37. PubMed PMID: 23356739. Pubmed Central PMCID: PMC3583671. Epub 2013/01/30. eng.

85. Bora-Tatar G, Dayangac-Erden D, Demir AS, Dalkara S, Yelekci K, Erdem-Yurter H. Molecular modifications on carboxylic acid derivatives as potent histone deacetylase inhibitors: Activity and docking studies. *Bioorganic & Medicinal Chemistry*. 2009;17(14):5219–28. PubMed PMID: 19520580. Epub 2009/06/13. eng.

86. Chen Y, Shu W, Chen W, Wu Q, Liu H, Cui G. Curcumin, both histone deacetylase and p300/CBP-specific inhibitor, represses the activity of nuclear factor kappa B and Notch 1 in Raji cells. *Basic & Clinical Pharmacology & Toxicology*. 2007;101(6):427–33. PubMed PMID: 17927689. Epub 2007/10/12. eng.

87. Kleer CG, Cao Q, Varambally S, Shen R, Ota I, Tomlins SA, et al. EZH2 is a marker of aggressive breast cancer and promotes neoplastic transformation of breast epithelial cells. *Proceedings of the National Academy of Sciences of the United States of America*. 2003;100(20):11606–11. PubMed PMID: 14500907. Pubmed Central PMCID: PMC208805. Epub 2003/09/23. eng.

88. Hua WF, Fu YS, Liao YJ, Xia WJ, Chen YC, Zeng YX, et al. Curcumin induces downregulation of EZH2 expression through the MAPK pathway in MDA-MB-435 human breast cancer cells. *European Journal of Pharmacology*. 2010;637(1–3):16–21. PubMed PMID: 20385124. Epub 2010/04/14. eng.

89. Bao B, Ali S, Banerjee S, Wang Z, Logna F, Azmi AS, et al. Curcumin analogue CDF inhibits pancreatic tumor growth by switching on suppressor microRNAs and attenuating EZH2 expression. *Cancer Research*. 2012;72(1):335–45. PubMed PMID: 22108826. Pubmed Central PMCID: PMC3792589. Epub 2011/11/24. eng.

90. Balasubramanyam K, Varier RA, Altaf M, Swaminathan V, Siddappa NB, Ranga U, et al. Curcumin, a novel p300/CREB-binding protein-specific inhibitor of acetyltransferase, represses the acetylation of histone/nonhistone proteins and histone acetyltransferase-dependent chromatin transcription. *The Journal of Biological Chemistry*. 2004;279(49):51163–71. PubMed PMID: 15383533. Epub 2004/09/24. eng.

91. Satyamoorthy K, Li G, Gerrero MR, Brose MS, Volpe P, Weber BL, et al. Constitutive mitogen-activated protein kinase activation in melanoma is mediated by both BRAF mutations and autocrine growth factor stimulation. *Cancer Research*. 2003;63(4):756–9. PubMed PMID: 12591721. Epub 2003/02/20. eng.

92. Pandey M, Shukla S, Gupta S. Promoter demethylation and chromatin remodeling by green tea polyphenols leads to re-expression of GSTP1 in human prostate cancer cells. *International Journal of Cancer*. 2010;126(11):2520–33. PubMed PMID: 19856314. Pubmed Central PMCID: PMC2874465. Epub 2009/10/27. eng.

93. Nandakumar V, Vaid M, Katiyar SK. (-)-Epigallocatechin-3-gallate reactivates silenced tumor suppressor genes, Cip1/p21 and p16INK4a, by reducing DNA methylation and increasing histones acetylation in human skin cancer cells. *Carcinogenesis*. 2011;32(4):537–44. PubMed PMID: 21209038. Pubmed Central PMCID: PMC3066414. Epub 2011/01/07. eng.

94. Deb G, Thakur VS, Limaye AM, Gupta S. Epigenetic induction of tissue inhibitor of matrix metalloproteinase-3 by green tea polyphenols in breast cancer cells. *Molecular Carcinogenesis*. 2015;54(6):485–99. PubMed PMID: 24481780. Epub 2014/02/01. eng.

95. Lee WJ, Shim JY, Zhu BT. Mechanisms for the inhibition of DNA methyltransferases by tea catechins and bioflavonoids. *Molecular Pharmacology*. 2005;68(4):1018–30. PubMed PMID: 16037419. Epub 2005/07/23. eng.

96. Fang M, Chen D, Yang CS. Dietary polyphenols may affect DNA methylation. *The Journal of Nutrition*. 2007;137(1 Suppl):223S–8S. PubMed PMID: 17182830. Epub 2006/12/22. eng.

97. Meeran SM, Patel SN, Chan TH, Tollefsbol TO. A novel prodrug of epigallocatechin-3-gallate: Differential epigenetic hTERT repression in human breast cancer cells. *Cancer Prevention Research (Philadelphia, PA)*. 2011;4(8):1243–54. PubMed PMID: 21411498. Pubmed Central PMCID: PMC3128170. Epub 2011/03/18. eng.

98. Li Y, Yuan YY, Meeran SM, Tollefsbol TO. Synergistic epigenetic reactivation of estrogen receptor-alpha (ERalpha) by combined green tea polyphenol and histone deacetylase inhibitor in ERalpha-negative breast cancer cells. *Molecular Cancer.* 2010;9:274. PubMed PMID: 20946668. Pubmed Central PMCID: PMC2967543. Epub 2010/10/16. eng.

99. Thakur VS, Gupta K, Gupta S. Green tea polyphenols causes cell cycle arrest and apoptosis in prostate cancer cells by suppressing class I histone deacetylases. *Carcinogenesis.* 2012;33(2):377–84. PubMed PMID: 22114073. Pubmed Central PMCID: PMC3499108. Epub 2011/11/25. eng.

100. Balasubramanian S, Lee K, Adhikary G, Gopalakrishnan R, Rorke EA, Eckert RL. The Bmi-1 polycomb group gene in skin cancer: Regulation of function by (-)-epigallocatechin-3-gallate. *Nutrition Reviews.* 2008;66 Suppl 1:S65–8. PubMed PMID: 18673494. Pubmed Central PMCID: PMC3120230. Epub 2008/08/21. eng.

101. Choudhury SR, Balasubramanian S, Chew YC, Han B, Marquez VE, Eckert RL. (-)-Epigallocatechin-3-gallate and DZNep reduce polycomb protein level via a proteasome-dependent mechanism in skin cancer cells. *Carcinogenesis.* 2011;32(10):1525–32. PubMed PMID: 21798853. Pubmed Central PMCID: PMC3179425. Epub 2011/07/30. eng.

102. Balasubramanian S, Adhikary G, Eckert RL. The Bmi-1 polycomb protein antagonizes the (-)-epigallocatechin-3-gallate-dependent suppression of skin cancer cell survival. *Carcinogenesis.* 2010;31(3):496–503. PubMed PMID: 20015867. Pubmed Central PMCID: PMC2832547. Epub 2009/12/18. eng.

103. Banerjee S, Kong D, Wang Z, Bao B, Hillman GG, Sarkar FH. Attenuation of multi-targeted proliferation-linked signaling by 3,3′-diindolylmethane (DIM): From bench to clinic. *Mutation research.* 2011;728(1–2):47–66. PubMed PMID: 21703360. Pubmed Central PMCID: PMC4120774. Epub 2011/06/28. eng.

104. Fang MZ, Chen D, Sun Y, Jin Z, Christman JK, Yang CS. Reversal of hypermethylation and reactivation of p16INK4a, RARbeta, and MGMT genes by genistein and other isoflavones from soy. *Clinical Cancer Research: An Official Journal of the American Association for Cancer Research.* 2005;11(19 Pt 1):7033–41. PubMed PMID: 16203797. Epub 2005/10/06. eng.

105. Xie Q, Bai Q, Zou LY, Zhang QY, Zhou Y, Chang H, et al. Genistein inhibits DNA methylation and increases expression of tumor suppressor genes in human breast cancer cells. *Genes, Chromosomes & Cancer.* 2014;53(5):422–31. PubMed PMID: 24532317. Epub 2014/02/18. eng.

106. Zheng S, Wang Z, Pan Y-X. Oral intake of genistein changes DNA methylation at the promoters of rat colon genes. *The FASEB Journal.* 2008;22(1 Supplement):885.6.

107. Hong T, Nakagawa T, Pan W, Kim MY, Kraus WL, Ikehara T, et al. Isoflavones stimulate estrogen receptor-mediated core histone acetylation. *Biochemical and Biophysical Research Communications.* 2004;317(1):259–64. PubMed PMID: 15047177. Epub 2004/03/30. eng.

108. Majid S, Dar AA, Ahmad AE, Hirata H, Kawakami K, Shahryari V, et al. BTG3 tumor suppressor gene promoter demethylation, histone modification and cell cycle arrest by genistein in renal cancer. *Carcinogenesis.* 2009;30(4):662–70. PubMed PMID: 19221000. Pubmed Central PMCID: PMC2664457. Epub 2009/02/18. eng.

109. Kikuno N, Shiina H, Urakami S, Kawamoto K, Hirata H, Tanaka Y, et al. Genistein mediated histone acetylation and demethylation activates tumor suppressor genes in prostate cancer cells. *International Journal of Cancer.* 2008;123(3):552–60. PubMed PMID: 18431742. Epub 2008/04/24. eng.

110. Phillip CJ, Giardina CK, Bilir B, Cutler DJ, Lai Y-H, Kucuk O, et al. Genistein cooperates with the histone deacetylase inhibitor vorinostat to induce cell death in prostate cancer cells. *BMC Cancer.* 2012;12(1):1.

The Influence of Dietary Components on Gene Expression 265

111. Wang H, Li Q, Chen H. Genistein affects histone modifications on Dickkopf-related protein 1 (DKK1) gene in SW480 human colon cancer cell line. *PLoS One.* 2012;7(7):e40955.
112. Chen D, Li Q, Chen H. Genistein-induced histone modifications on ATF3 may contribute to cell cycle arrest and apoptosis in human colon cancer cell line SW620 (800.8). *The FASEB Journal.* 2014;28(1 Supplement):800.8.
113. Li Y, Liu L, Andrews LG, Tollefsbol TO. Genistein depletes telomerase activity through cross-talk between genetic and epigenetic mechanisms. *International Journal of Cancer.* 2009;125(2):286–96.
114. Qin W, Zhang K, Clarke K, Weiland T, Sauter ER. Methylation and miRNA effects of resveratrol on mammary tumors vs. normal tissue. *Nutrition and Cancer.* 2014;66(2):270–7. PubMed PMID: 24447120. Epub 2014/01/23. eng.
115. Lou XD, Wang HD, Xia SJ, Skog S, Sun J. Effects of resveratrol on the expression and DNA methylation of cytokine genes in diabetic rat aortas. *Archivum Immunologiae et Therapiae Experimentalis.* 2014;62(4):329–40. PubMed PMID: 24496569. Epub 2014/02/06. eng.
116. Wang RH, Zheng Y, Kim HS, Xu X, Cao L, Luhasen T, et al. Interplay among BRCA1, SIRT1, and Survivin during BRCA1-associated tumorigenesis. *Molecular Cell.* 2008;32(1):11–20. PubMed PMID: 18851829. Pubmed Central PMCID: PMC2577018. Epub 2008/10/15. eng.
117. Higashida K, Kim SH, Jung SR, Asaka M, Holloszy JO, Han D-H. Correction: Effects of resveratrol and SIRT1 on PGC-1α activity and mitochondrial biogenesis: A reevaluation. *PLoS Biology.* 2014;12(1):10.1371/annotation/900c9397-eeb9-4d4e-9a05-ff18d657be79.
118. Venturelli S, Berger A, Böcker A, Busch C, Weiland T, Noor S, et al. Correction: Resveratrol as a Pan-HDAC inhibitor alters the acetylation status of jistone proteins in human-derived hepatoblastoma cells. *PLoS One.* 2013;8(9):10.1371/annotation/5b9a8614-1009-40ca-b90b-db817fe445c9.
119. Han S, Uludag MO, Usanmaz SE, Ayaloglu-Butun F, Akcali KC, Demirel-Yilmaz E. Resveratrol affects histone 3 lysine 27 methylation of vessels and blood biomarkers in DOCA salt-induced hypertension. *Molecular Biology Reports.* 2015;42(1):35–42. PubMed PMID: 25234650. Epub 2014/09/23. eng.
120. Wong CP, Hsu A, Buchanan A, Palomera-Sanchez Z, Beaver LM, Houseman EA, et al. Effects of sulforaphane and 3, 3′-diindolylmethane on genome-wide promoter methylation in normal prostate epithelial cells and prostate cancer cells. *PLoS One.* 2014;9(1):e86787.
121. Meeran SM, Patel SN, Tollefsbol TO. Sulforaphane causes epigenetic repression of hTERT expression in human breast cancer cell lines. *PLoS One.* 2010;5(7):e11457.
122. Lubecka-Pietruszewska K, Kaufman-Szymczyk A, Stefanska B, Cebula-Obrzut B, Smolewski P, Fabianowska-Majewska K. Sulforaphane alone and in combination with clofarabine epigenetically regulates the expression of DNA methylation-silenced tumour suppressor genes in human breast cancer cells. *Journal of Nutrigenetics and Nutrigenomics.* 2015;8(2):91–101.
123. Myzak MC, Dashwood WM, Orner GA, Ho E, Dashwood RH. Sulforaphane inhibits histone deacetylase in vivo and suppresses tumorigenesis in Apc-minus mice. *FASEB Journal: Official Publication of the Federation of American Societies for Experimental Biology.* 2006;20(3):506–8. PubMed PMID: 16407454. Pubmed Central PMCID: PMC2373266. Epub 2006/01/13. eng.
124. Ho E, Clarke JD, Dashwood RH. Dietary sulforaphane, a histone deacetylase inhibitor for cancer prevention. *The Journal of Nutrition.* 2009;139(12):2393–6. PubMed PMID: 19812222. Pubmed Central PMCID: PMC2777483. Epub 2009/10/09. eng.
125. Myzak MC, Karplus PA, Chung F-L, Dashwood RH. A novel mechanism of chemoprotection by sulforaphane inhibition of histone deacetylase. *Cancer Research.* 2004;64(16):5767–74.

126. Yuanfeng W, Gongnian X, Jianwei M, Shiwang L, Jun H, Lehe M. Dietary sulforaphane inhibits histone deacetylase activity in B16 melanoma cells. *Journal of Functional Foods*. 2015;18:182–9.

127. Atwell LL, Zhang Z, Mori M, Farris PE, Vetto JT, Naik AM, et al. Sulforaphane bioavailability and chemopreventive activity in women scheduled for breast biopsy. *Cancer Prevention Research (Philadelphia, PA)*. 2015;8(12):1184–91. PubMed PMID: 26511489. Pubmed Central PMCID: PMC4670794. Epub 2015/10/30. eng.

128. Cortez MA, Bueso-Ramos C, Ferdin J, Lopez-Berestein G, Sood AK, Calin GA. MicroRNAs in body fluids—The mix of hormones and biomarkers. *Nature Reviews Clinical Oncology*. 2011;8(8):467–77.

129. Ortega FJ, Mercader JM, Catalán V, Moreno-Navarrete JM, Pueyo N, Sabater M, et al. Targeting the circulating microRNA signature of obesity. *Clinical Chemistry*. 2013;59(5):781–92.

130. Prats-Puig A, Ortega FJ, Mercader JM, Moreno-Navarrete JM, Moreno M, Bonet N, et al. Changes in circulating microRNAs are associated with childhood obesity. *The Journal of Clinical Endocrinology and Metabolism*. 2013;98(10):E1655–60. PubMed PMID: 23928666. Epub 2013/08/10. eng.

131. Wang R, Hong J, Cao Y, Shi J, Gu W, Ning G, et al. Elevated circulating microRNA-122 is associated with obesity and insulin resistance in young adults. *European Journal of Endocrinology/European Federation of Endocrine Societies*. 2015;172(3):291–300. PubMed PMID: 25515554. Epub 2014/12/18. eng.

132. Subramaniam D, Ponnurangam S, Ramamoorthy P, Standing D, Battafarano RJ, Anant S, et al. Curcumin induces cell death in esophageal cancer cells through modulating Notch signaling. *PLoS One*. 2012;7(2):e30590.

133. Ali S, Ahmad A, Aboukameel A, Bao B, Padhye S, Philip PA, et al. Increased Ras GTPase activity is regulated by miRNAs that can be attenuated by CDF treatment in pancreatic cancer cells. *Cancer Letters*. 2012;319(2):173–81. PubMed PMID: 22261338. Pubmed Central PMCID: PMC3326199. Epub 2012/01/21. eng.

134. Yang J, Cao Y, Sun J, Zhang Y. Curcumin reduces the expression of Bcl-2 by upregulating miR-15a and miR-16 in MCF-7 cells. *Medical Oncology (Northwood, London, England)*. 2010;27(4):1114–18. PubMed PMID: 19908170. Epub 2009/11/13. eng.

135. Tsang WP, Kwok TT. Epigallocatechin gallate up-regulation of miR-16 and induction of apoptosis in human cancer cells. *The Journal of Nutritional Biochemistry*. 2010;21(2):140–6. PubMed PMID: 19269153. Epub 2009/03/10. eng.

136. Zhong Z, Dong Z, Yang L, Chen X, Gong Z. Inhibition of proliferation of human lung cancer cells by green tea catechins is mediated by upregulation of let-7. *Experimental and Therapeutic Medicine*. 2012;4(2):267–72.

137. Majid S, Dar AA, Saini S, Chen Y, Shahryari V, Liu J, et al. Regulation of minichromosome maintenance gene family by microRNA-1296 and genistein in prostate cancer. *Cancer Research*. 2010;70(7):2809–18. PubMed PMID: 20332239. Epub 2010/03/25. eng.

138. Zaman MS, Shahryari V, Deng G, Thamminana S, Saini S, Majid S, et al. Up-regulation of microRNA-21 correlates with lower kidney cancer survival. *PLoS One*. 2012;7(2):e31060. PubMed PMID: 22347428. Pubmed Central PMCID: PMC3275568. Epub 2012/02/22. eng.

139. Sun Q, Cong R, Yan H, Gu H, Zeng Y, Liu N, et al. Genistein inhibits growth of human uveal melanoma cells and affects microRNA-27a and target gene expression. *Oncology Reports*. 2009;22(3):563.

140. Xia J, Duan Q, Ahmad A, Bao B, Banerjee S, Shi Y, et al. Genistein inhibits cell growth and induces apoptosis through up-regulation of miR-34a in pancreatic cancer cells. *Current Drug Targets*. 2012;13(14):1750–6.

141. Xie J, Wang J, Zhu B. Genistein inhibits the proliferation of human multiple myeloma cells through suppression of nuclear factor-kappaB and upregulation of microRNA-29b. *Molecular Medicine Reports*. 2016;13(2):1627–32. PubMed PMID: 26718793. Epub 2016/01/01. eng.

142. Sheth S, Jajoo S, Kaur T, Mukherjea D, Sheehan K, Rybak LP, et al. Resveratrol reduces prostate cancer growth and metastasis by inhibiting the Akt/MicroRNA-21 pathway. *PLoS One*. 2012;7(12):e51655.

143. Mukhopadhyay P, Das S, Ahsan MK, Otani H, Das DK. Modulation of microRNA 20b with resveratrol and longevinex is linked with their potent anti-angiogenic action in the ischaemic myocardium and synergestic effects of resveratrol and gamma-tocotrienol. *Journal of Cellular and Molecular Medicine*. 2012;16(10):2504–17. PubMed PMID: 22050707. Pubmed Central PMCID: PMC3823443. Epub 2011/11/05. eng.

144. Tome-Carneiro J, Larrosa M, Yanez-Gascon MJ, Davalos A, Gil-Zamorano J, Gonzalvez M, et al. One-year supplementation with a grape extract containing resveratrol modulates inflammatory-related microRNAs and cytokines expression in peripheral blood mononuclear cells of type 2 diabetes and hypertension patients with coronary artery disease. *Pharmacological Research*. 2013;72:69–82. PubMed PMID: 23557933. Epub 2013/04/06. eng.

145. Venkatadri R, Muni T, Iyer A, Yakisich J, Azad N. Role of apoptosis-related miRNAs in resveratrol-induced breast cancer cell death. *Cell Death & Disease*. 2016;7(2):e2104.

146. Shan Y, Zhang L, Bao Y, Li B, He C, Gao M, et al. Epithelial-mesenchymal transition, a novel target of sulforaphane via COX-2/MMP2, 9/Snail, ZEB1 and miR-200c/ZEB1 pathways in human bladder cancer cells. *The Journal of Nutritional Biochemistry*. 2013;24(6):1062–9. PubMed PMID: 23159064. Epub 2012/11/20. eng.

147. Liu CM, Peng CY, Liao YW, Lu MY, Tsai ML, Yeh JC, et al. Sulforaphane targets cancer stemness and tumor initiating properties in oral squamous cell carcinomas via miR-200c induction. *Journal of the Formosan Medical Association*. 2017;116(1):41–48.

148. An YW, Jhang KA, Woo SY, Kang JL, Chong YH. Sulforaphane exerts its anti-inflammatory effect against amyloid-beta peptide via STAT-1 dephosphorylation and activation of Nrf2/HO-1 cascade in human THP-1 macrophages. *Neurobiology of Aging*. 2016;38:1–10. PubMed PMID: 26827637. Epub 2016/02/02. eng.

149. Tobi EW, Lumey LH, Talens RP, Kremer D, Putter H, Stein AD, et al. DNA methylation differences after exposure to prenatal famine are common and timing- and sex-specific. *Human Molecular Genetics*. 2009;18(21):4046–53. PubMed PMID: 19656776. Pubmed Central PMCID: PMC2758137. Epub 2009/08/07. eng.

150. Heijmans BT, Tobi EW, Stein AD, Putter H, Blauw GJ, Susser ES, et al. Persistent epigenetic differences associated with prenatal exposure to famine in humans. *Proceedings of the National Academy of Sciences of the United States of America*. 2008;105(44):17046–9. PubMed PMID: 18955703. Pubmed Central PMCID: PMC2579375. Epub 2008/10/29. eng.

151. Petry CJ, Dorling MW, Pawlak DB, Ozanne SE, Hales CN. Diabetes in old male offspring of rat dams fed a reduced protein diet. *International Journal of Experimental Diabetes Research*. 2001;2(2):139–43. PubMed PMID: 12369717. Pubmed Central PMCID: PMC2478537. Epub 2002/10/09. eng.

152. Han R, Li A, Li L, Kitlinska JB, Zukowska Z. Maternal low-protein diet up-regulates the neuropeptide Y system in visceral fat and leads to abdominal obesity and glucose intolerance in a sex- and time-specific manner. *FASEB Journal: Official Publication of the Federation of American Societies for Experimental Biology*. 2012;26(8):3528–36. PubMed PMID: 22539639. Pubmed Central PMCID: PMC3405267. Epub 2012/04/28. eng.

153. Lillycrop KA, Phillips ES, Torrens C, Hanson MA, Jackson AA, Burdge GC. Feeding pregnant rats a protein-restricted diet persistently alters the methylation of specific cytosines in the hepatic PPAR alpha promoter of the offspring. *The British Journal of Nutrition*. 2008;100(2):278–82. PubMed PMID: 18186951. Pubmed Central PMCID: PMC2564112. Epub 2008/01/12. eng.

154. Burdge GC, Slater-Jefferies J, Torrens C, Phillips ES, Hanson MA, Lillycrop KA. Dietary protein restriction of pregnant rats in the F0 generation induces altered methylation of hepatic gene promoters in the adult male offspring in the F1 and F2 generations. *The British Journal of Nutrition*. 2007;97(3):435–9. PubMed PMID: 17313703. Pubmed Central PMCID: PMC2211514. Epub 2007/02/23. eng.

155. Lillycrop KA, Phillips ES, Jackson AA, Hanson MA, Burdge GC. Dietary protein restriction of pregnant rats induces and folic acid supplementation prevents epigenetic modification of hepatic gene expression in the offspring. *The Journal of Nutrition*. 2005;135(6):1382–6. PubMed PMID: 15930441. Epub 2005/06/03. eng.

156. Lillycrop KA, Slater-Jefferies JL, Hanson MA, Godfrey KM, Jackson AA, Burdge GC. Induction of altered epigenetic regulation of the hepatic glucocorticoid receptor in the offspring of rats fed a protein-restricted diet during pregnancy suggests that reduced DNA methyltransferase-1 expression is involved in impaired DNA methylation and changes in histone modifications. *The British Journal of Nutrition*. 2007;97(6):1064–73. PubMed PMID: 17433129. Pubmed Central PMCID: PMC2211425. Epub 2007/04/17. eng.

157. Zheng S, Rollet M, Pan YX. Protein restriction during gestation alters histone modifications at the glucose transporter 4 (GLUT4) promoter region and induces GLUT4 expression in skeletal muscle of female rat offspring. *The Journal of Nutritional Biochemistry*. 2012;23(9):1064–71. PubMed PMID: 22079207. Epub 2011/11/15. eng.

158. Zeng Y, Gu P, Liu K, Huang P. Maternal protein restriction in rats leads to reduced PGC-1alpha expression via altered DNA methylation in skeletal muscle. *Molecular Medicine Reports*. 2013;7(1):306–12. PubMed PMID: 23117952. Epub 2012/11/03. eng.

159. Frantz ED, Aguila MB, Pinheiro-Mulder Ada R, Mandarim-de-Lacerda CA. Transgenerational endocrine pancreatic adaptation in mice from maternal protein restriction in utero. *Mechanisms of Ageing and Development*. 2011;132(3):110–16. PubMed PMID: 21291904. Epub 2011/02/05. eng.

160. Sandovici I, Smith NH, Nitert MD, Ackers-Johnson M, Uribe-Lewis S, Ito Y, et al. Maternal diet and aging alter the epigenetic control of a promoter-enhancer interaction at the Hnf4a gene in rat pancreatic islets. *Proceedings of the National Academy of Sciences of the United States of America*. 2011;108(13):5449–54. PubMed PMID: 21385945. Pubmed Central PMCID: PMC3069181. Epub 2011/03/10. eng.

161. Jia Y, Cong R, Li R, Yang X, Sun Q, Parvizi N, et al. Maternal low-protein diet induces gender-dependent changes in epigenetic regulation of the glucose-6-phosphatase gene in newborn piglet liver. *The Journal of Nutrition*. 2012;142(9):1659–65. PubMed PMID: 22833655. Epub 2012/07/27. eng.

162. Zheng S, Rollet M, Pan YX. Maternal protein restriction during pregnancy induces CCAAT/enhancer-binding protein (C/EBPbeta) expression through the regulation of histone modification at its promoter region in female offspring rat skeletal muscle. *Epigenetics*. 2011;6(2):161–70. PubMed PMID: 20930553. Epub 2010/10/12. eng.

163. Torrens C, Poston L, Hanson MA. Transmission of raised blood pressure and endothelial dysfunction to the F2 generation induced by maternal protein restriction in the F0, in the absence of dietary challenge in the F1 generation. *The British Journal of Nutrition*. 2008;100(4):760–6. PubMed PMID: 18304387. Epub 2008/02/29. eng.

164. Harrison M, Langley-Evans SC. Intergenerational programming of impaired nephrogenesis and hypertension in rats following maternal protein restriction during pregnancy. *The British Journal of Nutrition*. 2009;101(7):1020–30. PubMed PMID: 18778527. Pubmed Central PMCID: PMC2665257. Epub 2008/09/10. eng.

165. Goyal R, Goyal D, Leitzke A, Gheorghe CP, Longo LD. Brain renin-angiotensin system: Fetal epigenetic programming by maternal protein restriction during pregnancy. *Reproductive Sciences (Thousand Oaks, CA)*. 2010;17(3):227–38. PubMed PMID: 19923380. Epub 2009/11/20. eng.

166. Vucetic Z, Totoki K, Schoch H, Whitaker KW, Hill-Smith T, Lucki I, et al. Early life protein restriction alters dopamine circuitry. *Neuroscience.* 2010;168(2): 359–70. PubMed PMID: 20394806. Pubmed Central PMCID: PMC2873068. Epub 2010/04/17. eng.

167. Burdge GC, Dunn RL, Wootton SA, Jackson AA. Effect of reduced dietary protein intake on hepatic and plasma essential fatty acid concentrations in the adult female rat: Effect of pregnancy and consequences for accumulation of arachidonic and docosahexaenoic acids in fetal liver and brain. *The British Journal of Nutrition.* 2002;88(4):379–87. PubMed PMID: 12323087. Epub 2002/09/27. eng.

168. Torres N, Bautista CJ, Tovar AR, Ordaz G, Rodriguez-Cruz M, Ortiz V, et al. Protein restriction during pregnancy affects maternal liver lipid metabolism and fetal brain lipid composition in the rat. *American Journal of Physiology Endocrinology and Metabolism.* 2010;298(2):E270–7. PubMed PMID: 19920218. Pubmed Central PMCID: PMC2822484. Epub 2009/11/19. eng.

169. Altobelli G, Bogdarina IG, Stupka E, Clark AJ, Langley-Evans S. Genome-wide methylation and gene expression changes in newborn rats following maternal protein restriction and reversal by folic acid. *PLoS One.* 2013;8(12):e82989. PubMed PMID: 24391732. Pubmed Central PMCID: PMC3877003. Epub 2014/01/07. eng.

170. Torrens C, Brawley L, Anthony FW, Dance CS, Dunn R, Jackson AA, et al. Folate supplementation during pregnancy improves offspring cardiovascular dysfunction induced by protein restriction. *Hypertension.* 2006;47(5):982–7. PubMed PMID: 16585422. Epub 2006/04/06. eng.

171. Engeham SF, Haase A, Langley-Evans SC. Supplementation of a maternal low-protein diet in rat pregnancy with folic acid ameliorates programming effects upon feeding behaviour in the absence of disturbances to the methionine-homocysteine cycle. *The British Journal of Nutrition.* 2010;103(7):996–1007. PubMed PMID: 19941678. Epub 2009/11/28. eng.

172. Jackson AA, Dunn RL, Marchand MC, Langley-Evans SC. Increased systolic blood pressure in rats induced by a maternal low-protein diet is reversed by dietary supplementation with glycine. *Clinical Science (London, England: 1979).* 2002;103(6):633–9. PubMed PMID: 12444916. Epub 2002/11/26. eng.

173. Mortensen OH, Olsen HL, Frandsen L, Nielsen PE, Nielsen FC, Grunnet N, et al. A maternal low protein diet has pronounced effects on mitochondrial gene expression in offspring liver and skeletal muscle; protective effect of taurine. *Journal of Biomedical Science.* 2010;17 Suppl 1:S38. PubMed PMID: 20804614. Pubmed Central PMCID: PMC2994375. Epub 2010/09/11. eng.

174. Altmann S, Murani E, Schwerin M, Metges CC, Wimmers K, Ponsuksili S. Maternal dietary protein restriction and excess affects offspring gene expression and methylation of non-SMC subunits of condensin I in liver and skeletal muscle. *Epigenetics.* 2012;7(3):239–52. PubMed PMID: 22430800. Epub 2012/03/21. eng.

175. Drake AJ, McPherson RC, Godfrey KM, Cooper C, Lillycrop KA, Hanson MA, et al. An unbalanced maternal diet in pregnancy associates with offspring epigenetic changes in genes controlling glucocorticoid action and foetal growth. *Clinical Endocrinology.* 2012;77(6):808–15. PubMed PMID: 22642564. Epub 2012/05/31. eng.

176. Krasnow SM, Nguyen ML, Marks DL. Increased maternal fat consumption during pregnancy alters body composition in neonatal mice. *American Journal of Physiology Endocrinology and Metabolism.* 2011;301(6):E1243–53. PubMed PMID: 21900122. Pubmed Central PMCID: PMC3233776. Epub 2011/09/09. eng.

177. Chen JR, Zhang J, Lazarenko OP, Kang P, Blackburn ML, Ronis MJ, et al. Inhibition of fetal bone development through epigenetic down-regulation of HoxA10 in obese rats fed high-fat diet. *FASEB Journal: Official Publication of the Federation of American Societies for Experimental Biology.* 2012;26(3):1131–41. PubMed PMID: 22131269. Epub 2011/12/02. eng.

178. Liang C, Oest ME, Jones JC, Prater MR. Gestational high saturated fat diet alters C57BL/6 mouse perinatal skeletal formation. *Birth Defects Research Part B, Developmental and Reproductive Toxicology.* 2009;86(5):362–9. PubMed PMID: 19750487. Epub 2009/09/15. eng.
179. Dunn GA, Bale TL. Maternal high-fat diet promotes body length increases and insulin insensitivity in second-generation mice. *Endocrinology.* 2009;150(11):4999–5009. PubMed PMID: 19819967. Pubmed Central PMCID: PMC2775990. Epub 2009/10/13. eng.
180. Dunn GA, Bale TL. Maternal high-fat diet effects on third-generation female body size via the paternal lineage. *Endocrinology.* 2011;152(6):2228–36. PubMed PMID: 21447631. Pubmed Central PMCID: PMC3100614. Epub 2011/03/31. eng.
181. Kelsall CJ, Hoile SP, Irvine NA, Masoodi M, Torrens C, Lillycrop KA, et al. Vascular dysfunction induced in offspring by maternal dietary fat involves altered arterial polyunsaturated fatty acid biosynthesis. *PLoS One.* 2012;7(4):e34492. PubMed PMID: 22509311. Pubmed Central PMCID: PMC3317992. Epub 2012/04/18. eng.
182. Hoile SP, Irvine NA, Kelsall CJ, Sibbons C, Feunteun A, Collister A, et al. Maternal fat intake in rats alters 20:4n-6 and 22:6n-3 status and the epigenetic regulation of Fads2 in offspring liver. *The Journal of Nutritional Biochemistry.* 2013;24(7):1213–20. PubMed PMID: 23107313. Pubmed Central PMCID: PMC3698442. Epub 2012/10/31. eng.
183. Masuyama H, Hiramatsu Y. Effects of a high-fat diet exposure in utero on the metabolic syndrome-like phenomenon in mouse offspring through epigenetic changes in adipocytokine gene expression. *Endocrinology.* 2012;153(6):2823–30. PubMed PMID: 22434078. Epub 2012/03/22. eng.
184. Suter MA, Sangi-Haghpeykar H, Showalter L, Shope C, Hu M, Brown K, et al. Maternal high-fat diet modulates the fetal thyroid axis and thyroid gene expression in a nonhuman primate model. *Molecular Endocrinology (Baltimore, MD).* 2012;26(12):2071–80. PubMed PMID: 23015752. Pubmed Central PMCID: PMC3517714. Epub 2012/09/28. eng.
185. Sedova L, Seda O, Kazdova L, Chylikova B, Hamet P, Tremblay J, et al. Sucrose feeding during pregnancy and lactation elicits distinct metabolic response in offspring of an inbred genetic model of metabolic syndrome. *American Journal of Physiology Endocrinology and Metabolism.* 2007;292(5):E1318–24. PubMed PMID: 17213469. Epub 2007/01/11. eng.
186. Buckley AJ, Keseru B, Briody J, Thompson M, Ozanne SE, Thompson CH. Altered body composition and metabolism in the male offspring of high fat-fed rats. *Metabolism: Clinical and Experimental.* 2005;54(4):500–7. PubMed PMID: 15798958. Epub 2005/03/31. eng.
187. Guo F, Jen KL. High-fat feeding during pregnancy and lactation affects offspring metabolism in rats. *Physiology & Behavior.* 1995;57(4):681–6. PubMed PMID: 7777603. Epub 1995/04/01. eng.
188. Rodriguez L, Otero P, Panadero MI, Rodrigo S, Alvarez-Millan JJ, Bocos C. Maternal fructose intake induces insulin resistance and oxidative stress in male, but not female, offspring. *Journal of Nutrition and Metabolism.* 2015;2015:158091. PubMed PMID: 25763281. Pubmed Central PMCID: PMC4339788. Epub 2015/03/13. eng.
189. Tain YL, Wu KL, Lee WC, Leu S, Chan JY. Maternal fructose-intake-induced renal programming in adult male offspring. *The Journal of Nutritional Biochemistry.* 2015;26(6):642–50. PubMed PMID: 25765514. Epub 2015/03/15. eng.
190. Yajnik CS, Deshpande SS, Jackson AA, Refsum H, Rao S, Fisher DJ, et al. Vitamin B12 and folate concentrations during pregnancy and insulin resistance in the offspring: The Pune Maternal Nutrition Study. *Diabetologia.* 2008;51(1):29–38. PubMed PMID: 17851649. Pubmed Central PMCID: PMC2100429. Epub 2007/09/14. eng.
191. Kumar KA, Lalitha A, Reddy U, Chandak GR, Sengupta S, Raghunath M. Chronic maternal vitamin B12 restriction induced changes in body composition & glucose metabolism in the Wistar rat offspring are partly correctable by rehabilitation. *PLoS One.* 2014;9(11):e112991. PubMed PMID: 25398136. Pubmed Central PMCID: PMC4232526. Epub 2014/11/15. eng.

192. Waterland RA, Travisano M, Tahiliani KG, Rached MT, Mirza S. Methyl donor supplementation prevents transgenerational amplification of obesity. *International Journal of Obesity (2005)*. 2008;32(9):1373–9. PubMed PMID: 18626486. Pubmed Central PMCID: PMC2574783. Epub 2008/07/16. eng.

193. Liu J, Yu B, Mao X, Huang Z, Zheng P, Yu J, et al. Effects of maternal folic acid supplementation and intrauterine growth retardation on epigenetic modification of hepatic gene expression and lipid metabolism in piglets. *Journal of Animal and Plant Sciences*. 2014;24(1):63–70.

194. Kovacheva VP, Mellott TJ, Davison JM, Wagner N, Lopez-Coviella I, Schnitzler AC, et al. Gestational choline deficiency causes global and Igf2 gene DNA hypermethylation by up-regulation of Dnmt1 expression. *The Journal of Biological Chemistry*. 2007;282(43):31777–88. PubMed PMID: 17724018. Epub 2007/08/29. eng.

195. Niculescu MD, Craciunescu CN, Zeisel SH. Dietary choline deficiency alters global and gene-specific DNA methylation in the developing hippocampus of mouse fetal brains. *FASEB Journal: Official Publication of the Federation of American Societies for Experimental Biology*. 2006;20(1):43–9. PubMed PMID: 16394266. Pubmed Central PMCID: PMC1635129. Epub 2006/01/06. eng.

196. Zeisel SH. Epigenetic mechanisms for nutrition determinants of later health outcomes. *The American Journal of Clinical Nutrition*. 2009;89(5):1488S–93S. PubMed PMID: 19261726. Pubmed Central PMCID: PMC2677001. Epub 2009/03/06. eng.

197. Dolinoy DC, Weidman JR, Waterland RA, Jirtle RL. Maternal genistein alters coat color and protects Avy mouse offspring from obesity by modifying the fetal epigenome. *Environmental Health Perspectives*. 2006;114(4):567–72. PubMed PMID: 16581547. Pubmed Central PMCID: PMC1440782. Epub 2006/04/04. eng.

198. Venu L, Harishankar N, Krishna TP, Raghunath M. Does maternal dietary mineral restriction per se predispose the offspring to insulin resistance? *European Journal of Endocrinology/European Federation of Endocrine Societies*. 2004;151(2):287–94. PubMed PMID: 15296486. Epub 2004/08/07. eng.

199. Venu L, Padmavathi IJ, Kishore YD, Bhanu NV, Rao KR, Sainath PB, et al. Long-term effects of maternal magnesium restriction on adiposity and insulin resistance in rat pups. *Obesity (Silver Spring, Md)*. 2008;16(6):1270–6. PubMed PMID: 18369337. Epub 2008/03/29. eng.

200. Venu L, Kishore YD, Raghunath M. Maternal and perinatal magnesium restriction predisposes rat pups to insulin resistance and glucose intolerance. *The Journal of Nutrition*. 2005;135(6):1353–8. PubMed PMID: 15930437. Epub 2005/06/03. eng.

201. Padmavathi IJ, Kishore YD, Venu L, Ganeshan M, Harishankar N, Giridharan NV, et al. Prenatal and perinatal zinc restriction: Effects on body composition, glucose tolerance and insulin response in rat offspring. *Experimental Physiology*. 2009;94(6):761–9. PubMed PMID: 19251982. Epub 2009/03/03. eng.

202. Padmavathi IJ, Rao KR, Venu L, Ganeshan M, Kumar KA, Rao Ch N, et al. Chronic maternal dietary chromium restriction modulates visceral adiposity: Probable underlying mechanisms. *Diabetes*. 2010;59(1):98–104. PubMed PMID: 19846803. Pubmed Central PMCID: PMC2797950. Epub 2009/10/23. eng.

203. Lodish H, Berk A, Kaiser CA, Krieger M, Bretscher A, Ploegh H, et al. *Molecular cell biology*. 7th edn. New York, Freeman; 2012.

204. Faustino NA, Cooper TA. Pre-mRNA splicing and human disease. *Genes & Development*. 2003;17(4):419–37.

205. Mor A, Suliman S, Ben-Yishay R, Yunger S, Brody Y, Shav-Tal Y. Dynamics of single mRNP nucleocytoplasmic transport and export through the nuclear pore in living cells. *Nature cell Biology*. 2010;12(6):543–52.

206. Zaret KS, Carroll JS. Pioneer transcription factors: Establishing competence for gene expression. *Genes & Development*. 2011;25(21):2227–41.

207. Mangelsdorf DJ, Thummel C, Beato M, Herrlich P, Schutz G, Umesono K, et al. The nuclear receptor superfamily: The second decade. *Cell.* 1995;83(6):835–9. PubMed PMID: 8521507. Epub 1995/12/15. eng.

208. Sever R, Glass CK. Signaling by nuclear receptors. *Cold Spring Harbor Perspectives in Biology.* 2013;5(3):a016709. PubMed PMID: 23457262. Pubmed Central PMCID: PMC3578364. Epub 2013/03/05. eng.

209. McGee SL, van Denderen BJ, Howlett KF, Mollica J, Schertzer JD, Kemp BE, et al. AMP-activated protein kinase regulates GLUT4 transcription by phosphorylating histone deacetylase 5. *Diabetes.* 2008;57(4):860–7. PubMed PMID: 18184930. Epub 2008/01/11. eng.

210. Aranda A, Pascual A. Nuclear hormone receptors and gene expression. *Physiological Reviews.* 2001;81(3):1269–304. PubMed PMID: 11427696. Epub 2001/06/28. eng.

211. Echeverria PC, Picard D. Molecular chaperones, essential partners of steroid hormone receptors for activity and mobility. *Biochimica et Biophysica Acta.* 2010;1803(6):641–9. PubMed PMID: 20006655. Epub 2009/12/17. eng.

212. Glass CK, Rosenfeld MG. The coregulator exchange in transcriptional functions of nuclear receptors. *Genes & Development.* 2000;14(2):121–41. PubMed PMID: 10652267. Epub 2000/02/01. eng.

213. Berrabah W, Aumercier P, Lefebvre P, Staels B. Control of nuclear receptor activities in metabolism by post-translational modifications. *FEBS Letters.* 2011;585(11):1640–50. PubMed PMID: 21486568. Epub 2011/04/14. eng.

214. Germain P, Staels B, Dacquet C, Spedding M, Laudet V. Overview of nomenclature of nuclear receptors. *Pharmacological Reviews.* 2006;58(4):685–704. PubMed PMID: 17132848. Epub 2006/11/30. eng.

215. Mark M, Ghyselinck NB, Chambon P. Function of retinoic acid receptors during embryonic development. *Nuclear Receptor Signaling.* 2009;7:e002. PubMed PMID: 19381305. Pubmed Central PMCID: PMC2670431. Epub 2009/04/22. eng.

216. Rossetto DdB, Kiyomoto EN, Carvalho CEBD, Zanelli CF, Valentini SR. New ligands of the Cellular Retinoic Acid-Binding Protein 2 (CRABP2) suggest a role for this protein in chromatin remodeling. *Revista de Ciências Farmacêuticas Básica e Aplicada.* 2014;25(3):371–7.

217. Bastien J, Rochette-Egly C. Nuclear retinoid receptors and the transcription of retinoid-target genes. *Gene.* 2004;328:1–16. PubMed PMID: 15019979. Epub 2004/03/17. eng.

218. Gudas LJ, Wagner JA. Retinoids regulate stem cell differentiation. *Journal of Cellular Physiology.* 2011;226(2):322–30. PubMed PMID: 20836077. Pubmed Central PMCID: PMC3315372. Epub 2010/09/14. eng.

219. Li G, Margueron R, Hu G, Stokes D, Wang YH, Reinberg D. Highly compacted chromatin formed in vitro reflects the dynamics of transcription activation *in vivo. Molecular Cell.* 2010;38(1):41–53. PubMed PMID: 20385088. Pubmed Central PMCID: PMC3641559. Epub 2010/04/14. eng.

220. Zhou X, Kong N, Wang J, Fan H, Zou H, Horwitz D, et al. Cutting edge: All-trans retinoic acid sustains the stability and function of natural regulatory T cells in an inflammatory milieu. *Journal of Immunology (Baltimore, MD: 1950).* 2010;185(5):2675–9. PubMed PMID: 20679534. Pubmed Central PMCID: PMC3098624. Epub 2010/08/04. eng.

221. Hosler BA, Rogers MB, Kozak CA, Gudas LJ. An octamer motif contributes to the expression of the retinoic acid-regulated zinc finger gene Rex-1 (Zfp-42) in F9 teratocarcinoma cells. *Molecular and Cellular Biology.* 1993;13(5):2919–28. PubMed PMID: 8474450. Pubmed Central PMCID: PMC359685. Epub 1993/05/01. eng.

222. Gianni M, Bauer A, Garattini E, Chambon P, Rochette-Egly C. Phosphorylation by p38MAPK and recruitment of SUG-1 are required for RA-induced RAR gamma degradation and transactivation. *The EMBO Journal.* 2002;21(14):3760–9. PubMed PMID: 12110588. Pubmed Central PMCID: PMC126119. Epub 2002/07/12. eng.

223. Marchildon F, St-Louis C, Akter R, Roodman V, Wiper-Bergeron NL. Transcription factor Smad3 is required for the inhibition of adipogenesis by retinoic acid. *The Journal of Biological Chemistry.* 2010 3;285(17):13274–84. PubMed PMID: 20179325. Pubmed Central PMCID: PMC2857127. Epub 2010/02/25. eng.

224. Whitfield GK, Jurutka PW, Haussler CA, Hsieh J-C, Barthel TK, Jacobs ET, et al. CHAPTER 13—Nuclear vitamin D receptor: Structure-function, molecular control of gene transcription, and novel bioactions A2—FELDMAN, DAVID. *Vitamin D (Second Edition). Burlington: Academic Press;* 2005. pp. 219–61.

225. Haussler MR, Haussler CA, Whitfield GK, Hsieh JC, Thompson PD, Barthel TK, et al. The nuclear vitamin D receptor controls the expression of genes encoding factors which feed the "Fountain of Youth" to mediate healthful aging. *The Journal of Steroid Biochemistry and Molecular Biology.* 2010;121(1–2):88–97. PubMed PMID: 20227497. Pubmed Central PMCID: PMC2906618. Epub 2010/03/17. eng.

226. Bouillon R, Carmeliet G, Verlinden L, van Etten E, Verstuyf A, Luderer HF, et al. Vitamin D and human health: Lessons from vitamin D receptor null mice. *Endocrine Reviews.* 2008;29(6):726–76. PubMed PMID: 18694980. Pubmed Central PMCID: PMC2583388. Epub 2008/08/13. eng.

227. Liu M, Lee MH, Cohen M, Bommakanti M, Freedman LP. Transcriptional activation of the Cdk inhibitor p21 by vitamin D3 leads to the induced differentiation of the myelomonocytic cell line U937. *Genes & Development.* 1996;10(2):142–53. PubMed PMID: 8566748. Epub 1996/01/15. eng.

228. Fleet JC, DeSmet M, Johnson R, Li Y. Vitamin D and cancer: A review of molecular mechanisms. *The Biochemical Journal.* 2012;441(1):61–76. PubMed PMID: 22168439. Pubmed Central PMCID: PMC4572477. Epub 2011/12/16. eng.

229. Guzey M, Kitada S, Reed JC. Apoptosis induction by 1alpha,25-dihydroxyvitamin D3 in prostate cancer. *Molecular Cancer Therapeutics.* 2002;1(9):667–77. PubMed PMID: 12479363. Epub 2002/12/14. eng.

230. Grygiel-Gorniak B. Peroxisome proliferator-activated receptors and their ligands: Nutritional and clinical implications—A review. *Nutrition Journal.* 2014;13:17. PubMed PMID: 24524207. Pubmed Central PMCID: PMC3943808. Epub 2014/02/15. eng.

231. Huang TH, Teoh AW, Lin BL, Lin DS, Roufogalis B. The role of herbal PPAR modulators in the treatment of cardiometabolic syndrome. *Pharmacological Research.* 2009;60(3):195–206. PubMed PMID: 19646659. Epub 2009/08/04. eng.

232. Mandard S, Muller M, Kersten S. Peroxisome proliferator-activated receptor alpha target genes. *Cellular and Molecular Life Sciences.* 2004;61(4):393–416. PubMed PMID: 14999402. Epub 2004/03/05. eng.

233. Fernandez-Alvarez A, Alvarez MS, Gonzalez R, Cucarella C, Muntane J, Casado M. Human SREBP1c expression in liver is directly regulated by peroxisome proliferator-activated receptor alpha (PPARalpha). *The Journal of Biological Chemistry.* 2011;286(24):21466–77. PubMed PMID: 21540177. Pubmed Central PMCID: PMC3122206. Epub 2011/05/05. eng.

234. Hertz R, Bishara-Shieban J, Bar-Tana J. Mode of action of peroxisome proliferators as hypolipidemic drugs. Suppression of apolipoprotein C-III. *The Journal of Biological Chemistry.* 1995;270(22):13470–5. PubMed PMID: 7768950. Epub 1995/06/02. eng.

235. Delerive P, De Bosscher K, Besnard S, Berghe WV, Peters JM, Gonzalez FJ, et al. Peroxisome proliferator-activated receptor α negatively regulates the vascular inflammatory gene response by negative cross-talk with transcription factors NF-κB and AP-1. *Journal of Biological Chemistry.* 1999;274(45):32048–54.

236. Zhou J, Zhang S, Xue J, Avery J, Wu J, Lind SE, et al. Activation of peroxisome proliferator-activated receptor α (PPARα) suppresses hypoxia-inducible factor-1α (HIF-1α) signaling in cancer cells. *Journal of Biological Chemistry.* 2012;287(42):35161–9.

237. Thomas M, Burk O, Klumpp B, Kandel BA, Damm G, Weiss TS, et al. Direct transcriptional regulation of human hepatic cytochrome P450 3A4 (CYP3A4) by peroxisome proliferator-activated receptor alpha (PPARalpha). *Molecular Pharmacology.* 2013;83(3):709–18. PubMed PMID: 23295386. Epub 2013/01/09. eng.

238. Barish GD, Narkar VA, Evans RM. PPAR delta: A dagger in the heart of the metabolic syndrome. *The Journal of Clinical Investigation.* 2006;116(3):590–7. PubMed PMID: 16511591. Pubmed Central PMCID: PMC1386117. Epub 2006/03/03. eng.

239. Wang YX, Lee CH, Tiep S, Yu RT, Ham J, Kang H, et al. Peroxisome-proliferator-activated receptor delta activates fat metabolism to prevent obesity. *Cell.* 2003;113(2):159–70. PubMed PMID: 12705865. Epub 2003/04/23. eng.

240. Beyaz S, Mana MD, Roper J, Kedrin D, Saadatpour A, Hong SJ, et al. High-fat diet enhances stemness and tumorigenicity of intestinal progenitors. *Nature.* 2016;531(7592):53–8. PubMed PMID: 26935695. Pubmed Central PMCID: PMC4846772. Epub 2016/03/05. eng.

241. Sugii S, Evans RM. Epigenetic codes of PPARgamma in metabolic disease. *FEBS Letters.* 2011;585(13):2121–8. PubMed PMID: 21605560. Pubmed Central PMCID: PMC3129683. Epub 2011/05/25. eng.

242. Lehrke M, Lazar MA. The many faces of PPARgamma. *Cell.* 2005;123(6):993–9. PubMed PMID: 16360030. Epub 2005/12/20. eng.

243. Ricote M, Glass CK. PPARs and molecular mechanisms of transrepression. *Biochimica et Biophysica Acta.* 2007;1771(8):926–35. PubMed PMID: 17433773. Pubmed Central PMCID: PMC1986735. Epub 2007/04/17. eng.

244. Pascual G, Fong AL, Ogawa S, Gamliel A, Li AC, Perissi V, et al. A SUMOylation-dependent pathway mediates transrepression of inflammatory response genes by PPAR-gamma. *Nature.* 2005;437(7059):759–63. PubMed PMID: 16127449. Pubmed Central PMCID: PMC1464798. Epub 2005/08/30. eng.

245. Puigserver P. Tissue-specific regulation of metabolic pathways through the transcriptional coactivator PGC1-alpha. *International Journal of Obesity (2005).* 2005;29 Suppl 1:S5–9. PubMed PMID: 15711583. Epub 2005/02/16. eng.

246. Reka AK, Kurapati H, Narala VR, Bommer G, Chen J, Standiford TJ, et al. Peroxisome proliferator-activated receptor-γ activation inhibits tumor metastasis by antagonizing Smad3-mediated epithelial-mesenchymal transition. *Molecular Cancer Therapeutics.* 2010;9(12):3221–32.

247. Yamauchi T, Kamon J, Waki H, Murakami K, Motojima K, Komeda K, et al. The mechanisms by which both heterozygous peroxisome proliferator-activated receptor gamma (PPARgamma) deficiency and PPARgamma agonist improve insulin resistance. *The Journal of Biological Chemistry.* 2001;276(44):41245–54. PubMed PMID: 11533050. Epub 2001/09/05. eng.

248. Rosen ED, Hsu CH, Wang X, Sakai S, Freeman MW, Gonzalez FJ, et al. C/EBPalpha induces adipogenesis through PPARgamma: A unified pathway. *Genes & Development.* 2002;16(1):22–6. PubMed PMID: 11782441. Pubmed Central PMCID: PMC155311. Epub 2002/01/10. eng.

249. Hinnebusch AG, Ivanov IP, Sonenberg N. Translational control by 5'-untranslated regions of eukaryotic mRNAs. *Science (New York, NY).* 2016;352(6292):1413–16.

250. Chrzanowska-Lightowlers ZMA, Pajak A, Lightowlers RN. Termination of protein synthesis in mammalian mitochondria. *Journal of Biological Chemistry.* 2011;286(40):34479–85.

251. Sengupta S, Peterson TR, Sabatini DM. Regulation of the mTOR complex 1 pathway by nutrients, growth factors, and stress. *Molecular Cell.* 2010;40(2):310–22. PubMed PMID: PMC2993060.

252. Jewell JL, Russell RC, Guan K-L. Amino acid signalling upstream of mTOR. *Nature Reviews Molecular Cell Biology.* 2013;14(3):133–9.

253. Laplante M, Sabatini DM. mTOR signaling at a glance. *Journal of Cell Science.* 2009;122(20):3589–94.

254. Guertin DA, Sabatini DM. Defining the role of mTOR in cancer. *Cancer Cell.* 2007;12(1):9–22.

255. Pause A, Methot N, Svitkin Y, Merrick WC, Sonenberg N. Dominant negative mutants of mammalian translation initiation factor eIF-4A define a critical role for eIF-4F in cap-dependent and cap-independent initiation of translation. *The EMBO Journal.* 1994;13(5):1205–15. PubMed PMID: 8131750. Pubmed Central PMCID: PMC394930. Epub 1994/03/01. eng.

256. Feldman ME, Apsel B, Uotila A, Loewith R, Knight ZA, Ruggero D, et al. Active-site inhibitors of mTOR target rapamycin-resistant outputs of mTORC1 and mTORC2. *PLoS Biology.* 2009;7(2):e38. PubMed PMID: 19209957. Pubmed Central PMCID: PMC2637922. Epub 2009/02/13. eng.

257. Zoncu R, Sabatini DM, Efeyan A. mTOR: From growth signal integration to cancer, diabetes and ageing. *Nature Reviews Molecular Cell Biology.* 2011;12(1):21–35. PubMed PMID: PMC3390257.

258. Laplante M, Sabatini DM. mTOR signaling in growth control and disease. *Cell.* 2012;149(2):274–93. PubMed PMID: 22500797. Pubmed Central PMCID: PMC3331679. Epub 2012/04/17. eng.

259. Gwinn DM, Shackelford DB, Egan DF, Mihaylova MM, Mery A, Vasquez DS, et al. AMPK phosphorylation of raptor mediates a metabolic checkpoint. *Molecular Cell.* 2008;30(2):214–26. PubMed PMID: 18439900. Pubmed Central PMCID: PMC2674027. Epub 2008/04/29. eng.

260. Zheng X, Boyer L, Jin M, Kim Y, Fan W, Bardy C, et al. Alleviation of neuronal energy deficiency by mTOR inhibition as a treatment for mitochondria-related neurodegeneration. *eLife.* 2016;5:e13378.

261. Nobukuni T, Joaquin M, Roccio M, Dann SG, Kim SY, Gulati P, et al. Amino acids mediate mTOR/raptor signaling through activation of class 3 phosphatidylinositol 3OH-kinase. *Proceedings of the National Academy of Sciences of the United States of America.* 2005;102(40):14238–43. PubMed PMID: PMC1242323.

262. Duran RV, Oppliger W, Robitaille AM, Heiserich L, Skendaj R, Gottlieb E, et al. Glutaminolysis activates Rag-mTORC1 signaling. *Molecular Cell.* 2012;47(3):349–58. PubMed PMID: 22749528. Epub 2012/07/04. eng.

263. Bauchart-Thevret C, Cui L, Wu G, Burrin DG. Arginine-induced stimulation of protein synthesis and survival in IPEC-J2 cells is mediated by mTOR but not nitric oxide. *American Journal of Physiology Endocrinology and Metabolism.* 2010;299(6):E899–909. PubMed PMID: 20841502. Epub 2010/09/16. eng.

264. Kim E, Goraksha-Hicks P, Li L, Neufeld TP, Guan KL. Regulation of TORC1 by Rag GTPases in nutrient response. *Nat Cell Biol.* 2008;10(8):935–45. PubMed PMID: 18604198. Pubmed Central PMCID: PMC2711503. Epub 2008/07/08. eng.

265. Sancak Y, Peterson TR, Shaul YD, Lindquist RA, Thoreen CC, Bar-Peled L, et al. The Rag GTPases bind raptor and mediate amino acid signaling to mTORC1. *Science (New York, NY).* 2008;320(5882):1496–501.

266. Sancak Y, Bar-Peled L, Zoncu R, Markhard AL, Nada S, Sabatini DM. Ragulator-Rag complex targets mTORC1 to the lysosomal surface and is necessary for its activation by amino acids. *Cell.* 2010;141(2):290–303. PubMed PMID: PMC3024592.

267. Johnson SC, Rabinovitch PS, Kaeberlein M. mTOR is a key modulator of ageing and age-related disease. *Nature.* 2013;493(7432):338–45. PubMed PMID: 23325216. Pubmed Central PMCID: PMC3687363. Epub 2013/01/18. eng.

268. Longo VD, Antebi A, Bartke A, Barzilai N, Brown-Borg HM, Caruso C, et al. Interventions to slow aging in humans: Are we ready? *Aging Cell.* 2015;14(4): 497–510. PubMed PMID: 25902704. Pubmed Central PMCID: PMC4531065. Epub 2015/04/24. eng.

269. Lamming DW, Ye L, Sabatini DM, Baur JA. Rapalogs and mTOR inhibitors as anti-aging therapeutics. *The Journal of Clinical Investigation.* 2013;123(3):980–9. PubMed PMID: 23454761. Pubmed Central PMCID: PMC3582126. Epub 2013/03/05. eng.

270. Baur JA, Pearson KJ, Price NL, Jamieson HA, Lerin C, Kalra A, et al. Resveratrol improves health and survival of mice on a high-calorie diet. *Nature.* 2006;444(7117):337–42. PubMed PMID: 17086191. Epub 2006/11/07. eng.

271. Rajapakse AG, Yepuri G, Carvas JM, Stein S, Matter CM, Scerri I, et al. Hyperactive S6K1 mediates oxidative stress and endothelial dysfunction in aging: Inhibition by resveratrol. *PLoS One.* 2011;6(4):e19237. PubMed PMID: 21544240. Pubmed Central PMCID: PMC3081344. Epub 2011/05/06. eng.

13

Nutrigenomic Aspects of Vitamins

Fatemeh Rezaiian, Bahareh Nikooyeh, and Tirang R. Neyestani
Shahid Beheshti University of Medical Sciences
Tehran, Iran

Contents

13.1 Introduction 280
13.2 Fat-soluble vitamins...280
    13.2.1 Vitamin A, retinoids, and carotenoids 280
        13.2.1.1 General characteristics and metabolism 280
        13.2.1.2 Health implications of vitamin A deficiency...........281
        13.2.1.3 Health implications of vitamin A toxicity 281
        13.2.1.4 Receptor-mediated retinoid signaling....................281
        13.2.1.5 Vitamin A-associated gene-expression mechanisms.. 282
        13.2.1.6 Regulation of methylation by vitamin A 283
        13.2.1.7 Regulation of mt gene expression 284
        13.2.1.8 The role of Vitamin A in chronic disorders 284
        13.2.1.9 Lipid metabolism and energy balance....................285
        13.2.1.10 Retinoids and hepatic gluconeogenesis..................286
        13.2.1.11 Carotenoids..288
    13.2.2 Vitamin D 289
        13.2.2.1 General characteristics and metabolism 289
        13.2.2.2 Health implications of vitamin D deficiency...........290
        13.2.2.3 Health implications of vitamin D toxicity 290
        13.2.2.4 Vitamin D genomic actions...................................290
        13.2.2.5 Histone modifications 291
        13.2.2.6 Regulation of immune system by vitamin D...........291
        13.2.2.7 Proliferation: Cell-cycle control 292
        13.2.2.8 Apoptosis..293
        13.2.2.9 Vitamin D, cell adhesion molecules, and loss of
                    contact inhibition 293
        13.2.2.10 Vitamin D and diseases 294
13.3 Water-soluble vitamins 297
    13.3.1 Folate and cobalamins..297
        13.3.1.1 General characteristics and metabolism 297

279

		13.3.1.2	Health implications of folate deficiency	298
		13.3.1.3	Health implications of folate toxicity	298
		13.3.1.4	Vitamin B_{12}: Health implications	299
		13.3.1.5	Gene expression	299
		13.3.1.6	Cancer prevention	299
	13.3.2	Folate, cobalamins, and human diseases		300
		13.3.2.1	Insulin resistance and obesity	300
		13.3.2.2	Oxidative stress, hypertension, endothelial function, and CVD	301
		13.3.2.3	CNS development and function	301
13.4	Summary			303
13.5	Future insights			304
References				305

13.1 Introduction

Both fat-soluble and water-soluble vitamins affect genome stability. Vitamin A and retinoids, for instance, have crucial roles in histone modifications and gene expression. Vitamin A is necessary for mitochondrial (mt) function and the amount needed for optimal mt function is genotype specific [1]. On the contrary, vitamin D is involved in methylation reaction and gene expression, which affects carcinogenesis [2]. Vitamin D has been attributed to alter cellular proliferation through multiple mechanisms, primarily via effects on cell cycle progression, apoptosis, and differentiation [3].

Folate and vitamin B_{12} are among the most-cited micronutrients, which affect genomic stability by serving as a cofactor for one-carbon transfer reactions involved in DNA methylation, and their deficiency leads to a wide range of cancers, central nervous system (CNS)-related disease and cardiovascular disease (CVD). Rapidly dividing cells of the bone marrow, such as leucocytes and platelets, are especially sensitive to folate deficiency due to disturbed DNA synthesis. Due to its roles in DNA synthesis, transcription, methylation, and gene expression, folate deficiency affects brain growth, differentiation, development, and repair especially in the CNS [4]. Furthermore, several cancers including those of the colon, breast, pancreas, stomach, cervix, bronchus, and blood have been associated with poor folate status [5]. Vitamin B_{12} is an essential coenzyme for methionine synthase and is involved in folate pathway via the action of methionine biosynthesis and the formation of DNA [6].

13.2 Fat-soluble vitamins

13.2.1 Vitamin A, retinoids, and carotenoids

13.2.1.1 General characteristics and metabolism

Vitamin A is a lipophilic micronutrient that is found in animal sources (mainly as retinyl esters [RE]) or plant sources (as provitamin A and carotenoids) [7,8]. It exists in four main forms within the body: retinol (circulating form), RE (storage form), retinal, and retinoic acid (RA), which represents its most active form. As a group, the various forms of vitamin A are called *retinoids* [9,10]. Being a fat-soluble vitamin, 70%–90% of the vitamin is physiologically absorbed with the aid of intestinal juice and bile salts [8,11]. Ingested RE are broken down to retinol in the small intestine or the intestinal mucosa and then retinol is re-esterified to RE. Provitamin A carotenoids first form retinaldehyde and then retinol. Secreted chylomicrons are transported via the lymphatic system to the blood and taken up by hepatocytes and hydrolyzed again. The free retinol must bind to specific proteins to perform its necessary functions. Plasma retinol-binding protein (RBP) and epididymal RA binding protein carry retinoids in bodily fluids, while cellular retinol-binding proteins (CRBPs) and cellular RA-binding proteins carry retinoids within cells. CRBP-1 is necessary to solubilize retinol in the aqueous environment of the cell [12].

Vitamin A (also known as *retinol*) is necessary for human survival from development of the embryo to adulthood. Although its roles in vision, immunity, spermatogenesis, fertilization, pregnancy maintenance, morphogenesis, organogenesis, and fetal and perinatal growth have been well described, new functions such as lipid metabolism, insulin resistance and response, energy homeostasis and the nervous system remain open issues [9,13,14].

13.2.1.2 Health implications of vitamin A deficiency

Vitamin A deficiency leads to growth retardation and a large spectrum of congenital malformations known as *fetal vitamin A deficiency syndrome* [11,13,15]. Vitamin A deficiency correlates with dryness and keratinization of epithelial cells of the skin, dryness of the conjunctiva epithelium, night blindness, severe anemia, wasting, alterations in dendritic cell and neutrophil development, inflammatory cytokine release by macrophages, and the production of T lymphocytes and natural killer cells, all of which lead to impaired immunity and increased risk of mortality [16–19].

13.2.1.3 Health implications of vitamin A toxicity

The clinical symptoms of excessive intake of vitamin A, also known as *hypervitaminosis A* or *vitamin A toxicity*, include nausea, vomiting, vision changes, headache and dizziness, and occasionally bone pain [20,21]. Regarding the role of retinoids in embryogenesis and organ differentiation, high prenatal exposures of the fetus to therapeutic doses of retinoids may lead to teratogenicity [22].

13.2.1.4 Receptor-mediated retinoid signaling

RA interacts with retinoic acid receptor (RAR) and other transcriptional factors, including RXR, peroxisome proliferator activated receptor δ (PPARδ), and redox-sensitive factors, that are involved in RA-mediated transcription [23]. These receptors act as transcription factors by binding to specific DNA sequences (retinoic acid response element [RARE] or retinoid X response element) found in the promoter region of retinoid target genes either as RAR–RXR or RXR–RXR dimers. All-trans retinoic acid (atRA) can bind RARs only, whereas 9-cis RA is a ligand for both. Unlike other nuclear receptors, RXRs heterodimerize with other nuclear receptors such as PPARs, liver X receptor (LXR), farnesoid X receptor and pregnane X receptor, RARs, thyroid hormone receptor, and vitamin D receptor (VDR), which explains the extensive role of RA in the regulation of expression of several genes [10]. It has been shown that most of the pleiotropic functions are not exerted by retinol itself. Indeed, the expression of most of the target genes involved in cell growth and differentiation, development, and homeostasis is regulated by atRA, which is the main endogenous active metabolite of vitamin A [13].

Despite the fact that liver is the major place for vitamin A metabolism and storage in mammals, studies have demonstrated that adipose tissue also plays a key role in the metabolism and vitamin A through taking up circulatory chylomicron-bound (by lipoprotein lipase) and RBP4-bound (by STRA6) retinol [23]. Besides, all the enzymes necessary for vitamin A transport and metabolism can be expressed in adipose tissue. Several isomers of retinol, including all-trans, 9-cis, and 13-cis isomers, have been found in white adipose tissue (WAT) [10].

The metabolism of retinol is catalyzed by different enzymes. Alcohol dehydrogenases and retinol dehydrogenases convert retinol to retinaldehyde. Retinaldehyde produces RA by the cytosolic aldehyde dehydrogenase-1 (Aldh1) [24,25]. RBP4 is secreted mainly by adipose tissue and the liver. RBP4 is the main transport protein for retinol (vitamin A) in the circulation and is encoded by the *RBP4* gene [26].

It has been shown that most of the pleiotropic functions of vitamin A are not exerted by retinol itself. Indeed, the expression of most of the target genes involved in cell growth, development, differentiation, and homeostasis is regulated by atRA, which is the main endogenous active metabolite [13].

13.2.1.5 Vitamin A-associated gene-expression mechanisms

It has long been recognized that many biological activities of RA are mediated by RA receptors (RARα, RARβ, and RARδ). However, recent observations have demonstrated that RA also has extranuclear nontranscriptional effects, including the activation of the mitogen-activated protein kinase (MAPK) signaling pathway, which influences the expression of RA target genes via phosphorylation processes. Moreover, other studies have revealed that RA activates not only RARs but also other nuclear receptors, such as the PPARs, and recently it was proved that vitamin A/retinol activates the Janus kinase/STAT5 signaling pathway. These last two recently discovered effects lead to the regulation of genes that are not direct RAR targets, thus confirming the extensive biological functions of vitamin A/RA, especially in energy balance [13]. Retinoids have crucial roles in histone modification as follows:

- In the absence of ligand, transcription is turned off by RXR/RAR heterodimers and the DNA-bound RARα subtype is associated with corepressors. These corepressors will subsequently recruit histone deacetylase (HDAC). These complexes deacetylate lysine residues in the N-terminal tails of histones and maintain chromatin in a condensed, silenced state over the target promoter [13].
- Binding of ligand (RA) to the RAR partner of the DNA-bound induces conformational changes on RARα, which triggers the release of corepressor and coactivator binding. Then, like corepressors, the coactivators initiate the recruitment of large complexes with different enzymatic activities, such as histone acetyl transferases (HAT), histone methyl transferases, histone demethylases (HDM), and DNA-dependent ATPases. All these complexes alter the chromatin structure surrounding the promoter of target genes and create tags or binding sites that form a "histone code" read by particular effectors, which in turn mediate distinct outcomes [8,13].
- The phosphorylation of RARs and RXRs occurs when the kinases are activated in response to RA. This will result in the recruitment of RARα target promotors, which in turn phosphorylate histones and contribute to chromatin remodeling and promoter recruitment of RXR/RAR heterodimers and the transcriptional machinery [13].

13.2.1.6 Regulation of methylation by vitamin A

Studies on rats showed that the cytosolic enzyme, glycine N-methyltransferase (GNMT), functions to optimize transmethylation reactions by regulating the S-adenosylmethionine (SAM)/S-adenosylhomocysteine (SAH) ratio and is critical for the optimal supply of methyl groups necessary for SAM-dependent transmethylation reactions. It seems that all three retinoids can induce the synthesis and activation of GNMT, which consequently results in the protein existing mainly in its enzymatically active homotetrameric state. Understanding the exact mechanisms by which retinoids regulate GNMT remains to be elucidated in future research. These findings demonstrate that upregulation of GNMT leads to important alterations in methyl group metabolism. The decrease in levels of methyl groups due to the activation of GNMT by retinoids appeared to compromise SAM-dependent transmethylation reactions, particularly the methylation of DNA. atRA-treated rats exhibited the greatest activation of GNMT and the greatest decrease in endogenous methylation status of hepatic DNA, suggesting functional deficiency of methyl groups. Considering the regulatory roles of DNA methylation status on important processes such as gene expression and development, retinoid-induced DNA hypomethylation can potentially have significant implications [27].

13.2.1.7 Regulation of mt gene expression

Previous studies have suggested that vitamin A is necessary for mt function and that the level needed for optimal mt function is genotype specific. Mitochondria contain their own double-stranded closed circular DNA (mtDNA) [1]. Two nuclear transcription factors have been detected in mitochondria:

1. Mitochondrial transcription factor A (mtTFA), which is involved in transcription and replication initiation as well as maintenance of mtDNA levels. Its upregulation can upregulate mt transcription.
2. Mitochondrial transcription termination factor (mTERF), which is involved in termination of the heavy strand after the rRNAs are formed [1,28].

Furthermore, mitochondria transcription can be regulated via a second mechanism that involves the direct binding of gene active substances to their cognate receptors, which in turn bind to specific elements in the mt promoter region, the D-loop. Studies have demonstrated that vitamin A is essential for mt function through its potential to regulate the mt encoded genes. These include regulation of NADH dehydrogenase subunit 5 (ND5), cytochrome c oxidase subunit I mRNA, and 16srRNA; the upregulation of mRNA levels of the ATPase 6, ATPase 6, 8, and ND1; as well as protein levels of ATPase subunit a (6 gene) in a dose-dependent manner [1].

The regulation of mt gene expression is managed through three possible mechanisms. First, insulin-stimulated glucose flux is shown to upregulate mt gene expression. RA has been found to regulate several key enzymes in glucose metabolism and also to affect insulin production and release, indicating the possible indirect impact of RA on mt gene expression via its influence on glucose flux. The second level of regulation of mt gene expression by RA possibly occurs through the regulation of the nuclear encoded mtTFA. The evidence shows that increased dietary vitamin A can upregulate mtTFA protein expression. Whether this is a direct effect on mtTFA transcription or via posttranscriptional regulation of mtTFA by increased mtDNA levels is yet unclear. Third, RA bound to its cognate receptor may bind mtDNA and directly regulate mt gene expression, which is the most controversial and has to be elucidated in future research.

In conclusion, these studies suggest that low levels (10^{-9}M) of RA are needed for mt function by regulating mt gene expression, which could be obtained by consumption of an adequate dietary level of vitamin A. Future studies will clarify the exact mechanism(s) of this effect [1].

13.2.1.8 The role of Vitamin A in chronic disorders

The role of retinoids in regulation of lipid and energy metabolism has recently been an area of great interest, particularly in chronic disorders such as obesity, diabetes, nonalcoholic fatty liver disease, and atherosclerosis. Evidence suggests that specific retinoids, notably RA, have significant regulatory roles in developmental and biochemical processes influencing mammalian adiposity, including adipocyte differentiation (adipogenesis) and lipogenesis, adaptive thermogenesis, lipolysis, and fatty acid oxidation in tissues.

13.2.1.9 Lipid metabolism and energy balance

Lipid metabolism is controlled by interaction among hormones, transcription factors, and energy substrates. Insulin and glucose work together in proceeding hepatic lipogenesis through inducing glycolytic and lipogenic gene expression and by exerting short-term stimulatory effects on these pathways. The induction or activation of transcription factors LXR, sterol regulatory element binding protein-1c (SREBP-1c), and carbohydrate response element binding protein in response to glucose and insulin is significant. RA modulates the expression of retinoid target genes through multiple mechanisms, including binding of RA isomers to the RARs and the RXRs. RAR:RXR heterodimers bind to RAREs in the gene promoter and modulate transcription control and subsequent recruitment of cofactor complexes. Several genes encoding proteins in lipid metabolism appear to be regulated by RAR-dependent pathways, including the genes for phosphoenolpyruvate carboxykinase, (glyceroneogenesis and gluconeogenesis), stearoyl-CoA desaturase 1 (promoting fatty acid synthesis but decreasing oxidation); UCP1 gene; UCP3 gene; and possibly the gene encoding medium-chain acyl-CoA dehydrogenase (involved in mt β-oxidation) [29].

The results of a study revealed that RA treatment of obese mice leads to depletion of adipose lipid stores, induction of weight loss, reversal of hepatic steatosis, increase of muscle mt content, improvement of glucose tolerance, and reactivation of the FABP5/PPARβ/δ pathway. These results provide evidence that vitamin A might have regulatory roles in energy balance and be effective in suppressing obesity and insulin resistance [30].

Low vitamin A status favors fat deposition. A growing body of evidence has demonstrated that RAR and RXR are involved in controlling adipogenesis. RA is formed from its sole precursor, Rald, through an irreversible oxidation mediated by retinaldehyde dehydrogenase (Raldh). However, a recent study showed that Rald exists in adipose tissue and may have potential effects independent of its conversion to RA [31]. Mice lacking Raldh1 are resistant to diet-induced obesity and diabetes. Rald appears to inhibit RXR:PPARγ activation. A novel mechanism has recently been proposed for the exclusive effect of RA on lipid metabolism that is mediated by differential effects on activating RARs versus PPARβ/δ [31]. Furthermore, available data suggest that both PPARs and RARs may regulate uncoupling protein 1 (UCP1), a protein that mediates energy dissipation, and apolipoprotein A1 (apo A1), which is implicated in plasma transport of cholesterol and other lipids. RA is a proposed ligand for PPARβ/δ, a receptor involved in energy balance, lipid metabolism, and glucose homeostasis and through its activation promotes lipid catabolism in skeletal muscle and adipose tissue, preventing the development of obesity [30].

In diet-induced obesity, RA treatment forwarded weight loss through the expression of RAR and PPARβ/δ target genes involved in regulation of lipid homeostasis. In addition to PPAR β/δ, the classical RARs may also be involved in regulating lipid and energy homeostasis [32]. For example, available information suggests that UCP1 (a mt protein that uncouples respiration from ATP production, resulting in heat production) [10] and apo A1, which is involved in plasma transport of cholesterol and other lipids, may be regulated by both PPARs and RARs [30].

Another mechanism through which vitamin A amends the metabolic profile is via its inhibitory effects on leptin expression. Interestingly, this effect is mainly mediated by the direct effects of RA on leptin gene expression. Furthermore, it has been shown that leptin expression is increased in the brown adipose tissue of mice fed a vitamin A–deficient diet [10]. In accord with this finding, a more recent study reported that vitamin A supplementation reduced serum leptin in rats [33].

13.2.1.10 Retinoids and hepatic gluconeogenesis

Abnormal hepatic lipid and glucose metabolism leads to insulin resistance and metabolic derangements. The main key abnormalities are the altered expression of genes involved in lipid and glucose metabolism. Glucokinase (GK) is an enzyme exclusively expressed in hepatocytes that facilitates phosphorylation of glucose to glucose-6 phosphate, which is the first step of both glycogen synthesis and glycolysis. GK is exclusively expressed in hepatocytes, and when the glucose level is high, GK serves as a central metabolic switch to shift hepatic carbohydrate metabolism between fed and fasting states. Retinoids act synergistically with insulin to induce GK expression by the activation of both RAR and RXR [31]. The *in vivo* study with Zucker lean rats fed with a vitamin A–deficient diet demonstrated that hepatic GK activity and GK mRNA levels were significantly lower than those of rats fed with a vitamin A sufficient diet. These results suggest that retinoids synergize with insulin to induce hepatic GK expression [34].

13.2.1.10.1 Retinoids and insulin sensitivity

Several studies have been conducted on the relationship between insulin resistance and the components of retinoid metabolism, mainly on the effect of RXR on glucose metabolism. Among the three RXR subtypes, RXRγ is mainly expressed in the skeletal muscle, and its expression is dependent on nutritional status. Overexpression of RXRγ in mice was associated with higher glucose disposal than in control mice in an insulin-independent manner. Furthermore, an increase in GLUT1 expression was seen in skeletal muscle from mice overexpressing RXRγ in an insulin-independent manner [35]. Chronic feeding of a vitamin A–rich diet to obese adult male rats for 2 weeks decreased body weight gain and visceral WAT mass [36]. However, fasting plasma glucose and insulin sensitivity were not affected by vitamin A. In another study on lean and obese 50-day-old male rats subsequently fed with either stock diet or vitamin A-enriched diet for 3 months, decreased body weight gain, visceral adiposity, and improved insulin sensitivity were seen in vitamin A–enriched diet–fed obese rats compared with stock diet–fed obese rats. These alterations were accompanied by decreased fasting plasma insulin and unaltered glucose levels [37].

Binding of retinol-bound RBP (holoRBP) to STRA6 induces the phosphorylation of a tyrosine residue in the receptor C-terminus, leading to the activation of a JAK/STAT signaling cascade [31]. STRA6-mediated retinol transport and cell signaling are interrelated, and it is believed that STRA6 suppresses insulin responses. This is a possible explanation for obesity-induced insulin resistance [38].

13.2.1.10.2 Retinoids and insulin secretion

The effects of RA on the function of β-cells are follows [31]:

1. Restoring insulin secretion in vitamin-deficient rats
2. Inducing both first and second phase insulin secretory responses to glucose in explants of human fetal pancreas
3. Increasing insulin production in insulin-secreting cell lines
4. Increasing pancreatic GK activity and mRNA levels in the insulinoma cell line and primary rat pancreatic islets

Moreover, 9cRA reduces glucose-stimulated insulin secretion in mouse islets by rapid reduction of GLUT2 and GK activity [39]. Induction of the expression of SREBP-1c results in the elevation of its target gene, fatty acid synthase. RXR, but not RAR, is involved in induction of SREBP-1c expression. The studies had previously identified the RA-responsive elements in the SREBP-1c promoter as two LXR elements responsible for mediating insulin action. These findings imply a potential role of vitamin A in the regulation of hepatic gene expression [31].

13.2.1.10.3 Effects of retinoids on the prevention of type 1 diabetes

Type 1 diabetes is a chronic disorder that results in the selective autoimmune destruction of the beta cells in the pancreas [40]. Studies have suggested an important immunomodulatory role for vitamin A in progression of type 1 diabetes, and a deficiency status of vitamin A in these patients [41–43]. The results of a study demonstrated that atRA treatment has immunomodulatory effects on the prevention of type 1 diabetes, mediated by effects on T-regulatory (Treg) cells and T-effector cells [44]. Another study revealed that the effectiveness of T1DM suppression by retinoids depends on the presence of Tregs, which down-modulate immunoinflammatory events [45]. These results suggest that atRA exerts a protective effect on type 1 diabetes development through the modulation of immune function, especially through the expansion of Treg cells [31].

13.2.1.10.4 Retinoids and prevention of cancer

Decreased cellular proliferation is considered to be a good anticancer biomarker. Many transcriptional target genes of retinoids are involved in this effect, since several inhibitors of cell cycle progression are the direct targets of retinoids. The inhibitory effect of RA on cell proliferation is mainly mediated by the upregulation of RARβ2 by atRA and the acyclic retinoid effect of RA on cell. Additionally, RA induces the ubiquitin-mediated degradation of cyclin D1, which results in suppression of cyclin-dependent kinase (CDK) activities, interfering with retinoblastoma phosphorylation and cyclin E expression. All these events lead to the transition of a cell to S-phase. Retinoids increase the tendency of cells to a more differentiated status. However, these changes will not always cause the net suppression of tumor formation in various tissues treated with retinoids. Another novel ability of retinoids is the potential to modulate effectively the inflammatory pathways critical for carcinogenesis, which may offer applicable targets for chemoprevention. Furthermore, increasing data show that reprogramming of stromal cells, fibroblasts, adipocytes, and immune cells are among the factors that might be affected by retinoids in modulating tumorigenesis in a number of tissues [22].

RA-regulated tumor suppressor genes, when expressed, can inhibit tumor growth. Among the three RAR subtypes, RARβ has been well established for its tumor suppressive effects in epithelial cells. Exogenous expression of the RARβ gene can lead to RA-dependent and RA-independent apoptosis and growth arrest. RARβ induced growth arrest and apoptosis in a RARα-dependent manner [46]. Binding of RA ligand-bound RARα to the RARE on the RARβ promoter attracts several activator proteins and results in the upregulation of the RARβ gene. The expression of RARβ induces the transactivation and expression of a number of its target genes that contribute to cell differentiation and death. It is becoming an area of interest that RARβ expression is disturbed early in carcinogenesis or is epigenetically silenced in many solid tumors, providing future novel treatment strategies to be further investigated using retinoids together with epigenetic modifiers to re-express the silenced genes [46].

13.2.1.11 Carotenoids

Carotenoids are lipophilic isoprenoids pigments that are found in plants and microorganisms [47,48]. Carotenoids primarily act as the precursors of vitamin A–associated retinoids, including retinol, retinal, and RA and are involved in visual cycle, gene regulation, and physiological processes. Several animal studies have demonstrated that carotenoids and carotenoid derivatives exert their anti-obesity and anti-inflammatory actions through suppressive effects on PPAR/δ and adipogenesis and activating effects on lipid oxidation and thermogenesis [48].

The anticancer and/or cancer chemopreventive activities of carotenoids are mediated through their effects on (1) gap junctional intercellular communication, (2) growth factors (suppression of Insulin-like Growth Factor-1-signaling by lycopene), (3) cell cycle progression (reduction in cyclin D1 protein levels by lycopene, lycopene-induced delay in progression through the G1 and S phases, induction of a cell cycle delay in the G1 phase in normal human fibroblasts by β-carotene), (4) Wnt/β-catenin pathway (inhibition by lycopene), and (5) inflammatory cytokines (inhibitory effects on NF-κB, etc.) [49].

13.2.2 Vitamin D
13.2.2.1 General characteristics and metabolism

Vitamin D is a fat-soluble secosterol that is essential for bone formation and the maintenance of calcium homeostasis [50]. The active form of vitamin D, calcitriol, is a steroid hormone that plays a critical role in a various range of biological actions including the regulation of cell growth and cell cycle, cellular differentiation, apoptosis, and immune modulation and the integration of hormonal and cellular signaling pathways [51]. More recently, vitamin D has received huge attention as an antioxidant [52].

Both forms of vitamin D (i.e., D2 and D3) in the circulatory system, bind to plasma α1-globulin (D-binding protein), which are then converted in the liver by the enzyme 25-hydroxylase (CYP2R1) to 25-hydroxy vitamin D (25(OH)D or calcidiol). Calcidiol is enzymatically converted in the kidney to the active form, $1,25(OH)_2D3$ (calcitriol), by 25(OH)D 1α-hydroxylase (CYP27B1), a cytochrome P450 protein. This active form of the vitamin is then transported in the blood to the tissues that need it. The presence of the extrarenal 1α-OHase allows $1,25(OH)_2D$ thus produced to act as a paracrine or autocrine hormone [51,53]. Another component of cytochrome P450, 24-hydroxylase (CYP24A1), is involved in vitamin D degradation by hydroxylation of 25(OH)D and 1, 25(OH)2D to their hydroxylated derivatives [54]. It has been reported that CYP24A1 deficiency contributes to nephrolithiasis [55]. Calcitriol is a pleiotropic hormone with several regulatory actions. Traditionally, vitamin D deficiency has been linked to impaired intestinal calcium absorption and bone formation (rickets in children, osteomalacia in adults). However, several other roles have been proposed for vitamin D deficiency, including a higher risk of developing colon cancer and perhaps other neoplasias, autoimmune disorders like multiple sclerosis (MS), and certain infectious diseases such as tuberculosis [56]. At the cellular level, it can modulate proliferation, differentiation, survival, and metabolism and enhances the antitumoral activity of certain chemotherapeutic agents, in a cell type– and context-dependent manner [57]. Cellular conditions such as low serum calcium or phosphorus levels determine the need for the synthesis of 1,25(OH)$_2$D, which is tightly regulated and stimulated by serum parathyroid hormone, and circulating fibroblast growth factor (FGF) 23 produced by osteocytes inhibits its synthesis [58].

13.2.2.2 Health implications of vitamin D deficiency

Several factors impact 25(OH)D levels including race, vitamin D intake, sun exposure, adiposity, age, and physical activity. The duration of vitamin D insufficiency, the responsiveness of the VDR, dietary calcium intake, and individual calcium requirements are among the factors that modify the clinical consequences of vitamin D deficiency or insufficiency [58–61]. Vitamin D deficiency causes rickets among children and osteoporosis among adults and leads to the painful bone disease osteomalacia. Risk of many cancers, CVD, MS, rheumatoid arthritis, and type 1 diabetes mellitus are also associated with vitamin D deficiency [56,62–66].

13.2.2.3 Health implications of vitamin D toxicity

Vitamin D toxicity is a rare condition that may occur following ingestion of large amounts of vitamin D (>10,000 IU/d) for prolonged periods. Vitamin D toxicity is recognized not only on the basis of an elevated circulating 25(OH)D level but also as a clinical syndrome of both hypervitaminosis D and hypercalcemia, which might be accompanied by hyperphosphatemia and hypercalciuria [67]. Early clinical presentations of vitamin D toxicity include nausea, dehydration, anorexia, vomiting, and constipation, commonly due to hypercalcemia. Bone pain, drowsiness, continuous headaches, irregular heartbeat, loss of appetite, and muscle and joint pain might also occur within a few days or weeks. Frequent urination, especially at night, excessive thirst, weakness, nervousness and itching, and kidney stones are other symptoms of hypervitaminosis D [67,68].

13.2.2.4 Vitamin D genomic actions

VDR is a nuclear receptor superfamily involved in the actions of 1,25(OH)$_2$D$_3$ signaling in calcium homeostasis, control of cell growth and differentiation, cell adhesion, and apoptosis (programmed cell death) [51]. It is expressed by at least 38 cell types in the human body. In the absence of its ligand (i.e., calcitriol), VDR is mainly located in the cytoplasm. Following binding of the ligand, VDR heterodimerizes with the RXR and translocates to the nucleus, where it binds to vitamin D response element and regulates the transcription of 1,25(OH)$_2$D$_3$ target genes [51,69]. It is believed that VDR has two ligand binding sites, including genomic pocket (VDR-GP) and an alternative pocket (VDR-AP). VDR-GP is involved in gene transcription, whereas VDR-AP is responsible for rapid responses [70].

Having large CpG islands in their promoter regions, the genes coding for VDR and for the enzymes CYP2R1, CYP27B1, and CYP24A1 can be silenced by DNA methylation. Moreover, certain genes, like HDMs of the Jumonji C (JmjC) domain–containing proteins and lysine-specific demethylase families that code for chromatin modifiers and remodelers, are primary targets of VDR and its ligands [71]. Moreover, 1,25(OH)2D3 has regulatory effects on genes lacking VDR binding sites and has shown posttranslational gene regulatory effects through controlling the expression of multiple proteases and protease inhibitors [57]. Histone modifications exert a complex regulatory role in gene transcription, which is influenced by a various chromatin modification enzymes. The recent evidence shows that $1,25(OH)_2D_3$ induces the accumulation of VDR and upregulates histone H4 acetylation at conserved regions in the human VDR gene. VDR/RXR dimer interacts with transcriptional coactivators, such as the HATs in order to regulate transcription. VDR regulates FOXOs. Moreover, FOXO proteins also interact with other epigenetic regulators, such as sirtuin-1 (silent mating type information regulation 2 homolog), or SIRT1. VDR has inhibitory effects on NF-κB function through SIRT1 and $1,25(OH)_2D$ signaling, which indicates the role of calcitriol-mediated deacetylation of NF-κB through its interaction with SIRT1. VDR and its ligand are also involved in regulation of cell cycle arrest through regulating the p21(waf1/cip1) gene [71].

13.2.2.5 Histone modifications

A recent study demonstrated that vitamin D intake is involved in hypomethylation and hence activation of Dickkopf-related protein 1 (DKK1) promoter in CRC patients. This negative association implies the expression of DKK1 in CRC patients with high vitamin D intake [2]. Data obtained from colon cancer patients indicates that JMJD3 (the largest group of HDM enzymes that contains a JmjC) is a $1,25(OH)_2D_3$ target gene that in turn partially mediates the antitumoral effects of $1,25(OH)_2D_3$ on human colon cancer cells. JMJD3 may be recruited to the regulatory region of $1,25(OH)_2D_3$ target genes, such as CYP24A1, CDH1/E-cadherin, and CST5/cystatin D, and subsequently exert epigenetic changes that would lead to gene transcription activation [57].

13.2.2.6 Regulation of immune system by vitamin D

Recently there has been much interest in the immunomodulatory role of vitamin D against respiratory pathogens, opportunistic infections, and environmental agents [72–76].

Calcitriol affects maturation and migration of dendritic cells and has a tolerogenic function [75]. *In vitro* treatment of murine bone marrow–derived dendritic cells with calcitriol caused promotion of Treg production over cytotoxic T cells [77]. Calcitriol also upregulates immunoglobulin-like transcript 3 (an inhibitory receptor that modulates immune response), especially on monocytes [78].

Treg cells have a crucial role in immune homeostasis. Forkhead box P3 (Foxp3) is a transcription factor that is essential for Treg cell development as well as survival [79]. There is *in vitro* evidence that calcitriol enhances production of both IL-10[(+)] and Foxp3[(+)] Treg cells [80] through direct binding of VDR to the Foxp3 gene, which seems axial for inhibitory functions of Treg cells [81]. In a study on HIV-1–infected subjects on suppressive antiretroviral therapy, though no significant association was found between vitamin D deficiency and distribution of T cells and B cells subsets, vitamin D supplementation in vitamin D–deficient subjects caused immune alterations consistent with longer survival [82].

Innate immune cells identify microbes, mostly through pattern recognition receptors, including Toll-like receptors (TLRs) [83]. It has been shown that treatment of blood and tissue CD3[+] T cells with 1, 25(OH)$_2$D$_3$ results in overexpression of TLR9 by Treg IL-10+ cells. In accord with this finding, calcitriol supplementation in healthy subjects also resulted in upregulation of both IL-10 and TLR9 by CD3[+]CD4[+] T cells [84]. Vitamin D has an inhibitory effect on T-cell proliferation and modulates the profile of cytokines secreted by T helper (Th) 1 and Th2; it inhibits Th1-driven IFN-γ and IL-17 but enhances Th2 IL-4 [85].

In a recent study, higher intake of vitamin D during pregnancy was associated with some reduction in the risk of persistent wheeze in children at age 5 years [86]. Modification of Th effector cell cytokine production and Treg cell function may contribute to this effect [87]. Vitamin D–induced reduction of differentiation and expansion of pro-inflammatory Th17 cells has been shown in both asthmatic and healthy children [88].

13.2.2.7 Proliferation: Cell-cycle control

Vitamin D compounds have been implicated in alteration of cellular proliferation through multiple mechanisms, primarily via effects on cell cycle progression, apoptosis, and differentiation [3]. Suppression or activation of the transcription genes regulating cell growth by VDR is mediated through direct or indirect mechanisms that involve interaction of the associated genes. It has been shown that the growth of primary cell cultures from normal prostate and other tissues is inhibited by 1,25(OH)$_2$D and vitamin D analogues. In the case of cultured murine keratinocytes, the administration of low doses of 1,25(OH)$_2$D increased cellular proliferation, while growth inhibition occurred at high concentrations. Due to its effects in decreasing proliferation and promoting differentiation of keratinocytes, calcitriol has been proven to improve hyperproliferative skin conditions and psoriasis. Vitamin D secosteroids downregulate the expression of several factors involved in cell proliferation, such as the epidermal growth factor receptor, c-myc proto-oncogene, and keratin [89]. The antiproliferative potential of vitamin D is also associated with the suppressed expression of antiapoptotic proteins such as Bcl2 in cancer cells and arrest of cell cycle in G0/G1 [90].

Calcitriol affects cyclin pathways by regulating gene expression of the proteins p27 and p21 and the consequent inhibition of CDK. The entry and passage through the cell cycle is regulated by the binding and changing levels of p21 and p27. Calcitriol exerts regulatory effects on cell cycle checkpoints through p53 and also affects genes involved in apoptosis, including heat shock proteins Hsp70 and Hsp90 and Apaf1 [51].

13.2.2.8 Apoptosis

Calcitriol or its analogues affect the levels of pro-apoptotic (bax, bak) and/or anti-apoptotic (Bcl-2, Bcl-XL) proteins, proceeding the balance toward apoptosis rather than cell survival [91]. The findings of a study showed that vitamin D treatment suppressed the apoptosis rate in the PBMCs of systemic lupus erythematosus patients, increased the DNA content in G0/G1, and downregulated the expression rate of FasL and Bax, while upregulating the expression of Bcl-2 [91]. Further research revealed that there are at least two pathways involved in prostate cells including transforming growth factor β and insulin-like growth factor 3 pathways [92]. The apoptosis-inducing property of vitamin D has led to development of vitamin D analogues as potential therapeutic agents for malignancies [93,94].

On the contrary, some studies have shown anti-apoptotic effects of vitamin D. In a murine model, vitamin D attenuated development of colitis induced by a chemical, 2,4,6-trinitrobenzene sulfonic acid. The proposed mechanism was through downregulation of p53-upregulated modulator of apoptosis expression and hence inhibition of intestinal epithelial cell apoptosis [95].

13.2.2.9 Vitamin D, cell adhesion molecules, and loss of contact inhibition

E-cadherin is essential for the adherens junction, the intercellular structure needed for the correct formation of compact epithelial layers. Loss of E-cadherin expression is seen in cellular deadhesion and migration during the epithelial to mesenchymal transition, a common finding in carcinomas [96]. E-cadherin, induced by the nongenomic rapid action of $1\alpha,25(OH)_2D_3$, can suppress cell growth by inhibiting β-catenin transcriptional activity [97].

Almost all colon tumors present a deregulated β-catenin signaling pathway. $1\alpha,25(OH)2D3$ inhibits the transcriptional activity of β-catenin by two mechanisms. First, a rapid increase in the amount of VDR bound to β-catenin blocks the interaction of this catenin with transcription factor 4. Secondly, in human colon carcinoma cells, changes in β-catenin transcriptional activity caused by $1\alpha,25(OH)_2D_3$ are followed by the nuclear export of β-catenin, causing its relocalization to the plasma membrane, which occurs concomitantly to E-cadherin protein expression. In summary, the protective effects of $1\alpha,25(OH)_2D_3$ in colon carcinoma cells are accompanied by a panel of mutations in critical genes such as p53, Ras, and APC and expressing negligible amounts of E-cadherin but overexpressing c-Myc and in other human colon cell lines expressing functional VDR. These findings indicate the key role of VDR expression in colon carcinogenesis [98].

Nutrigenomic Aspects of Vitamins   **293**

The results of another study demonstrated that since VDR is expressed in metaplastic carcinomas, they may respond to 1α,25(OH)(2)D(3) and that 1α,25(OH)(2)D(3) enhances *de novo* E-cadherin expression in breast cancer cells through promoter demethylation [99].

It was demonstrated that calcitriol is capable of inducing cells to be more adhesive to each other [100]. The results of a recent study revealed the role of $1α,25(OH)_2D_3$ in upregulating E-cadherin in a metastatic, triple-negative breast cancer cell line, indicating that vitamin D is potent to decrease the aggressiveness of this subtype of breast cancer, leading to better outcomes [99].

It has been reported that the calcitriol–VDR signaling pathway with anticancer effects, which are not mediated just through canonical vitamin D response element signaling, is highly conserved between mouse and human [101].

13.2.2.10 Vitamin D and diseases
13.2.2.10.1 Obesity

Circulating 25(OH)D concentrations tend to be lower in obese individuals who are at risk of developing the metabolic syndrome and diabetes [102]. The expression of VDR in adipocytes justifies the role of $1,25(OH)_2D$ in promoting lipogenesis and decreased lipolysis [103]. While calcitriol and its metabolites have an inhibitory effect against adipocyte formation in the 3T3-L1 cell line, 1, 25(OH)2D3 enhances human preadipocyte differentiation. Transgenic animal models have given evidence of the role of vitamin D in adipose tissue. It has been shown that VDR and CYP27BI mice fail to gain weight through high energy intake, while overexpression of VDR in adipose tissue results in increased fat mass [104]. In adipose tissue obtained from vitamin D–deficient rats, the expression of uncoupling proteins (UCP1 and UCP2) is increased, indicating elevated energy expenditure, whereas p160 steroid receptor coactivator 3, a regulator of adipogenesis, is downregulated [105].

Contrary to these findings, recently a strong inhibitory effect of calcitriol on fat deposition in mature 3T3-L1 was reported, suggesting a metabolic promoting role and anti-adiposity role for vitamin D. This effect of calcitriol may be related to nicotinamide adenine dinucleotide concentration and SIRT1 activity [106].

The evidence indicates the role of matrix metalloproteinases (MMPs) in the pathogenesis of obesity. Increased MMP-2 and MMP-9 levels are found in obese subjects. Data show that MMP-9 correlates with BMI [107]. In one study, higher activity of MMP-8, lower plasma tissue inhibitor of metalloproteinase 1 (TIMP-1) concentrations, and higher MMP-8/TIMP-1 ratios were seen in obese children and adolescents compared with nonobese controls [108].

Prostaglandins (PGs) play a role in the inflammatory processes. Cyclooxygenase (COX) is involved in the conversion of arachidonic acid into PGs. The role of

PGE2 and PGD2/PGJ2 have been demonstrated in adiposity promotion in mice through the inhibition of lipolysis and the induction of adipogenesis, respectively. PGF2α was shown to be a potent inhibitor of adipocyte differentiation and increased lipid accumulation in hepatocytes, leading to the development of hepatic steatosis in *in vivo* models of obesity [107]. Calcitriol has been found to have regulatory effects on the expression of several genes involved in the PG pathway, such as selective inhibition of COX-2, which leads to a decrease in PG production. All these indicate the modulatory effect of vitamin D on the inflammatory process seen in obesity [107].

13.2.2.10.2 Insulin resistance and type 2 diabetes

Since the activation of inflammatory pathways disturbs normal insulin metabolism and proper insulin signaling, it is likely that vitamin D could affect glucose homeostasis through modulating inflammatory response [109]. Vitamin D has anti-inflammatory actions through suppressing the release of TNF-α and IL-6 while upregulating synthesis of the anti-inflammatory cytokine IL-10 [110–113]. Plasma MMP are inflammatory markers involved in vascular damage and unstable angina. MMP2 and MMP9 are negatively associated with vitamin D status [114]. Modified function of β cells due to β-cell apoptosis can develop through the presence of elevated cytokines in systemic inflammation, commonly found in diabetes, and can also induce insulin resistance directly. Vitamin D has subsiding effects on systemic inflammation through interaction with components in the region of promotion of cytokine genes [115]. In particular, in the case of insulin sensitivity, it was shown that vitamin D can downregulate the activation of NF-κB (which plays a regulatory role for genes of pro-inflammatory cytokines involved in insulin resistance) [116]. Furthermore, vitamin D exerts regulatory effects on the insulin signaling cascade. A vitamin D response element has been recognized on the human insulin receptor (InR) gene promoter, and treatment with 1,25-dihydroxyvitamin D3 causes an increased transcription of the InR gene, leading to improved insulin-dependent glucose transport. Moreover, $1,25(OH)_2D_3$ shows stimulatory effects on glucose oxidation either via the activation of InR transcription or by a direct regulation of phosphatidylinositol 3-kinase activity [114]. Improvement of glycemic status following vitamin D supplementation has been already reported [117]. The presence of VDRs in skeletal muscles, stimulation of expression of InR in bone marrow cells, and vitamin D activation of PPAR-γ are among the direct mechanisms by which vitamin D may improve insulin action. The indirect role of vitamin D is mediated through the regulation of pools of intracellular and extracellular calcium and control of normal influx of calcium within the membranes of cells [115]. Some mechanisms for the effects of vitamin D on insulin resistance and the subsequent diabetes can be summarized as follows [116]:

1. Presence of VDRs on pancreatic β cells
2. Expression of 1α-hydroxylase in pancreatic β cells

3. Presence of vitamin D response element in the insulin gene
4. Presence of VDR in skeletal muscle
5. Increase in the transcription of insulin receptor genes 1,25(OH)D
6. Suppression of the renin gene and thus blockade of renin–angiotensin activity

13.2.2.10.3 Autoimmune diseases

Several studies have demonstrated the potential role of vitamin D in the pathogenesis of certain systemic and organ-specific autoimmune diseases, such as type 1 diabetes mellitus, MS, rheumatoid arthritis, and Crohn's disease [118,119]. Current data indicate a link between poor vitamin D status and the prevalence of autoimmune disorders [120,121].

VDR exists in immune-competent cells, including macrophages and activated T-lymphocytes, which indicates the immunomodulatory effects of 1,25(OH)$_2$D in these cells [122]. Vitamin D effects on the innate and adaptive immune systems are mediated by TLRs and T-cell differentiation, respectively. By regulating the differentiation and activity of CD4$^+$ T cells, vitamin D has suppressive effects in autoimmune disease pathology, resulting in a more balanced Th1/Th2 response, followed by a decrement in development of self-reactive T cells and consequent autoimmunity [118].

Rheumatoid arthritis is a chronic autoimmune disorder defined by systemic features and joint involvement that affects 1% of the world's adults [123]. Calcitriol is capable of declining the expression of pro-inflammatory cytokines (IL-1β, IL-6, and TNF-α) in human activated macrophages by decreasing the aromatase activity, particularly in the presence of an estrogenic milieu, such as in rheumatoid arthritis synovial tissue [124]. A recent meta-analysis revealed the lower serum vitamin D levels in rheumatoid arthritis patients and their inverse association with disease activity, particularly in low-latitude and developing nations [123]. In a recent cohort study on rheumatoid arthritis patients, a high prevalence of vitamin D deficiency was observed, which was associated with disease severity [125].

MS, another prevalent autoimmune disease, is a common cause of neurological disability in young adults. Epidemiological studies have shown that the prevalence of MS depends on the geographical region, with higher prevalence in higher latitude regions that have lower levels of sunlight exposure. Therefore, it has been speculated that poor vitamin D status may be the causal risk factor mediating this latitudinal gradient [126]. Low concentration of circulating calcidiol, 25(OH)D, has also been correlated with higher rates of MS relapse and higher MS-specific disease activity and disability. The immunomodulatory effects of vitamin D have been observed in multiple cell-culture experiments, implying the possible mechanisms by which vitamin D may affect MS risk [126]. There is a growing body of evidence that supports a protective role for vitamin D in MS risk and progression. Several studies have demonstrated that high 25(OH)D levels at the time of a first demyelinating event predicts a lower MS risk and a decreased risk of MS in offspring with mothers having high 25(OH)D levels. 25(OH)D levels were negatively correlated with exacerbation risk in relapsing–remitting MS [118].

Future well-designed studies will clarify the interactive effects of vitamin D supplementation and the host genotypes on prevention and treatment of autoimmune disorders [61,127].

13.3 Water-soluble vitamins

13.3.1 Folate and cobalamins

13.3.1.1 General characteristics and metabolism

Folate is a water-soluble B vitamin found in foods, including fresh green leafy vegetables, citrus fruits, wheat bread, legumes, and liver [128,129]. It exists in the reduced form (e.g., 5-methyltetrahydrofolate [5-MTHF]), the predominant form in foods and the human body. Humans are not able to produce folate. Much folate (up to 70%) can be lost during the cooking process [129,130]. After ingestion of polyglutamate folate and synthetic monoglutamate folic acid (FA), both are absorbed by the cells of the upper small intestine. FA can be absorbed directly, while folate has to be converted to its monoglutamate form by the enzyme folate conjugase (gamma-glutamyl hydrolase). In order to be metabolically active, FA must first be converted to dihydrofolate (DHF) and in the next step to tetrahydrofolate (THF) by enzymatic reductions catalyzed by the enzyme DHF reductase (DHFR). Then, THF can be converted to the biologically active l-methylfolate by the enzyme methylenetetrahydrofolate reductase (MTHFR). This is the main process required to supply l-methylfolate for the one-carbon transfer reactions necessary for purine/pyrimidine synthesis during DNA and RNA assembly, for DNA methylation for the synthesis of SAM, which is the major methyl group donor for the majority of genomic and nongenomic methylation reactions, and to regulate homocysteine (Hcy) metabolism. MTHFR is the critical enzyme for almost all biologic processes involved in the metabolism of folate and methionine [4,129,131,132]. In the brain, these reactions are necessary for the synthesis of neurotransmitters (serotonin, dopamine, norepinephrine, and acetylcholine), hormones (melatonin), membrane phospholipids, and myelin, and also for the epigenetic control of gene expression [4]. Folate is necessary for human health and development and its persistent deficiency during pregnancy leads to adverse pregnancy outcomes affecting public health worldwide [133].

Vitamin B_{12} is a common name for a group of compounds (also named cobalamins) with more or less similar chemical and biological characteristics. It is a water-soluble essential vitamin containing the metal cobalt core. Vitamin B_{12} is synthesized by bacteria and is found mainly in meat, egg, and dairy products. Plant sources commonly lack vitamin B_{12} [134]. Since methionine synthase, the enzyme catalyzing the transfer of a methyl group from 5-MTHF to Hcy, thereby generating methionine (the precursor of SAM), requires vitamin B_{12} as a cofactor, this vitamin also plays a critical role in methylation reactions [4,132].

13.3.1.2 Health implications of folate deficiency

Folate is necessary for human health and development and its persistent deficiency during pregnancy may lead to adverse pregnancy outcomes through epigenomic effects [133]. Folate and vitamin B12 deficiencies are accompanied by a reduction in methionine synthase activity, decreasing SAM levels and increasing the levels of Hcy–hyperhomocysteinemia and S-adenosylhomocysteine (a potent inhibitor of methyltransferases) and also disturbing nucleotide synthesis, particularly thymidine, leading to an increase in dUMP:dTMP ratio. Rapidly dividing cells of the bone marrow, such as leucocytes and platelets, are especially sensitive to folate deficiency due to disturbed DNA synthesis. Because of its roles in DNA synthesis, transcription, methylation, and gene expression, folate deficiency affects brain growth, differentiation, development, and repair especially in the CNS [4]. Folate deficiency and genetic folate metabolism alterations have been associated with conditions including megaloblastic anemia, mood alterations, Alzheimer's disease (AZD), and thrombogenetic and atherogenetic vascular disease, including hypertension [6]. Folate deficiency has also been implicated in the etiology of Down syndrome, neural tube defects (NTDs), pregnancy complications, and male infertility, making it an important factor at the reproductive phase of the lifecycle. Furthermore, several cancers including those of the colon, breast, pancreas, stomach, cervix, bronchus, and blood have been associated with poor folate status [5].

13.3.1.3 Health implications of folate toxicity

Observational studies have shown chemopreventive properties of high folate intake or high plasma levels against cancer and CVD. However, folate supplementation might induce an increased risk for individuals at a higher risk of these chronic diseases. Although not proven and still controversial, high folate status may increase the risk of some chronic diseases in certain individuals, possibly through disturbing the balance of one-carbon metabolism [135]. A prospective study demonstrated a positive association of folate status with risk of developing premenopausal breast cancer and estrogen receptor or progesterone receptor tumors [136]. Similarly, another study showed an increased risk of postmenopausal breast cancer with high intake of folate, usually attributable to supplemental FA [137]. High intake of FA could have antagonistic effects through the accumulation of DHF, since it has inhibitory effects on thymidylate synthase and MTHFR, by which high concentrations of FA could inhibit the formation of 5-methyl THF [135]. Intensification of B_{12} deficiency symptoms, increased insulin resistance in the offspring of mothers with high red blood cell folate, suppressed natural killer cell activity in elderly women, fourfold increased risk of unilateral retinoblastoma in the newborns born to women who were homozygous for the 19 bp deletion in the DHFR gene and who were folate supplemented during pregnancy, and lower mental functions in the elderly carrying similar polymorphism are among the other side effects controversially attributed to high folate intakes [138].

13.3.1.4 Vitamin B_{12}: Health implications

Vitamin B_{12} is an essential coenzyme for methionine synthase and is involved in folate pathway via the action of methionine biosynthesis and the formation of DNA [6]. This step is especially necessary for cell multiplication and hence fetal development during pregnancy. Low vitamin B_{12} status leads to hyperhomocysteinemia, which is related to clinical conditions including placental vasculopathy, which impacts fetal growth. Vitamin B_{12} deficiency also leads to pernicious megaloblastic anemia, characterized by symptoms including vomiting, diarrhea, and pyrexia, with edema and albuminuria occurring most often in the later stages. Due to its roles in metabolism of neural tissue, vitamin B_{12} deficiency can cause anencephaly. Increased Hcy and decreased THF levels, as well as secondary elevation of guanidinoacetate (neurotoxic) have been proposed in the pathogenesis of encephalopathy [139,140]. Vitamin B_{12} deficiency is also involved in development of fetal NTDs by elevation in plasma total Hcy [141,142]. No adverse effects due to high vitamin B_{12} intake have been reported to date [132].

13.3.1.5 Gene expression

As mentioned earlier, a growing body of evidence indicates that folate regulates the epigenetic and epigenomic mechanisms involved in intrauterine growth retardation, fetal programming, and embryo-fetal brain development [133]. Folate, in the form of 5-MTHF, is implicated in remethylation of Hcy to methionine, which is a precursor of SAM, the principal methyl group donor for most biological methylation reactions, including DNA synthesis [143]. Methylation of the genes at specific sites makes them not transcribed or transcribed at a reduced rate; thereby gene expression and ultimately protein synthesis are controlled. Folate deficiency can interfere with this function by inhibiting normal DNA methylation [144].

13.3.1.6 Cancer prevention

Hypomethylation seems to be a crucial determinant of cancer involved in chromosomal stability and specific gene targets [145]. A deficiency in cellular folate and also vitamin B_{12} leads to abnormal DNA methylation, point mutations, chromosome breakage, increased frequency of micronuclei, defective chromosome recombination, and aneuploidy [145,146]. As mentioned above, MTHFR is a key enzyme in folate metabolism, which is involved in catalyzing the reconversion of 5,10-methylene THF to 5-methyl THF. The enzyme THF synthetase converts 5,10-methylene THF to 10-formyl THF, which then donates a formyl group at positions C8 and C2 for purine ring synthesis, through which THF is regenerated. In folate deficiency, these reactions are impaired, leading to double-strand breakages during excision of uracil and increased chromosome instability, a mechanism usually predisposed to carcinogenesis [147]. Several studies have demonstrated the protective effect of folate in a wide range of cancers, including breast, prostate, pancreatic, and colorectal cancers [130].

13.3.2 Folate, cobalamins, and human diseases

13.3.2.1 Insulin resistance and obesity

Studies have provided evidence that mild hyperhomocysteinemia leads to target organ damage and hypertension and that folate supplementation can reverse these adverse effects. However, the relationships between folate deficiency/hyperhomocysteinemia and insulin resistance have not been conclusive [148]. In a 6-year follow-up study of pregnant Indian women, higher maternal erythrocyte folate concentration was associated with higher offspring adiposity and increased insulin resistance, as judged by HOMA-IR (homeostatic model assessment for insulin resistance), while low maternal vitamin B_{12} predicted higher HOMA-IR in the children. The offspring of mothers with a combination of high folate and low vitamin B_{12} concentrations were the most insulin resistant [149]. A study showed that reduced dietary intake of folate leads to low serum folate levels and hyperhomocysteinemia accompanied by glucose tolerance; increased ectopic fat accumulation in liver; oxidative tissue damage in liver, heart, and kidneys; and increased blood pressure [148]. Hyperhomocysteinemia with concomitant elevated concentrations of asymmetric di-methyl arginine and resulting increased production of pro-inflammatory prooxidant peroxynitrite may have a role in folate deficiency–induced vascular damage and increased insulin resistance [150–152]. Impaired insulin signaling due to homocyteine has also been observed in a cell culture model [153].

Supplementing the maternal diet with folate, vitamin B_{12}, choline, or betaine increases DNA methylation of the agouti gene in the offspring, which leads to low agouti expression and therefore the prevention of obesity [149]. Studies have demonstrated that vitamin B_{12} deficiency is associated with altered lipid profile and metabolic disorder, and it has been speculated that this might result from DNA methylation changes. A study found that vitamin B_{12} plays a critical role in biosynthesis of cholesterol through induction of SREBP expression in human adipocytes and DNA hypomethylation, which is mediated by limited availability of SAM. The other important observation was significant hypomethylated regions in two cholesterol-regulating genes, SREBF1 and low density lipoprotein receptor, in cells cultured in low or no B_{12} media compared with cells cultured in control media containing high B_{12}. These findings provided molecular evidence for the critical role of vitamin B_{12} in the metabolism of adipocytes and increased Hcy and total cholesterol in B_{12} deficiency [154].

300 Nutrigenomics and Nutraceuticals

13.3.2.2 Oxidative stress, hypertension, endothelial function, and CVD

Oxidative stress is involved in the pathogenesis of both hypertension and certain metabolic disorders, but the underlying mechanisms are not fully elucidated. Induction of oxidative stress by increasing Hcy levels that are associated with oxidation and auto-oxidation of Hcy and reduction of antioxidant enzyme activities, such as superoxide dismutase and glutathione peroxidase, are among the plausible mechanisms in this regard. Folate deficiency accompanied by hyperhomocysteinemia is also considered to be correlated with hypertension, at least in part through disruption of endothelial and vascular function associated with impaired bioavailability of tetrahydrobiopterin, an essential cofactor of endothelial nitric oxide synthase (eNOS) [148]. The main mechanism of the effect of FA on endothelial function has been proposed to be a reduction in plasma Hcy concentrations by remethylation of Hcy back to methionine [155]. Hypertension has been shown to be associated with impaired nitric oxide (NO) production and an imbalance in antioxidant status. Hyperhomocysteinemia is considered to be an independent risk factor for CVD. The mechanisms involved in the effect of high-dose FA supplementation on endothelial dysfunction are not fully understood but may be related to the superoxide anion scavenging function of folate and enhanced NO production through induction of eNOS [155].

13.3.2.3 CNS development and function

Insufficient folate and B_{12} status is associated with impaired DNA development and repair mechanisms in neurons. Increased apoptosis and cell death were observed in hippocampus cells cultured in folate-deficient medium. The possible mechanism could be uracil misincorporation and the subsequent disrupted repair process for amyloid beta peptide-induced oxidative modification of DNA bases. Moreover, folate deficiency decreases the one-carbon supply necessary for methylation-dependent pathways in the CNS, leading to neurological deficiency disorders. Folate is also involved in neurotransmitter synthesis including dopamine, serotonin, and norepinephrine [6].

NTDs are the most prevalent congenital abnormality of the CNS [129,156]. Sufficient folate intake has been shown to be crucial for protecting against these defects. Malformation or failed closure of the neural tube during CNS development in the third and fourth weeks of gestation leads to the NTDs. The characteristics include anencephaly, a failed closure of the neural tube at the cerebral cortex, and spina bifida [130]. The etiology of NTDs is complex and multifactorial; genetic predisposition, chromosomal abnormalities, and environmental factors could be involved. However, some evidence has indicated that increased FA intake before conception is negatively associated with the prevalence of NTDs. Moreover, sufficient levels of total folate may also protect against congenital heart defects, oral clefts, and neurodevelopmental problems [130]. A percentage of NTDs in the populations with sufficient folate intake might be due to poor maternal B_{12} status [157]. The lower activity of

MTHFR enzyme leads to a decrease in the production of 5-MTHF and an increase in the plasma Hcy level, which results in a delay in the closure of the neural tube. Furthermore, reduced MTHFR activity may also limit the amount of SAM available for critical methylation reactions, disturbing the proliferation of cells at the site of neural-tube closure [129].

Autism spectrum disorder (ASD) is another neurological condition related to folate and B_{12}. Periconceptional FA supplements have been suggested to be protective against ASD. There have been elevated levels of plasma Hcy, adenosine, and SAM in mothers with ASD children. Moreover, elevated pteroylglutamate (PteGlu) levels may lead to the aberrant expression of multiple genes related to early brain development, and elevated PteGlu intake may be associated with increased expression of γ-aminobutyric acid (type A) beta 1 receptor and disrupt inhibitory synaptic transmission of neuron development in the embryo [6].

Most recently, cobalamin status has also been associated with ASD [158,159]. In subjects with ASD, the brain levels of methylcobalamin and adenosylcobalamin, which are accompanied by decreased MS activity and increased Hcy levels, can be as low as 30% of normal subjects. Decreased total cobalamins and methylcobalamin in glutamate-cysteine ligase modulatory subunit knockout mice are accompanied by low glutathione level, which has been associated with both ASD and schizophrenia [159]. These findings were endorsed by a recent clinical trial that reported improvement of clinical symptoms as well as methionine metabolism and cellular methylation capacity in ASD children following 8 weeks' supplementation with 75 µg/kg methyl cobalamin [160].

Epilepsy is another condition related to both folate and B_{12} [161]. In animals, systemic administration of high doses of Hcy induces convulsive seizures [162]. The mechanism of the association between Hcy and epilepsy is not fully understood but the evidence from animal studies shows that Hcy sequesters adenosine, an endogenous anticonvulsant, leading to the decreased seizure threshold. Other mechanisms, including oxidative stress, DNA damage, inhibition of NA/K-ATPase, and activation of caspases, might be implicated in Hcy-induced neuronal excitotoxicity [163]. Intriguingly, antiseizure medications may cause altered folate and B_{12} metabolism and consequent elevated Hcy and asymmetric dimethyl arginine levels [164–167]. Anti-epileptic therapy–induced elevated Hcy levels had no association with C677T variants of the MTHFR gene [168,169].

Studies have shown that hyperhomocysteinemia and low folate levels are independent risk factors for depression and particularly dementia, including both AZD and vascular dementia. The results of the prospective Framingham community study demonstrated that a high plasma Hcy concentration doubled the risk of developing either AZD or other dementias [170]. Hyperhomocysteinemia has also been suggested to exert a neurotoxic action independent of its vascular effects through overstimulation of N-methyl d-aspartate receptors or by

302   Nutrigenomics and Nutraceuticals

increasing hippocampal neuron vulnerability to excitotoxic insults and amyloid-β peptide toxicity. Moreover, the direct adverse effect of folate deficiency on the cortical neurons is another possible factor in developing AZD [171].

A few studies have investigated the effect of vitamin B_{12} supplementation on cognitive function in humans and no improvement was observed in the majority of them [172]. In contrast, a study examined the effects of FA supplementation, with or without vitamin B_{12}, on healthy and demented elderly people, in prevention of cognitive impairment or retarding its progress. Administration of FA alone showed no beneficial effect while cosupplementation with FA and vitamin B_{12} was effective in reducing serum Hcy concentrations [173].

Elevated plasma Hcy level has been observed in up to 30% of patients with severe depression [172]. In an Australian study, low circulating FA and high Hcy levels were associated with increased depressive symptoms, while serum concentrations of vitamin B_{12} did not show such a significant association [174]. Evidence from the NHANES and Framingham cohort studies indicates that it is unmetabolized FA that is responsible for poor cognitive function. The findings of a study showed that low vitamin B_{12} levels are associated with cognitive decline and that this risk is aggravated in the presence of high folate levels [175]. Low circulating concentration of B_{12} with high serum folate levels has also been reported as an unusual cause of a case of generalized tonic–clonic seizure [161].

A meta-analysis demonstrated that low serum levels of folate were correlated with general and specific impairments in cognitive functions. Despite the inconclusive data, the evidence indicates that folate deficiency may be an independent risk factor for the development of depression in the older population. The most relevant mechanisms relating folate deficiency to the development of depression can be summarized as below: (1) hyperhomocysteinemia; (2) lower occurrence of methylation reactions and tetrahydrobiopterin availability; (3) increased incorporation of uracil into DNA; and (4) shorter telomere length [4].

13.4 Summary

Nutrigenomics is the study of the effects of nutrients and bioactive food compounds on an individual's genetic makeup and genome integrity, which will help us better understand the etiology of nutrition-related disease and find remedies for the prevention of modern diseases such as diabetes, obesity, CVD, cancer, inflammatory disorders, cognitive disorders, etc. Folate and vitamin B12 are among the most cited micronutrients that affect genomic stability by serving as a cofactor for one-carbon transfer reactions involved in DNA methylation, and their deficiency leads to a wide range of cancers, CNS-related disease, and CVD. Vitamin A is also involved in different aspects of human health including vision, immunity, fertilization, fetal development, insulin resistance, etc. It exerts its biological effects on gene expression through RA receptors and also signaling pathways such as MAPK, PPARs, and Janus kinase/STAT5. Vitamin D as a steroid hormone plays a critical role in a various range of biological actions including the regulation of cell growth and the cell cycle, cellular differentiation, apoptosis, immune modulation, and in the integration of hormonal and cellular signaling pathways. It exerts its modulatory effects on gene expression through its nuclear receptor (VDR), which impacts histone modifications, FOXOs, SIRT, NF-κB function, and regulation of cell cycle.

Deficit in the supply of methyl groups leads to the disruption of purine, thymidine, nucleotide, DNA synthesis and transcription, gene expression, and other epigenetic mechanisms affecting growth, differentiation, and repair. Folates and vitamin B_{12} are critical for CNS function at all ages. Proper DNA methylation patterns are essential for normal genome function and aberrant DNA methylation patterns lead to the development of several human diseases like cancer, cognitive decline, dementia, and depression in individuals. Maternal folate deficiency can increase the risk of NTDs in a fetus in comparison with pregnancies of normal folate status. The evidence implies that folate and vitamin B_{12} deficiency are correlated with decreases in global DNA methylation. However, the specific regions of the genome affected by high or low folate intake are not well defined.

13.5 Future insights

The study of the interaction between food and human biology is of great interest and important to develop more efficient nutritional interventions to promote health outcomes through reducing risk factors for chronic disease like obesity and metabolic syndrome, CVDs, and cancer. Elucidating the molecular mechanisms by which the bioactive components of diet exert their effects is the main goal of current nutrigenomics investigations and could lead to the discovery of novel biomarkers. At least four distinct processes are involved in epigenetics: DNA methylation, histone modifications, microRNAs as well as other noncoding regulatory RNA, and chromatin modelling. In case of folate, understanding DNA methylation patterns and genomic regions affected by folate and B_{12} along with sufficient doses appropriate to alter these patterns can create a new pathway for both prevention and treatment of the related diseases. Furthermore, randomized clinical trials with long follow-up periods and large sample sizes need to be performed to determine a more precise supplementation dose to prevent the associated diseases. Vitamin D impacts the expression of approximately 250 genes. The role of vitamin D in CVD and cancer is still an important area of ongoing research, and future studies with an emphasis on high-quality observational and experimental designs are needed to further elucidate the role and potential public health impacts that vitamin D may offer for both traditionally associated roles such as bone health and more recent potential benefits for diseases such as cancer and CVD. The function of vitamin A in regulating energy balance is poorly understood and more studies need to be performed to define the exact mechanism by which RA suppresses obesity and insulin resistance. Furthermore, the roles of retinoids have been investigated extensively in cancer prevention and treatment. Future prevention trials will provide strong evidence for planning combined therapies like using retinoids in combination with epigenetic modifiers such as the HDAC inhibitors, as well as standard cytotoxic agents, tyrosine kinase inhibitors, and other novel agents that have clinical benefits for patients. Moreover, clinical trials should be performed to accurately investigate the biomarkers of response to retinoid therapy.

Although the impacts of folate deficiency on DNA methylation status have been extensively studied, little is known about the effects of high folate intake in this area. It also remains unclear whether folate/FA intake dependently affects DNA methylation and whether there is an interaction with other micronutrients such as other 1-carbon sources (e.g., betaine, choline) or genetic variation. The impact of FA fortification and supplementation on reducing NTDs is studied and has led to mandatory food fortification in most countries. Concerns that folate supplementation increases the risk of cancer or masks vitamin B_{12} deficiency remains a controversy, and more studies should be designed to provide a safe dose recommended for women of childbearing age. Since there is little evidence that FA supplementation, alone or in combination with other B vitamins, can hinder neuropsychiatric diseases in healthy older individuals or slow cognitive decline in older patients, more studies need to be performed. In particular, RCTs with long follow-up periods and large sample sizes need to be performed to determine a more precise supplementation dose to prevent the diseases mentioned above. As mentioned earlier, understanding DNA methylation patterns and genomic regions affected by folate and B_{12} along with sufficient doses appropriate to alter these patterns can create a new pathway for both prevention and treatment of the related diseases.

References

1. Everts HB, Berdanier CD. Regulation of mitochondrial gene expression by retinoids. *IUBMB life*. 2002;54(2):45–9.
2. Rawson JB, Sun Z, Dicks E, Daftary D, Parfrey PS, Green RC, et al. Vitamin D intake is negatively associated with promoter methylation of the Wnt antagonist gene DKK1 in a large group of colorectal cancer patients. *Nutrition and Cancer*. 2012;64(7):919–28.
3. Díaz L, Díaz-Muñoz M, García-Gaytán AC, Méndez I. Mechanistic effects of calcitriol in cancer biology. *Nutrients*. 2015;7(6):5020–50.
4. Araujo JR, Martel F, Borges N, Araujo JM, Keating E. Folates and aging: Role in mild cognitive impairment, dementia and depression. *Ageing Research Reviews*. 2015;22:9–19.
5. Williams JD, Jacobson EL, Kim H, Kim M, Jacobson MK. Folate in skin cancer prevention. *Sub-cellular Biochemistry*. 2012;56:181–97.

6. Choi JH, Yates Z, Veysey M, Heo YR, Lucock M. Contemporary issues surrounding folic acid fortification initiatives. *Preventive Nutrition and Food Science.* 2014;19(4):247–60.
7. McLaren DS, Kraemer K. Vitamin A in nature. *World Review of Nutrition and Dietetics.* 2012;103:7–17.
8. Conaway HH, Henning P, Lerner UH. Vitamin a metabolism, action, and role in skeletal homeostasis. *Endocrine Reviews.* 2013;34(6):766–97.
9. Jeyakumar SM, Vajreswari A. Vitamin A as a key regulator of obesity & its associated disorders: Evidences from an obese rat model. *The Indian Journal of Medical Research.* 2015;141(3):275–84.
10. Landrier JF, Marcotorchino J, Tourniaire F. Lipophilic micronutrients and adipose tissue biology. *Nutrients.* 2012;4(11):1622–49.
11. McLaren DS, Kraemer K. Vitamin A in health. *World Review of Nutrition and Dietetics.* 2012;103:33–51.
12. Zhang YR, Zhao YQ, Huang JF. Retinoid-binding proteins: Similar protein architectures bind similar ligands via completely different ways. *PloS One.* 2012;7(5):e36772.
13. Al Tanoury Z, Piskunov A, Rochette-Egly C. Vitamin A and retinoid signaling: Genomic and nongenomic effects. *Journal of Lipid Research.* 2013;54(7):1761–75.
14. Zhang R, Wang Y, Li R, Chen G. Transcriptional factors mediating retinoic acid signals in the control of energy metabolism. *International Journal of Molecular Sciences.* 2015;16(6):14210–44.
15. Wiseman EM, Bar-El Dadon S, Reifen R. The vicious cycle of vitamin A deficiency: A review. *Critical Reviews in Food Science and Nutrition.* 2016;29:0.
16. Beijer MR, Kraal G, den Haan JM. Vitamin A and dendritic cell differentiation. *Immunology.* 2014;142(1):39–45.
17. Ross AC. Vitamin A and retinoic acid in T cell-related immunity. *The American Journal of Clinical Nutrition.* 2012;96(5):1166S–72S.
18. Albahrani AA, Greaves RF. Fat-Soluble Vitamins: Clinical indications and current challenges for chromatographic measurement. *The Clinical Biochemist Reviews / Australian Association of Clinical Biochemists.* 2016;37(1):27–47.
19. Akhtar S, Ahmed A, Randhawa MA, Atukorala S, Arlappa N, Ismail T, et al. Prevalence of vitamin A deficiency in South Asia: Causes, outcomes, and possible remedies. *Journal of Health, Population, and Nutrition.* 2013;31(4):413–23.
20. Russell RM. The vitamin A spectrum: From deficiency to toxicity. *The American Journal of Clinical Nutrition.* 2000;71(4):878–84.
21. Baineni R, Gulati R, Delhi CK. Vitamin A toxicity presenting as bone pain. *Archives of Disease in Childhood.* 2016. Published Online First: 06 June 2016. doi: 10.1136/archdischild-2016-310631.
22. Uray IP, Dmitrovsky E, Brown PH. Retinoids and rexinoids in cancer prevention: From laboratory to clinic. *Seminars in Oncology.* 2016;43(1):49–64.
23. Yasmeen R, Jeyakumar SM, Reichert B, Yang F, Ziouzenkova O. The contribution of vitamin A to autocrine regulation of fat depots. *Biochimica et Biophysica Acta.* 2012;1821(1):190–7.
24. Duester G. Retinoic acid synthesis and signaling during early organogenesis. *Cell.* 2008;134(6):921–31.
25. Ziouzenkova O, Plutzky J. Retinoid metabolism and nuclear receptor responses: New insights into coordinated regulation of the PPAR-RXR complex. *FEBS Letters.* 2008;582(1):32–8.
26. Esteve E, Ricart W, Fernandez-Real JM. Adipocytokines and insulin resistance: The possible role of lipocalin-2, retinol binding protein-4, and adiponectin. *Diabetes Care.* 2009;32 Suppl 2:S362–7.
27. Rowling MJ, McMullen MH, Schalinske KL. Vitamin A and its derivatives induce hepatic glycine N-methyltransferase and hypomethylation of DNA in rats. *The Journal of Nutrition.* 2002;132(3):365–9.

28. Everts HB, Claassen DO, Hermoyian CL, Berdanier CD. Nutrient-gene interactions: Dietary vitamin A and mitochondrial gene expression. *IUBMB Life*. 2002;53(6):295–301.
29. Bonet ML, Ribot J, Palou A. Lipid metabolism in mammalian tissues and its control by retinoic acid. *Biochimica et Biophysica Acta*. 2012;1821(1):177–89.
30. Berry DC, Noy N. All-trans-retinoic acid represses obesity and insulin resistance by activating both peroxisome proliferation-activated receptor beta/delta and retinoic acid receptor. *Molecular and Cellular Biology*. 2009;29(12):3286–96.
31. Rhee EJ, Plutzky J. Retinoid metabolism and diabetes mellitus. *Diabetes & Metabolism Journal*. 2012;36(3):167–80.
32. Berry DC, DeSantis D, Soltanian H, Croniger CM, Noy N. Retinoic acid upregulates preadipocyte genes to block adipogenesis and suppress diet-induced obesity. *Diabetes*. 2012;61(5):1112–21.
33. Xiong RB, Li Q, Wan WR, Guo JQ, Luo BD, Gan L. Effects and mechanisms of vitamin A and vitamin E on the levels of serum leptin and other related cytokines in rats with rheumatoid arthritis. *Experimental and Therapeutic Medicine*. 2014;8(2):499–504.
34. Chen G, Zhang Y, Lu D, Li NQ, Ross AC. Retinoids synergize with insulin to induce hepatic Gck expression. *The Biochemical Journal*. 2009;419(3):645–53.
35. Sugita S, Kamei Y, Akaike F, Suganami T, Kanai S, Hattori M, et al. Increased systemic glucose tolerance with increased muscle glucose uptake in transgenic mice overexpressing RXRgamma in skeletal muscle. *PloS One*. 2011;6(5):e20467.
36. Jeyakumar SM, Vajreswari A, Giridharan NV. Chronic dietary vitamin A supplementation regulates obesity in an obese mutant WNIN/Ob rat model. *Obesity (Silver Spring, Md)*. 2006;14(1):52–9.
37. Jeyakumar SM, Vijaya Kumar P, Giridharan NV, Vajreswari A. Vitamin A improves insulin sensitivity by increasing insulin receptor phosphorylation through protein tyrosine phosphatase 1B regulation at early age in obese rats of WNIN/Ob strain. *Diabetes, Obesity & Metabolism*. 2011;13(10):955–8.
38. Noy N. Vitamin A in regulation of insulin responsiveness: Mini review. *The Proceedings of the Nutrition Society*. 2016;75(2):212–5.
39. Kane MA, Folias AE, Pingitore A, Perri M, Obrochta KM, Krois CR, et al. Identification of 9-cis-retinoic acid as a pancreas-specific autacoid that attenuates glucose-stimulated insulin secretion. *Proceedings of the National Academy of Sciences of the United States of America*. 2010;107(50):21884–9.
40. Zendehdel K, Nyren O, Ostenson CG, Adami HO, Ekbom A, Ye W. Cancer incidence in patients with type 1 diabetes mellitus: A population-based cohort study in Sweden. *Journal of the National Cancer Institute*. 2003;95(23):1797–800.
41. Baena RM, Campoy C, Bayes R, Blanca E, Fernandez JM, Molina-Font JA. Vitamin A, retinol binding protein and lipids in type 1 diabetes mellitus. *European Journal of Clinical Nutrition*. 2002;56(1):44–50.
42. Takahashi N, Takasu S. A close relationship between type 1 diabetes and vitamin A-deficiency and matrix metalloproteinase and hyaluronidase activities in skin tissues. *Experimental Dermatology*. 2011;20(11):899–904.
43. Yosaee S, Akbari Fakhrabadi M, Shidfar F. Positive evidence for vitamin A role in prevention of type 1 diabetes. *World Journal of Diabetes*. 2016;7(9):177–88.
44. Van YH, Lee WH, Ortiz S, Lee MH, Qin HJ, Liu CP. All-trans retinoic acid inhibits type 1 diabetes by T regulatory (Treg)-dependent suppression of interferon-gamma-producing T-cells without affecting Th17 cells. *Diabetes*. 2009;58(1):146–55.
45. Stosic-Grujicic S, Cvjeticanin T, Stojanovic I. Retinoids differentially regulate the progression of autoimmune diabetes in three preclinical models in mice. *Molecular Immunology*. 2009;47(1):79–86.
46. Connolly RM, Nguyen NK, Sukumar S. Molecular pathways: Current role and future directions of the retinoic acid pathway in cancer prevention and treatment. *Clinical Cancer Research*. 2013;19(7):1651–9.

47. Tanaka Y, Sasaki N, Ohmiya A. Biosynthesis of plant pigments: Anthocyanins, betalains and carotenoids. *The Plant Journal.* 2008;54(4):733–49.
48. Bonet ML, Canas JA, Ribot J, Palou A. Carotenoids and their conversion products in the control of adipocyte function, adiposity and obesity. *Archives of Biochemistry and Biophysics.* 2015;572:112–25.
49. Tanaka T, Shnimizu M, Moriwaki H. Cancer chemoprevention by carotenoids. *Molecules.* 2012;17(3):3202–42.
50. de Paula FJ, Rosen CJ. Vitamin D safety and requirements. *Archives of Biochemistry and Biophysics.* 2012;523(1):64–72.
51. Ingraham BA, Bragdon B, Nohe A. Molecular basis of the potential of vitamin D to prevent cancer. *Current Medical Research and Opinion.* 2008;24(1):139–49.
52. Nikooyeh B, Neyestani TR. Oxidative stress, type 2 diabetes and vitamin D: Past, present and future. *Diabetes/Metabolism Research and Reviews.* 2016;32(3):260–7.
53. Judd SE, Tangpricha V. Vitamin D deficiency and risk for cardiovascular disease. *The American Journal of the Medical Sciences.* 2009;338(1):40–4.
54. Jones G, Prosser DE, Kaufmann M. 25-Hydroxyvitamin D-24-hydroxylase (CYP24A1): Its important role in the degradation of vitamin D. *Archives of Biochemistry and Biophysics.* 2012;523(1):9–18.
55. Nesterova G, Malicdan MC, Yasuda K, Sakaki T, Vilboux T, Ciccone C, et al. 1,25-(OH)2D-24 Hydroxylase (CYP24A1) Deficiency as a cause of nephrolithiasis. *Clinical Journal of the American Society of Nephrology: CJASN.* 2013;8(4):649–57.
56. Neyestani TR. Is multiple sclerosis a sun deprivation disease? In: Watson RR, Preedy VR, editors. *Bioactive Nutraceuticals and Dietary Supplements in Neurological and Brain Disease, Prevention and Therapy.* Waltham, MA: Elsevier; 2015. pp. 481–94.
57. Pereira F, Barbachano A, Singh PK, Campbell MJ, Munoz A, Larriba MJ. Vitamin D has wide regulatory effects on histone demethylase genes. *Cell cycle (Georgetown, Tex).* 2012;11(6):1081–9.
58. Thacher TD, Clarke BL. Vitamin D insufficiency. *Mayo Clinic Proceedings.* 2011;86(1):50–60.
59. Neyestani TR, Djazayery A, Shab-Bidar S, Eshraghian MR, Kalayi A, Shariatzadeh N, et al. Vitamin D receptor fok-I polymorphism modulates diabetic host response to vitamin D intake: Need for a nutrigenetic approach. *Diabetes Care.* 2013;36(3): 550–6.
60. Shab-Bidar S, Neyestani TR, Djazayery A. Vitamin D receptor Cdx-2-dependent response of central obesity to vitamin D intake in the subjects with type 2 diabetes: A randomised clinical trial. *The British Journal of Nutrition.* 2015;114(9):1375–84.
61. Shab-Bidar S, Neyestani TR, Djazayery A. The interactive effect of improvement of vitamin D status and VDR FokI variants on oxidative stress in type 2 diabetic subjects: A randomized controlled trial. *European Journal of Clinical Nutrition.* 2015;69(2):216–22.
62. Neyestani TR. Vitamin D and Skin Cancer: Meet Sunshine Halfway. In: *Bioactive Dietary Factors and Plant Extracts in Dermatology.* Watson RR and Zibadi S (Eds.). New York: Springer; 2013. pp. 257–268.
63. Lange NE, Litonjua A, Hawrylowicz CM, Weiss S. Vitamin D, the immune system and asthma. *Expert Review of Clinical Immunology.* 2009;5(6):693–702.
64. Holick MF. Sunlight, ultraviolet radiation, vitamin D and skin cancer: How much sunlight do we need? *Advances in Experimental Medicine and Biology.* 2014;810:1–16.
65. Ghandchi Z, Neyestani TR, Yaraghi AA, Eshraghian MR, Gharavi A, Shariatzadeh N, et al. Vitamin D status and the predictors of circulating T helper 1-type immunoglobulin levels in Iranian subjects with type 1 diabetes and their siblings: A case-control study. *Journal of Human Nutrition and Dietetics.: The Official Journal of the British Dietetic Association.* 2012;25(4):365–72.

308 Nutrigenomics and Nutraceuticals

66. Neyestani TR. Vitamin D, oxidative stress and diabetes: Is there a link. In: *Diabetes: Oxidative Stress and Dietary Antioxidants.* Preedy VR, (editor). Waltham, MA: Elsevier/Academic Press, 2014. pp.111–120.
67. Kennel KA, Drake MT, Hurley DL, editors. Vitamin D deficiency in adults: When to test and how to treat. *Mayo Clinic Proceedings.* 2010;85:752–8.
68. Alshahrani F, Aljohani N. Vitamin D: Deficiency, sufficiency and toxicity. *Nutrients.* 2013;5(9):3605–16.
69. Fetahu IS, Hobaus J, Kallay E. Vitamin D and the epigenome. *Frontiers in Physiology.* 2014;5:164.
70. Haussler MR, Jurutka PW, Mizwicki M, Norman AW. Vitamin D receptor (VDR) mediated actions of 1α,25(OH)(2)vitamin D(3): Genomic and non-genomic mechanisms. *Best Practice & Research Clinical Endocrinology & Metabolism.* 201125(4):543–59.
71. Sundar IK, Rahman I. Vitamin d and susceptibility of chronic lung diseases: Role of epigenetics. *Frontiers in Pharmacology.* 2011;2:50.
72. de Sa Del Fiol F, Barberato-Filho S, Lopes LC, de Cassia Bergamaschi C. Vitamin D and respiratory infections. *Journal of Infection in Developing Countries.* 2015;9(4): 355–61.
73. Cegielski P, Vernon A. Tuberculosis and vitamin D: What's the rest of the story? *The Lancet Infectious Diseases.* 2015;15(5):489–90.
74. Das BK, Panda AK. Vitamin D: The unexplored immunomodulator. *International Journal of Rheumatic Diseases.* 2016;19(4):332–4.
75. Barragan M, Good M, Kolls JK. Regulation of dendritic cell function by vitamin D. *Nutrients.* 2015;7(9):8127–51.
76. Trochoutsou AI, Kloukina V, Samitas K, Xanthou G. Vitamin-D in the immune system: Genomic and non-genomic actions. *Mini Reviews in Medicinal Chemistry.* 2015;15(11):953–63.
77. Ferreira GB, van Etten E, Verstuyf A, Waer M, Overbergh L, Gysemans C, et al. 1,25-Dihydroxyvitamin D3 alters murine dendritic cell behaviour in vitro and in vivo. *Diabetes/Metabolism Research and Reviews.* 2011;27(8):933–41.
78. Waschbisch A, Sanderson N, Krumbholz M, Vlad G, Theil D, Schwab S, et al. Interferon beta and vitamin D synergize to induce immunoregulatory receptors on peripheral blood monocytes of multiple sclerosis patients. *PloS One.* 2014;9(12):e115488.
79. Li X, Zheng Y. Regulatory T cell identity: Formation and maintenance. *Trends in Immunology.* 2015;36(6):344–53.
80. Urry Z, Chambers ES, Xystrakis E, Dimeloe S, Richards DF, Gabrysova L, et al. The role of 1alpha,25-dihydroxyvitamin D3 and cytokines in the promotion of distinct Foxp3+ and IL-10+ CD4+ T cells. *European Journal of Immunology.* 2012;42(10): 2697–708.
81. Kang SW, Kim SH, Lee N, Lee WW, Hwang KA, Shin MS, et al. 1,25-Dihyroxyvitamin D3 promotes FOXP3 expression via binding to vitamin D response elements in its conserved noncoding sequence region. *Journal of Immunology.* 2012;188(11):5276–82.
82. Fabre-Mersseman V, Tubiana R, Papagno L, Bayard C, Briceno O, Fastenackels S, et al. Vitamin D supplementation is associated with reduced immune activation levels in HIV-1-infected patients on suppressive antiretroviral therapy. *AIDS.* 2014;28(18):2677–82.
83. Thompson MR, Kaminski JJ, Kurt-Jones EA, Fitzgerald KA. Pattern recognition receptors and the innate immune response to viral infection. *Viruses.* 2011;3(6):920–40.
84. Urry Z, Xystrakis E, Richards DF, McDonald J, Sattar Z, Cousins DJ, et al. Ligation of TLR9 induced on human IL-10-secreting Tregs by 1alpha,25-dihydroxyvitamin D3 abrogates regulatory function. *The Journal of Clinical Investigation.* 2009;119(2):387–98.
85. Cantorna MT, Snyder L, Lin YD, Yang L. Vitamin D and 1,25(OH)2D regulation of T cells. *Nutrients.* 2015;7(4):3011–21.
86. Litonjua AA. Childhood asthma may be a consequence of vitamin D deficiency. *Current Opinion in Allergy and Clinical Immunology.* 2009;9(3):202–7.

87. Lovinsky-Desir S, Miller RL. Epigenetics, asthma, and allergic diseases: A review of the latest advancements. *Current Allergy and Asthma Reports.* 2012;12(3):211–20.
88. Hamzaoui A, Berraies A, Hamdi B, Kaabachi W, Ammar J, Hamzaoui K. Vitamin D reduces the differentiation and expansion of Th17 cells in young asthmatic children. *Immunobiology.* 2014;219(11):873–9.
89. Samuel S, Sitrin MD. Vitamin D's role in cell proliferation and differentiation. *Nutrition Reviews.* 2008;66(10 Suppl 2):S116–24.
90. Lai Y-H, Fang T-C. The pleiotropic effect of vitamin D. *ISRN Nephrology.* 2013;2013: 898125.
91. Tabasi N, Rastin M, Mahmoudi M, Ghoryani M, Mirfeizi Z, Zamani Taghizadeh Rabe S, et al. Influence of vitamin D on cell cycle, apoptosis, and some apoptosis related molecules in systemic lupus erythematosus. *Iranian Journal of Basic Medical Sciences.* 2015;18(11):1107–11.
92. Murthy S, Weigel NL. 1α,25-dihydroxyvitamin D3 induced growth inhibition of PC-3 prostate cancer cells requires an active transforming growth factor beta signaling pathway. *The Prostate.* 2004;59(3):282–91.
93. Berkovich L, Ben-Shabat S, Sintov AC. Induction of apoptosis and inhibition of prostate and breast cancer growth by BGP-15, a new calcipotriene-derived vitamin D3 analog. *Anti-cancer Drugs.* 2010;21(6):609–18.
94. Berkovich L, Sintov AC, Ben-Shabat S. Inhibition of cancer growth and induction of apoptosis by BGP-13 and BGP-15, new calcipotriene-derived vitamin D3 analogs, in-vitro and in-vivo studies. *Investigational New Drugs.* 2013;31(2):247–55.
95. Zhu T, Liu TJ, Shi YY, Zhao Q. Vitamin D/VDR signaling pathway ameliorates 2,4,6-trinitrobenzene sulfonic acid-induced colitis by inhibiting intestinal epithelial apoptosis. *International Journal of Molecular Medicine.* 2015;35(5):1213–8.
96. Ordonez-Moran P, Larriba MJ, Palmer HG, Valero RA, Barbachano A, Dunach M, et al. RhoA-ROCK and p38MAPK-MSK1 mediate vitamin D effects on gene expression, phenotype, and Wnt pathway in colon cancer cells. *The Journal of Cell Biology.* 2008;183(4):697–710.
97. Campbell FC, Xu H, El-Tanani M, Crowe P, Bingham V. The yin and yang of vitamin D receptor (VDR) signaling in neoplastic progression: Operational networks and tissue-specific growth control. *Biochemical Pharmacology.* 2010;79(1):1–9.
98. Palmer HG, Gonzalez-Sancho JM, Espada J, Berciano MT, Puig I, Baulida J, et al. Vitamin D(3) promotes the differentiation of colon carcinoma cells by the induction of E-cadherin and the inhibition of beta-catenin signaling. *The Journal of Cell Biology.* 2001;154(2):369–87.
99. Lopes N, Carvalho J, Duraes C, Sousa B, Gomes M, Costa JL, et al. 1α,25-Dihydroxyvitamin D3 induces de novo E-cadherin expression in triple-negative breast cancer cells by CDH1-promoter demethylation. *Anticancer Research.* 2012;32(1):249–57.
100. Pendas-Franco N, Gonzalez-Sancho JM, Suarez Y, Aguilera O, Steinmeyer A, Gamallo C, et al. Vitamin D regulates the phenotype of human breast cancer cells. *Differentiation.* 2007;75(3):193–207.
101. Keith ME, LaPorta E, Welsh J. Stable expression of human VDR in murine VDR-null cells recapitulates vitamin D mediated anti-cancer signaling. *Molecular Carcinogenesis.* 2014;53(4):286–99.
102. Salekzamani S, Neyestani TR, Alavi-Majd H, Houshiarrad A, Kalayi A, Shariatzadeh N, et al. Is vitamin D status a determining factor for metabolic syndrome? A case-control study. *Diabetes, Metabolic Syndrome and Obesity : Targets and Therapy.* 2011;4:205–12.
103. Bikle DD. Vitamin D metabolism, mechanism of action, and clinical applications. *Chemistry & Biology.* 2014;21(3):319–29.
104. Mutt SJ, Hypponen E, Saarnio J, Jarvelin MR, Herzig KH. Vitamin D and adipose tissue-more than storage. *Frontiers in Physiology.* 2014;5:228.

105. Bhat M, Noolu B, Qadri SS, Ismail A. Vitamin D deficiency decreases adiposity in rats and causes altered expression of uncoupling proteins and steroid receptor coactivator3. *The Journal of Steroid Biochemistry and Molecular Biology.* 2014;144 Pt B:304–12.

106. Chang E, Kim Y. Vitamin D decreases adipocyte lipid storage and increases NAD-SIRT1 pathway in 3T3-L1 adipocytes. *Nutrition.* 2016;32(6):702–8.

107. vinh quoc Lu'o'ng K, Nguyen LT. The beneficial role of vitamin D in obesity: Possible genetic and cell signaling mechanisms. *Nutrition Journal.* 2013;12:89.

108. Belo VA, Souza-Costa DC, Lana CM, Caputo FL, Marcaccini AM, Gerlach RF, et al. Assessment of matrix metalloproteinase (MMP)-2, MMP-8, MMP-9, and their inhibitors, the tissue inhibitors of metalloproteinase (TIMP)-1 and TIMP-2 in obese children and adolescents. *Clinical Biochemistry.* 2009;42(10–11):984–90.

109. Chagas CE, Borges MC, Martini LA, Rogero MM. Focus on vitamin D, inflammation and type 2 diabetes. *Nutrients.* 2012;4(1):52–67.

110. Shab-Bidar S, Neyestani TR, Djazayery A. Efficacy of vitamin D3-fortified-yogurt drink on anthropometric, metabolic, inflammatory and oxidative stress biomarkers according to vitamin D receptor gene polymorphisms in type 2 diabetic patients: A study protocol for a randomized controlled clinical trial. *BMC Endocrine Disorders.* 2011;11:12.

111. Shab-Bidar S, Neyestani TR, Djazayery A, Eshraghian MR, Houshiarrad A, Gharavi A, et al. Regular consumption of vitamin D-fortified yogurt drink (Doogh) improved endothelial biomarkers in subjects with type 2 diabetes: A randomized double-blind clinical trial. *BMC Medicine.* 2011;9:125.

112. Neyestani TR, Nikooyeh B, Alavi-Majd H, Shariatzadeh N, Kalayi A, Tayebinejad N, et al. Improvement of vitamin D status via daily intake of fortified yogurt drink either with or without extra calcium ameliorates systemic inflammatory biomarkers, including adipokines, in the subjects with type 2 diabetes. *The Journal of Clinical Endocrinology and Metabolism.* 2012;97(6):2005–11.

113. Shab-Bidar S, Neyestani TR, Djazayery A, Eshraghian MR, Houshiarrad A, Kalayi A, et al. Improvement of vitamin D status resulted in amelioration of biomarkers of systemic inflammation in the subjects with type 2 diabetes. *Diabetes/Metabolism Research and Reviews.* 2012;28(5):424–30.

114. von Hurst PR, Stonehouse W, Coad J. Vitamin D supplementation reduces insulin resistance in South Asian women living in New Zealand who are insulin resistant and vitamin D deficient—A randomised, placebo-controlled trial. *The British Journal of Nutrition.* 2010;103(4):549–55.

115. Al-Shoumer KA, Al-Essa TM. Is there a relationship between vitamin D with insulin resistance and diabetes mellitus? *World journal of Diabetes.* 2015;6(8):1057–64.

116. Talaei A, Mohamadi M, Adgi Z. The effect of vitamin D on insulin resistance in patients with type 2 diabetes. *Diabetology & Metabolic Syndrome.* 2013;5(1):1–5.

117. Nikooyeh B, Neyestani TR, Farvid M, Alavi-Majd H, Houshiarrad A, Kalayi A, et al. Daily consumption of vitamin D–or vitamin D+ calcium–fortified yogurt drink improved glycemic control in patients with type 2 diabetes: A randomized clinical trial. *The American Journal of Clinical Nutrition.* 2011;93(4):764–71.

118. Hossein-nezhad A, Holick MF. Vitamin D for health: A global perspective. *Mayo Clinic Proceedings.* 2013;88(7):720–55.

119. Broder AR, Tobin JN, Putterman C. Disease-specific definitions of vitamin D deficiency need to be established in autoimmune and non-autoimmune chronic diseases: A retrospective comparison of three chronic diseases. *Arthritis Research & Therapy.* 2010;12(5):R191.

120. Agmon-Levin N, Theodor E, Segal RM, Shoenfeld Y. Vitamin D in systemic and organ-specific autoimmune diseases. *Clinical Reviews in Allergy & Immunology.* 2013;45(2):256–66.

121. Yang CY, Leung PS, Adamopoulos IE, Gershwin ME. The implication of vitamin D and autoimmunity: A comprehensive review. *Clinical Reviews in Allergy & Immunology.* 2013;45(2):217–26.
122. Di Rosa M, Malaguarnera M, Nicoletti F, Malaguarnera L. Vitamin D3: A helpful immuno-modulator. *Immunology.* 2011;134(2):123–39.
123. Lin J, Liu J, Davies ML, Chen W. Serum vitamin D level and rheumatoid arthritis disease activity: Review and meta-analysis. *PloS One.* 2016;11(1):e0146351.
124. Villaggio B, Soldano S, Cutolo M. 1,25-dihydroxyvitamin D3 downregulates aromatase expression and inflammatory cytokines in human macrophages. *Clinical and Experimental Rheumatology.* 2012;30(6):934–8.
125. Kostoglou-Athanassiou I, Athanassiou P, Lyraki A, Raftakis I, Antoniadis C. Vitamin D and rheumatoid arthritis. *Therapeutic Advances in Endocrinology and Metabolism.* 2012;3(6):181–7.
126. Mokry LE, Ross S, Ahmad OS, Forgetta V, Smith GD, Leong A, et al. Vitamin D and risk of multiple sclerosis: A Mendelian randomization study. *PLoS Medicine.* 2015;12(8):e1001866.
127. Antico A, Tampoia M, Tozzoli R, Bizzaro N. Can supplementation with vitamin D reduce the risk or modify the course of autoimmune diseases? A systematic review of the literature. *Autoimmunity Reviews.* 2012;12(2):127–36.
128. Beydoun MA, Fanelli Kuczmarski MT, Beydoun HA, Shroff MR, Mason MA, Evans MK, et al. The sex-specific role of plasma folate in mediating the association of dietary quality with depressive symptoms. *The Journal of Nutrition.* 2010;140(2):338–47.
129. Czeizel AE, Dudas I, Vereczkey A, Banhidy F. Folate deficiency and folic acid supplementation: The prevention of neural-tube defects and congenital heart defects. *Nutrients.* 2013;5(11):4760–75.
130. Ami N, Bernstein M, Boucher F, Rieder M, Parker L. Folate and neural tube defects: The role of supplements and food fortification. *Paediatrics & Child Health.* 2016;21(3):145–54.
131. Greenberg JA, Bell SJ, Guan Y, Yu Y-h. Folic acid supplementation and pregnancy: More than just neural tube defect prevention. *Reviews in Obstetrics and Gynecology.* 2011;4(2):52–9.
132. Stover PJ. Physiology of folate and vitamin B12 in health and disease. *Nutrition reviews.* 2004; 62(s1).
133. Gueant JL, Namour F, Gueant-Rodriguez RM, Daval JL. Folate and fetal programming: A play in epigenomics? *Trends in Endocrinology and Metabolism: TEM.* 2013;24(6):279–89.
134. Hanna S, Lachover L, Rajarethinam R. Vitamin B12 deficiency and depression in the elderly: Review and case report. *Primary Care Companion to the Journal of Clinical Psychiatry.* 2009;11(5):269.
135. Sauer J, Mason JB, Choi SW. Too much folate: A risk factor for cancer and cardiovascular disease? *Current Opinion in Clinical Nutrition and Metabolic Care.* 2009;12(1):30–6.
136. Lin J, Lee IM, Cook NR, Selhub J, Manson JE, Buring JE, et al. Plasma folate, vitamin B-6, vitamin B-12, and risk of breast cancer in women. *The American Journal of Clinical Nutrition.* 2008;87(3):734–43.
137. Stolzenberg-Solomon RZ, Chang SC, Leitzmann MF, Johnson KA, Johnson C, Buys SS, et al. Folate intake, alcohol use, and postmenopausal breast cancer risk in the prostate, lung, colorectal, and ovarian cancer screening trial. *The American Journal of Clinical Nutrition.* 2006;83(4):895–904.
138. Selhub J, Rosenberg IH. Excessive folic acid intake and relation to adverse health outcome. *Biochimie.* 2016;126:71–8.
139. Hunt A, Harrington D, Robinson S. Vitamin B12 deficiency. *BMJ.* 2014;349:g5226.

140. Lachner C, Steinle NI, Regenold WT. The neuropsychiatry of vitamin B12 deficiency in elderly patients. *Journal of Neuropsychiatry and Clinical Neurosciences.* 2012;24(1):5–15.

141. Wilson RD, Wilson RD, Audibert F, Brock JA, Carroll J, Cartier L, et al. Pre-conception folic acid and multivitamin supplementation for the primary and secondary prevention of neural tube defects and other folic acid-sensitive congenital anomalies. *Journal of obstetrics and gynaecology Canada: JOGC = Journal d'obstetrique et gynecologie du Canada: JOGC.* 2015;37(6):534–52.

142. Molloy AM, Kirke PN, Troendle JF, Burke H, Sutton M, Brody LC, et al. Maternal vitamin B12 status and risk of neural tube defects in a population with high neural tube defect prevalence and no folic Acid fortification. *Pediatrics.* 2009;123(3):917–23.

143. Kim YI. Nutritional epigenetics: Impact of folate deficiency on DNA methylation and colon cancer susceptibility. *The Journal of Nutrition.* 2005;135(11):2703–9.

144. McNeil CJ, Beattie JH, Gordon MJ, Pirie LP, Duthie SJ. Differential effects of nutritional folic acid deficiency and moderate hyperhomocysteinemia on aortic plaque formation and genome-wide DNA methylation in vascular tissue from ApoE-/- mice. *Clinical Epigenetics.* 2011;2(2):361–8.

145. Haslberger A, Varga F, Karlic H. Recursive causality in evolution: A model for epigenetic mechanisms in cancer development. *Medical Hypotheses.* 2006;67(6):1448–54.

146. Coppedè F. Epigenetic biomarkers of colorectal cancer: Focus on DNA methylation. *Cancer Letters.* 2014;342:238–47.

147. Luo WP, Li B, Lin FY, Yan B, Du YF, Mo XF, et al. Joint effects of folate intake and one-carbon-metabolizing genetic polymorphisms on breast cancer risk: A case-control study in China. *Scientific Reports.* 2016;6:29555.

148. Pravenec M, Kozich V, Krijt J, Sokolova J, Zidek V, Landa V, et al. Folate deficiency is associated with oxidative stress, increased blood pressure, and insulin resistance in spontaneously hypertensive rats. *American Journal of Hypertension.* 2013;26(1):135–40.

149. Wang J, Wu Z, Li D, Li N, Dindot SV, Satterfield MC, et al. Nutrition, epigenetics, and metabolic syndrome. *Antioxidants & Redox Signaling.* 2012;17(2):282–301.

150. Pacher P, Beckman JS, Liaudet L. Nitric oxide and peroxynitrite in health and disease. *Physiological Reviews.* 2007;87(1):315–424.

151. Dupont LL, Glynos C, Bracke KR, Brouckaert P, Brusselle GG. Role of the nitric oxide-soluble guanylyl cyclase pathway in obstructive airway diseases. *Pulmonary Pharmacology & Therapeutics.* 2014;29(1):1–6.

152. Mangge H, Becker K, Fuchs D, Gostner JM. Antioxidants, inflammation and cardiovascular disease. *World Journal of Cardiology.* 2014;6(6):462–77.

153. Najib S, Sanchez-Margalet V. Homocysteine thiolactone inhibits insulin signaling, and glutathione has a protective effect. *Journal of Molecular Endocrinology.* 2001;27(1):85–91.

154. Adaikalakoteswari A, Finer S, Voyias PD, McCarthy CM, Vatish M, Moore J, et al. Vitamin B12 insufficiency induces cholesterol biosynthesis by limiting s-adenosylmethionine and modulating the methylation of SREBF1 and LDLR genes. *Clinical Epigenetics.* 2015;7:14.

155. McRae MP. High-dose folic acid supplementation effects on endothelial function and blood pressure in hypertensive patients: A meta-analysis of randomized controlled clinical trials. *Journal of Chiropractic Medicine.* 2009;8(1):15–24.

156. Zaganjor I, Sekkarie A, Tsang BL, Williams J, Razzaghi H, Mulinare J, et al. Describing the prevalence of neural tube defects worldwide: A systematic literature review. *PloS One.* 2016;11(4):e0151586.

157. Ray JG, Wyatt PR, Thompson MD, Vermeulen MJ, Meier C, Wong PY, et al. Vitamin B12 and the risk of neural tube defects in a folic-acid-fortified population. *Epidemiology.* 2007;18(3):362–6.

158. Fluegge K. Methyl B12 and autism spectrum disorders: Any clues to etiology? *Journal of Child and Adolescent Psychopharmacology.* 2016;26:853.
159. Zhang Y, Hodgson NW, Trivedi MS, Abdolmaleky HM, Fournier M, Cuenod M, et al. Decreased brain levels of vitamin B12 in aging, autism and schizophrenia. *PloS One.* 2016;11(1):e0146797.
160. Hendren RL, James SJ, Widjaja F, Lawton B, Rosenblatt A, Bent S. Randomized, Placebo-controlled trial of methyl B12 for children with autism. *Journal of Child and Adolescent Psychopharmacology.* 2016;26:774–83.
161. Lubana SS, Alfishawy M, Singh N, Atkinson S. Vitamin B12 deficiency and elevated folate levels: An unusual cause of generalized tonic-clonic seizure. *The American Journal of Case Reports.* 2015;16:386–9.
162. Baldelli E, Leo G, Andreoli N, Fuxe K, Biagini G, Agnati LF. Homocysteine potentiates seizures and cell loss induced by pilocarpine treatment. *Neuromolecular Medicine.* 2010;12(3):248–59.
163. Eldeen ON, Abd Eldayem SM, Shatla RH, Omara NA, Elgammal SS. Homocysteine, folic acid and vitamin B12 levels in serum of epileptic children. *Egyptian Journal of Medical Human Genetics.* 2012;13(3):275–80.
164. Kurul S, Unalp A, Yis U. Homocysteine levels in epileptic children receiving antiepileptic drugs. *Journal of Child Neurology.* 2007;22(12):1389–92.
165. Linnebank M, Moskau S, Semmler A, Widman G, Stoffel-Wagner B, Weller M, et al. Antiepileptic drugs interact with folate and vitamin B12 serum levels. *Annals of Neurology.* 2011;69(2):352–9.
166. Ozdemir O, Yakut A, Dinleyici EC, Aydogdu SD, Yarar C, Colak O. Serum asymmetric dimethylarginine (ADMA), homocysteine, vitamin B(12), folate levels, and lipid profiles in epileptic children treated with valproic acid. *European Journal of Pediatrics.* 2011;170(7):873–7.
167. Sharma TK, Vardey SK, Sitaraman S. Evaluate the effect of valproate monotherapy on the serum homocysteine, folate and vitamin B12 levels in epileptic children. *Clinical Laboratory.* 2015;61(8):933–40.
168. Vurucu S, Demirkaya E, Kul M, Unay B, Gul D, Akin R, et al. Evaluation of the relationship between C677T variants of methylenetetrahydrofolate reductase gene and hyperhomocysteinemia in children receiving antiepileptic drug therapy. *Progress in Neuro-Psychopharmacology & Biological Psychiatry.* 2008;32(3):844–8.
169. Coppola G, Ingrosso D, Operto FF, Signoriello G, Lattanzio F, Barone E, et al. Role of folic acid depletion on homocysteine serum level in children and adolescents with epilepsy and different MTHFR C677T genotypes. *Seizure.* 2012;21(5):340–3.
170. Reynolds EH. The neurology of folic acid deficiency. *Handbook of Clinical Neurology.* 2014;120:927–43.
171. Agarwal R, Chhillar N, Kushwaha S, Singh NK, Tripathi CB. Role of vitamin B(12), folate, and thyroid stimulating hormone in dementia: A hospital-based study in north Indian population. *Annals of Indian Academy of Neurology.* 2010;13(4):257–62.
172. Agarwal R. Vitamin B(1)(2) deficiency & cognitive impairment in elderly population. *The Indian Journal of Medical Research.* 2011;134:410-2.
173. Malouf M, Grimley EJ, Areosa SA. Folic acid with or without vitamin B12 for cognition and dementia. *The Cochrane Database of Systematic Reviews.* 2003(4):CD004514.
174. Sachdev PS, Parslow RA, Lux O, Salonikas C, Wen W, Naidoo D, et al. Relationship of homocysteine, folic acid and vitamin B12 with depression in a middle-aged community sample. *Psychological Medicine.* 2005;35(4):529–38.
175. Moore EM, Ames D, Mander AG, Carne RP, Brodaty H, Woodward MC, et al. Among vitamin B12 deficient older people, high folate levels are associated with worse cognitive function: Combined data from three cohorts. *Journal of Alzheimer's Disease: JAD.* 2014;39(3):661–8.

14

Nutrigenomic Aspects of Trace Elements

Sudabeh Motamed, Bahareh Nikooyeh, and Tirang R. Neyestani
Shahid Beheshti University of Medical Sciences
Tehran, Iran

Contents

14.1 Introduction 316
14.2 Iron 317
    14.2.1 Iron regulation mechanisms 318
    14.2.2 Iron functions 319
        14.2.2.1 Iron-dependent cofactors 319
        14.2.2.2 Iron-dependent enzymes 319
        14.2.2.3 Iron and the cell cycle 320
        14.2.2.4 Iron and epigenetics 321
    14.2.3 Iron and nutrigenomics 322
        14.2.3.1 Iron and gene instability 323
        14.2.3.2 Iron overload and genome instability 323
        14.2.3.3 Iron deficiency and genome instability.................. 325
        14.2.3.4 Genomic effect of iron on metabolism.................. 326
        14.2.3.5 Iron and cancer 327
        14.2.3.6 Iron and aging.. 329
14.3 Zinc 330
    14.3.1 Zinc deficiency 331
    14.3.2 Zinc overload 332
    14.3.3 Zinc and genome 332
        14.3.3.1 Zinc and the immune/inflammatory system 333
        14.3.3.2 Zinc and gene stability.. 335
        14.3.3.3 Zinc and telomere length 337
    14.3.4 Zinc and epigenetics 337
    14.3.5 Zinc and apoptosis.. 339
    14.3.6 Zinc and signaling 341
    14.3.7 Zinc and metabolism 341

	14.3.8 Zinc and disease	342
	14.3.8.1 Zinc and cancer	342
	14.3.8.2 Zinc and aging	344
	14.3.8.3 Zinc and obesity	344
	14.3.8.4 Zinc and type 2 diabetes	345
	14.3.8.5 Zinc and atherosclerosis	346
14.4	Selenium	347
	14.4.1 Selenium deficiency	348
	14.4.2 Selenium toxicity	349
	14.4.3 Selenium and epigenetics	349
	14.4.4 Selenium and nutrigenomics	350
	14.4.5 Selenium and genomic stability	352
	14.4.6 Selenium and diseases	354
	14.4.6.1 Selenium and cancer	355
	14.4.6.2 Selenium and age-related diseases	359
14.5	Summary	360
14.6	Future insights	361
References		362

14.1 Introduction

The effect of the nutritional milieu on health begins long before a human is born and takes the first breath. It has been shown that poor maternal nutrition status, either under- or overnutrition, can determine the metabolic fate of the child in his or her adulthood [1–3]. Evidence from experimental studies has revealed that nutritional insults during pregnancy will result in fetal programming for future morbidities with aging [4]. The effects of developmental programming may be transferred even to further generations [5]. Interestingly, it has recently been reported that the nutritional status of the father may also have a role in programming the offspring's phenotype. Increased fat mass in a fat father may induce genetic changes in his sperm that predispose his unborn child to obesity later in life [6]. Indeed, the interaction of nutrients and genes determines the health outcomes.

Among all nutrients and bioactive compounds, micronutrients, including vitamins and minerals, deserve special attention. Though the human body needs only minute amounts of micronutrients, usually acquired through a balanced diet, they affect almost all aspects of life. Though overt micronutrient deficiency may be uncommon in many countries, marginal deficiency affects billions of people worldwide. Consequently, though the stomach may be full, the cells are "hungry." Hence subclinical micronutrient deficiency is often referred to as "hidden hunger," a situation that has no clinical symptoms but still has genomic effects.

Zinc, iron, and selenium, for instance, are essential trace elements in the diet that are related to altered biological functions during aging, potentially through affecting antioxidant capacity or the expression of proteins responsible for biological functions. It has been proposed that deficiencies or excess of these trace elements can influence genomic stability, which in turn is associated with aging and cancer risk [7–9].

Zinc, iron, and selenium deficiencies and ionizing radiation have been found to convey similar effects on oxidative stress-induced DNA damage, reactive oxygen species (ROS) production, and the associated DNA instability [7]. Trace elements affect genome stability directly or indirectly, as a component of the enzymes affecting the genomic network [7].

According to the results of a systematic review, an appropriate serum concentration of trace elements (mainly zinc, copper, and selenium) in human centenarians was associated with satisfactory immune functions, increased antioxidant capabilities, and slight inflammation. Furthermore, through a nutrigenomic approach, these trace elements were suggested to influence the expression of genes encoding pro- and anti-inflammatory cytokines, as well as proteins involved in trace element homeostasis, such as metallothioneins (MTs), which are all involved in age-related disorders [10]. It has been proposed that deficiencies or excess of trace elements can influence genomic stability, which in turn is associated with aging and cancer risk [7–9].

Regarding the association between trace elements and DNA damage response pathways, fighting hidden hunger could potentially be a preventive strategy against genome instability–related disorders [11] like cancers [11–13].

This chapter is not intended to cover all trace elements but just those that have been more widely studied by the nutrigenomic approach and whose deficiencies are more prevalent than other trace elements.

14.2 Iron

Iron is the most abundant and essential trace element in the human body and most eukaryotic cells. Iron-deficiency anemia (IDA) is the world's most common nutritional deficiency disease despite the wide availability of iron-rich foods. IDA mostly occurs in children and pregnant women [14].

The total iron content of the human body exists in two major pools: (1) functional iron, or heme iron, which is the essential constituent for oxygen transport in hemoglobin, oxygen storage in myoglobin, and the function of enzymes involved in aerobic respiration (cytochromes) and signal transduction (nitric oxide synthase and guanylyl cyclase); and (2) storage iron in ferritin, hemosiderin, and transferrin. Total iron in the body in healthy men is estimated at 3.6 g, whereas women have approximately 2.4 g. The amount of iron storage in adult women is much lower than men. Iron metabolism is subject to a high degree of conservation; approximately 90% is captured for reutilization in the production of new erythrocytes and the rest is excreted, in feces (0.6 mg/day), urine (0.1 mg/day), and sweat (0.3 mg/day). The average blood loss during the menstrual period is approximately 40 mL/cycle or 0.4 to 0.5 mg/day [15].

There are two concerns about iron nutritional status. It has been shown that iron deficiency (ID) and also its excess increase mitochondrial DNA damage and subsequently mitochondrial dysfunction, which results in increased generation of reactive ROS. Moreover, elevated ROS production has been suggested to be associated with increased risk of several physiological disorders including chronic diseases and cancer risk [16,17].

14.2.1 Iron regulation mechanisms

The mechanism of iron regulation can be defined by the following steps:

1. Following digestion, heme iron from animal sources enters the cytosol of intestinal absorbing cells via vesicle formation around the heme. Following enzymatic digestion, Fe^{2+} is removed from heme.
2. Nonheme iron, which is found predominantly in plant foods and some animal foods, is reduced from Fe^{3+} to Fe^{2+} by duodenal cytochrome b (DcytB) and then absorbed across the brush border of intestinal absorbing cells at duodenal enterocytes via divalent metal transporter 1 (DMT1).
3. Free ions from nonheme iron and heme iron combine with apoferritin to form ferritin complexes that move across the cell to the basolateral membrane for absorption across the basolateral membrane.
4. The final step of absorption that is common for heme and nonheme iron is active transportation of iron ions into the circulation.
5. Active transport of iron ions from the basolateral membrane into the blood is controlled by ferroportin, whose activity and stability is regulated by a hepatic hormone known as *hepcidin*.
6. Absorbed iron is bound to transferrin. Then, transferrin-bound iron circulates in the body and is taken up by the transferrin receptors in peripheral tissues for storage or utilization.
7. Iron transferrin-transferrin receptor 1 (TfR1) on the cell membrane enters the cell via the process of endocytosis.
8. Iron transferrin complex (known as *holo-Tf*) is acidified in the endosome to release Fe^{3+}.
9. Apo-Tf is then released from TfR1 and goes back to the cell membrane for another cycle. A metalloreductase, STEAP3, reduces the released Fe^{3+} to Fe^{2+}. Then DMT1 or transient receptor potential protein (TRPML1) transports Fe^{2+} into the cytoplasm, where it goes into the redox-active labile iron pool [18–20].

It is worth mentioning that two iron regulatory proteins (IRPs), namely, IRP1 and IRP2, regulate cellular iron balance post-transcriptionally. Indeed, under ID conditions, IRPs bind to iron-responsive elements (IREs) in 3′- or 5′-UTR of the mRNAs of TfR1, ferritin (H chain and L chain), and DMT1 to enhance iron uptake and to decrease iron sequestration [18,21].

14.2.2 Iron functions

14.2.2.1 Iron-dependent cofactors

Iron participates in the structure of organic cofactors such as heme and inorganic cofactors such as iron–sulfur clusters (ISCs) [18]. Additionally, it contributes to the metallation of mononuclear and di-iron enzymes such as methane monooxygenase (MMO), which transforms methane into the methanol via di-oxygen as the oxidant [22].

14.2.2.1.1 Heme iron cofactors

Heme is a cofactor containing Fe^{2+} (ferrous) ion and as a prosthetic group that binds to the heme protein covalently or noncovalently [23]. Heme proteins such as hemoglobin and myoglobin carry out essential roles in the storage and transport of oxygen in mammals [23]. Other hemeproteins, including cytochromes a, b, and c, are essential for electron transfer functions [24].

14.2.2.1.2 Nonheme iron cofactors

Proteins and enzymes with nonheme iron cores are widespread in nature and display important functions. Iron cores with primarily sulfur ligation are involved in the following:

- Electron transfer
- Electrophilic activation of hydroxyl groups
- Fixation of n_2
- Regulation of gene expression

Mononuclear and di-iron centers with oxygen and nitrogen ligation are involved in various reactions with O_2 and also in hydrolysis [25].

14.2.2.2 Iron-dependent enzymes

Iron-requiring proteins are mainly present in mitochondria, the cytosol, and the nucleus. Thereby, iron status is associated with most of the major metabolic processes, including electron transfer, ribosome maturation, DNA replication/repair, cell cycle control, oxidation, and reduction reactions in the cell [18].

Iron plays an important role as a cofactor of peroxidases such as catalase (a key antioxidant enzyme), ribonucleotide reductase (RR) (which is involved in DNA synthesis and repair), mitochondrial cytochromes (performing oxidation and reduction), myeloperoxidases (involved in killing pathogens) [26], three DNA polymerases (Pol α, Pol δ, and Pol ε) [18], and DNA helicases, which all are involved in preserving genome stability and are genetically related to diseases caused by DNA repair defects [18]. It has been reported that mutations in iron-containing DNA repair enzymes such as XPD, FANCJ, MUTYH, and NTHL1 are associated with increased risk of cancers. For instance, mutated MUTYH is involved in familial adenomatous colon polyposis [27]. Furthermore, FANCJ mutations have been shown to be associated with breast cancer and also related to Fanconi anemia [28]. The eukaryotic RNR is another iron-requiring enzyme whose expression and activity are strictly regulated during the cell cycle to initiate nucleotide reduction and maintain the proper dNTP pools for DNA synthesis and repair [29].

14.2.2.3 Iron and the cell cycle

Heme and hemoproteins, as iron-containing organic cofactors, are involved in controlling the expressions of cell cycle regulators and cell growth in mammals (18). It has been revealed that Fe depletion leads to G(1)/S arrest and apoptosis [30]. During the study of related mechanisms, it was found that numerous molecules that mediate cell cycle control, namely p53, p27(Kip1), cyclin D1, and cyclin-dependent kinase 2(cdk2), are influenced by iron [31]. It has been suggested that Fe depletion–induced downregulation of p21(CIP1/WAF1) may occur through inhibiting translocation of p21(CIP1/WAF1) mRNA from the nucleus to cytosol and increasing its proteasomal degradation in a ubiquitin-independent manner [32]. Upregulation of p38 mitogen-activated protein kinase (MAPK) in response to Fe depletion revealed another mechanism that confirmed the antiproliferative effect and apoptosis induction caused by iron depletion [31]. These findings were further supported by the results of studies suggesting that using Fe chelators might suppress the growth of aggressive tumors such as neuroblastoma and proposing that iron chelation could be an important therapeutic strategy [33]. According to the systematic time studies of neuroblastoma cell growth, it has been shown that iron chelation prevents Src kinase activity, which is needed for cellular proliferation [34]. It has been shown that using iron chelators halts the cell cycle through G1/S arrest [30,32]. However, more investigations are needed to clarify the positive effect of iron chelators on tumor suppression due to several reasons, including:

1. The inhibitory effect of iron chelators on DNA synthesis through inactivating the R2 subunit of RR, which converts ribonucleotides into deoxyribonucleotides (dNTPs). Moreover, its defect leads to elevated mutation rates during DNA replication/repair and subsequently genomic instability [29].
2. Fe depletion possibly inhibits p53R2 (contains similar iron-binding sites as R2), which provides dNTPs needed for the DNA repair process.
3. Iron chelation could decrease phosphorylation of the retinoblastoma protein (pRb) and downregulation of cyclins A, B and D, which play an important role in cell cycle progression.
4. Iron depletion leads to decreased activity of hypoxia inducible factor (HIF)-α prolyl hydroxylase, an iron-dependent enzyme involved

in controlling HIF-1α activity. Therefore, HIF-α prolyl hydroxylase suppression results in HIF-1α stabilization and affects downstream targets essential for angiogenesis and tumor growth.

5. Although iron chelation significantly increases the transcription levels of the p53-inducible cdk inhibitor, p21(WAF1/CIP1), increased p21(WAF1/CIP1) mRNA is not followed by increased protein level and this may bring about some sort of dysregulation of the normal cell cycle [33].

Overall, the evidence regarding the antiproliferative effect of iron depletion is not as yet sufficient, and further studies are needed to determine clearly the effects of Fe depletion on the expression of cell cycle control molecules and its effectiveness in cancer treatment [31].

14.2.2.4 Iron and epigenetics

Epigenetics is defined as transient but biologically important changes including histone modification, DNA modification, and RNA interference (RNAi) that are unrelated to DNA code and caused by environmental exposures such as diet, physical activity, and tobacco and alcohol use. These inheritable changes can influence the gene expression profiles and phenotypes, as well as portions of the DNA transcribed [35,36]. An increasing number of studies have shown that several small molecules such as iron, adenosine triphosphate, S-adenosylmethionine, nicotinamide adenine dinucleotide, flavin adenine dinucleotide, folate, acetyl coenzyme A, and α-ketoglutarate that are involved in controlling metabolic status have great importance in epigenetic regulation of the cells [37,38].

As mentioned earlier, iron is an essential trace element for controlling a variety of cellular processes, including proliferation, DNA synthesis/repair, and mitochondrial electron transport, which are all essential for the accurate maintenance of normal cellular homeostasis. Furthermore, iron plays an important role in regulating DNA function and histone modifying proteins [35,39], including histone demethylases such as the Jumonji domain-containing histone demethylase (JHDM) family (catalyzes demethylation of tri- and dimethylated lysine 9 and lysine 36 residues in histone H3) [35,40], and 10–11 translocation methylcytosine dioxygenase 1-3 (TET1-3). TET1-3 catalyzes the hydroxylation of 5-methylcytosine to form 5-hydroxymethylcytosine, which has been proposed as the initial step of active DNA demethylation in mammals [41,42]. Moreover, enzymes with the Fe^{2+} and 2-oxoglutarate (2OG)-dependent dioxygenase domain modulate transcription factor stability and have a coactivator function [35]. The HIF-prolyl hydroxylases (HIF PHDs), as members of 2-oxoglutarate-dependent dioxygenases, have important roles in the stability of the stress-response activity of HIF-1 [43].

There is a considerable link between the regulation of epigenetic mechanisms and the status of cellular iron metabolism. Both of these processes are tightly controlled in normal cells, though in cancer cells they may both be profoundly disturbed [35]. Limited evidence indicates that during human cancer development, the expression level of endogenous antioxidants such as superoxide dismutase (SOD)2 and glutathione peroxidase (GPx) is partly affected by epigenetic mechanisms including histone methylation, histone acetylation, and DNA methylation [36].

Hitchler et al. showed that the absence of these histone modifications leads to creating a repressive chromatin structure at *SOD2*, which influences the binding of SP-1, AP-1, and NFκB to *SOD2* regulatory cis-elements *in vivo*. They also reported that using trichostatin A and sodium butyrate to inhibit histone deacetylase potentially reactivates *SOD2* expression in breast cancer cell lines. Therefore, the epigenetic silencing of *SOD2* could be facilitated by changes in histone modifications, leading to altered expression of manganese superoxide dismutase (MnSOD), which is commonly decreased in many breast cancers [44]. Decreased expression of GPx3 resulting from promoter hypermethylation is associated with head and neck cancer (HNC) chemoresistance. Therefore, GPx3 methylation affects chemotherapy response and clinical manifestations in HNC patients [45].

In the same vein, Yara et al. suggested that Fe/Asc may play a role in altered methylation, which leads to changes in SOD2 and GPx activity that are concomitant with a significant alteration in antioxidant defense inflammatory processes, as manifested by the elevated NF-κB, IL-6, cycloxygenase-2, and the reduced level of IκB [36].

Novel therapeutic approaches related to the disruption of iron metabolism using iron-chelating agents (desferrioxamine [DFO]) for correcting cancer may act through several mechanisms, including inhibition of DNA synthesis, G(1)–S phase arrest, inhibition of epithelial-to-mesenchymal transition, and epigenetic alterations at the global and gene-specific levels. These alterations, all together, activate apoptosis and intensify the effect of the chemotherapeutic agents doxorubicin and cisplatin, with enhancement of the sensitivity of cancer cells [39]. It has also been reported that DFO treatment of wild-type TP53 MCF-7 and mutant TP53 MDA-MB-231 human breast cancer cells leads to downregulation of Jumonji domain-containing protein 2A (JMJD2A), histone demethylase, and lysine-specific demethylase 1 (LSD1), followed by changes in expression patterns of histone H3K9, H3K36, and H3K4 methyltransferase genes [39].

14.2.3 Iron and nutrigenomics

According to the concept of nutrigenomics, dietary nutrient intake can affect gene expression through binding to specific nucleotide sequences (response elements) within a gene's regulatory region as ligands and then result in changes in regulating transcription and consequently changes in gene expression [46,47]. It is therefore important to find out what amount of iron intake would be the most appropriate and safe to prevent unwanted alterations in gene expression and its potential outcomes [47].

14.2.3.1 Iron and gene instability

Maintenance of genome stability is of great importance because the instability of the nuclear genome and mitochondrial genome (mtDNA) is the fundamental contributor to a wide range of human diseases such as cancer and aging [11,48,49]. Cells have the ability to maintain genome stability by developing an intricate network of mechanisms contributing to cell cycle control and DNA repair [49,50]. Nevertheless, there are several factors including radiation, chemical agents, nutrient deficiency or excess, and mitochondrial dysfunction (leads to a defect in the biogenesis of (ISC), which is required for maintenance of genome stability) [49,51], as well as exposure to the accelerated iron ions [52], that defect genome integrity through overproduction of ROS and cause human diseases.

For instance, iron is capable of catalyzing the slow Haber–Weiss reaction, which generates hydroxyl radicals as a member of ROS [50,53]. Through this reaction, iron plays a role in production of hydroxyl radicals, which in turn contribute to 8-hydroxydeoxyguanosine (8OH-dG) formation and its related lesions, including DNA strand breaks, telomere shortening, DNA hypermethylation, and point mutations [50]. Iron has also the capacity of inducing DNA damage directly and independent of hydroxyl radical formation. In fact, iron plays a pivotal role in some processes, including (1) antioxidant defense through the expression of CAT gene (encodes peroxidase), (2) DNA distortion repair within FancJ expression (encodes helicase), and (3) DNA repair and base excision using the expression of ERCC2 (encodes helicase), NTHL1 (encodes endonuclease), and MUTYH (encodes glycosylase) [50].

14.2.3.2 Iron overload and genome instability

Iron overload is involved in generating iron-mediated oxidative stress, point mutations, DNA single and double strand breaks, mtDNA impairment, and mitochondrial respiratory dysfunction, as well as genetic and epigenetic alterations, including DNA and histone modification and chromatin remodeling. These may eventually lead to genomic instability and a significant increase in cancer risk [18,53], as well as other oxidative stress-related diseases such as coronary heart disease [16].

Chronic ingestion of excessive doses of iron, alcoholism, inherited autosomal recessive blood disorder (e.g., thalassemia), and/or using blood transfusions for such a disease are the leading causes for iron accumulation [50]. Hereditary hemochromatosis (HH) is another abnormal iron accumulation condition that results from disorders of the mechanisms involved in iron regulation such as upregulation of genes mediating iron absorption and downregulation of genes for hepcidin, which inhibits transportation of iron from the intestine [54,55]. This abnormally high accumulation of iron in the body is usually accompanied by increased risk of cancer [55,56], cardiovascular disease [57,58], and neurodegenerative disease [59]. Pancreatic dysfunction and other clinical signs like arthritis, abnormal skin pigmentation, diabetes, fatigue, and abdominal pain are commonly found in hemochromatosis [50].

Cardiomyopathy is one of the pathological manifestations of HH and is caused by the effects of iron overload on the heart tissue. In a study, the effects of iron overload on gene expression in the skeletal muscle and the heart were investigated using a genome-wide expression analysis of genes in the skeletal muscle and heart of iron-loaded mice and those of the control group. The results revealed that the expression of several genes involved in glucose and lipid metabolism, transcription, and cellular stress responses were down- or upregulated in response to iron overload. These results partly clarified the mechanisms through which iron overload in HH induces pathological manifestations such as cardiomyopathy and diabetes [54]. In this study, iron overload was indicated to increase the expression of two genes of the EF-hand family, a helix-loop-helix structural domain or *motif* found in a large family of calcium-binding proteins, such as myosin light polypeptide 4 (Myl4) (encoding the alkali atrial essential light chain [ELCa], which is important in the interaction between myosin and actin) and myosin light polypeptide 7 (Myl7) (encoding the regulatory light chain [RLC-A]) in the cardiac muscle up to tenfold. Furthermore, the expression of skeletal muscle and smooth muscle isoforms of actin (acta1 and acta2) in the heart, as well as the cardiac isoform (actc1) in skeletal muscle, has been shown to be related to iron overload. A link between iron overload and a remarkable upregulation of a stearoyl-coenzyme A desaturase 1 (*Scd1*), up to 1.75 fold in the skeletal muscle, and its downregulation up to –2.40 times in the heart was also observed [54].

In an experimental study, 2.49-fold elevation in the levels of Scd1 mRNA in the liver of iron-overloaded mice was reported [60]. The overexpression of Scd1 has been suggested to increase the risk of hepatocarcinogenesis [61].

According to a rat study conducted to find the effect of iron overload on the expression of stress-responsive proteins such as acute phase reactants (APRs) and heat shock proteins (HSPs), the expression levels of Hsp32 (heme oxygenase-1; 12-fold increase versus controls) and MT-1 and -2 (both increased approximately sixfold), as well as α1-AGP (the major rat APR), increased significantly in the iron-loaded rats compared to controls. Therefore, in response to chronic iron administration, hepatic tissue damage would be limited through the altered expression of stress response proteins [62]. Unexpectedly, this study suggested iron had no effect on the mRNA levels for several HSPs, and the amounts of Hsp25, Hsp70, and Hsp90 proteins were even uniformly decreased in the iron-loaded livers through an unclear mechanism [62]. Therefore, more studies are needed to unravel the underlying mechanism.

The results of another study aimed at investigating the effect of two distinct doses of Fe(II)/ascorbate (15 and 50 microM) on intestinal cells (Caco-2) showed an increased expression of two genes involved in cell response to stress, including HSP70 and MT 2A, although the severity of response was dependent on the dose of treatment [63]. Therefore, these contradictory results indicate the necessity for further studies in this regard.

Telomeres as noncoding fragments are placed at the end of chromosomes and are naturally shortened during each DNA replication period. Telomerase is the enzyme that inhibits progressive shortening of telomeres during chromosome replications. Oxidative stress caused by iron accumulation in the bodies of patients with primary hemochromatosis, and also in patients taking iron supplementation, may lead to decreased activity of telomerase. This may subsequently result in exacerbation of telomere shortening. Accordingly, a relationship between the length of chromosome at telomere parts of leukocytes and increased level of transferrin saturation has been suggested [64]. It has been reported that individuals with higher than normal levels of transferrin saturation and serum ferritin (phenotype positive) but not HFE genotype* have shorter telomeres [65]. Nevertheless, further investigations will be required to clarify the association between telomere length and iron overload.

In order to find the effects of systemic iron overload on the brain, Johnstone et al. investigated brain gene expression pattern in mice after short-term iron supplementation via microarray analysis. They found altered expression of 287 genes, although most changes were not remarkable. They also showed increased mRNA levels of iron storage protein ferritin light chain by 20% ($p = 0.002$) and decreased transcription level of IRP1, which downregulated ferritin expression by 28% ($p = 0.048$). In addition they revealed that iron is also related to the altered expression of genes involved in neurotransmission and nitric oxide signaling but the changes related to ROS, inflammation, or apoptosis were not considerable. Furthermore, altered expression of genes responsible for neurological disorders such as Charcot–Marie–Tooth disease, neuronal ceroid lipofuscinosis, and mucolipidosis were observed. These results proposed that iron overload may potentially influence the genes related to brain function [66].

Iron overload seems to be associated with elevated lipid peroxidation and increased cardiovascular risk through its role in oxidative reactions [67,68]. On the contrary, a possible relationship between IDA and cardiovascular disease has been proposed as well [56].

14.2.3.3 Iron deficiency and genome instability

Considering the existing evidence for direct preventive effect of micronutrients against gene mutations, or indirect effects as enzyme cofactors in cellular processes, dietary micronutrient deficiency is likely to be a possible cause

---

* Individuals with either homozygous or compound heterozygous status for C282Y and/or H63D HFE mutations were defined as genotype positive, or G+.

for DNA damage and increased cancer risk [11]. It is well established that even in the lack of IDA, for instance, iron depletion (without impairments of iron function and transportation) tends to damage genome integrity and to increase the risk of cancer by several mechanisms [39,50].

Iron is an important cofactor for enzymes having basic functions in human physiology. It is, therefore, not surprising that ID can lead to several pathologic consequences including brain development disorder, cognitive impairment, depression of immune system, and decreased work capacity [14,69]. Furthermore, ID increases oxidative stress and decreases antioxidant capacity, which is associated with the risk of oxidative stress-related diseases such as cancer, aging, and most neurodegenerative diseases [14,17,50]. Moreover, ID can affect the electron transport chain and reduce the amount of protein complexes that transfer electrons [18]. Some studies, using the budding yeast *Saccharomyces cerevisiae*, have revealed that ID impairs the function of iron-dependent enzymes, hemoproteins, and Fe-S proteins, resulting in the altered metabolism of glucose, amino acids, and lipids [70,71].

Studies have also indicated that iron, as an important part of cytochrome C oxidase, has a significant role in the apoptotic cascade. Therefore, ID can lead to decreased apoptosis rate [55]. Also, ID can affect the function of other mitochondrial cytochrome enzymes, such as P450, that are involved in detoxification of xenobiotics and chemical drugs. Thereby, ID can lead to increased DNA damage and cancer risk [50].

The results of an experimental study in rats showed that an *ad libitum* iron-deficient diet (3 ppm iron) for 16 days against similar rats with pair-fed control diet containing normal amounts of iron (48 ppm iron) is related to the following:

1. Upregulation of 600 genes that contribute to cholesterol, amino acid, and glucose metabolism
2. Upregulation of genes for caspases 3 and 12, which mediate endoplasmic reticulum (ER)-specific apoptosis
3. Downregulation of 500 genes linked to lipid metabolism

Thus ID exerts various impacts on both nutrient metabolism and apoptosis as a result of ER stress in the liver [55].

14.2.3.4 Genomic effect of iron on metabolism

As mentioned earlier, an experimental study using a murine model has already reported the genomic effects of iron on the expression of genes responsible for glucose, lipid, and protein metabolism [55]. Along the same line of evidence and in the same study, it was shown that ID leads to a decline in cholesterol levels, potentially due to the elevated gene expression of Cyp51 (cytochrome *P*-450 subfamily 51) and Cyp7a1, which are key factors in cholesterol metabolism. In response to decreased cholesterol levels, SREBP2, a transcription factor that enhances the expression of cholesterol biosynthetic enzymes, is activated, thereby increasing the expression of genes encoding for cholesterol biosynthetic enzymes [55].

To evaluate the effects of iron dextran on lipid metabolism, Silva et al. conducted an experimental study. They divided Fischer rats into two groups who were either on a standard diet (control) or a standard diet together with injections of iron dextran (supplement). They found higher serum levels of cholesterol and triglycerides in iron-supplemented rats as compared with the control group. Moreover, an inverse relationship between iron dextran and mRNA levels of PPAR-α, and its downstream targeted gene, cpt1a (known to be involved in lipid oxidation), was observed. Also, transcription levels of apoB-100, microsomal triglyceride transfer protein (MTP), and liver-type fatty acid binding protein (L-FABP) increased in response to iron dextran, which in turn resulted in changes in lipid secretion. A significant positive association between oxidative stress products, L-FABP expression, and iron stores and a negative correlation between PPAR-α expression, thiobarbituric acid reactive substances (TBARS), carbonyl protein, and iron stores was observed as well [72].

14.2.3.5 Iron and cancer

The association of iron and cancer has been reviewed in detail elsewhere (72–75). Some epidemiologic and experimental studies have shown the association between inadequate iron intake or low somatic iron stores and elevated risk of gastrointestinal (GI) cancer. Inconsistently, according to the results of a systematic review and meta-analysis, a higher intake of heme iron (1 mg/day) was associated with increased risk of GI cancer [76]. Overall, there are some controversies in this regard; for instance the findings of a cohort study with 49,654 Canadian women did not confirm the association between heme iron intake and the increased risk of GI cancer [77]. These contradictory results can be explained partly by the fact that meat contains other carcinogenic compounds such as high levels of saturated fat, preservatives, and/or cooking by-products that attenuate the association between heme iron intake and cancer risk. In fact, determining the independent toxic effect of each ingredient of cooked meat is very difficult. Furthermore, the interaction between dietary intake and genetic background can affect the association between dietary intake of iron and risk of cancer. Additionally, ID is often concomitant with other nutrient deficiencies during malnourishment. Thus, the impairment of the immune system and DNA integrity can hardly be attributed just to ID [14,50]. Therefore, more research is needed to determine the causal relationship between ID and increased risk of cancer.

It has been shown that taking approximately 15 mg/day of iron is associated with significantly (50%) lower risk of genetic instability and subsequently lower cancer risk in subjects (aged 7–17 years) compared with the recommended daily allowance (RDA), which is only 8 mg/day [17]. With regard to these results, approximately 20 mg/day of iron has been suggested as a proxy in order to decrease the risk of colorectal cancer (CRC) in adults. Nevertheless, it is noteworthy that there is a U-shaped dose–response pattern (Bertrand's rule) between iron intake and the risk of CRC in adults [50].

Iron has been suggested to be involved in CRC development. However, the association between the expression level of iron-related genes and cancer progression is not fully understood. It has been revealed that there is an association between the level of divalent metal transporter 1 transcript and mRNA levels of IRPs in tumor specimens. Moreover, it has been shown that IRP2 mediates stabilization of other iron transporter-transferrin receptor 1 (TfR1) mRNA early in the course of disease, but in the late stages of CRC, the mRNA level of TfR1 is correlated with the miR-31 level. It has also been observed that the ferroportin concentration is markedly related to the miR-194 level, which leads to a decreased amount of this transporter in the tumor tissues of patients with end-stage CRC. Altered expression of miR-31, miR-133a, miR-141, miR-145, miR-149, miR-182, and miR-194 was detected even in the early stage of disease. Generally, these iron-related genes were proposed as potential biomarkers for diagnosis and/or prognosis of CRC [78]. Although dietary iron intake may influence the initiation and progression of CRC risk, this effect might be modified by various single nucleotide polymorphisms (SNPs), such as three SNPs of HEPHL1, including carriers of the AA genotype at rs7946162, the TT genotype at rs2460063, and the GG genotype at rs7127348. A positive association between heme iron intake and CRC in subjects with GG genotypes for ACO1 rs10970985 has been reported. However, this significant association diminished after disappeared after adjustment for several covariates [79].

Oxidative stress has been repeatedly shown as a promoting factor for carcinogenesis, including prostate cancer [80, 81]. On the contrary, iron overload may be related to increased risk of prostate cancer due to augmentation of oxidative stress. This notion has been examined in the Carotene and Retinol Efficacy Trial cohort in a nested case-control study. It was discovered that the risk of clinically aggressive prostate cancer was associated with higher iron intake. However, these associations could be modified by endogenous antioxidant capabilities [82]. Consistently, it is becoming clear that elevated levels of ROS or decreased antioxidant capacity, which leads to oxidative stress, are an important risk factor for the occurrence of breast cancer. A nested case-control study of postmenopausal women (505 cases and 502 controls) from the American Cancer Society Prevention II Nutrition Cohort investigated the association between breast cancer risk and genetic polymorphisms of enzymes (including Nrf2 (11108C>T), NQO1 (609C>T), NOS3 (894G>T), and HO-1 [(GT)(n) dinucleotide length polymorphism]), responsible for providing a well balance of iron-mediated ROS. The results showed that lower antioxidant capacity, as judged by total number of putative "at risk" alleles in Nrf2, NQO1, NOS3, and HO-1, in the presence of high dietary iron intake (near supplemental iron intake) may result in elevated risk for postmenopausal breast cancer among women [83]. Retrograde menstruation may result in genome instability and endometriosis as a consequence of oxidative stress induced by iron and heme accumulation, which initiates the Fenton chemical reaction [53]. Heme is also shown to possess pro-inflammatory properties, which increase the risk of cellular impairment and DNA damage [53].

14.2.3.6 Iron and aging

Unhealthy aging and its related mental disorders and cognitive impairment such as Parkinson's disease and Alzheimer's disease (AD) are associated with alteration in DNA integrity and gene expression. Altered DNA integrity and gene expression may resulte from oxidative stress as a consequence of nutrient deficiency or excess [84]. The relationship between iron accumulation and both aging and neurodegenerative disorders such as AD and Parkinson's disease has already been well established [85].

Though iron is an essential element, its free form contributes to the production of free radicals and increased oxidative stress, which is associated with several disorders. With regard to this fact, a rat study evaluated the effects of iron-restricted and iron-enriched diets on oxidative stress and aging biomarkers. Iron-restricted diet correlated with a decline in iron concentrations in skeletal muscle and decreased level of tissue damage and also with weight loss, whereas iron-enriched diet was linked to increased hematocrit values, serum iron, gamma-glutamyl transferase, iron concentrations, and oxidative stress in most tissues. These findings proposed that iron supplementation in adult rats is possibly associated with an accelerated aging process through enhancing oxidative stress, while iron restriction might bring reverse outcomes [86].

Vasudevaraju et al. assessed the levels of copper (Cu), iron (Fe), and zinc (Zn) in three age groups (group I: below 40 years; group II: between 41 and 60 years; and group III: above 61 years) in the hippocampus and frontal cortex regions of normal brains. Each group consisted of eight samples. Genomic DNA was isolated and DNA integrity was evaluated by nick translation studies and presented as single and double strand breaks. The number of single strand breaks correspondingly increased with aging compared with double strand breaks. The strand breaks were more in the frontal cortex against the hippocampus. They observed that the levels of Cu and Fe were significantly elevated, while Zn was significantly depleted, as one progressed from group I to group III, indicating changes with aging in the frontal cortex and hippocampus. However, the elevation of metals was more in the frontal cortical region compared with the hippocampal region. There was a clear correlation between Cu and Fe levels and strand breaks in aging brain regions. This indicates that genomic instability is progressive along with aging and induces changes in gene expression [84].

14.3 Zinc

Zinc (Zn) an essential trace element with widespread distribution throughout the human body, is needed for optimum health because of its involvement in the structure or function of a number of macromolecules. Zn is considered to be a crucial factor for over 300 different enzymatic reactions responsible for many cellular processes, including growth and development, immune function, and antioxidant response [87–89]. In addition, zinc can be found abundantly in the cell nucleus, where it mediates storage, synthesis, and maintenance of chromatins and is also involved in transcription, replication, the gene expression process [89], DNA repair, and genetic stability [90].

Previous studies indicated that alterations in body Zn status could immediately lead to changes in the expression of genes, especially those involved in anti- and pro-inflammatory processes [10], the genes encoding MT, p53, and retinal binding protein [90]. Therefore, tight control of Zn homeostasis in mammalian organisms is unavoidable when its pivotal role in mediating cellular processes is taken into account [91].

A well-balanced body Zn status results from intestinal uptake of dietary Zn and body Zn loss mainly through intestinal secretion and urinary excretion. This latter could be dramatically increased in response to inflammation, leading to severe imbalanced Zn status. It is important to note that diet is commonly responsible for daily replenishment of 1% of the total body Zn in humans. Finally, Zn is delivered to the tissues and cells and diffused to intracellular areas in a tightly regulated manner [92,93].

MTs are cysteine-rich proteins that are rich in Zn and contain lesser amounts of copper, iron, cadmium, and mercury. MTs are involved in the absorption and intracellular reservoir of Zn. Additionally, they have a vital role in the availability of intracellular zinc through binding to and transferring it to other apoenzymes or apoproteins under specific conditions such as temporal stress or inflammatory status [94]. Therefore, MTs may have a role in antioxidant defense [15].

Disturbed intracellular Zn status is mainly attributed to overexpression of MT and defects in Zn transporters, which leads to increased accumulation of MT-bound Zn and decreased intracellular free Zn content. It is becoming evident that Zn release from MT decreases during aging; thus concomitantly the activity of Zn-dependent antioxidant enzymes and those proteins involved in immune functions are prone to be defective. On the contrary, Zn accumulation may also become toxic and possibly result in abnormal activation of some zinc-dependent enzymes [88].

In common with other micronutrients, the status of total body Zn is determined via the interaction between nutritional intake of Zn and genotype. The genes involved in modulating Zn status dominantly include the *Slc39A* gene family encoding specialized membrane proteins such as ZRT/IRT-related proteins (ZIP), which are involved in Zn uptake, as well as the Slc30A genes encoding zinc transporter (ZnT) families, which regulate intracellular traffic and/or excretion of Zn. It is important to note that the expression of both ZnTs and ZIPs are tissue-specific. Additionally, they have a distinguished response to dietary Zn deficiency and excess, as well as to physiological provocations induced by hormones and cytokines [95]. Alteration and mutation of ZIP4 (SLC39A4) importer gene has been shown to cause inborn errors such as acrodermatitis enteropathica with consequent severe zinc deficiency [76].

Furthermore, gene polymorphisms for pro-inflammatory cytokines (e.g., interleukin [IL]-6 and tumor necrosis factor [TNF]-α) may result in differences in Zn status. Dietary habits are another contributing factor in Zn absorption and availability through its interaction with other nutrients and trace elements in a diet [95].

14.3.1 Zinc deficiency

The essentiality of Zn was reported over half a century ago [96] when short stature, low circulating concentrations of Zn, anemia, and immune dysfunction in some areas of the Middle East, notably Iran, were associated with the high consumption of a sort of unleavened bread, *toonok* [97]. It is believed that the high phytate content of cereals interferes with intestinal Zn absorption [98,99].

In spite of the critical roles played by Zn, its total body content is limited (2–3 g). It is easily depleted in response to alterations in its intake, retention, sequestration, or secretion, and can hardly compensate for zinc deficiency condition over long periods of time [100]. Furthermore, Zn deficiency during infections will be more severe because of zinc sequestration into liver cells caused by pro-inflammatory cytokines [101]. It is noteworthy that Zn imbalance can be caused by insufficient dietary intake, insufficient intestinal uptake, and disorders of proteins involved in Zn metabolism [95].

Zinc deficiency is accompanied by augmented DNA oxidation and DNA breaks, as well as increased chromosome damage [87]. A substantial body of persuasive evidence indicates that Zn has an important role in the onset and/ or progression of multifactorial diseases. Therefore, with regard to the widespread functions of Zn in several organs, imbalance of it in specific tissues is prone to increase the risk of several diseases [95].

Poor Zn status in humans and experimental animals is manifested by clinical features including skin lesions, immune deficiency, impaired appetite, abnormal development, growth retardation, delayed sexual maturation, hypogonadism and hypospermia, alopecia, and delayed wound healing [90]. Furthermore, long-term Zn deprivation induces membrane lipid peroxidation and increases susceptibility to oxidative stress [89]. Increased oxidative stress in the state of dietary Zn deficiency may have a role in the incidence of a variety of chronic diseases such as diabetes, cardiovascular disease, and age-related disease [89,95].

Both innate and acquired immune functions are considerably influenced by Zn deficiency (genetic or nutritional). This may subsequently lead to promotion of systemic inflammation and impaired antioxidant capacity [88,102]. Although the mechanisms involved in the effect of Zn deficiency on clinical outcomes are not fully understood, the consequences might occur in relation to significantly altered gene expression [90].

Zn supplementation during Zn deficiency has been suggested at physiological doses (10–12 mg zinc/day) for 1 month in sequential periods. These doses provide an optimum balance among minerals (copper and iron), which normally have a close interaction [103]. Zn supplementation at a dosage of 10 mg/d for children younger than 6 months and 20 mg/d for children 6 months and over for 10–14 days has also been recommended for clinical management of acute diarrhea [104,105].

Several lines of evidence have suggested that Zn supplementation could be effective to improve immunity in the presence of Zn deficiency, especially during aging. This effect may be due to altered regulation of MTs [89]. Zn supplementation was found to enhance the activation of T cells and natural killer (NK) cells and subsequently to reduce the incidence of infections. However, Zn supplementation with high doses (100–300 mg/day) or in individuals (generally in young individuals) with normal Zn status may bring about such adverse effects as copper depletion and immune function impairment [89].

14.3.2 Zinc overload

Zinc toxicity due to oral ingestion of toxic amounts (100–300 mg/day) may induce copper deficiency [106], possibly through reduced expression of the genes encoding ATP7A protein (mediator of intestinal copper absorption), as is evident in Menkes disease [107]. Furthermore, through suppression of some DNA repair proteins, namely N-methylpurine–DNA glycosylase and DNA ligase 1, Zn toxicity may induce carcinogenesis [88]. The effect of zinc toxicity on neurodegenerative disease occurrence has been indicated, as well [88].

According to some evidence, zinc toxicity may occur as a result of the sequestering activity of postsynaptic zinc proteins, such as MT-III. These proteins sequester and immediately release zinc under oxidative provocation and subsequently activate neuronal apoptotic processes, as seen in Alzheimer-type dementia (AD). In AD, zinc may also be associated with β-amyloid accumulation in the senile plaques. In order to inhibit the toxic effects of Zn, chelating agents may be used in AD and the related neurodegenerative disorders [88].

14.3.3 Zinc and genome

Considering the fact that approximately 25% of the total amount of cellular zinc is localized in the nucleus, there is no wonder that it plays a critical role in maintenance of genetic stability and regulation of gene expression.

Zinc finger proteins, which participate in DNA replication and protein synthesis, are crucial for various processes, including cell proliferation, cell differentiation, cell growth arrest, cell division, signal transmission, growth factor production, chemokine production, and for the expression of nuclear receptor superfamily as well as nuclear transcription factor activation [88]. It is important to point out that zinc, independent of zinc finger proteins, may influence the expression of a variety of genes responsible for controlling the metabolism, oxidative stress, and inflammatory/immune response by different mechanisms [104].

14.3.3.1 Zinc and the immune/inflammatory system

The main reason why Zn deficiency induces impairment of immune function is partly attributed to the thymus involution caused by increased apoptosis of lymphocyte precursors and also by decreased activity of thymulin, a Zn-dependent hormone that is needed for differentiation, maturation, and function of T cells [10]. Zinc deficiency–induced cellular and humoral immune suppression is accompanied by a significant loss of pre-T cells and a decline in the number of naive mature T cells in circulation [88].

Zinc deficiency is related to reduced T-cell proliferation upon mitogen stimulation, a decline in the number activity of $CD8^+$ cytotoxic T cells, and dysfunction of $CD4^+$ helper T cells. These alterations may lead to an imbalance of Th1/Th2 cytokine secretion [88], as reflected by decreased IFN-γ, IL-2, and TNF-α production and increased production of IL-6 by Th2 cells and macrophages [88].

In vitro studies have suggested that zinc supplementation can modulate adaptive immune function through cytokine-mediated T-cell activation. In contrast, toxic levels of Zn appeared to directly suppress T-cell function via reducing IL-1-dependent T-cell stimulation caused by the inhibition of interleukin-1 receptor associated kinase-1[88].

Animal and human investigations revealed that Zn has a significant effect on signal transduction for immune cell functions. Furthermore, it plays an important role in proper functioning of both innate and adaptive immunity and subsequently optimal inflammatory/immune response [10,101].

In response to antigenic stimulation, Zn-regulated transcription factors (NF-κB, STAT, HSF-1, Kruppel zinc finger family), in combination with certain inhibitory transcription factors (Egr-1, Sp1, A20), regulate the expression of pro-inflammatory cytokines (IL-6, TNF-α) and HSP70 [88].

Through preventing phosphorylation and degradation of the inhibitory proteins (A20) that normally arrest NF-κB in the cytoplasm, Zn influences the translocation of NF-κB. This would be an explanation for the involvement of Zn deficiency in chronic inflammation as observed in elderly individuals [108]. On the contrary, most of the genes encoding cytokines are polymorphic and related to atherosclerosis and type 2 diabetes. Thus, in individuals genetically susceptible to an impaired regulation of the inflammatory/immune response, zinc turnover (via MT homeostasis) potentially plays a key role in the incidence of events with the characteristic of chronic and age-related diseases [108].

To find the possible mechanisms by which Zn deficiency may result in systemic inflammation, an experimental study using a small animal model of sepsis suggested that zinc deficiency induces NF-κB activity in vital organs, including the lungs [109]. At the molecular level, it has been shown that NF-κB p65 DNA-binding activity increased in response to Zn deficiency resulting from polymicrobial sepsis. Additionally, Zn deficiency enhances the expression of the NF-κB-targeted genes including IL-1β, TNF-α, and ICAM-1, as well as the acute phase response gene SAA1/2. Moreover, in Zn-deficient mice an increased level of NF-κB p65 mRNA and protein in the alveolar epithelia accompanied by a significant increase in the activity of caspase-3 was shown within 24 hours from the beginning of sepsis relative to the control group. However, these effects was counteracted by short-term zinc supplementation. The investigators concluded that Zn supplementation has the capacity to provide protective effects against sepsis-related morbidity and mortality through attenuation of inflammation and resulting lung injury [109].

Among the transcription factors, the Kruppel zinc-finger family (highly conserved zinc-finger transcription factors) has received considerable attention. These factors contribute to the expression or suppression of genes involved in proliferation, differentiation, apoptosis, and development and to regulating the inflammatory/immune response and antioxidant activity [110]. For instance, Klf2, a member of the Kruppel zinc-finger family, has a significant role in T-cell proliferation, IFN-γ regulation, and TNF-α production via NF-κB [63]. Thus it is involved in controlling inflammatory response. This issue was supported by finding an increased formation of TNF-α in mutant mice lacking Kfl2 (ZFP36), which resulted in severe generalized inflammation [110].

Recently it was found that KLF2 transcription factor could restrict the generation T follicular helper (Tfh) cells. This effect is exerted by decreasing the expression of S1PR (needed for efficient Tfh cell production) and also by increasing the expression of the transcription factor Blimp-1 (involved in Bcl-6 suppression). Furthermore, KLF2 deficiency was shown to increase the activation of CD4[+] T cells resulting in increased Tfh cell generation and B cell priming [111]. Another example of Zn-finger-containing transcription factors is the BTB/POZ domain containing zinc finger (ZF) transcription factor family (BTB-ZF), which is involved in T cell development [112].

During zinc deficiency, expression of genes encoding pro-inflammatory cytokines (IL-6, TNF-α) and chemokines (CXCL3) is increased. Meanwhile, expression of peroxisome proliferator activated receptor (PPAR), especially PPAR-α, is downregulated [89]. PPAR-α downregulates inflammatory response gene expression in a NF-κB-dependent manner (113,114).

Overall, zinc finger proteins are involved in the maintenance of Th1/Th2 balance through mediating signal transition from cytokine receptors to the responsible genes [88].

14.3.3.2 Zinc and gene stability

As mentioned earlier, Zn is an essential constituent of Zn finger proteins and, as a cofactor of many enzymes, is essential for cellular metabolism and genome stability.

Previous studies have shown that Zn depleted cells have impaired DNA repair mechanisms and thus an elevated rate of DNA damage. There are numerous Zn-dependent proteins involved in antioxidant response and DNA damage response. For instance, proteins with antioxidant activity such as Cu/Zn SOD removes superoxide anion. MTs are Zn proteins that scavenge hydroxyl radicals. DNA repair and/or DNA damage response may also be mediated by such Zn proteins as poly (ADP-ribose)-polymerase (PARP). It recognizes and binds to DNA single strand breaks during base excision repair. Oxoguanine glycosylase (OGG)-1 during base excision repair recognizes and removes 8-hydroxy-2-deoxyguanosine. Apurinic/apyrimidinic endonuclease (APE) is an endonuclease that cleavages damage sites in DNA. Activator protein (AP)-1 is involved in controlling stress responses, cell proliferation, and apoptosis. Nuclear factor (NF)κB is responsible for controlling oxidative stress responses, cell proliferation, and apoptosis. Finally, some Zn-proteins display apoptosis and DNA repair functions such as p53, which through induction of G1 arrest provides an opportunity for the cell to induce DNA repair processes and also coordinates events, which leads to proper DNA repair [115,116].

Zn is believed to boost the antioxidant capacity possibly through activating zinc sensory transcription factors involved in the expression of several proteins, namely MTs, methionine sulfoxide reductase (MsR), HSPs, PARP-1, SOD, GPx (GSH-px) [103,117], OGG1, and APE [117]. It has been shown that Zn may both directly and indirectly upregulate these genes [101].

Zn may also be involved in the activity of the enzyme betaine-homocysteine methyltransferase (BHMT), which in turn mediates methylation reactions in the folate–methionine cycle [117].

In order to determine the effect of Zn on expression of various genes responsible for encoding antioxidant enzymes, in an experimental study, different levels of dietary zinc (6.69, 33.8, 710.6, and 3,462.5 mg/kg) were applied in the hepatopancreas of abalone *Haliotis discus hannai* for 20 weeks. The antioxidant enzymes and proteins studied were Cu/Zn-SOD, manganese superoxide dismutase (Mn-SOD), catalase (CAT), mu-glutathione-S-transferase (mu-GST), and thioredoxin peroxidase (TPx), as well as HSPs. It was found that dietary zinc of 33.8 mg/kg was associated with an increased level of mRNA expression of the antioxidant enzymes, but after reaching maximum the expression level dropped gradually. Furthermore, at first, the increased expression levels of the HSPs (HSP26, HSP70, and HSP90) were achieved by adding 33.8 mg/kg dietary Zn and reached the maximum at 710.6 mg/kg. Thereafter, it dropped at 3,462.5 mg/kg. However, the toxic level of dietary Zn (710.6 and 3,462.5 mg/kg) had a negative effect and significantly decreased the total antioxidant capacity (TAC) in hepatopancreas. Therefore, the expression of antioxidant enzymes and HSPs was found to be upregulated in the presence of dietary Zn at 33.8 mg/kg. However, oxidative stress was augmented in response to excessive Zn intake (710.6 and 3,462.5 mg/kg) [118].

It has been demonstrated that arsenic may inhibit DNA repair through targeting PARP-1, a zinc-finger DNA repair protein. Considering the fact that cellular PARP-1 activity has a positive relationship with zinc status in cells, arsenic-induced zinc loss and subsequent altered conformation of zinc finger structure (including PARP-1 and Kfl5, an important member of the Kruppel zinc-finger family) [119] can result in DNA repair inhibition, a condition similar to Zn deficiency. Zn supplementation can reverse these detrimental consequences [120].

Zn deficiency appeared to reduce the ability of the transcription factors p53, NFκB, and AP1 to bind to the targeted DNA sequence. It was shown previously that low intracellular Zn status induced oxidative DNA damage and defects in p53, NFκB, and AP1 DNA binding and influenced DNA repair in a rat glioma cell line [121]. Again, here, Zn replenishment could reverse these DNA damage process [121].

In a study using a rat model, an extremely zinc-depleted diet, as compared with Zn-adequate diet, resulted in severe DNA damage in peripheral blood cells and also higher plasma F(2)-isoprostane concentrations. However, these changes reversed in response to zinc repletion. Furthermore, p53 DNA binding and activation of the base excision repair proteins 8-oxoguanine glycosylase and poly ADP ribose polymerase, which are all involved in the DNA repair process, were also impaired in response to Zn depletion [122].

Considering the fact that Zn is an important cofactor for enzymes involved in maintaining DNA stability, the effect of deficient or excess amounts of two Zn compounds, Zn sulfate ($ZnSO_4$) and Zn carnosine (ZnC), on genomic instability and proliferation of the WIL2-NS human lymphoblastoid cell line was evaluated. The findings suggested that Zn has a crucial role in genomic stability and the range of 4–16 µM would be an optimal concentration of Zn to inhibit DNA damage and cytotoxicity [123]. These findings were further supported by the findings of the same research group [116,117,124].

Both *in vitro* and *in vivo* studies have proposed that Zn supplementation may attenuate the hypoxic phenotype in cancer cells. To evaluate this notion, genome-wide analyses of colon cancer cells treated with combinations of cobalt and zinc were performed. It was found that zinc considerably

336   Nutrigenomics and Nutraceuticals

inverted the altered gene expression caused by cobalt. Moreover, it reactivated transcription of the pro-apoptotic genes induced by drugs. Indeed, cobalt ions stabilize HIF-1α. Since HIF-1α overexpression is associated with increased risk of drug resistance and cancer mortality, it could be concluded that the hypoxia pathway could be targeted by zinc as a potential therapeutic approach through influencing tumor cell response to anticancer drugs [125].

Taken together, interactions among zinc deficiency, DNA integrity, oxidative stress, and DNA repair suggest that Zn is an essential nutrient for maintenance of DNA stability [122].

14.3.3.3 Zinc and telomere length

Telomeres, which cap the ends of chromosomes, play a crucial role in inhibition of chromosomal end-to-end fusion [116]. Therefore, telomere length has a key role in chromosome stability and its degradation may contribute to increased rate of cellular aging and cancer risk [126].

The activity of telomerase, which mediates telomere elongation, was found to be inhibited by terminal restriction fragment (TRF)1 (TTAGGG repeat binding factor 1), a telomere-binding protein that regulates the telomere length negatively. By contrast, tankyrase-1 (TNKS1), a Zn-containing enzyme that belongs to the growing family of PARPs, poly-ADP-ribosylates TRF1 and displaces it from telomeric DNA, thereby increasing the accessibility of the telomeres to telomerase [126].

Telomere shortening and the consequent high percentage of cells with short telomeres is more frequent among old individuals. This tends to be related to impaired intracellular zinc homeostasis and MTs expression, which in turn is linked to an enhanced inflammatory response [127].

It has been suggested that Zn-finger protein 637 (Zfp637), a member of the Kruppel-like protein family, plays a role in oxidative stress, which itself contributes to cellular senescence and aging. It seems that the overexpression of Zfp637 significantly induces the expression of mouse telomerase reverse transcriptase (mTERT) and telomerase activity. This in turn results in telomere length maintenance and prevents senescence induced by H2O2, D-galactose, and ROS production. However, it has been shown that the beneficial effects of Zfp637 can only be provided in the presence of mTERT. Therefore Zfp637 has a protective role against oxidative stress-induced senescence through upregulation of mTERT [128].

14.3.4 Zinc and epigenetics

Increasing evidence suggests that Zn and Zn-dependent proteins are essential factors that contribute to several pathways related to epigenetic regulation and modifications [129].

Based on analysis of the chromatin structure, the increased production of interleukin (IL)-1β and tumor necrosis factor (TNF)-α in HL-60 cells in response to Zn deficiency is attributed to the increased availability of IL-1β and TNF-α promoters in Zn-deficient cells [130]. Moreover, Zn deficiency can lead to increased levels of nicotinamide adenine dinucleotide phosphate (NADPH) oxidase-produced ROS, which results in the phosphorylation of p38 MAPK. The p38 MAPK activity seems to be essential for post-transcriptional modification in the process of IL-1β and TNF-α synthesis. Therefore, Zn deficiency alters the expression of IL-1β and TNF-α via epigenetic and redox-mediated mechanisms [130].

Data from experimental studies have suggested a role for Zn in the regulation of meiotic cell cycle and ovulation. A study using a Zn-deficient diet (ZDD) for 3–5 days before ovulation (preconception) showed a significant disruption in oocyte chromatin methylation and pre-implantation development due to inducing the transcription of repetitive elements (Iap, Line1, Sineb1, Sineb2) and suppressing Gdf9, Zp3, Figla, Igf2, and H19 mRNA production as well as histone H3K4 trimethylation. Moreover, general DNA methylation decreased in Zn-deficient oocytes. Thus these alterations, influenced by zinc availability, affected the final oocyte development [131].

It has been proposed that *in utero* Zn deficiency may cause a series of fetal epigenetic alterations, resulting in disease occurrence among children of developing countries. In an animal study, a low-Zn (IU-LZ, 5.0 μg Zn/g) or control (IU-CZ, 35 μg Zn/g) *ad libitum* diet was applied in pregnant mice at gestation day 8 until delivery, with a regular diet afterwards. It was discovered that Zn deficiency was associated with histone modification in the MT2 promoter region having metal responsive elements (MREs). It is, therefore, likely fetal epigenetic alterations induced *in utero* may be permanent until adulthood [132].

Immunoblotting and densitometric analyses of human neuronal M17 cells elucidated that enhanced Zn concentration was associated with increased deacetylation, methylation, and phosphorylation combined with a decrease in acetylation of H3. These alterations are highly associated with the apoptotic process, as judged by reduced production Bcl-2 (an anti-apoptotic marker) and increased levels of caspase-3 (an apoptotic marker), as well as cell viability assays [133]. However, docosahexaenoic acid (DHA) stabilized the imbalance of acetylation homeostasis, representing its capacity to improve neurodegenerative diseases. Taken together, histone modification was altered in response to zinc and DHA treatment and resulted in the epigenetic regulation of neuronal cell gene expression. Nonetheless, zinc and DHA metabolism appeared to be dependent on each other in part. For instance, DHA may attenuate the epigenetic alterations caused by increased zinc levels and thereby contribute to neuroprotection [133].

Zn has an important role in MT-I gene transcription via recruitment of metal response element-binding transcription factor-1 (MTF-1) to the promoter of

338   Nutrigenomics and Nutraceuticals

the MT-I gene. Using chromatin immunoprecipitation assays, Okumura et al. examined alterations in the chromatin structure of the MT-I promoter and suggested that zinc treatment immediately resulted in [1] reduced Lys(4)-trimethylated histone H3 (H3K4me3) and Lys(9)-acetylated histone H3 (H3K9Ac) in the promoter, besides reducing total histone H3, and [2] increased micrococcal nuclease sensitivity of the MT-I promoter. It is important to note that these results were not observed in the absence of MTF-1. Therefore, MTF-1-coactivator complex, in a Zn-dependent manner, induces a quick impairment of nucleosome structure at the promoter of MT-I [134].

Methylation of cytosine in CpG sequences is another form of epigenetic modification and plays an important role in controlling gene expression [116]. There is still limited information about the effect of Zn concentration on methylation status. According to the results of some studies, Zn deficiency (<1 mg/kg Zn in diet) led to a reduction in the utilization of methyl groups from SAM in rat liver. This change was found to result in hypomethylation of both genomic DNA and histone [116].

Furthermore, betaine-homocysteine-S-methyltransferase (BHMT), a Zn metalloenzyme that transfers methyl groups from betaine to homocysteine for synthesizing SAM precursor (dimethylglycine and methionine), may also affect SAM generation, which is needed for DNA methyl transferases activity during zinc deficiency [116]. It is important to point that Zn is essential for methionine synthase reaction through enabling the active site conformational changes that are needed for homocysteine activation and methyl transfer. Therefore, due to Zn deficiency the function of both BHMT and the enzymes mediating methionine synthesis tend to be impaired, which subsequently relates to hypomethylation [116].

High levels of zinc oxide (1,000–3,000 mg zinc oxide per kg feed) are usually applied in the diet of weaned pigs to improve their battening and health status. However, according to recent studies, this approach may disturb Zn homeostasis. Therefore, Karweina et al. conducted an experimental study to unravel the effect of Zn-dependent epigenetic modification (DNA methylation) on the expression of Zn transporter (ZIP)4 gene (which contains frequent CpG sites) in the small intestine of piglets exposed to different dietary zinc intakes (including 57, 164, or 2,425 mg Zn/kg feed for 1 or 4 weeks). Interestingly, the level of DNA methylation in almost all checked regions were dependent on dose and duration of supplementation in all groups. Indeed, DNA methylation served as a precise mechanism for maintenance of zinc homeostasis through regulating the ZIP4 gene [129].

14.3.5 Zinc and apoptosis

Zinc plays a critical role in many types of apoptosis through activation of the p53 pathway [101]. Zn deficiency can increase cell apoptosis through inhibition of MT expression, which results in enhanced reactive oxygen species production, impaired mitochondrial function, and inhibition of cytochrome C oxidase activity [135]. According to some studies, Zn deficiency induces apoptosis of neuronal precursor cells via translocation of phosphorylated p53 into the mitochondria [136]. This leads to overexpression of pro-apoptotic mitochondrial protein BAX and disrupted mitochondrial membrane integrity, which results in release of apoptosis inducing factor (AIF) from the mitochondria and translocation of it to the nucleus. These events are accompanied by an increment in ROS formation following 24 hours of Zn deficiency [136].

Zn deficiency may induce apoptosis via activation of caspases 2, 3, 6, and 7. Then, the activated caspases target nuclear structure proteins, lamins, and polyADP ribose polymerase (PARP) and cleave them. Using a p53 inhibitor, pifithrin-mu, confirmed the role of p53 in mediating these alterations [136]. A recent study revealed that Zn at concentrations in the range 33.7–75 μM induces apoptosis of human melanoma cells through increasing the intracellular levels of ROS, which results in activating p53 and FAS ligand proteins [137].

The protective effect of zinc against diabetes-induced osteoporosis could also be explained by its role in preventing MC3T3E1 cell apoptosis induced by advanced glycation end products (AGE). The proposed mechanisms include decreasing ROS production, inhibiting the activation of caspase3 and caspase9, and inhibiting cytochrome c release from the mitochondria as well via the MAPK/extracellular signal-regulated kinase and phosphoinositide 3-kinase/AKT signaling pathways [137].

An investigation revealed that Zn supplementation has the capacity to reduce the apoptosis and cytotoxicity of cultured renal tubular epithelial cells (NRK-52E) caused by high glucose (HG). This effect is mediated by decreasing the production of ROS, preventing the translocation of cytochrome C from mitochondria to the cytosol, and inactivation of caspase-3 and caspase-9. Furthermore, Zn supplementation increases nuclear translocation of NF-E2-related factor 2 (Nrf2), through which two antioxidant enzymes including hemeoxygenase-1 and glutamate cysteine ligase are upregulated. Via its anti-apoptotic property, Zn activates the Akt and ERK signal pathways, which results in Nrf2 activation, inducing the Nrf2 target gene, and subsequently protecting the NRK-52E cells against HG-induced apoptosis [139].

Consistently, the results of another study revealed the protective effects of Zn supplementation against HG-induced apoptosis in rat peritoneal mesothelial cells (PMCs). In fact, Zn supplementation attenuated ROS production, which resulted in preventing HG-induced sFasR and sFasL overexpression, preventing caspase-8 and caspase-3 activation, and also preventing cytochrome c release from mitochondria to the cytosol. Moreover, cell survival resulting from Zn supplementation could be mediated by the activity of the phosphatidylinositol 3-kinase/Akt signaling pathway and MAPK/ERK pathways [140].

340 Nutrigenomics and Nutraceuticals

14.3.6 Zinc and signaling

There are several genetic networks and functional canonical pathways that are responsive to the Zn status. Amongst them are tryptophan metabolism, eicosanoid signaling, p38 MAPK signaling, integrin signaling, purine metabolism, G-protein–coupled receptor signaling, protein kinase C (PKC) [90], and, most significantly, peroxisome proliferator-activated receptor (PPAR) signaling with different regulation among young and elderly individuals [88].

In the context of zinc–gene network regulation, MTs have a critical role in intracellular zinc homeostasis. In fact, the metal responsive transcription factor 1 (MTF-1), which is a Zn sensory transcription factor, firstly binds to zinc-sensing gene promoter elements (MRE) and subsequently induces the expression of MT-I and MT-II (the best known isoforms of MT) [88]. Therefore, MTF-1 is of great importance for regulating the expression of Zn target inflammatory genes, including IL-6, TNF-a, RANTES, IL-8, MCP-1, PPAR-α, and PPAR-γ [89]. These findings clarified that the zinc–MT–gene interaction plays a key role in controlling inflammation and longevity [88].

14.3.7 Zinc and metabolism

Zinc as a trace element is essential for controlling metabolism through a variety of pathways. Both dietary zinc deficiency (ZD) and overload (ZO) can upregulate two genes involved in glutamine metabolism: glutaminase and tissue-type transglutaminase. It has been shown that both ZD and ZO alter the expressions of several genes responsible for transcription and translation processes. ZO upregulated the enzymes (except zinc-finger protein) involved in DNA replication and transcription in rats, whereas ZD considerably downregulated the expression of DNA polymerase and fork-head-like transcription factor, which are positive regulators. On the contrary, transcription repressors and transcription elongation regulators (the negative regulators) were upregulated in response to Zn deficiency. In both ZD and ZO groups, Zn-finger proteins genes were downregulated unexpectedly. However, factors involved in translation (except ribosomal protein in ZD rats) were upregulated in both groups [90].

The results of a rat study suggested that dietary ZO decreased the expression level of serine-threonine kinase 39, which leads to considerable changes in a particular signaling pathway due to its role in signaling cascades, involved in protein metabolism and cell signaling [90].

Considering the vast array of its vital functions, it is no surprise that ZD is often accompanied by several signs and symptoms involving skin, immune response, growth, appetite, and gonads. Since Zn is needed for DNA and protein synthesis as well as cell division, growth retardation is often a consequence of ZD [141]. Dysregulation of Zn homeostasis may have a role in metabolic changes and the related consequences of cancer cachexia [142].

On the contrary, supplemental Zn may affect the genes responsible for blood glucose and lipid homeostasis in a favorable manner. Recent meta-analysis studies supported the beneficial effect of Zn on circulating glucose and lipids [143,144].

In summary, Zn plays a crucial role in genetic stability through modifying chromatin structure, regulating DNA replication, and also transcription via transcription factors and DNA polymerase. Furthermore, different concentrations of Zn in the diet may influence the levels of hepatic gene expression involved in a wide range of metabolic pathways. Nevertheless, further investigations are needed to clarify the exact mechanisms through which the different concentrations of Zn affect the levels of transcription/translation and their clinical consequences.

14.3.8 Zinc and disease

14.3.8.1 Zinc and cancer

Given the fact that Zn is an important cofactor of enzymes involved in DNA metabolism and genomic integrity, its impaired homeostasis may possibly result in chromosomal mutations and genomic instability, as the main indicators for the elevated risk of cancer. Since the current chemotherapeutic agents, such as anthracycline, which includes doxorubicin and idarubicin, have been revealed to be associated with several side effects, using potentially protective agents such as Zn as an adjuvant chemotherapy has received increasing attention in recent years [145,146].

It has been suggested that Zn would be a useful agent for attenuating anthracycline toxicity to normal cells during chemotherapy of acute lymphocytic leukemia (ALL) [146].

Low blood Zn concentration is usually detected in ALL. It is becoming clear that Zn supplementation accompanied by chemotherapy may have the capability to accelerate recovery from and treatment of ALL. To test this hypothesis, an experimental study used an acute lymphoblastic leukemia cell line (CCRF-CEM) and lymphocytes from the peripheral blood of healthy adult individuals to evaluate the effect of Zn on DNA damage induced by therapeutic agents such as doxorubicin and idarubicin, two anthracyclines used in ALL treatment. Interestingly, the results of the study revealed that Zn exerted different response to DNA damage in normal and cancer cells. Zn significantly increased DNA damage in cancer cells, whereas it did not induce the same effect in normal cells. Therefore, Zn may have a two-sided protective effect in normal and cancer cells [146]. In the same vein, a study investigated the cyto- and genotoxicity effects of zinc sulfate ($ZnSO_4$) in normal human lymphocytes and human myelogenous leukemia K562 cancer cells in the presence of hydrogen peroxide (H_2O_2). The viability of cancer cells (especially those with low Zn levels) exposed to Zn concentrations ranging from 10 to 1000 μM decreased significantly relative to normal cells. Zn induced DNA damage only in cancer cells but not in normal cells. It also counteracted the DNA repair induced by H_2O_2 in cancer cells, whereas it exhibited protective effects against DNA damage in normal cells. Thus the dual effect of Zn treatment in cancer cells should be taken into consideration in cancer therapy [147].

p53 is a single zinc-ion–containing transcription factor that binds to site-specific DNA binding and mediates transcription initiation from a correct site. Furthermore, it plays an important role as a tumor suppressor. Due to the fact that Zn has a significant role in proper folding of p53, its deficiency or excess results in p53 misfolding and hence improper binding of p53 to DNA. This may result in loss of its function, which subsequently leads to mutation, genetic instability, and consequently increased cancer risk [148].

Increasing evidence suggests that Zn ions may be able to stabilize the p53/DNA binding to induce canonical target genes. To evaluate this, the effect of two different antitumor interventions, including high doses of the chemotherapeutic agent adriamycin and adriamycin combined with $ZnCl_2$, on wild-type p53-carrying colon cancer were investigated. The findings showed that low-dose adriamycin failed to induce p53 activation in wtp53-carrying colon cancer cells. In contrast, the second treatment, which was the combination of adriamycin and $ZnCl_2$, induced tumor regression via activating endogenous wtp53. Thus, $ZnCl_2$ should be taken into account as a valuable adjuvant of chemotherapeutic agents applied in CRC carrying wild-type p53, which has been linked to reduction in drugs needed for antitumor purposes [149].

Zn might carry cancer-protective properties in the secretory organs, notably the pancreas, prostate, and breast. This might be due to its role in the physiology and pathology of these organs, which have unusual Zn requirements [150]. Lower hair Zn levels in patients with breast cancer compared with the control group with no significant difference in serum Zn levels was reported by a recent meta-analysis [151].

Both *in vitro* and *in vivo* studies have shown that zinc protoporphyrin (ZnPP) has anticancer properties potentially through diminishing the expression of beta-catenin protein in cancer cells, which is probably mediated by the lysosome protein degradation pathway. In addition, suppression of the activity of proteasome is another mechanism suggested for the effects of ZnPP. However, the existence of cross-talk between the ubiquitin–proteasome system and the lysosome pathway remains to be understood [152]. Protective effects of Zn against gastric cancer have also been suggested [153].

In Iran, a positive relationship between imbalanced level of Cu and Zn concentrations and increased risk of CRC was reported. It seems that changed levels of these trace elements might be an effective factor in cancer development among Iranians [154].

14.3.8.2 Zinc and aging

Aging is commonly associated with progressively biochemical and physiological alterations associated with the increased predisposition to diseases and physical inactivity. During aging, both innate (natural) and adaptive (acquired) immune functions decrease gradually. Zn is considered as a fundamental nutritional factor in aging due to its involvement in the regulation of genes related to inflammatory/immune response and antioxidant activity [88,101]. Accumulating lines of evidence point to an insufficient dietary Zn intake (lower than 50% of the recommended dietary allowance) among old people. This might be due to poor diet quality, periodontal disease, or physiological factors (decreased intestinal absorption, impaired Zn transporters including the Zip and ZnT family, divalent metal transporter 1, and altered MT production). Therefore, low body Zn status during aging might result in immune function disorders and decreased antioxidant capacity [10,155], followed by an increased risk of degenerative age-related diseases such as cancer, infections, and atherosclerosis [10].

Several investigations have indicated that Zn supplementation in the elderly may induce beneficial effects, including reduced occurrence of infections and increased immune function through optimizing the activity of thymic endocrine activity, lymphocyte mitogen proliferative response, CD4$^+$ T cell number, Th1/Th2 ratio, and NK cell cytotoxicity [88]. Moreover, Zn supplementation may lead to a reduction in age-related pro-inflammatory markers, including C-reactive protein and inflammatory cytokines [109]. Zn also appears to improve the DNA repair process, possibly through increasing the antioxidant activity of MT and subsequently decreasing production of ROS [88]. However, differences in doses and duration of Zn supplementation used by elderly subjects in various studies has led to considerable controversy regarding its effect on immune function [101]. Furthermore, the presence of specific MT and IL-6 polymorphisms may influence the response of older subjects to Zn supplementation [88].

Using a cDNA microarray, it has been shown that the expression levels of genes belonging to diencephalons changed remarkably during Zn deficiency. However, Zn replenishment by 6-day supplementation resulted in recovered expression of the noted genes. Thus, gene expression patterns in the diencephalon respond rapidly to the altered levels of Zn observed during aging [156].

14.3.8.3 Zinc and obesity

Several investigations have established the contribution of overweight and obesity to the occurrence of chronic disease (insulin resistance, type 2 diabetes, and cardiovascular disease). It is believed that increased body fat can induce chronic inflammatory response characterized by enhanced inflammatory markers including C-reactive protein (CRP), pro-inflammatory cytokines [157,158], as well as adipose-derived cytokines such as leptin, TNF-α, and IL-6 [159]. However, these alterations were shown to be normalized by weight loss [158].

The ZIP family of Zn transporters contributes to the regulation of Zn metabolism. In a study, the associations among obesity, Zn transporter gene expression, and inflammatory markers in young Korean women were investigated. Significantly lower expression levels of ZnT4, ZnT5, ZnT9, Zip1, Zip4, and Zip6, as well as increased levels of CRP and TNF-α, were found among obese women relative to the normal weight group. Therefore the altered expression of Zn transporters that potentially occurs in obese individuals may be responsible for the inflammatory state associated with obesity [160]. However, Zn supplementation may restore the altered gene expression levels of ZnT transporters in obese women [160].

The association between dietary Zn intake and development of obesity or deteriorating preexisting obesity status has been found by a few studies [161]. Zn was shown to be involved in the decreased expression of leptin, which modulates appetite and energy intake via decreasing the expression of neuropeptide Y [158,161]. Due to its involvement in decreasing the expression of leptin, TNF-α, and IL-6, Zn may potentially attenuate obesity-induced complications [155].

14.3.8.4 Zinc and type 2 diabetes

Diabetes is a chronic disease characterized by impaired glucose homeostasis and eventually hyperglycemia. Plentiful Zn can be found in the pancreas, with a higher concentration in the secretory vesicles of cells, where it stabilizes the structure of insulin and contributes to its biological activities. According to human and animal studies, Zn status may play an important role in the inception and/or progression of diabetes. ZnT8 is known as the only pancreas-specific Zn transporter. Surprisingly, overexpression of ZnT8 in INS-1E cells resulted in increased intracellular Zn content and boosted insulin secretion. ZnT5 is another transporter with a marked expression in beta cells.

MTs, which are released by acinar cells in the pancreatic juice and also expressed in the endocrine part of the pancreas, were found to have an important role in pancreatic Zn excretion. Upregulation of MT genes following Zn supplementation was suggested to induce protective effects against streptozotocin-induced diabetes [95].

Persistent low-grade inflammation in patients suffering from type 2 diabetes mellitus (T2D) may be related to changes in Zn homeostasis. To elucidate this issue, a 12-week randomized controlled trial was conducted to elucidate the effect of Zn supplementation (40 mg/day) on the gene expression of cytokines, Zn transporters, and MT in women with T2D. According to the results, the expression of the TNF-α gene markedly increased after 12 weeks in the Zn-supplemented group. However, no significant alterations were found in the expression of IL-1β or IL-6 in the Zn-treated group. Furthermore, the association observed between Zn transporters, MT, and cytokines confirmed close interactions between Zn homeostasis and inflammation [162]. The relationship among inflammatory cytokines, Zn transporters, and MT gene expression in T2D reported by another study further supports these findings [163].

T2D is generally accompanied by Zn depletion. Zn supplementation, therefore, may induce therapeutic benefits in diabetes. To find the underlying mechanism, the effect of Zn supplementation (40 mg/day) and flaxseed oil (FSO; 2 g/day) on the expression of Zn transporters (ZnT1, ZnT5, ZnT6, ZnT7, ZnT8, Zip1, Zip3, Zip7, and Zip10), MT (MT-1A and MT-2A), and markers of glycemic control (glucose, insulin, glycated hemoglobin [HbA1c]) among postmenopausal women (n = 48) with T2D was investigated in a 12-week trial. Changes in glycemic indicators, HOMA-IR, and altered expression of Zn transporters and MT were not significant during the 12 weeks. A significant predictive association among Zip10, ZnT6, serum glucose, and HOMA-IR and between HbA1c and ZnT8 was observed. These findings further endorsed a relationship between Zn homeostasis and T2D [164].

The results of a case-control study among 1,796 participants suggested that the C allele of rs13266634 is associated with elevated risk of T2D, and higher plasma Zn is inversely associated with the lower odds of T2D. However, the negative association between plasma Zn concentrations and T2D was attenuated by SLC30A8 rs13266634. Further studies are needed to support this finding and explain the mechanisms of the interaction between plasma Zn and the SLC30A8 gene in relation to T2D [165].

14.3.8.5 Zinc and atherosclerosis

It has been established that augmented oxidative stress, inflammation, and genetic background are the main factors in the pathogenesis of atherosclerosis (AT) and cardiovascular disease (CVD). According to the mechanistic data, Zn is involved in providing a well-balanced inflammatory/immune response and protecting biological structures from oxidative damages [89]. This effect is potentially exerted through enhancing the antioxidant activity resulting from increased expression of antioxidant proteins including MTs [89], chaperones [89], ApoJ [89], Poly (ADP-ribose) polymerase-1 (PARP-1) [103], methionine sulfoxide reductase (Msr) [103], and SOD [11]. Moreover, Zn as a "second messenger" appears to activate Nrf-2 transcription factor and the Zn-finger protein A20, which in turn are involved in NF-κB suppression via the TRAF pathway and finally improve antioxidant activity and immune function [166]. Therefore, Zn could display a protective role against atherogenesis and endothelial cell instability caused by oxidative stress [167].

MT dysfunction frequently occurs during aging (inability to release Zn) and is followed by impaired antioxidant activity [168]. For this reason, Zn deficiency has been considered an environmental risk factor for AT [94]. *In vitro* evidence points to the effect of Zn (50 mM) on the enhanced expression of the PPAR-α gene from the PBMCs of elderly people (age range 69–79 years) [89], which resulted in modulation of lipid profile. However, the results of a trial revealed that Zn supplementation (150 mg/day) induced no significant effects on the oxidation and concentration of low-density lipoprotein (LDL). Inconsistently, Zn supplementation higher than 50 mg/day lowered plasma high-density lipoprotein (HDL)–cholesterol concentrations [169]. Thus, the effect of Zn supplementation might be dose- and time-dependent. In addition, age-related alterations such as altered inflammatory/immune response and lipid profile may in part explain the existent controversies regarding the effect of Zn supplementation on lipid profile [89,94].

14.4 Selenium

Selenium (Se) is an essential trace element for human health. Se status can vary considerably across different populations and regions of the world. This may be due to different concentrations of Se in the soil, which enters crops and fodder and subsequently the food chain, resulting in variations in dietary Se among individuals around the world [170,171]. Apart from geographical region and Se content of the soil, there are several other factors that influence Se status and Se requirement of individuals, amongst which are intense exercise, smoking, and intake of nutritional antioxidants including vitamin C and E (172–174).

The discovery of Keshan cardiomyopathy disease in a severely selenium-deficient population was the key step towards consideration of the essentiality of Se for optimal health. This resulted in Se supplementation in Keshan, where severe selenium deficiency was first reported in a human population [171].

Selenium, with a recommended dietary allowance of 55 µg/day in humans, has a fundamental significance in different metabolic pathways and physiological processes related to human health [175]. A growing body of evidence indicates that Se plays an important role in normal growth, immune function, thyroid function, and reproduction [171,175]. A typical diet or dietary supplement contains various kinds of Se [176], including the inorganic forms (selenite, SeO3; selenate, SeO4), which are in the oxidized state, and the organic ones (selenomethionine [SM] and selenocysteine), which are in the reduced state [11].

As an essential nutrient, selenium is required for the expression of selenium-containing proteins known as *selenoproteins*, which are essential for physiological functions and influence oxidative and inflammatory processes [170,177]. Selenium contributes to the structure of 25 selenoproteins as unusual amino acids, such as selenomethionine (Se-Met), which randomly incorporates into selenoproteins by replacing methionine [176,178], and selenocysteine (Sec) which specifically enters selenoprotein compounds [11]. Sec [179,180] incorporates into the polypeptide chain during selenoprotein translation at specific UGA codons. UGA codons normally signal the termination of translation. Incorporation of Sec into the peptide chain, therefore, requires the recoding of these UGA codons from stop to Sec [171].

Approximately half of the selenoproteins, including five GPXs (GPx1-GPx4, GPx6), three thioredoxin reductases (TR1–TR3), selenoprotein P, and three deiodinases (IDI), have been shown to catalyze reactions of redox balance and are predicted to protect the cell against oxidative stress [170,177]. It has been reported that knockout mice without both GPx1 and GPx2 are more prone to oxidative damage [171]. The evidence provided using GPx1 knockout mice fed with a selenium-deficient or selenium-normal diet revealed that GPx1 is the major form of body selenium and protects the body against acute ROS-induced lethality [11]. Moreover, Se through GPx4 also has a role in lipoxygenase metabolism and sperm function [171].

The TR1–3 along with thioredoxin provides a redox complex with several functions, including the reduction of ribonucleotides to deoxyribonucleotides, maintenance of redox state, and regulation of transcription factor activity. Furthermore, it reduces ubiquinone-10 in order to reproduce the antioxidant ubiquinol-10 [171,181].

Selenoprotein P (SePP), with at least two isoforms of 50 and 60 kDa molecular weight, exists in the blood and constitutes nearly 50% of the total plasma Se content. It contains up to 10 Sec residues that mostly reside in a Sec-rich C-terminal domain and appears to have antioxidant function (182–184). SePP is also a critical factor in the regulation of Se transportation to other tissues [170,185].

Regulation of inflammatory responses is the other pivotal activity of Se conducted by selenoproteins, particularly selenoprotein S (Se-S), possibly through the regulation of pro-inflammatory cytokines such as interleukin-1β (IL-1β), interleukin-6 (IL-6), and tumor necrosis factor-α (TNF-α). Three other selenoproteins, including GPx-4, SePP, and selenoprotein 15 (Sep-15), have been shown to be related to the inflammatory processes during 5-lipoxygenase (5-LO) metabolism, cytokine regulation, and ER stress, through a genotype-dependent modulation [186–188].

14.4.1 Selenium deficiency

Although severe deficiency of Se and the resulting clinical presentation, for example, Keshan disease (KD), is very rare [171], suboptimal intake of Se is commonly observed in many populations and has been reported to be associated with inadequate synthesis of selenoproteins and also induction of nuclear factor erythroid 2–related factor 2 (Nrf2), both of which are key components of the cellular redox and antioxidant systems [175,176,189]. For instance, induced Nrf2 has been suggested to be associated with upregulation of GPx2 and thioredoxin reductase 1 (TrxR1) [189].

Regarding the known functions of selenoproteins, suboptimal intakes of Se may contribute to the development and severity of a number of human chronic diseases, such as cancer and inflammatory diseases, as well as suboptimal physiological functions, including thyroid and muscle function and spermatogenesis [176].

14.4.2 Selenium toxicity

Although high Se intake counteracts the carcinogenesis process through upregulation of a few selenoproteins, it could also be toxic based on various end points, including formation of selenium metabolites and free radical by-products, which may cause cellular adverse effects like other chemical compounds [190].

The mechanism for Se toxicity may be related to its role in the promotion of genome instability, likely through the induction of ROS formation [11]. Excessive Se induced histone H3 acetylation in a rat model with colorectal carcinogenesis and also phosphorylation of histone H2AX in CRC cells, as well as inhibition of histone deacetylase activity in B-cell lymphoma [190].

It has been reported that diabetes is one of the adverse health outcomes of Se toxicity [190]. Therefore, like many other trace elements, both too much and low intake of Se could be harmful and bring about adverse health outcomes [11,176,191].

14.4.3 Selenium and epigenetics

The epigenetic effect is another mechanism affecting genome integrity through direct methylation and demethylation of cytosine bases, known as *cis-epigenetics*, and chromatin modification, known as *trans-epigenetics*. An increasing body of evidence has revealed a link between Se and epigenetic regulation and consequently gene regulation [190]. Therefore, some of the effects of Se compounds on gene expression could be explained by epigenetic effects, including regulation of DNA methylation or prevention of histone deacetylation [170,176].

To investigate the epigenetic effects of selenium, DNA methylation, histone modifications, and gene expression were evaluated in LNCaP cells in response to selenite treatment. It was found that the levels of DNMT1* and methylated H3-Lys 9 associated with the pi-class glutathione-S-transferase (GSTP1) promoter decreased, whereas the levels of acetylated H3-Lys 9 associated with this promoter increased in response to the treatment. Generally, selenite treatment induced a reduction in DNA methylation and led to partial promoter demethylation and re-expression of APC. Therefore, Se may be involved in cancer prevention via epigenetic modifications [192]. In the same

---

* The DNMT1 gene encodes the enzyme DNA (cytosine-5)-methyltransferase 1.

vein, a rat study showed that long-term consumption of a supranutritional dose of Se (4 mg) not only affects global genomic DNA methylation but also enhances exon-specific DNA methylation of the p53 gene (exons 5–8) in a Se-dose-dependent manner in rat liver and colon mucosa compared with the Se-deficient group [193]. Furthermore, supranutritional Se provoked histone H3 acetylation in a rat model of colorectal carcinogenesis and histone H2AX phosphorylation in CRC cells. It also suppressed histone deacetylation in B-cell lymphoma [190]. Uthus et al. employed a DNA methylation array (Panomics) in a human colonic epithelial Caco-2 cell model showed that low-SeMSC media induced promoter region hypermethylation of the von Hippel–Lindau (VHL) gene (a tumor suppressor), followed by downregulation of it in cells grown in low SeMSC compared to those grown in 250 nM SeMSC. They also reported a significant reduction in VHL gene expression in mucosa from rats who consumed low diet selenium [194]. Taken together, the existing data strongly supports the epigenetic effects of selenium and its possible role in cancer prevention.

A strong body of evidence for the epigenetic effects of Se has come from severe Se deficiency syndrome, that is, KD.

14.4.4 Selenium and nutrigenomics

It is becoming clear that antioxidant nutrients such as Se not only have overt health effects but also influence every single cell at all levels, including a complex network of genes [88,195]. Therefore, extreme Se deficiency or excess can affect cellular functions through genetic, genomic, or epigenomic regulation [170]. It seems that various effects of different chemical forms of selenium on molecular-level and downstream Se-targeted pathways could be evaluated via nutrigenomic approaches [196–198]. Nutrigenomics is also considered a key tool in determining sensitive biomarkers for the optimal Se status at which individual or population health can be provided [170].

According to a rat study, maternal Se/folate deficiency during pregnancy and lactation is linked to an alteration in the patterns of gene expression in the offspring after weaning [199]. Some studies have proposed that the kind of selenium (organic or inorganic) does not contribute to diversity in gene expression or activity of selenoproteins [197]. However, some other studies have indicated that inorganic selenium (selenite or selenate) compounds have less influence on the genomic levels than organic compounds [197,200,201]. In the same vein, Barger et al. examined the gene expression profiles in the intestine, gastrocnemius, cerebral cortex, and liver of weanling mice who were fed either a selenium-deficient (SD) diet (<0.01 mg/kg diet) or a diet supplemented with one of three selenium sources (1 mg/kg diet, as either SM, sodium selenite [SS], or yeast-derived selenium [YS]) for 100 days. The results showed a similar influence of all types of selenium on the expression of genes encoding selenoproteins (Gpx1 and Txnrd2) and selenoenzyme (GPX1) activity. However, when overall gene expression patterns were taken into account, the effect of SM was different from other types of Se (SS and YS). Furthermore, only YS significantly inhibited DNA damage by means of the reduced expression of Gadd45b (growth arrest and DNA-damage-inducible, beta) in all four tissues and also reduced GADD45B protein levels in liver [197].

The analysis of gene expression in the oviduct of hens supplemented with SP (Sel-Plex®, SP) and SS (sodium selenite, SS) revealed the upregulation of several subunits of the mitochondrial respiratory complexes, ubiquinone production, and ribosomal subunits in the SP group. However, in the SS group, the expression of genes associated with respiratory complexes, ATP synthesis, and protein translation and metabolism was significantly lower than in the control group [201]. Thus, the source of Se seems to be important during gene expression in the oviduct of hens.

In a human study, a year after supplementation of 16 healthy men with 300 μg Se/day as high-Se yeast or placebo yeast, a prominent cluster of protein kinases involved in protein phosphorylation in leukocytes of the high-Se yeast group was upregulated. Therefore, protein phosphorylation in leukocytes responds to the Se supplementation. Another important finding was highly ranked clusters of genes that were involved in processing of RNA and transportation of proteins. This finding implied the role of dietary Se in post-transcriptional and post-translational modification of proteins expressed in leukocytes. The increased expression of genes involved in FAS apoptosis signaling and T-cell and natural killer cell cytotoxicity was observed, as well. These findings suggest an anti-inflammatory effect for Se through its role in regulation of protein kinase activities and immune reactions [202].

During cell exposure to DNA damaging agents, the process of DNA damage reactions including checkpoint responses and DNA repair mechanisms is rapidly activated to halt the cell progression into the next phase and thus to inhibit proliferation of cells containing defective DNA. For instance, during S-phase, cells are sensitive to agents that lead to DNA damage and induce DNA replication fork arrest. Ataxia-telangiectasia mutated (ATM), activated through the MRN (Mre11-Rad50-Nbs1)–ATM pathway [11], is an essential kinase in early response to DNA damage, chromatin remodeling, and oxidative stress. It acts via phosphorylation of several downstream substrates, leading to the activation of DNA repair, cell cycle arrest, senescence, and/or apoptosis [190]. Consequently, DNA damage fixation and maintenance of genome integrity will be provided, while defective DNA damage responses result in genome instability.

Se is associated with increased apoptosis, particularly in combination with a damage-inducing agent like doxorubicin. It may also govern the cell cycle through the induction of adenomatous polyposis coli (APC) gene expression. APC is a key tumor suppressor gene involved in assembly, stability, and activity of the Wnt signaling destruction complex [203], epithelial cell polarization, and three-dimensional morphogenesis [204]. It also promotes transcription-independent apoptosis [205]. It has been shown that Se at concentrations of 5, 50, and 500 ng/mL has no cytotoxicity and has no effect on cell proliferation in an intestinal adenocarcinoma cell (HT29) model. However, elevated expression of CASP9 as well as lower expression of BCL-XL was found in the selenium (500 ng/mL) and doxorubicin treatment group. Moreover, APC gene expression increased in the Se group without doxorubicin [206].

Methylselenol, as one of the Se metabolites, may exert anticancer effects *in vivo*. In a study, methylselenol at submicromolar value, provided by incubating methionase with seleno-L-methionine, inhibited HT1080 tumor cell migration and invasion. Real-time RT-PCR showed the increased expression of cdk inhibitor 1C (CDKN1C), heme oxygenase 1, platelet/endothelial cell adhesion molecule, and PPARg genes up to 2.8- to 5.7-fold of the control. Downregulation of the Bcl-2-related protein A1, hedgehog interacting protein, and p53 target Zn-finger protein genes up to 26%–52% of the control during exposure to methylselenol were observed. All these genes are directly involved in the regulation of the cell cycle and apoptosis. Methylselenol increased apoptotic cells up to 3.4-fold of the control and inhibited the extracellular-regulated kinase 1/2 (ERK1/2) signaling and cellular myelocytomatosis oncogene (c-Myc) expression. Therefore, through the regulation of the aforementioned genes, the G1 cell cycle is arrested and apoptosis, which may lead to inhibition of tumor cell invasion, ensues [207]. However, the previous findings of the same authors showed that low concentrations of methylselenol had a stronger capacity to induce cell cycle arrest than to cause apoptosis [207].

14.4.5 Selenium and genomic stability

Increasing evidence indicates that Se metabolites and selenoproteins play a crucial role in the maintenance of genome stability, either indirectly through antioxidant activity or more directly through elevated cellular DNA repair capacity and epigenetic alterations [170,177,190]. Both these procedures can be analyzed in the DNA from white blood cells using the single-cell gel electrophoresis (COMET) assay, which has been used to show a U-shaped curve for Se requirements [208]. Indeed, Se intake higher than nutritional needs can activate early barriers of tumorigenesis, such as DNA damage response and cellular senescence, which are mostly dependent upon ATM, oxidative stress, p53, and DNA-PKcs [209]. It has been suggested that serum Se concentrations up to 100 ng/mL are associated with lower DNA damage and increase in the activity of GPx-1 and TR enzymes, which are related to DNA repair [170]. Until now, only five selenoproteins—namely selenoprotein H, methionine-R-sulfoxide reductase 1, GPx4, thioredoxin reductase-1, and thioredoxin glutathione reductase—were known to have potential roles in redox balance and genome integrity [190].

SelH as a nuclear selenoprotein seems to carry redox and transactivation domains through which yields protection against oxidative stress and thus maintains genome stability [190,209]. The homologue of human SelH in the fruit fly, *Drosophila*, has been proposed as essential for embryogenesis through its antioxidant activity [209]. Consistently, the results of studies of human SelH in HT22 mouse neuronal cells indicated that selenoprotein protects against oxidative stress through acting as a transactivator for GSH biosynthesis and also by limitation of cellular senescence [209]. Generally, it seems that augmented oxidative stress and consequently DNA damage observed in SelH-deficient cells can result in activated ATM–p53 pathway along with decreased expression of phase II antioxidant enzymes [209].

Given the fact that lead as an environmental toxin contributes to decreased antioxidant capacity and subsequently increases ROS generation and genome instability, McKelvey et al. evaluated lead nitrate detoxification in HepG2 cells, under various compounds of Se (organic and inorganic). They used the COMET assay to quantify DNA damage and also determined gene expression patterns related to DNA damage and signaling using PCR arrays. They found that the organic-type selenium compounds (selenium yeast and SM) protect DNA damage in HepG2 cells caused by DNA-damaging agents like lead [200].

The most important dietary form of Se is seleno-L-methionine (Se-Met), whose effect on genome stability was evaluated to demonstrate the effective and safety limit of intake. Accordingly, Se, as Se-Met, at concentrations up to 430 µg Se/L, potentially increases genome stability but higher doses (≥1880 µg Se/L) may display cytotoxic effects, suppress cell division, and enhance cell deterioration [210]. Results obtained from a study that investigated the effects of Se-Met on bleomycin (BLM)-induced DNA damage in human leukocytes showed a decline in BLM-induced strand breaks in response to treatment with SeMet. In fact, these findings indicated the protective effect of SeMet against the genotoxic effect caused by BLM [211]. However, it is of great importance to determine a cautious approach for SeMet supplementation to provide optimal genome integrity without cytotoxic effects [210].

A randomized trial analyzed the effect of one Brazil nut containing nearly 290 µg of Se per day on blood Se status, erythrocyte GPx activity, and levels of DNA damage in morbidly obese women. After 8 weeks, an improvement in plasma Se, erythrocyte Se, and GPx activity were observed. Furthermore, DNA damage level was significantly less than baseline data. However, the evaluated biomarkers showed that responses to supplementation were distinct regarding the different polymorphisms. In other words, more decrement in DNA damage in Leu/Leu subjects, as compared with Pro/Pro (wild-type genotype) subjects, was observed [212].

Chronic kidney disease (CKD) is usually accompanied by a decline in Se status, augmented oxidative stress, and hence increased DNA damage [213]. In a supplementation study in CKD subjects on hemodialysis, daily intake of 200 µg Se (as Se-rich yeast) for 3 months resulted in a significant decrease in DNA damage (including single-strand breaks and oxidative base lesions) in white blood cells [213].

A growing body of evidence has indicated that high selenium status is likely to increase the activity of serum SOD, GPx, and catalase and also to reduce the levels of malondialdehyde, thereby enhancing DNA repair and genome integrity [214].

14.4.6 Selenium and diseases

Selenium deficiency has been revealed to be the major cause of KD, and a predisposing factor for Kashin–Beck disease (KBD). KD is a fatal dilated cardiomyopathy, whereas KBD is a type of osteochondropathy with altered metabolism of proteoglycan chondroitin sulfate [215,216].

Several studies have proposed a critical role of selenium deficiency in DNA methylation during KD [217]. A study to elucidate the epigenetic impacts of Se on DNA methylation and gene expression in KD showed two inflammatory-related genes (toll-like receptor [TLR] 2 and intercellular adhesion molecule [ICAM] 1), with different methylation and expression among KD cases compared to normal subjects. Moreover, decreased CpG island methylation in the promoter regions of TLR2 and ICAM1 along with their upregulation occurred in response to Se deficiency. However, selenite treatment was linked to increased methylation of TLR2 and ICAM1 promoter, which led to silencing the expression of these genes and reducing myocardial inflammatory cell infiltration [217]. In accordance with these findings, in a cell culture model of KD, selenite treatment resulted in suppression of Gadd45alpha, TLR2, and ICAM1 gene expression in a dose-dependent manner, whereas selenium deficiency was associated with upregulation of Gadd45alpha, TLR2, and ICAM1 and reduced methylation of the TLR2 and ICAM1 promoters in a time-dependent manner. Therefore, the TLR2–ICAM1–Gadd45alpha axis is possibly involved in gene-specific active DNA demethylation during inflammatory response in the myocardium [217]. Additionally, it has been shown that severe selenium or GPx1 deficiency has an important role in elevating the virulence of coxsackie virus B, which induces myocarditis occurred in KD [11].

Increasing evidence over the past two decades has suggested that suboptimal Se intake and low circulating selenium concentrations are associated with a wide range of diseases [218], including cancer, especially CRC, heart disease, and diabetes [170]. Through defined mechanisms, Se and selenoproteins seem to be involved in colorectal function and play a role in cancer prevention in humans and in animal and cell models [171].

It has also been proposed that selenium levels are inversely associated with IBD [172], and a number of other health problems, including poor prognosis in HIV-positive people, epileptic seizures in children and adults, as well as a number of age-related neurological disorders [172]. Furthermore, based on numerous studies, Se deficiency contributes to several reproductive and obstetric complications, including male and female infertility, miscarriage,

354 Nutrigenomics and Nutraceuticals

preeclampsia, fetal growth restriction, preterm labor, gestational diabetes, and obstetric cholestasis [175].

14.4.6.1 Selenium and cancer

Extensive epidemiological and some nutritional trials and meta-analysis studies suggest an inverse association between supranutritional intake of Se and the incidence of several types of cancer [11,219].

According to animal studies, anticarcinogenic effects would be provided by Se intake at >1 mg/kg diet, that is, at least 10 times higher than that needed for the inhibition of clinical manifestations of deficiency and to support near-maximal tissue activities of selenoenzymes [207].

Overproduction of ROS and the consequent augmented oxidative stress that results from metabolic disorders in tumor cells may be associated with several types of cancer [220]. Selenium has been suggested to reduce the risk of cancer due to its presence in selenoproteins such as GPx and thioredoxin reductase, which possess antioxidant and antimutagenic activities [219–221]. Therefore, Se supplementation is considered a public health policy in regions with poor Se status [175]. It is important to note that, apart from dietary intake of Se, genetic variants of selenoenzymes may also affect their activities and consequently directly or indirectly impact cancer risk [221].

It has become clear that redox active forms of Se, including selenite and Se-methylselenocysteine as well as selenocystine, are pro-oxidants, and their highly cytotoxic effects target tumor cells and prevent their growth and proliferation [191]. These redox active compounds of Se have, therefore, received considerable attention for possible use in chemotherapy against cancer for their anticancer effects with a mechanism that is not fully understood [191,219].

According to the Nutritional Prevention of Cancer (NPC) Trial, a prospective, double-blinded, randomized, placebo-controlled trial involving 1,312 patients, yeast-derived Se, specifically seleno-L-methionine (SeMet) 6 and other sources of Se, can decrease overall cancer morbidity by approximately 50% [207].

The anticarcinogenic effects of higher-than-usual intakes of Se could be explained by several mechanisms, including prevention of DNA damage, oxidative stress, and inflammation and also activation of phase II enzymes, increasing immune response, halting cell cycle and angiogenesis, and induction of apoptosis [222]. Se supplementation may contribute to the DNA damage repair response potentially through induction of the activity of repair enzymes, including DNA glycosylases, and also provocation of DNA damage repair pathways, including p53, BRCA1, and Gadd45, and thus reduction of DNA lesions and chromosome breaks, which in turn results in reducing the potential detrimental mutations that are ultimately involved in carcinogenesis [219].

SM can induce p53-dependent and BRCA1/APE1-associated cell death [11]. BRCA1 (breast cancer-1), as a major tumor suppressor gene, plays a key role in genome integrity through controlling DNA damage checkpoints [11].

Selenium has also been indicated to increase the sensitivity of cancer cells to apoptotic agents such as TNF-related apoptosis-inducing ligand (TRAIL) and doxorubicin [11].

Selenite has been proposed to possess cytotoxic effects on cancer cells, likely through its metabolites, such as endogenous selenium nanoparticles (SeNPs), which bind to glycolytic enzymes, insoluble tubulin, and HSP90. SeNPs, through binding to glycolytic enzymes and sequestration of them, inhibit ATP generation and subsequently disrupt the function and structure of mitochondria. Transcriptome sequencing demonstrated considerable downregulation of mitochondrial respiratory NADH dehydrogenase (complex I), cytochrome c oxidase (complex IV), and ATP synthase (complex V) due to mitochondrial dysfunction caused by glycolytic enzyme sequestration [223]. Sequestration of insoluble tubulin seems to be associated with microtubule depolymerization and dynamic changes of it. Moreover, HSP90 sequestration by SeNPs results in disruption of downstream effectors through autophagy, which consequently initiates a cell-signaling that mediates apoptosis. Selenite-induced cytotoxicity is thought to be induced by endogenous SeNPs [223].

Low doses of such Se compounds as 30 nM SS or 10 μM SeMet, through activation of GPx1 and TrxR, have been shown to have protective effects against oxidative stress (UVA or H_2O_2)-induced cell toxicity and genotoxicity. Therefore, the benefits of Se could be explained by a combination of antioxidant activity, reduction in DNA damage, and enhancement of the oxidative DNA repair capacity [224]. However, the beneficial effects of Se compounds are significantly related to the chemical forms [224,225]. For instance, the protective effect of SS against oxidative stress and DNA damage is 300-fold higher than SeMet [224].

14.4.6.1.1 Colorectal cancer

Limited epidemiological evidence has suggested that Se deficiency could be considered a risk factor in CRC [171,221]. It has been shown that Se supplementation exerts a protective effect against CRC, possibly through increasing the expression of rectal selenoproteins [226]. Additionally, a genetic variant of the selenoprotein S gene has been linked to CRC risk. Therefore, a combination of low Se intake and single nucleotide polymorphisms (SNPs) in selenoprotein genes may potentially increase the risk of genome instability and then elevate the risk of colon cancer [171].

Selenium intake governs the expression of colon selenoproteins, namely selenoproteins W, H, M, 15kDa selenoprotein, and GPx1, and also regulates downstream targets, including stress response via ER, oxidative stress, and inflammatory pathways. Selenium is hypothesized to increase the responsiveness of colonic epithelial cells to microbial and oxidative challenges [171]. Low dietary Se intake has been suggested to be associated with the mTOR and insulin signaling pathways and hence protein biosynthesis, inflammatory response, and Wnt signaling pathways in the colons of mice [8].

In support of findings from animal studies, an inverse association between serum selenium concentrations and colorectal adenoma risk was found during the Prostate, Lung, Colorectal and Ovarian Cancer Screening Trial [221]. The results of the SELGEN study showed the effect of Se supplementation on the protein biosynthetic pathways among healthy individuals [8,227] and also the effect of selenoprotein P SNPs on response to Se supplementation [228].

A defective DNA mismatch repair (MMR) is considered a main cause of the majority of CRCs. In this regard, an investigation on the MMR-deficient HCT 116 CRC cells and the MMR-proficient HCT 116 cells with hMLH1 complementation was performed to find the role of hMLH1 in selenium-induced DNA damage response. It was found that Se can attenuate tumorigenesis, possibly through increasing the relationship between hMLH1 and hPMS2 proteins, a heterodimer essential for the function of MMR, in a manner dependent on ATM protein, responsive to DNA damage, and ROS. For more explanation, hMLH1 complementation increases the susceptibility of HCT 116 cells to methylseleninic acid, methylselenocysteine, and SS in a manner dependent on ROS and facilitates selenium-induced oxidative 8-oxoguanine damage, DNA breaks, the activation of the G2/M checkpoint, and ATM kinase activation [229]. Furthermore, it has been hypothesized that Se compounds stimulate DNA damage response at any stage of colorectal tumorigenesis differentially. At the first step, sublethal doses of selenium compounds insert DNA damage followed by senescence response, through which the cancer progression is inhibited at a very early stage. Selenium compounds at lethal doses during tumorigenesis progression can halt cells in the G2/M phase and can induce hMLH1-dependent cell death [230].

The human selenium-binding protein 1 (SBP1, SELENBP1) is another group of selenoproteins (selenium-containing proteins), made of 472 amino acids with a molecular weight of 56 kDa, in which Se tightly binds to the peptide but not incorporating co-translationally. These proteins are encoded by genes in the liver, heart, lung, and kidney tissues and placed in the nucleus and/or cytoplasm [231]. Numerous studies have shown decreased expression of SBP1 in various cancer cell lines, and poor prognosis in several type of cancers including liver, prostate, breast, lung, esophageal, gastric, and CRC has been linked to decreased levels of SBP1 [231].

In vivo induction of SBP1 in nude mice via the inducible system and mouse xenograft model revealed cancer-protective effects including suppression of colorectal cell growth and metastasis. The relationship between tumor suppressor effects of SBP1 and changes of proteins linked to lipid/glucose metabolism, as well as those involved in glycolysis, MAPK, Wnt, NOTCH, and epithelial–mesenchymal transition (EMT) signaling pathways such as DKK1, ANXA4, or NF-κB, has been observed as well. It is likely that these altered proteins have an important role in regulating downstream targets involved in carcinogenesis and progression [231]. SBP1 may also interact with other proteins, such as von Hippel–Lindau (pVHL), which catalyzes ubiquitination and deubiquitination in protein degradation pathways [232]. Overall, previous studies implicated the tumorigenesis barrier property of both endogenous and ectopic SBP1 [231].

14.4.6.1.2 Prostate cancer

Prostate cancer is one of the main causes of mortality among men worldwide [233]. There are several studies that have shown a significantly inversely association between Se status and the prostate cancer risk [170]. In the NPC study, Se supplementation in the form of Se yeast was related to the decrement of prostate cancer risk in subjects with nutritional Se deficiency [170]. However, there have also been some controversies in this regard. Even in the NPC study, the beneficial effects of Se supplementation was not shown in all subjects [11,170,207]. For instance, a high level of serum Se was observed to be related to a slightly increased risk of aggressive prostate cancer in subjects of a specific variant form of the SOD2 gene [170].

The potential mechanism for the protective effect of Se against DNA damage and subsequent cancer risk could be defined by the redox properties of selenoenzymes *in vivo* and Se-induced apoptosis [222]. Survivin is a member of the inhibitor of apoptosis (IAP) protein family, which is highly expressed in most cancers, especially prostate cancer, and plays a key role in protecting cells against apoptosis. The effect of selenium on survivin expression and subsequently sensitizing prostate cancer cells to chemotherapeutic agents has been evaluated in numerous hormone refractory prostate cancer cell lines [233]. Despite the inhibitory effect of Se on the growth of hormone-refractory prostate cancer cells *in vitro* and *in vivo*, the growth inhibition was not through decreasing the expression of survivin and the effect of Se on apoptosis was modest. However, survivin silencing considerably increased the growth inhibitory effects of Se [233]. The results of a nested case control study as a part of the Physicians Health Study (PHS), carried out in a large number (1,286 cases and 1,267 controls) of the US population, suggested that there is a relationship between Se status and the risk of prostate cancer. Additionally, the risk of prostate cancer mortality is much lower in those who have high serum concentration of Se combined with genetic variation on the 15 kDa selenoprotein (SEP15) gene, with carriers of the G allele [8].

A nested case-control study, which was part of the EPIC-Heidelberg cohort, analyzed serum selenium and selenoprotein P concentrations and GPx activity to determine their association with the risk of prostate cancer. The findings revealed that (1) poor status of Se can be modified by genetic variants in

358   Nutrigenomics and Nutraceuticals

selenoprotein genes; and (2) serum Se concentration had a borderline significant association with prostate cancer risk, which was modulated by rs1050450 in the GPX1 gene, indicating SePP and GPx1 play an important role in prostate function. Nevertheless, further studies are needed to determine the underlying biological mechanisms of the functional effects of these polymorphisms (e.g., measurements of GPx1 activity) in the prostate [222].

14.4.6.1.3 Breast cancer

Selenium supplementation has been shown to be associated with a reduction in chromosome breakage in BRCA1 mutation carriers who are at risk of breast cancer. In this scheme, in a study the relationship between toenail Se concentrations and DNA repair capacity in both BRCA1 carrier and noncarrier women was evaluated. The findings showed an inverse association between toenail selenium and the levels of chromosomal breakage induced by gamma-irradiation, as assessed by the micronucleus test. However, through application of the COMET assay or the number of gamma-H2AX foci, toenail selenium failed to predict DNA repair capacity, in either carriers or noncarriers. Therefore, these results suggested a potential breast cancer–protective effect of selenium in female BRCA1 mutation carriers [234].

14.4.6.2 Selenium and age-related diseases

It has been proposed that aging and longevity may be affected by the interaction between nutrigenomic and nutrigenetic approaches [88].

Pro- and anti-inflammatory cytokines are considered important factors for the major geriatric disorders [88]. Se insufficiency found to be prevalent during aging, maybe due to a limited intake of protein sources, such as red meat [234]. Se adequacy is suggested to be an effective anti-aging factor, possibly due to the fact that Se plays an important role in stimulating antibody synthesis and the activity of T cell and NK cells [235]. Moreover, it improves the function of leukocytes through reducing ROS formation during aging [236]. It has been suggested that several pathways, such as the mTOR pathway, which has been found to be associated with the aging process and age-related diseases through its involvement in cell senescence, could be affected by Se status [237].

With regard to the fact that oxidative stress has a major role in AD, Cardoso et al. investigated the frequency of the GPx1 Pro198Leu polymorphism and also its relationship with GPx activity and Se status in AD patients [238]. According to the findings, despite the null effect of different genotypes on GPx activity, Pro/Pro AD patients had lower blood Se levels in comparison to Pro/Pro control subjects. Moreover, the Pro198Leu genotype modified the association between the Se concentration of erythrocyte. Therefore, the Se status of AD patients was obviously influenced by this polymorphism, which seems to be associated with a lower activity of GPx [238]. The Epidemiology of Vascular Ageing (EVA) study has also shown that people with low plasma selenium are susceptible to cognitive decline [239].

Observational studies have proposed a protective effect of dietary antioxidant nutrients such as vitamin E and selenium against the development of cataracts. However, the Selenium and Vitamin E Cancer Prevention Trial (SELECT) Eye Endpoints Study, conducted among over 35,000 men aged 50 years and plus residing in the United States, Canada, and Puerto Rico, evaluated the long-term effects of Se (200 µg L-SM/day) and vitamin E (400 IU all rac-alpha-tocopheryl acetate/day) supplementation on the incidence of cataracts. The results showed that a considerable beneficial effect on age-related cataracts may not be provided by long-term daily supplementation with selenium and/or vitamin E [240]. Nevertheless, Se as an essential trace element may influence aging and its related disorders. Further approaches that consider the combination of nutrigenomics with longevity in humans seem to be necessary for identifying the mechanisms by which Se affects the aging process [8].

14.5 Summary

Although investigations have indicated that iron-requiring proteins have been implicated in DNA replication/repair and cell cycle control, limited information is available regarding their functional mechanisms. Several iron-requiring proteins, such as DNA polymerases/primases, DNA helicases, and RNRs, directly participate in DNA replication and repair. Disruption of some iron-requiring proteins, particularly hemoproteins, has been shown to be associated with the generation of ROS, which may cause DNA damage. Furthermore, ROS formation is associated with some diseases characterized by DNA repair defects and/or a poor response to replication stress in mammals. Thus, a detailed understanding of the mechanisms of Fe-requiring protein functions may provide insights into the related mutagenic diseases.

Zn contributes to genetic stability and cancer prevention through its role as a key part of enzymes involved in DNA repair and antioxidant activity. Zn displays crucial roles in preventing chronic diseases such as T2D, CVD, and also age-related diseases including inflammatory degenerative diseases through contribution to the antioxidant defense mechanism and also to providing a balanced immune function.

Zn deficiency resulting from malnutrition, aging, or disease considerably influences immune function and consequently increases the risk of infection. Enhanced production of ROS and pro-inflammatory cytokines in Zn deficiency may be due to epigenetic alterations. Various studies have demonstrated the altered expression of several genes associated with inflammation and oxidative stress in response to dietary Zn intake. Nevertheless, there are conflicting results regarding the beneficial effects of Zn supplementation during aging, because of the impact of several other factors such as dietary habits, genotype, gender, drug use, and frailty. Further well-designed prospective studies are needed to elucidate the possible effects of Zn on both genomic and clinical outcomes.

Dietary Se deficiency can induce DNA breaks and oxidation through mechanisms that have not been completely defined. Moreover, selenium in excess has also been suggested to increase oxidative stress, which leads to DNA breaks and oxidation. Therefore, both Se deficiency and overdose can promote genome instability through induction of oxidative damage. However, dietary intake of Se that is higher than nutritional intake but below toxic levels may be able to provide optimal health and attenuate carcinogenesis through apoptosis, DNA repair, and limiting endogenous ROS formation at an acceptable level by increased expression of selenoproteins such as GPx1. Many studies have indicated that Se-containing proteins are involved in maintaining genome stability in a catalytic and/or epigenetic manner. The role of Se in the stimulation of immune response, oxidative stress response, and DNA metabolism is majorly connected, directly or indirectly, with other micronutrients, including zinc, folate, and vitamins D, E, B2, B6, and B12.

It is important to mention that the bioavailability of Se, like other micronutrients, depends on its dose, source, chemical form, and physiological processes, including digestion, absorption, metabolism, and excretion. Therefore, the net effects of Se depend on the interaction among genes, gene products, and environmental factors.

Overall, because of the inconclusive results provided by epidemiological studies and also supplementation trials regarding the linkage between low Se intake and elevated risk of various cancers, as well as differences in baseline status of Se and the likelihood of genetic influences, indiscriminate use of Se supplements may not be recommended.

14.6 Future insights

There is a wide variety of health benefits provided by iron, Zn, and selenium that remain to be understood. Regarding the limited studies and also remarkable controversies about the beneficial effects of iron, Zn, and Se supplementation at the population level, further epidemiological and interventional studies using nutrigenomic and/or nutrigenetic approaches in different and larger populations are needed to determine an appropriate source and optimal dose of iron, Zn, and Se for each condition (sex, geographic location, and type of cancer) in order to prevent genomic instability, carcinogenesis, and age-related diseases. Furthermore, incorporation of nutrigenomic and nutrigenetic approaches will be helpful for determining the susceptible population subgroups who are more prone to suffer from iron, Zn, and Se deficiency and who will benefit more from supplementation.

More interventional studies using validated biomarkers of chromosome integrity may be able to clarify dietary reference values for iron, Zn, and Se intake based on their protective effects against DNA damage and genetic instability. On the contrary, the information regarding the relationship between iron, Zn, and Se status and DNA damage/chromosomal instability is still very limited. Therefore, there is a critical need for conducting robust and reproducible intervention *in vivo* studies with well-validated biomarkers of DNA integrity.

References

1. Heerwagen MJ, Miller MR, Barbour LA, Friedman JE. Maternal obesity and fetal metabolic programming: A fertile epigenetic soil. *American Journal of Physiology Regulatory, Integrative and Comparative Physiology.* 2010;299(3):R711–22.
2. Ford SP, Long NM. Evidence for similar changes in offspring phenotype following either maternal undernutrition or overnutrition: Potential impact on fetal epigenetic mechanisms. *Reproductive, Fertility and Development.* 2011;24(1):105–11.
3. Yajnik CS. Transmission of obesity-adiposity and related disorders from the mother to the baby. *Annals of Nutrition and Metabolism.* 2014;64 Suppl 1:8–17.
4. Langley-Evans SC. Fetal programming of CVD and renal disease: Animal models and mechanistic considerations. *The Proceedings of the Nutrition Society.* 2013;72(3):317–25.
5. Aiken CE, Ozanne SE. Transgenerational developmental programming. *Human Reproduction Update.* 2014;20(1):63–75.
6. McPherson NO, Fullston T, Aitken RJ, Lane M. Paternal obesity, interventions, and mechanistic pathways to impaired health in offspring. *Annals of Nutrition and Metabolism.* 2014;64(3–4):231–8.
7. Meramat A, Rajab NF, Shahar S, Sharif R. Cognitive impairment, genomic instability and trace elements. *The Journal of Nutrition, Health and Aging.* 2015;19(1):48–57.
8. Méplan C. Trace elements and ageing, a genomic perspective using selenium as an example. *Journal of Trace Elements in Medicine and Biology.* 2011;25 Suppl 1:S11–6.
9. Vural H, Demirin H, Kara Y, Eren I, Delibas N. Alterations of plasma magnesium, copper, zinc, iron and selenium concentrations and some related erythrocyte antioxidant enzyme activities in patients with Alzheimer's disease. *Journal of Trace Elements in Medicine and Biology: Organ of the Society for Minerals and Trace Elements (GMS).* 2010;24(3):169–73.
10. Mocchegiani E, Malavolta M, Giacconi R, Costarelli L. Dietary intake and impact of zinc supplementation on the immune functions in elderly: Nutrigenomic approach. *Immunology of Aging.* Berlin Heidelberg: Springer-Verlag; 2014. pp. 295–308. DOI: 10.1007/978-3-642-39495-9_22.
11. Cheng WH. Impact of inorganic nutrients on maintenance of genomic stability. *Environmental and Molecular Mutagenesis.* 2009;50(5):349–60.
12. Adeoti ML, Oguntola AS, Akanni EO, Agodirin OS, Oyeyemi GM. Trace elements; copper, zinc and selenium, in breast cancer afflicted female patients in LAUTECH Osogbo, Nigeria. *Indian Journal of Cancer.* 2015;52(1):106–9.
13. Singh BP, Dwivedi S, Dhakad U, Murthy RC, Choubey VK, Goel A, et al. Status and interrelationship of zinc, copper, iron, calcium and selenium in prostate cancer. *Indian Journal of Clinical Biochemistry.* 2016;31(1):50–6.
14. Pra D, Rech Franke SI, Pegas Henriques JA, Fenech M. A possible link between iron deficiency and gastrointestinal carcinogenesis. *Nutrition and Cancer.* 2009;61(4):415–26.
15. Ruttkay-Nedecky, Nejdl L, Gumulec J, Zitka O, Masarik M, Eckschlager T, et al. The role of metallothionein in oxidative stress. *International Journal of Molecular Sciences.* 2013;14:6044–66.

16. Tanaka T, Roy CN, Yao W, Matteini A, Semba RD, Arking D, et al. A genome-wide association analysis of serum iron concentrations. *Blood.* 2010;115(1):94–6.

17. Prá D, Bortoluzzi A, Müller LL, Hermes L, Horta JA, Maluf SW, et al. Iron intake, red cell indicators of iron status, and DNA damage in young subjects. *Nutrition.* 2011;27(3):293–7.

18. Zhang C. Essential functions of iron-requiring proteins in DNA replication, repair and cell cycle control. *Protein & Cell.* 2014;5(10):750–60.

19. Pantopoulos K, Porwal SK, Tartakoff A, Devireddy L. Mechanisms of mammalian iron homeostasis. *Biochemistry.* 2012;51(29):5705–24.

20. Dehghan M, López Jaramillo P, Dueñas R, Anaya LL, Garcia RG, Zhang X, et al. Development and validation of a quantitative food frequency questionnaire among rural- and urban-dwelling adults in Colombia. *Journal of Nutrition Education and Behavior.* 2012;44(6):609–13.

21. Rouault TA. The role of iron regulatory proteins in mammalian iron homeostasis and disease. *Nature Chemical Biology.* 2006;2(8):406–14.

22. Frey AG, Nandal A, Park JH, Smith PM, Yabe T, Ryu MS, et al. Iron chaperones PCBP1 and PCBP2 mediate the metallation of the dinuclear iron enzyme deoxyhypusine hydroxylase. *Proceedings of the National Academy of Sciences of the United States of America.* 2014;111(22):8031–6.

23. Hardison R. The Evolution of hemoglobin: Studies of a very ancient protein suggest that changes in gene regulation are an important part of the evolutionary story. *American Scientist.* 1990;87(2):126.

24. Caughey WS, Smythe GA, O'Keeffe DH, Maskasky JE, Smith MI. Heme A of cyto-chrome c oxicase. Structure and properties: Comparisons with hemes B, C, and S and derivatives. *The Journal of Biological Chemistry.* 1975;250(19):7602–22.

25. Muckenthaler MU, Rivella S, Hentze MW, Galy B. A Red Carpet for Iron Metabolism. *Cell.* 2017;168:344–61.

26. Fenech M. The Genome Health Clinic and Genome Health Nutrigenomics concepts: Diagnosis and nutritional treatment of genome and epigenome damage on an individual basis. *Mutagenesis.* 2005;20(4):255–69.

27. Hiom K. FANCJ: Solving problems in DNA replication. *DNA Repair.* 20102;9(3):250–6.

28. Bharti SK, Sommers JA, George F, Kuper J, Hamon F, Shin-ya K, et al. Specialization among iron-sulfur cluster helicases to resolve G-quadruplex DNA structures that threaten genomic stability. *The Journal of Biological Chemistry.* 2013;288(39):28217–29.

29. Sanvisens N, de Llanos R, Puig S. Function and regulation of yeast ribonucleotide reductase: Cell cycle, genotoxic stress, and iron bioavailability. *Biomedical Journal.* 2013;36(2):51–8.

30. Siriwardana G, Seligman PA. Two cell cycle blocks caused by iron chelation of neuro-blastoma cells: Separating cell cycle events associated with each block. *Physiological Reports.* 2013;1(7):e00176.

31. Yu Y, Kovacevic Z, Richardson DR. Tuning cell cycle regulation with an iron key. *Cell Cycle.* 2007;6(16):1982–94.

32. Fu D, Richardson DR. Iron chelation and regulation of the cell cycle: 2 mechanisms of posttranscriptional regulation of the universal cyclin-dependent kinase inhibitor p21CIP1/WAF1 by iron depletion. *Blood.* 2007;110(2):752–61.

33. Le NT, Richardson DR. The role of iron in cell cycle progression and the proliferation of neoplastic cells. *Biochimica et biophysica acta.* 2002 Oct 2;1603(1):31–46.

34. Siriwardana G, Seligman PA. Iron depletion results in Src kinase inhibition with associated cell cycle arrest in neuroblastoma cells. *Physiological Reports.* 2015;3(3):e12341.

35. Karuppagounder SS, Kumar A, Shao DS, Zille M, Bourassa MW, Caulfield JT, et al. Metabolism and epigenetics in the nervous system: Creating cellular fitness and resistance to neuronal death in neurological conditions via modulation of oxygen-, iron-, and 2-oxoglutarate-dependent dioxygenases. *Brain Research.* 2015;1628(Pt B):273–87.

36. Yara S, Lavoie JC, Beaulieu JF, Delvin E, Amre D, Marcil V, et al. Iron-ascorbate-mediated lipid peroxidation causes epigenetic changes in the antioxidant defense in intestinal epithelial cells: Impact on inflammation. *PloS One.* 2013;8(5):e63456.
37. Teperino R, Schoonjans K, Auwerx J. Histone methyl transferases and demethylases; can they link metabolism and transcription? *Cell Metabolism.* 2010;12(4):321–7.
38. Burgio G, Onorati MC, Corona DF. Chromatin remodeling regulation by small molecules and metabolites. *Biochimica et biophysica acta.* 2010;1799(10–12):671–80.
39. Pogribny IP, Tryndyak VP, Pogribna M, Shpyleva S, Surratt G, Gamboa da Costa G, et al. Modulation of intracellular iron metabolism by iron chelation affects chromatin remodeling proteins and corresponding epigenetic modifications in breast cancer cells and increases their sensitivity to chemotherapeutic agents. *International Journal of Oncology.* 2013;42(5):1822–32.
40. Shmakova A, Batie M, Druker J, Rocha S. Chromatin and oxygen sensing in the context of JmjC histone demethylases. *The Biochemical Journal.* 2014;462(3):385–95.
41. Ito IY, Junior FM, Paula-Silva FW, Da Silva LA, Leonardo MR, Nelson-Filho P. Microbial culture and checkerboard DNA-DNA hybridization assessment of bacteria in root canals of primary teeth pre- and post-endodontic therapy with a calcium hydroxide/chlorhexidine paste. *International Journal of Paediatric Dentistry/the British Paedodontic Society [and] the International Association of Dentistry for Children.* 2011;21(5):353–60.
42. Hahn MA, Qiu R, Wu X, Li AX, Zhang H, Wang J, et al. Dynamics of 5-hydroxymethylcytosine and chromatin marks in Mammalian neurogenesis. *Cell Reports.* 2013;3(2):291–300.
43. Bruick RK, McKnight SL. A conserved family of prolyl-4-hydroxylases that modify HIF. *Science (New York, NY).* 2001;294(5545):1337–40.
44. Hitchler MJ, Oberley LW, Domann FE. Epigenetic silencing of SOD2 by histone modifications in human breast cancer cells. *Free Radical Biology & Medicine.* 2008;45(11):1573–80.
45. Chen L, Guo G, Liu T, Guo L, Zhu R. Radiochemotherapy of hepatocarcinoma via lentivirus-mediated transfer of human sodium iodide symporter gene and herpes simplex virus thymidine kinase gene. *Nuclear Medicine and Biology.* 2011;38(5):757–63.
46. Dawson KA. Nutrigenomics: Feeding the genes for improved fertility. *Animal Reproduction Science.* 2006;96(3–4):312–22.
47. Keiko A. Studies on food functionality and safety in Japan—Evaluation by genomics. *Journal of Food and Drug Analysis.* 2012;20 Suppl 1:208–12.
48. Stehling O, Vashisht AA, Mascarenhas J, Jonsson ZO, Sharma T, Netz DJ, et al. MMS19 assembles iron-sulfur proteins required for DNA metabolism and genomic integrity. *Science (New York, NY).* 2012;337(6091):195–9.
49. Diaz de la Loza Mdel C, Gallardo M, Garcia-Rubio ML, Izquierdo A, Herrero E, Aguilera A, et al. Zim17/Tim15 links mitochondrial iron-sulfur cluster biosynthesis to nuclear genome stability. *Nucleic Acids Research.* 2011;39(14):6002–15.
50. Pra D, Franke SI, Henriques JA, Fenech M. Iron and genome stability: An update. *Mutation Research.* 2012;733(1–2):92–9.
51. Veatch JR, McMurray MA, Nelson ZW, Gottschling DE. Mitochondrial dysfunction leads to nuclear genome instability via an iron-sulfur cluster defect. *Cell.* 2009;137(7):1247–58.
52. Turker MS, Connolly L, Dan C, Lasarev M, Gauny S, Kwoh E, et al. Comparison of autosomal mutations in mouse kidney epithelial cells exposed to iron ions in situ or in culture. *Radiation Research.* 2009;172(5):558–66.
53. Kobayashi H, Imanaka S, Nakamura H, Tsuji A. Understanding the role of epigenomic, genomic and genetic alterations in the development of endometriosis (review). *Molecular Medicine Reports.* 2014;9(5):1483–505.
54. Rodriguez A, Hilvo M, Kytomaki L, Fleming RE, Britton RS, Bacon BR, et al. Effects of iron loading on muscle: Genome-wide mRNA expression profiling in the mouse. *BMC Genomics.* 2007;8:379.

55. Kamei A, Watanabe Y, Ishijima T, Uehara M, Arai S, Kato H, et al. Dietary iron-deficient anemia induces a variety of metabolic changes and even apoptosis in rat liver: A DNA microarray study. *Physiological Genomics.* 2010;42(2):149–56.
56. Toxqui L, De Piero A, Courtois V, Bastida S, Sanchez-Muniz FJ, Vaquero MP. Iron deficiency and overload. Implications in oxidative stress and cardiovascular health. *Nutricion Hospitalaria.* 2010;25(3):350–65.
57. Aursulesei V, Cozma A, Krasniqi A. Iron hypothesis of cardiovascular disease: Still controversial. *Revista medico-chirurgicala a Societatii de Medici si Naturalisti din Iasi.* 2014;118(4):901–9.
58. Merono T, Sorroche P, Brites FD. Increased iron store and its relationship with cardiovascular disease. *Medicina.* 2011;71(6):566–72.
59. Xu X, Pin S, Gathinji M, Fuchs R, Harris ZL. Aceruloplasminemia: An inherited neurodegenerative disease with impairment of iron homeostasis. *Annals of the New York Academy of Sciences.* 2004;1012:299–305.
60. Pigeon C, Legrand P, Leroyer P, Bouriel M, Turlin B, Brissot P, et al. Stearoyl coenzyme A desaturase 1 expression and activity are increased in the liver during iron overload. *Biochimica et biophysica acta.* 2001;1535(3):275–84.
61. Li L, Wang C, Calvisi DF, Evert M, Pilo MG, Jiang L, et al. SCD1 Expression is dispensable for hepatocarcinogenesis induced by AKT and Ras oncogenes in mice. *PloS One.* 2013;8(9):e75104.
62. Brown KE, Broadhurst KA, Mathahs MM, Weydert J. Differential expression of stress-inducible proteins in chronic hepatic iron overload. *Toxicology and Applied Pharmacology.* 2007;223(2):180–6.
63. Das M, Lu J, Joseph M, Aggarwal R, Kanji S, McMichael BK, et al. Kruppel-like factor 2 (KLF2) regulates monocyte differentiation and functions in mBSA and IL-1beta-induced arthritis. *Current Molecular Medicine.* 2012;12(2):113–25.
64. Kepinska M, Szyller J, Milnerowicz H. The influence of oxidative stress induced by iron on telomere length. *Environmental Toxicology and Pharmacology.* 2015;40(3):931–5.
65. Mainous AG 3rd, Wright RU, Hulihan MM, Twal WO, McLaren CE, Diaz VA, et al. Telomere length and elevated iron: The influence of phenotype and HFE genotype. *American Journal of Hematology.* 2013;88(6):492–6.
66. Johnstone D, Milward EA. Genome-wide microarray analysis of brain gene expression in mice on a short-term high iron diet. *Neurochemistry International.* 2010;56(6–7):856–63.
67. Abtahi M, Neyestani TR, Pouraram H, Siassi F, Dorosty AR, Elmadfa I, et al. Iron-fortified flour: Can it induce lipid peroxidation? *International Journal of Food Sciences and Nutrition.* 2014;65(5):649–54.
68. Pouraram H, Elmadfa I, Dorosty AR, Abtahi M, Neyestani TR, Sadeghian S. Long-term consequences of iron-fortified flour consumption in nonanemic men. *Annals of Nutrition and Metabolism.* 2012;60(2):115–21.
69. Paul VD, Lill R. Biogenesis of cytosolic and nuclear iron-sulfur proteins and their role in genome stability. *Biochimica et biophysica acta.* 2015;1853(6):1528–39.
70. Philpott CC, Leidgens S, Frey AG. Metabolic remodeling in iron-deficient fungi. *Biochimica et biophysica acta.* 2012;1823(9):1509–20.
71. Shakoury-Elizeh M, Protchenko O, Berger A, Cox J, Gable K, Dunn TM, et al. Metabolic response to iron deficiency in Saccharomyces cerevisiae. *The Journal of Biological Chemistry.* 2010;285(19):14823–33.
72. Silva M, da Costa Guerra JF, Sampaio AF, de Lima WG, Silva ME, Pedrosa ML. Iron dextran increases hepatic oxidative stress and alters expression of genes related to lipid metabolism contributing to hyperlipidaemia in murine model. *BioMed Research International.* 2015;2015:272617.
73. Richardson DR, Kalinowski DS, Lau S, Jansson PJ, Lovejoy DB. Cancer cell iron metabolism and the development of potent iron chelators as anti-tumour agents. *Biochimica et biophysica acta.* 2009;1790(7):702–17.

74. Torti SV, Torti FM. Iron and cancer: More ore to be mined. *Nature Reviews Cancer.* 2013;13(5):342–55.
75. Xiong W, Wang L, Yu F. Regulation of cellular iron metabolism and its implications in lung cancer progression. *Medical Oncology.* 2014;31(7):28.
76. Panzer R, Kury S, Schmitt S, Folster-Holst R. Identification of a novel mutation in the SLC39A4 gene in a case of acrodermatitis enteropathica. *Acta Dermato Venereology.* 2016;96(3):424–5.
77. Solomon J, Kamalammal R, Sait MY, Lohith H. Cow's milk protein allergy mimicking acrodermatitis enteropathica. *Journal of Clinical and Diagnostic Research.* 2014;8(3):160–1.
78. Hamara K, Bielecka-Kowalska A, Przybylowska-Sygut K, Sygut A, Dziki A, Szemraj J. Alterations in expression profile of iron-related genes in colorectal cancer. *Molecular Biology Reports.* 2013;40(10):5573–85.
79. Ruder EH, Berndt SI, Gilsing AM, Graubard BI, Burdett L, Hayes RB, et al. Dietary iron, iron homeostatic gene polymorphisms and the risk of advanced colorectal adenoma and cancer. *Carcinogenesis.* 2014;35(6):1276–83.
80. Durackova Z. Some current insights into oxidative stress. *Physiological Research/ Academia Scientiarum Bohemoslovaca.* 2010;59(4):459–69.
81. Paschos A, Pandya R, Duivenvoorden WC, Pinthus JH. Oxidative stress in prostate cancer: Changing research concepts towards a novel paradigm for prevention and therapeutics. *Prostate Cancer Prostatic Disease.* 2013;16(3):217–25.
82. Choi JY, Neuhouser ML, Barnett MJ, Hong CC, Kristal AR, Thornquist MD, et al. Iron intake, oxidative stress-related genes (MnSOD and MPO) and prostate cancer risk in CARET cohort. *Carcinogenesis.* 2008;29(5):964–70.
83. Hong CC, Ambrosone CB, Ahn J, Choi JY, McCullough ML, Stevens VL, et al. Genetic variability in iron-related oxidative stress pathways (Nrf2, NQ01, NOS3, and HO-1), iron intake, and risk of postmenopausal breast cancer. *Cancer Epidemiology, Biomarkers & Prevention: A Publication of the American Association for Cancer Research, Cosponsored by the American Society of Preventive Oncology.* 2007;16(9):1784–94.
84. Vasudevaraju P, Bharathi, TJ, Shamasundar NM, Subba Rao K, Balaraj BM, et al. New evidence on iron, copper accumulation and zinc depletion and its correlation with DNA integrity in aging human brain regions. *Indian Journal of Psychiatry.* 2010;52(2):140–4.
85. Hagemeier J, Geurts JJ, Zivadinov R. Brain iron accumulation in aging and neurodegenerative disorders. *Expert Review of Neurotherapeutics.* 2012;12(12):1467–80.
86. Arruda LF, Arruda SF, Campos NA, de Valencia FF, Siqueira EM. Dietary iron concentration may influence aging process by altering oxidative stress in tissues of adult rats. *PloS One.* 2013;8(4):e61058.
87. Fenech MF. Nutriomes and nutrient arrays—the key to personalised nutrition for DNA damage prevention and cancer growth control. *Genome Integrity.* 2010;1:11.
88. Mocchegiani E, Costarelli L, Giacconi R, Malavolta M, Basso A, Piacenza F, et al. Micronutrient-gene interactions related to inflammatory/immune response and antioxidant activity in ageing and inflammation. A systematic review. *Mechanisms of Ageing and Development.* 2014;136:29–49.
89. Mazzatti DJ, Malavolta M, White AJ, Costarelli L, Giacconi R, Muti E, et al. Differential effects of in vitro zinc treatment on gene expression in peripheral blood mononuclear cells derived from young and elderly individuals. *Rejuvenation Research.* 2007;10(4):603–20.
90. Sun JY, Wang JF, Zi NT, Jing MY, Weng XY. Gene expression profiles analysis of the growing rat liver in response to different zinc status by cDNA microarray analysis. *Biological Trace Element Research.* 2007;115(2):169–85.
91. Mocchegiani E. Zinc, metallothioneins, longevity: Effect of zinc supplementation on antioxidant response: A Zincage study. *Rejuvenation Research.* 2008;11(2):419–23.

92. Cousins RJ, Liuzzi JP, Lichten LA. Mammalian zinc transport, trafficking, and signals. *The Journal of Biological Chemistry*. 2006;281(34):24085–9.
93. Sekler I, Sensi SL, Hershfinkel M, Silverman WF. Mechanism and regulation of cellular zinc transport. *Molecular Medicine (Cambridge, Mass)*. 2007;13(7–8):337–43.
94. Giacconi R, Caruso C, Malavolta M, Lio D, Balistreri CR, Scola L, et al. Pro-inflammatory genetic background and zinc status in old atherosclerotic subjects. *Ageing Research Reviews*. 2008;7(4):306–18.
95. Devirgiliis C, Zalewski PD, Perozzi G, Murgia C. Zinc fluxes and zinc transporter genes in chronic diseases. *Mutation Research-Fundamental and Molecular Mechanisms of Mutagenesis*. 2007;622(1–2):84–93.
96. Prasad AS. Discovery of human zinc deficiency: 50 years later. *Journal of Trace Elements in Medicine and Biology: Organ of the Society for Minerals and Trace Elements (GMS)*. 2012;26(2–3):66–9.
97. Prasad AS. Discovery of human zinc deficiency: Its impact on human health and disease. *Advances in Nutrition (Bethesda, MD)*. 2013;4(2):176–90.
98. Prasad AS. Impact of the discovery of human zinc deficiency on health. *Journal of the American College of Nutrition*. 2009;28(3):257–65.
99. Sandstead HH. Human zinc deficiency: Discovery to initial translation. *Advances in Nutrition (Bethesda, MD)*. 2013;4(1):76–81.
100. King JC, Brown KH, Gibson RS, Krebs NF, Lowe NM, Siekmann JH, et al. Biomarkers of Nutrition for Development (BOND)-Zinc Review. *The Journal of Nutrition*. 2016;146(9):1816S–48S.
101. Mocchegiani E, Costarelli L, Giacconi R, Piacenza F, Basso A, Malavolta M. Zinc, metallothioneins and immunosenescence: Effect of zinc supply as nutrigenomic approach. *Biogerontology*. 2011;12(5):455–65.
102. Wong CP, Ho E. Zinc and its role in age-related inflammation and immune dysfunction. *Molecular Nutrition & Food Research*. 2012;56(1):77–87.
103. Mocchegiani E, Costarelli L, Giacconi R, Piacenza F, Basso A, Malavolta M. Micronutrient (Zn, Cu, Fe)-gene interactions in ageing and inflammatory age-related diseases: Implications for treatments. *Ageing Research Reviews*. 2012;11(2):297–319.
104. WHO. *Clinical Management of Acute Diarrhoea*. Geneva: World Health Organization; 2004.
105. WHO. *Implementing the New Recommendations of the Clinical Management of Diarrhoea*. Geneva: World Health Organization; 2006.
106. Maret W. Zinc coordination environments in proteins as redox sensors and signal transducers. *Antioxidants & Redox Signaling*. 2006;8(9–10):1419–41.
107. Llanos RM, Mercer JF. The molecular basis of copper homeostasis copper-related disorders. *DNA and Cell Biology*. 2002;21(4):259–70.
108. Vasto S, Mocchegiani E, Malavolta M, Cuppari I, Listi F, Nuzzo D, et al. Zinc and inflammatory/immune response in aging. *Annals of the New York Academy of Sciences*. 2007;1100:111–22.
109. Bao S, Liu MJ, Lee B, Besecker B, Lai JP, Guttridge DC, et al. Zinc modulates the innate immune response in vivo to polymicrobial sepsis through regulation of NF-kappaB. *American Journal of Physiology Lung Cellular and Molecular Physiology*. 2010;298(6):L744–54.
110. Pearson R, Fleetwood J, Eaton S, Crossley M, Bao S. Kruppel-like transcription factors: A functional family. *The International Journal of Biochemistry & Cell Biology*. 2008;40(10):1996–2001.
111. Lee JL, Lo CW, Inserra C, Bera JC, Chen WS. Ultrasound enhanced PEI-mediated gene delivery through increasing the intracellular calcium level and PKC-delta protein expression. *Pharmaceutical Research*. 2014;31(9):2354–66.
112. Ellmeier W, Taniuchi I. The role of BTB-zinc finger transcription factors during T cell development and in the regulation of T cell-mediated immunity. *Current Topics in Microbiology and Immunology*. 2014;381:21–49.

113. Vanden Berghe W, Vermeulen L, Delerive P, De Bosscher K, Staels B, Haegeman G. A paradigm for gene regulation: Inflammation, NF-kappaB and PPAR. *Advances in Experimental Medicine and Biology.* 2003;544:181–96.
114. Grygiel-Gorniak B. Peroxisome proliferator-activated receptors and their ligands: Nutritional and clinical implications—A review. *Nutrition Journal.* 2014;13:17.
115. Yan M, Song Y, Wong CP, Hardin K, Ho E. Zinc deficiency alters DNA damage response genes in normal human prostate epithelial cells. *The Journal of Nutrition.* 2008;138(4):667–73.
116. Sharif R, Thomas P, Zalewski P, Fenech M. The role of zinc in genomic stability. *Mutation Research.* 2012;733(1–2):111–21.
117. Sharif R, Thomas P, Zalewski P, Fenech M. Zinc deficiency or excess within the physiological range increases genome instability and cytotoxicity, respectively, in human oral keratinocyte cells. *Genes & Nutrition.* 2012;7(2):139–54.
118. Wu C, Zhang W, Mai K, Xu W, Zhong X. Effects of dietary zinc on gene expression of antioxidant enzymes and heat shock proteins in hepatopancreas of abalone Haliotis discus hannai. *Comparative Biochemistry and Physiology Toxicology & Pharmacology.* 2011;154(1):1–6.
119. Swamynathan SK. Kruppel-like factors: Three fingers in control. *Human Genomics.* 2010;4(4):263–70.
120. Sun X, Zhou X, Du L, Liu W, Liu Y, Hudson LG, et al. Arsenite binding-induced zinc loss from PARP-1 is equivalent to zinc deficiency in reducing PARP-1 activity, leading to inhibition of DNA repair. *Toxicology and Applied Pharmacology.* 2014;274(2):313–8.
121. Ho E, Ames BN. Low intracellular zinc induces oxidative DNA damage, disrupts p53, NFkappa B, and AP1 DNA binding, and affects DNA repair in a rat glioma cell line. *Proceedings of the National Academy of Sciences of the United States of America.* 2002;99(26):16770–5.
122. Song Y, Leonard SW, Traber MG, Ho E. Zinc deficiency affects DNA damage, oxidative stress, antioxidant defenses, and DNA repair in rats. *The Journal of Nutrition.* 2009;139(9):1626–31.
123. Sharif R, Thomas P, Zalewski P, Graham RD, Fenech M. The effect of zinc sulphate and zinc carnosine on genome stability and cytotoxicity in the WIL2-NS human lymphoblastoid cell line. *Mutation Research.* 2011;720(1–2):22–33.
124. Sharif R, Thomas P, Zalewski P, Fenech M. Zinc supplementation influences genomic stability biomarkers, antioxidant activity, and zinc transporter genes in an elderly Australian population with low zinc status. *Molecular Nutrition & Food Research.* 2015;59(6):1200–12.
125. Sheffer M, Simon AJ, Jacob-Hirsch J, Rechavi G, Domany E, Givol D, et al. Genome-wide analysis discloses reversal of the hypoxia-induced changes of gene expression in colon cancer cells by zinc supplementation. *Oncotarget.* 2011;2(12):1191–202.
126. Ha GH, Kim HS, Go H, Lee H, Seimiya H, Chung DH, et al. Tankyrase-1 function at telomeres and during mitosis is regulated by Polo-like kinase-1-mediated phosphorylation. *Cell Death and Differentiation.* 2012;19(2):321–32.
127. Cipriano C, Tesei S, Malavolta M, Giacconi R, Muti E, Costarelli L, et al. Accumulation of cells with short telomeres is associated with impaired zinc homeostasis and inflammation in old hypertensive participants. *The Journals of Gerontology Series A, Biological Sciences and Medical Sciences.* 2009;64(7):745–51.
128. Gao B, Li K, Wei YY, Zhang J, Li J, Zhang L, et al. Zinc finger protein 637 protects cells against oxidative stress-induced premature senescence by mTERT-mediated telomerase activity and telomere maintenance. *Cell Death & Disease.* 2014;5:e1334.
129. Karweina D, Kreuzer-Redmer S, Muller U, Franken T, Pieper R, Baron U, et al. The zinc concentration in the diet and the length of the feeding period affect the methylation status of the ZIP4 zinc transporter gene in piglets. *PloS One.* 2015;10(11):e0143098.

130. Wessels I, Haase H, Engelhardt G, Rink L, Uciechowski P. Zinc deficiency induces production of the proinflammatory cytokines IL-1beta and TNFalpha in promyeloid cells via epigenetic and redox-dependent mechanisms. *The Journal of Nutritional Biochemistry.* 2013;24(1):289–97.

131. Tian X, Diaz FJ. Acute dietary zinc deficiency before conception compromises oocyte epigenetic programming and disrupts embryonic development. *Developmental Biology.* 2013;376(1):51–61.

132. Kurita H, Ohsako S, Hashimoto S, Yoshinaga J, Tohyama C. Prenatal zinc deficiency-dependent epigenetic alterations of mouse metallothionein-2 gene. *The Journal of Nutritional Biochemistry.* 2013;24(1):256–66.

133. Sadli N, Ackland ML, De Mel D, Sinclair AJ, Suphioglu C. Effects of zinc and DHA on the epigenetic regulation of human neuronal cells. *Cellular Physiology and Biochemistry: International Journal of Experimental Cellular Physiology, Biochemistry, and Pharmacology.* 2012;29(1–2):87–98.

134. Okumura F, Li Y, Itoh N, Nakanishi T, Isobe M, Andrews GK, et al. The zinc-sensing transcription factor MTF-1 mediates zinc-induced epigenetic changes in chromatin of the mouse metallothionein-I promoter. *Biochimica et biophysica acta.* 2011;1809(1):56–62.

135. Kang M, Zhao L, Ren M, Deng M, Li C. Reduced metallothionein expression induced by Zinc deficiency results in apoptosis in hepatic stellate cell line LX-2. *International Journal of Clinical and Experimental Medicine.* 2015;8(11):20603–9.

136. Seth R, Corniola RS, Gower-Winter SD, Morgan TJ, Jr., Bishop B, Levenson CW. Zinc deficiency induces apoptosis via mitochondrial p53- and caspase-dependent pathways in human neuronal precursor cells. *Journal of Trace Elements in Medicine and Biology: Organ of the Society for Minerals and Trace Elements (GMS).* 2015;30:59–65.

137. Provinciali M, Pierpaoli E, Bartozzi B, Bernardini G. Zinc induces apoptosis of human melanoma cells, increasing reactive oxygen species, p53 and FAS ligand. *Anticancer Research.* 2015;35(10):5309–16.

138. Xiong M, Liu L, Liu Z, Gao H. Inhibitory effect of zinc on the advanced glycation end product-induced apoptosis of mouse osteoblastic cells. *Molecular Medicine Reports.* 2015;12(4):5286–92.

139. Zhang X, Zhao Y, Chu Q, Wang ZY, Li H, Chi ZH. Zinc modulates high glucose-induced apoptosis by suppressing oxidative stress in renal tubular epithelial cells. *Biological Trace Element Research.* 2014;158(2):259–67.

140. Zhang X, Liang D, Guo B, Yang L, Wang L, Ma J. Zinc inhibits high glucose-induced apoptosis in peritoneal mesothelial cells. *Biological Trace Element Research.* 2012;150(1–3):424–32.

141. Prasad AS. Clinical, endocrinological and biochemical effects of zinc deficiency. *The Journal of Clinical Endocrinology and Metabolism.* 1985;14(3):567–89.

142. Siren PM, Siren MJ. Systemic zinc redistribution and dyshomeostasis in cancer cachexia. *Journal of Cachexia Sarcopenia and Muscle.* 2010;1(1):23–33.

143. Jayawardena R, Ranasinghe P, Galappatthy P, Malkanthi R, Constantine G, Katulanda P. Effects of zinc supplementation on diabetes mellitus: A systematic review and meta-analysis. *Diabetology & Metabolic Syndrome.* 2012;4(1):13.

144. Ranasinghe P, Wathurapatha WS, Ishara MH, Jayawardana R, Galappatthy P, Katulanda P, et al. Effects of zinc supplementation on serum lipids: A systematic review and meta-analysis. *Nutrition & Metabolism.* 2015;12:26.

145. Jantas D, Lason W. Protective effect of memantine against Doxorubicin toxicity in primary neuronal cell cultures: Influence a development stage. *Neurotoxicity Research.* 2009;15(1):24–37.

146. Wysokinski D, Blasiak J, Wozniak K. Zinc differentially modulates DNA damage induced by anthracyclines in normal and cancer cells. *Experimental Oncology.* 2012;34(4):327–31.

Nutrigenomic Aspects of Trace Elements   369

147. Sliwinski T, Czechowska A, Kolodziejczak M, Jajte J, Wisniewska-Jarosinska M, Blasiak J. Zinc salts differentially modulate DNA damage in normal and cancer cells. *Cell Biology International.* 2009;33(4):542–7.
148. Loh SN. The missing zinc: p53 misfolding and cancer. *Metallomics: Integrated Biometal Science.* 2010;2(7):442–9.
149. Garufi A, Ubertini V, Mancini F, D'Orazi V, Baldari S, Moretti F, et al. The beneficial effect of Zinc(II) on low-dose chemotherapeutic sensitivity involves p53 activation in wild-type p53-carrying colorectal cancer cells. *Journal of Experimental & Clinical Cancer Research: CR.* 2015;34:87.
150. Hoang BX, Han B, Shaw DG, Nimni M. Zinc as a possible preventive and therapeutic agent in pancreatic, prostate, and breast cancer. *European Journal of Cancer Prevention: The Official Journal of the European Cancer Prevention Organisation (ECP).* 2015;25(5):457–61.
151. Wu X, Tang J, Xie M. Serum and hair zinc levels in breast cancer: A meta-analysis. *Scientific Reports.* 2015;5:12249.
152. Wang S, Hannafon BN, Lind SE, Ding WQ. Zinc protoporphyrin suppresses beta-catenin protein expression in human cancer cells: The potential involvement of lysosome-mediated degradation. *PloS One.* 2015;10(5):e0127413.
153. Khayyatzadeh SS, Maghsoudi Z, Foroughi M, Askari G, Ghiasvand R. Dietary intake of Zinc, serum levels of Zinc and risk of gastric cancer: A review of studies. *Advanced Biomedical Research.* 2015;4:118.
154. Khoshdel Z, Naghibalhossaini F, Abdollahi K, Shojaei S, Moradi M, Malekzadeh M. Serum copper and zinc levels among Iranian colorectal cancer patients. *Biological Trace Element Research.* 2016;170(2):294–9.
155. Mazzatti DJ, Malavolta M, White AJ, Costarelli L, Giacconi R, Muti E, et al. Effects of interleukin-6 –174C/G and metallothionein 1A +647A/C single-nucleotide polymorphisms on zinc-regulated gene expression in ageing. *Experimental Gerontology.* 2008;43(5):423–32.
156. Okada S, Abuyama M, Yamamoto R, Kondo T, Narukawa M, Misaka T. Dietary zinc status reversibly alters both the feeding behaviors of the rats and gene expression patterns in diencephalon. *BioFactors (Oxford, England).* 2012;38(3):203–18.
157. Noh H, Paik HY, Kim J, Chung J. The alteration of zinc transporter gene expression is associated with inflammatory markers in obese women. *Biological Trace Element Research.* 2014;158(1):1–8.
158. Costarelli L, Muti E, Malavolta M, Cipriano C, Giacconi R, Tesei S, et al. Distinctive modulation of inflammatory and metabolic parameters in relation to zinc nutritional status in adult overweight/obese subjects. *The Journal of Nutritional Biochemistry.* 2010;21(5):432–7.
159. Kralisch S, Sommer G, Deckert CM, Linke A, Bluher M, Stumvoll M, et al. Adipokines in diabetes and cardiovascular diseases. *Minerva Endocrinologica.* 2007;32(3):161–71.
160. Noh H, Paik HY, Kim J, Chung J. The changes of zinc transporter ZnT gene expression in response to zinc supplementation in obese women. *Biological Trace Element Research.* 2014;162(1–3):38–45.
161. El-Shazly AN, Ibrahim SA, El-Mashad GM, Sabry JH, Sherbini NS. Effect of zinc supplementation on body mass index and serum levels of zinc and leptin in pediatric hemodialysis patients. *International Journal of Nephrology and Renovascular Disease.* 2015;8:159–63.
162. Chu A, Foster M, Hancock D, Bell-Anderson K, Petocz P, Samman S. TNF-alpha gene expression is increased following zinc supplementation in type 2 diabetes mellitus. *Genes & Nutrition.* 2015;10(1):440.
163. Foster M, Petocz P, Samman S. Inflammation markers predict zinc transporter gene expression in women with type 2 diabetes mellitus. *The Journal of Nutritional Biochemistry.* 2013;24(9):1655–61.

164. Foster M, Chu A, Petocz P, Samman S. Zinc transporter gene expression and glycemic control in post-menopausal women with Type 2 diabetes mellitus. *Journal of Trace Elements in Medicine and Biology: Organ of the Society for Minerals and Trace Elements (GMS)*. 2014;28(4):448–52.

165. Shan Z, Bao W, Zhang Y, Rong Y, Wang X, Jin Y, et al. Interactions between zinc transporter-8 gene (SLC30A8) and plasma zinc concentrations for impaired glucose regulation and type 2 diabetes. *Diabetes*. 2014;63(5):1796–803.

166. Prasad AS. Zinc in human health: Effect of zinc on immune cells. *Molecular Medicine*. 2008;14(5–6):353–7.

167. Mariani E, Neri S, Cattini L, Mocchegiani E, Malavolta M, Dedoussis GV, et al. Effect of zinc supplementation on plasma IL-6 and MCP-1 production and NK cell function in healthy elderly: Interactive influence of +647 MT1a and -174 IL-6 polymorphic alleles. *Experimental Gerontology*. 2008;43(5):462–71.

168. Mocchegiani E, Bürkle A, Fulop T. Zinc and ageing (ZINCAGE Project). *Experimental Gerontology*. 2008;43(5):361–2.

169. Hughes S, Samman S. The effect of zinc supplementation in humans on plasma lipids, antioxidant status and thrombogenesis. *Journal of the American College of Nutrition*. 2006;25(4):285–91.

170. Ferguson LR, Karunasinghe N. Nutrigenetics, nutrigenomics, and selenium. *Frontiers in Genetics*. 2011;2:15.

171. Meplan C, Hesketh J. The influence of selenium and selenoprotein gene variants on colorectal cancer risk. *Mutagenesis*. 2012;27(2):177–86.

172. Gentschew L, Bishop KS, Han DY, Morgan AR, Fraser AG, Lam WJ, et al. Selenium, selenoprotein genes and Crohn's disease in a case-control population from Auckland, New Zealand. *Nutrients*. 2012;4(9):1247–59.

173. Fairweather-Tait SJ, Bao Y, Broadley MR, Collings R, Ford D, Hesketh JE, et al. Selenium in human health and disease. *Antioxidants & Redox Signaling*. 2011;14(7):1337–83.

174. Wastney ME, Combs GF, Jr., Canfield WK, Taylor PR, Patterson KY, Hill AD, et al. A human model of selenium that integrates metabolism from selenite and selenomethionine. *The Journal of Nutrition*. 2011;141(4):708–17.

175. Mistry HD, Broughton Pipkin F, Redman CWG, Poston L. Selenium in reproductive health. *American Journal of Obstetrics and Gynecology*. 2012;206(1):21–30.

176. Ferguson LR, Karunasinghe N, Zhu S, Wang AH. Selenium and its' role in the maintenance of genomic stability. *Mutation Research/Fundamental Molecular Mechanisms of Mutagenesis*. 2012;733(1–2):100–10.

177. Cheng WH, Holmstrom A, Li X, Wu RT, Zeng H, Xiao Z. Effect of dietary selenium and cancer cell xenograft on peripheral T and B lymphocytes in adult nude mice. *Biological Trace Element Research*. 2012;146(2):230–5.

178. Méplan C, Hesketh J. Selenium and cancer: A story that should not be forgotten-insights from genomics. *Cancer Treatment and Research*. 2014;159:145–66.

179. Bellinger FP, Raman AV, Reeves MA, Berry MJ. Regulation and function of selenoproteins in human disease. *The Biochemical Journal*. 2009;422(1):11–22.

180. Ferguson LR, Schlothauer RC. The potential role of nutritional genomics tools in validating high health foods for cancer control: Broccoli as example. *Molecular Nutrition & Food Research*. 2012;56(1):126–46.

181. Fenech M, El-Sohemy A, Cahill L, Ferguson LR, French TA, Tai ES, et al. Nutrigenetics and nutrigenomics: Viewpoints on the current status and applications in nutrition research and practice. *Journal of Nutrigenetics and Nutrigenomics*. 2011;4(2):69–89.

182. Burk RF, Hill KE. Selenoprotein P-expression, functions, and roles in mammals. *Biochimica et biophysica acta*. 2009;1790(11):1441–7.

183. Penney KL, Schumacher FR, Li H, Kraft P, Morris JS, Kurth T, et al. A large prospective study of SEP15 genetic variation, interaction with plasma selenium levels, and prostate cancer risk and survival. *Cancer Prevention Research*. 2010;3(5):604–10.

184. Higuchi A, Takahashi K, Hirashima M, Kawakita T, Tsubota K. Selenoprotein P controls oxidative stress in cornea. *PloS One.* 2010;5(3):e9911.
185. Meplan C, Nicol F, Burtle BT, Crosley LK, Arthur JR, Mathers JC, et al. Relative abundance of selenoprotein P isoforms in human plasma depends on genotype, se intake, and cancer status. *Antioxidants & Redox Signaling.* 2009;11(11):2631–40.
186. Schoenmakers E, Agostini M, Mitchell C, Schoenmakers N, Papp L, Rajanayagam O, et al. Mutations in the selenocysteine insertion sequence-binding protein 2 gene lead to a multisystem selenoprotein deficiency disorder in humans. *The Journal of Clinical Investigation.* 2010;120(12):4220–35.
187. Zhang J, Dhakal IB, Lang NP, Kadlubar FF. Polymorphisms in inflammatory genes, plasma antioxidants, and prostate cancer risk. *Cancer Causes & Control: CCC.* 2010;21(9):1437–44.
188. Zhang S, Rocourt C, Cheng WH. Selenoproteins and the aging brain. *Mechanisms of Ageing and Development.* 2010;131(4):253–60.
189. De Spirt S, Eckers A, Wehrend C, Micoogullari M, Sies H, Stahl W, et al. Interplay between the chalcone cardamonin and selenium in the biosynthesis of Nrf2-regulated antioxidant enzymes in intestinal Caco-2 cells. *Free Radical Biology and Medicine.* 2016;91:164–71.
190. Zhang X, Zhang L, Zhu JH, Cheng WH. Nuclear selenoproteins and genome maintenance. *IUBMB Life.* 2016;68(1):5–12.
191. Misra S, Boylan M, Selvam A, Spallholz JE, Bjornstedt M. Redox-active selenium compounds—From toxicity and cell death to cancer treatment. *Nutrients.* 2015;7(5):3536–56.
192. Xiang J, Li XY, Xu M, Hong J, Huang Y, Tan JR, et al. Zinc transporter-8 gene (SLC30A8) is associated with type 2 diabetes in Chinese. *The Journal of Clinical Endocrinology and Metabolism.* 2008;93(10):4107–12.
193. Zeng H, Yan L, Cheng WH, Uthus EO. Dietary selenomethionine increases exon-specific DNA methylation of the p53 gene in rat liver and colon mucosa. *The Journal of Nutrition.* 2011;141(8):1464–8.
194. Uthus E, Begaye A, Ross S, Zeng H. The von Hippel-Lindau (VHL) tumor-suppressor gene is down-regulated by selenium deficiency in Caco-2 cells and rat colon mucosa. *Biological Trace Element Research.* 2011;142(2):223–31.
195. Németh E, Feher J, Nagy V, Lengyel G, Fehér J. The role of antioxidants in prevention. *Orvosi Hetilap.* 2006;147(13):603–7.
196. Hesketh J. Nutrigenomics and selenium: Gene expression patterns, physiological targets, and genetics. *Annual Review of Nutrition.* 2008;28:157–77.
197. Barger JL, Kayo T, Pugh TD, Vann JA, Power R, Dawson K, et al. Gene expression profiling reveals differential effects of sodium selenite, selenomethionine, and yeast-derived selenium in the mouse. *Genes & Nutrition.* 2012;7(2):155–65.
198. Meplan C, Hesketh J. Selenium and cancer: A story that should not be forgotten-insights from genomics. *Cancer Treatment and Research.* 2014;159:145–66.
199. Barnett MP, Bermingham EN, Young W, Bassett SA, Hesketh JE, Maciel-Dominguez A, et al. Low folate and selenium in the mouse maternal diet alters liver gene expression patterns in the offspring after weaning. *Nutrients.* 2015;7(5):3370–86.
200. McKelvey SM, Horgan KA, Murphy RA. Chemical form of selenium differentially influences DNA repair pathways following exposure to lead nitrate. *Journal of Trace Elements in Medicine and Biology: Organ of the Society for Minerals and Trace Elements (GMS).* 2015;29:151–69.
201. Brennan KM, Burris WR, Boling JA, Matthews JC. Selenium content in blood fractions and liver of beef heifers is greater with a mix of inorganic/organic or organic versus inorganic supplemental selenium but the time required for maximal assimilation is tissue-specific. *Biological Trace Element Research.* 2011;144(1–3):504–16.

202. Hawkes WC, Richter D, Alkan Z. Dietary selenium supplementation and whole blood gene expression in healthy North American men. *Biological Trace Element Research.* 2013;155(2):201–8.
203. Kunttas-Tatli E, Roberts DM, McCartney BM. Self-association of the APC tumor suppressor is required for the assembly, stability, and activity of the Wnt signaling destruction complex. *Molecular Biology of the Cell.* 2014;25(21):3424–36.
204. Lesko AC, Goss KH, Yang FF, Schwertner A, Hulur I, Onel K, et al. The APC tumor suppressor is required for epithelial cell polarization and three-dimensional morphogenesis. *Biochimica et biophysica acta.* 2015;1853(3):711–23.
205. Steigerwald K, Behbehani GK, Combs KA, Barton MC, Groden J. The APC tumor suppressor promotes transcription-independent apoptosis in vitro. *Molecular Cancer Research.* 2005;3(2):78–89.
206. Mauro MO, Sartori D, Oliveira RJ, Ishii PL, Mantovani MS, Ribeiro LR. Activity of selenium on cell proliferation, cytotoxicity, and apoptosis and on the expression of CASP9, BCL-XL and APC in intestinal adenocarcinoma cells. *Mutation Research-Fundamental and Molecular Mechanisms of Mutagenesis.* 2011;715(1–2):7–12.
207. Zeng H, Wu M, Botnen JH. Methylselenol, a selenium metabolite, induces cell cycle arrest in G1 phase and apoptosis via the extracellular-regulated kinase 1/2 pathway and other cancer signaling genes. *The Journal of Nutrition.* 2009;139(9):1613–8.
208. Chiang EC, Shen S, Kengeri SS, Xu H, Combs GF, Morris JS, et al. Defining the Optimal Selenium Dose for Prostate Cancer Risk Reduction: Insights from the U-Shaped Relationship between Selenium Status, DNA Damage, and Apoptosis. *Dose-response: A Publication of International Hormesis Society.* 2009;8(3):285–300.
209. Wu RT, Cao L, Chen BP, Cheng WH. Selenoprotein H suppresses cellular senescence through genome maintenance and redox regulation. *The Journal of Biological Chemistry.* 2014;289(49):34378–88.
210. Wu J, Lyons GH, Graham RD, Fenech MF. The effect of selenium, as selenomethionine, on genome stability and cytotoxicity in human lymphocytes measured using the cytokinesis-block micronucleus cytome assay. *Mutagenesis.* 2009;24(3):225–32.
211. Laffon B, Valdiglesias V, Pasaro E, Mendez J. The organic selenium compound selenomethionine modulates bleomycin-induced DNA damage and repair in human leukocytes. *Biological Trace Element Research.* 2010;133(1):12–9.
212. Cominetti C, de Bortoli MC, Purgatto E, Ong TP, Moreno FS, Garrido Jr AB, et al. Associations between glutathione peroxidase-1 Pro198Leu polymorphism, selenium status, and DNA damage levels in obese women after consumption of Brazil nuts. *Nutrition.* 2011;27(9):891–6.
213. Zachara BA, Gromadzinska J, Palus J, Zbrog Z, Swiech R, Twardowska E, et al. The effect of selenium supplementation in the prevention of DNA damage in white blood cells of hemodialyzed patients: A pilot study. *Biological Trace Element Research.* 2011;142(3):274–83.
214. Xue W, Wang Z, Chen Q, Chen J, Yang H, Xue S. High selenium status in individuals exposed to arsenic through coal-burning in Shaanxi (PR of China) modulates antioxidant enzymes, heme oxygenase-1 and DNA damage. *Clinica Chimica Acta; International Journal of Clinical Chemistry.* 2010;411(17–18):1312–8.
215. Li S, Cao J, Caterson B, Hughes CE. Proteoglycan metabolism, cell death and Kashin-Beck disease. *Glycoconjugate Journal.* 2012;29(5–6):241–8.
216. Luo M, Chen J, Li S, Sun H, Zhang Z, Fu Q, et al. Changes in the metabolism of chondroitin sulfate glycosaminoglycans in articular cartilage from patients with Kashin-Beck disease. *Osteoarthritis and Cartilage/OARS, Osteoarthritis Research Society.* 2014;22(7):986–95.
217. Yang G, Zhu Y, Dong X, Duan Z, Niu X, Wei J. TLR2-ICAM1-Gadd45alpha axis mediates the epigenetic effect of selenium on DNA methylation and gene expression in Keshan disease. *Biological Trace Element Research.* 2014;159(1–3):69–80.

218. Gong J, Hsu L, Harrison T, King IB, Sturup S, Song X, et al. Genome-wide association study of serum selenium concentrations. *Nutrients*. 2013;5(5):1706–18.
219. Bera S, De Rosa V, Rachidi W, Diamond AM. Does a role for selenium in DNA damage repair explain apparent controversies in its use in chemoprevention? *Mutagenesis*. 2013;28(2):127–34.
220. Almondes KG, Leal GV, Cozzolino SM, Philippi ST, Rondo PH. The role of selenoproteins in cancer. *Revista da Associacao Medica Brasileira (1992)*. 2010;56(4):484–8.
221. Takata Y, Kristal AR, King IB, Song X, Diamond AM, Foster CB, et al. Serum selenium, genetic variation in selenoenzymes, and risk of colorectal cancer: Primary analysis from the Women's Health Initiative Observational Study and meta-analysis. *Cancer Epidemiology, Biomarkers & Prevention: A Publication of the American Association for Cancer Research, Cosponsored by the American Society of Preventive Oncology*. 2011;20(9):1822–30.
222. Steinbrecher A, Meplan C, Hesketh J, Schomburg L, Endermann T, Jansen E, et al. Effects of selenium status and polymorphisms in selenoprotein genes on prostate cancer risk in a prospective study of European men. *Cancer Epidemiology, Biomarkers & Prevention: A Publication of the American Association for Cancer Research, Cosponsored by the American Society of Preventive Oncology*. 2010;19(11):2958–68.
223. Bao P, Chen Z, Tai RZ, Shen HM, Martin FL, Zhu YG. Selenite-induced toxicity in cancer cells is mediated by metabolic generation of endogenous selenium nanoparticles. *Journal of Proteome Research*. 2015;14(2):1127–36.
224. de Rosa V, Erkekoglu P, Forestier A, Favier A, Hincal F, Diamond AM, et al. Low doses of selenium specifically stimulate the repair of oxidative DNA damage in LNCaP prostate cancer cells. *Free Radical Research*. 2012;46(2):105–16.
225. Wrobel JK, Choi JJ, Xiao R, Eum SY, Kwiatkowski S, Wolff G, et al. Selenoglycoproteins attenuate adhesion of tumor cells to the brain microvascular endothelium via a process involving NF-kappaB activation. *The Journal of Nutritional Biochemistry*. 2015;26(2):120–9.
226. Hu Y, McIntosh GH, Le Leu RK, Upton JM, Woodman RJ, Young GP. The influence of selenium-enriched milk proteins and selenium yeast on plasma selenium levels and rectal selenoprotein gene expression in human subjects. *The British Journal of Nutrition*. 2011;106(4):572–82.
227. Pagmantidis V, Meplan C, van Schothorst EM, Keijer J, Hesketh JE. Supplementation of healthy volunteers with nutritionally relevant amounts of selenium increases the expression of lymphocyte protein biosynthesis genes. *The American Journal of Clinical Nutrition*. 2008;87(1):181–9.
228. Meplan C, Crosley LK, Nicol F, Beckett GJ, Howie AF, Hill KE, et al. Genetic polymorphisms in the human selenoprotein P gene determine the response of selenoprotein markers to selenium supplementation in a gender-specific manner (the SELGEN study). *FASEB Journal: Official Publication of the Federation of American Societies for Experimental Biology*. 2007;21(12):3063–74.
229. Qi Y, Schoene NW, Lartey FM, Cheng WH. Selenium compounds activate ATM-dependent DNA damage response via the mismatch repair protein hMLH1 in colorectal cancer cells. *The Journal of Biological Chemistry*. 2010;285(43):33010–7.
230. Wu M, Kang MM, Schoene NW, Cheng WH. Selenium compounds activate early barriers of tumorigenesis. *The Journal of Biological Chemistry*. 2010;285(16):12055–62.
231. Ying Q, Ansong E, Diamond AM, Lu Z, Yang W, Bie X. Quantitative proteomic analysis reveals that anti-cancer effects of selenium-binding protein 1 in vivo are associated with metabolic pathways. *PloS One*. 2015;10(5):e0126285.
232. Jeong JY, Wang Y, Sytkowski AJ. Human selenium binding protein-1 (hSP56) interacts with VDU1 in a selenium-dependent manner. *Biochemical and Biophysical Research Communications*. 2009;379(2):583–8.
233. Liu X, Gao R, Dong Y, Gao L, Zhao Y, Zhao L, et al. Survivin gene silencing sensitizes prostate cancer cells to selenium growth inhibition. *BMC Cancer*. 2010;10:418.

234. Kotsopoulos J, Chen Z, Vallis KA, Poll A, Ghadirian P, Kennedy G, et al. Toenail selenium status and DNA repair capacity among female BRCA1 mutation carriers. *Cancer Causes & Control: CCC.* 2010;21(5):679–87.

235. Mehdi Y, Hornick JL, Istasse L, Dufrasne I. Selenium in the environment, metabolism and involvement in body functions. *Molecules.* 2013;18(3):3292–311.

236. Rayman MP. Selenium and human health. *The Lancet.* 2012;379(9822):1256–68.

237. Kipp A, Banning A, van Schothorst EM, Meplan C, Schomburg L, Evelo C, et al. Four selenoproteins, protein biosynthesis, and Wnt signalling are particularly sensitive to limited selenium intake in mouse colon. *Molecular Nutrition & Food Research.* 2009;53(12):1561–72.

238. Cardoso BR, Ong TP, Jacob-Filho W, Jaluul O, Freitas MI, Cominetti C, et al. Glutathione peroxidase 1 Pro198Leu polymorphism in Brazilian Alzheimer's disease patients: Relations to the enzyme activity and to selenium status. *Journal of Nutrigenetics and Nutrigenomics.* 2012;5(2):72–80.

239. Akbaraly TN, Hininger-Favier I, Carriere I, Arnaud J, Gourlet V, Roussel AM, et al. Plasma selenium over time and cognitive decline in the elderly. *Epidemiology.* 2007;18(1):52–8.

240. Christen WG, Glynn RJ, Gaziano JM, Darke AK, Crowley JJ, Goodman PJ, et al. Age-related cataract in men in the selenium and vitamin e cancer prevention trial eye endpoints study: A randomized clinical trial. *JAMA Ophthalmology.* 2015;133(1):17–24.

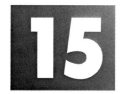

Prenatal Nutrition Exposure Leading to Adult Obesity, Diabetes, and Hypertension

Maryam Miraghajani and Rasoul Salehi
Isfahan University of Medical Sciences
Isfahan, Iran

Hossein Hajianfar
Flavarjan Islamic Azad University
and
Isfahan Islamic Azad University
Isfahan, Iran

Contents

15.1 Introduction 378
15.2 Prenatal nutrition exposure and obesity in adults 380
    15.2.1 The role of maternal diet on hypothalamo-pituitary-adrenal axis and programmed obesity 380
    15.2.2 The role of maternal diet on insulin and leptin and programmed obesity 383
    15.2.3 The role of maternal diet on white adipose tissue and programmed obesity 384
    15.2.4 The role of maternal diet on fetal growth and programmed obesity 384
15.3 Prenatal nutrition exposure and diabetes in adults 386
    15.3.1 The role of maternal diet on insulin-like growth factor 2 and development of diabetes 386
    15.3.2 The role of maternal diet on some nuclear receptors, signaling molecules, and transcription factors and development of diabetes 387
    15.3.3 The role of maternal diet on intrauterine growth restriction and development of diabetes 388
    15.3.4 The role of maternal diet on pancreatic β cell and development of diabetes 389

| | 15.3.5 | The role of maternal diet on insulin receptor and development of diabetes | 390 |

15.3.5 The role of maternal diet on insulin receptor and
development of diabetes...390
15.3.6 The role of maternal diet on mitochondrial function and
development of diabetes...390
15.4 Prenatal nutrition exposure and hypertension in adults 391
15.4.1 The role of maternal diet on renin–angiotensin system,
structure and function of glomeruli, and programmed
hypertension 391
15.4.2 The role of maternal diet on vascular changes and
programmed hypertension..392
15.4.3 The role of maternal diet on respiratory system and
sympathetic function and programmed hypertension...........393
15.4.4 The role of maternal diet on low birth weight and
programmed hypertension..393
15.4.5 The role of maternal diet on glucocorticoids and
programmed hypertension..394
References...396

15.1 Introduction

Some metabolic disorders including obesity, diabetes, and hypertension are becoming the most common chronic health problem worldwide and represent the main cause of mortality and morbidity [1,2]. As the importance of diet in health and disease has been established, the new field of "developmental origins of health and disease" discusses about epigenome programming during critical periods of early development following fetal nutrition exposure in pregnancy that permanently alters some metabolic status and organism's physiology in which consequences are often observed much later in adults [3]. These epigenetic modifications involve heritable or nonheritable changes in gene expression during this critical period [4,5].

A growing numbers of studies focusing on the great importance for the prevention of adult chronic diseases have identified links among early nutrition, epigenetic processes, and diseases in later life. As fetal life is characterized by a great plasticity and ability to respond to various environmental factors [6], nutrition by altering the compounds and certain energy metabolites that are essential cofactors for epigenetic enzymes can influence on susceptibility to disease [6,7].

Even monozygotic twins that are matched on their DNA sequence show an approximately 40% concordant rate in type 1 diabetes mellitus (DM), suggesting the important role of epigenetic modifications and environmental factors in disease development [8].

Alterations in DNA methylation is one of the important epigenetic events and mediators on chromatin structure and gene expression. Some maternal dietary factorssuch as folate, methionine, and choline through methyl-group

378 Nutrigenomics and Nutraceuticals

donors lead to modulation of DNA methylation and epigenome programming during this critical period [6,9].

Also, low-quality and low-quantity protein diet[10], methionine-deficient diet, high-fat [11], or high-glucose diet [6] induce epigenetic changes in the some specific genes.

A link between reduced fetal energy supply and the pattern of DNA remodeling has been appeared in the interaction of the programmed phenotype and development of metabolic disease with nutrition [12].

Other chromatin and epigenetic remodeling include alternation of the histone proteins that bind to DNA (acetylation, methylation, phosphorylation, ubiquitination, and sumoylation) and the nucleosome positioning along DNA and non-coding RNAs-mediated effects, suggesting significant controlling of gene silencing/unsilencing [13].

In addition, some phytochemicals such as sulforaphane compounds derived from cruciferous vegetables as a histone deacetylase (HDAC) inhibitor involve in controlling event for gene expression. Acetylation of histones by histone acetyl transferase is generally associated with "open" chromatin conformation, and transcriptionally active chromatin, whereas removal of acetyl groups by HDACs leads to condensation of chromatin, and inhibition of transcription [14]. Also, dietary fiber is metabolized by gut bacteria to butyrate as a short-chain fatty acid (SCFA), which acts as a HDAC inhibitor that epigenetically regulates some genes [15]. In this regard, probiotic foods have the efficient potential to restore the intestinal microbiota composition. Gut microbiota have a profound effect on program of later immunity and reduce the risk of developing some diseases through SCFA production affecting epigenetic modifications [7].

Besides the mentioned compounds, other vitamins, minerals, and bioactive compounds such as vitamin D, iron, and polyphenols are related to early origin of several non-communicable chronic diseases in adults.

It can be noted that poor in utero nutrition may be a major contributor to DNA methylation at genes involved in regulating cortisol levels, glucocorticoid action, blood pressure, and associated with cardiometabolic risk [16]. Also, the offspring's response to postnatal changes in leptinlevels, as a metabolic homeostasis hormone, which is present in the fetal brain can be explained by maternal diet. Nutrient availability during pregnancy can result in substantial modification in the development of endocrine and neuroendocrine systems involved in energy intake and expenditure. Taken together, maternal diet can substantially influence adult obesity, through the programming of leptin axis [17,18].

In addition to the direct effects of maternal nutrition on gene expression and the developmental origins of health and disease, impaired utero-placental blood flow caused by inadequate delivery of nutrients can lead to changes in placental development and function that consequently mediate fetal programming. As transportation of nutrients such as methyl donor components from mother to fetus is dependent on placental structure, function, and blood flow, abnormal development of the placenta can predispose to inappropriate fetal development and programming of later disease [19]. In this regards, the correlation between methylation of placental genes, placental oxidative/nitrative stress levels, and altered placental function indicates that sustained changes in maternal nutrition, especially peri-implantation embryo, are important in predicting the programming of endocrine metabolic control, cardiovascular disease, and later hypertension [20,21].

Further, recent evidence of disease risk factor programming by early diet showed that nutrient restriction can alter mRNA levels of leptin, insulin-like growth factors I/II, and glucocorticoid receptors (GRs) in kidney and fat mass and subsequently result in substantial changes in fetal organ development and function [22].

Although the identification of maternal dietary agents and target genes is an important area of developmental origins of health and disease, remodeling within tissues and organs that control metabolichomeostasis is beyond the responses of single genes to maternal nutritional status [12]. Moreover, these persistent changes in the imprinted and non-imprinted genes can be modified by the timing of malnutrition during gestation and sex [23].

15.2 Prenatal nutrition exposure and obesity in adults

Adipogenesis and fat storage which begin in utero are major candidates for developmental programming. Although the underlying mechanisms remain unclear, several studies contribute significantly to our understanding of the molecular mechanisms between the prenatal adverse nutritional conditions and obesity in adults.

Although inappropriate hormone levels, inflammation, modified glucocorticoid sensitivity, and epigenetic mechanisms are considered factors in the adipose tissue programming that is directly related to maternal nutrition, adverse nutritional effects on sympathetic outflow activity to offspring's adipose tissue and reduced noradrenergic innervations may contribute indirectly to programmed obesity in intrauterine. Overall, both mechanisms lead to increased adipogenesis and lipogenesis as well as reduced lipolysis and thermogenesis, resulting in predisposing to increased fat mass. However, epigenetic processes account for a central underlying mechanism of long-lasting programming of obesity [24].

15.2.1 The role of maternal diet on hypothalamo-pituitary-adrenal axis and programmed obesity

Some studies indicated that early dysregulation of the fetal hypothalamo-pituitary-adrenal (HPA) axis and abnormal development of the hypothalamus can affect maternalnutrition which is responsible for long-lasting programming of energy balance and obesityin offspring [25].

The hypothalamic arcuate (ARC) nucleus is a central regulator of energy homeostasis, specifically the feeding regulation. The ARC acts as an integrative center, with two major subgroups of neurons influencing appetite, primarily medial eating-stimulatory neuropeptide Y (NPY) and agouti-related peptide (AgRP) neurons and lateral eating-inhibitory pro-opiomelanocortin (POMC) neurons. So, identifying components that regulate hypothalamic development and function is important for prevention of hypothalamus-related obesity in adults [26].There was convincing evidence for the association between altered hypothalamic energy levels and sensor-mediated responses on neuro-proliferative and neuro-differentiation factors expression and ARC development during fetal life. When dams were fed a high-fat diet (HFD), obese phenotype among adult rats was demonstrated through the programming of hypothalamic ARC that resulted in enhanced expression and activity in AgRP relative to POMC neurons and induced hyperphagia [27]. Consistent with the mentioned data, offspring of overfed mothers predispose to become hyperphagic and increases the risk of later obesity via malprogramming of the appetite-regulating system and neurogenesis in the hypothalamus [28,29].

As a consequence of the maternal HFD, adult rats had significantly increased expression of hypothalamic energy sensors, phosphorylated 5′-adenosine monophosphate–activated protein kinase (pAMPK) and mammalian target of rapamycin (mTOR), and histone demethylase LSD1 than controls. Although hypothalamic expression of DNA methyltransferases 1 (DNMT1) was normal, ARC expression of HDAC SIRT and HDAC1 was significantly suppressed in the HFD group. In addition, sustained reduction in neurogenic factors (Hes1, Mash1, and Ngn3) is consistent with increased AgRP and decreased POMC. Hence, energy sensors and epigenetic responses modification that change gene expression likely promote hyperphagia and obesity in offspring [27]. Prenatal undernutrition also leads to increased mRNAexpression of NPY, AgRP, and leptin receptor (ObRb) neuroendocrines in the ARC [30].There is also substantial evidence in animal models to support that maternal reduced nutrition is associated with offspring's structural disorganization and malpro-gramming of the appetite-regulating system in the hypothalamus such as a greater volume of the ventral medial nucleus and paraventricular nucleus and appetite-regulating neuropeptide mRNA levels. Maternal low-protein (LP) diet during gestation can increase mRNA expression of NPY and decrease POMC. Maternal LP diet had a profound influence on the diurnal circadian rhythms that are important in metabolic functions. Disrupting this process through diet modification can lead to an increased risk of obesity [28].

Furthermore, studies in animals show that the increased hypothalamic pro-liferation of orexigenic peptide-expressing neurons may increase risk for overeating and obesity later in life following maternal HFD during the gesta-tion. Cafeteria feeding,highly palatable and energy-dense foods, in mothers induces alterations in preference for palatable and the motivation to consume the same range of foods, alters eating behavior, induces hyperphagia, and increases fat mass and weight gain in offspring [28].

Another investigation showed that acquired hypomethylation or hypermethyl-ation of CpG sites within the hypothalamic POMC promoter regions interfered with transcription factor binding and was associated with neonatal malnutrition in animals. This epigenetic programming of POMC by early-life nutrition is accompanied by obesity [31,32]. In addition, HFDs are associated with long-term alterations in hypothalamic dopamine and opioids gene expression and DNA hypomethylation as epigenetic markers in the rat offspring [33]. In this field, epigenetic mechanisms have been associated with long-term programming of gene expression after various in utero insults [33].

Also, increased cortisol production at the local tissue following the hypothalamic-pituitary-adrenal axis over-activation is associated with increased adipose and obesity [26]. Prenatal adverse nutritional conditions affect the gene expression and function of GRs and the glucocorticoid regulatory enzymes such as 11β-hydroxysteroid dehydrogenase 1 and 2 [25]. GR is a nuclear receptor that is important in the hypothalamic control of energy homeostasis by regulating the expression of neuropeptides such as POMC, NPY, and AgRP. Prolonged exposure to glucocorticoid that binds GR enhances adipogenesis [5].

The result of a cohort study which has focused on the impact of the maternal dietary habits and offspring epigenetic changes in glucocorticoid genes in human subjects revealed that unbalanced maternal diet in pregnancy was associated with elevated CpG methylation within GR (exon 1F), cortisol level, and adiposity in adult offspring [16]. In this way, the higher choline intake, as a methyl donor, in third-trimester pregnant women can program offspring elevation of placental promoter methylation of the cortisol-regulating genes, corticotropin releasing hormone (CRH), and glucocorticoid receptor and can lower placental CRH transcript abundance and cord plasma cortisol in human [34]. Furthermore, folic acid supplementation to an unbalanced maternal diet induces GR gene methylation and prevents altered mRNA expression in the GR gene in the liver of the offspring [35].

Programming epigenetic changes in the hypothalamic GR is also affected by maternal undernourishment and resulted in hypomethylation of GR promoter, and alterations in histone modifications associated with increased GR mRNA expression in the fetal hypothalamic regions involved in energy balance [36].

Normally, increased adipocyte responses to cortisol are affected by age that cause increase in fat mass among elder. However, such enhanced sensitivity is promoted in offspring born to mothers who were nutrient-restricted in utero associated with increased peroxisome proliferator-activated receptor alpha (PPAR α), and high fat mass accumulation could be an adaptive response to an increase in cortisol sensitivity. It has been described that PPAR α as a member of nuclear receptor family has an important role in the gene expression involving storage and mobilization of lipids and glucose metabolism [37]. Maternal low-fat diet throughout pregnancy had a significant effect on the body weight of the offspring when they were fed an obesogenic diet after weaning. Consequences of this maternal nutrition can affect gene expression, with a pronounced effect in liver. These modifications are mediated by defected retinoid X receptors (RXR) pathways via significant changes in the expression level of several key metabolic transcription factors such as PPARg, CAR (Nr1i3), PAR (Nr1i2) or REV-ERBα (Nr1d1), or REV-ERBα, which finally influence on the sterol regulatory element binding protein (SREBP) pathway and unlikely to be caused by DNA methylation differences in adult liver [38].

However, epigenetic processes account for a central underlying mechanism of long-lasting programming of obesity. As expression of lipogenic transcription factors, including PPARγ, CCAAT/enhancer-binding protein (C/EBPα), and GR, is changed by epigenetic modifications during adipogenesis, malnourished offspring in utero alter adipocyte commitment and differentiation following regulation of transcription factors due to epigenetic changes [24].

15.2.2 The role of maternal diet on insulin and leptin and programmed obesity

The functions of adipocyte-derived hormone, leptin, and the pancreatic beta-cell-derived hormone, insulin, as afferent signals to the hypothalamus in an endocrine feedback loop regulate body adiposity [39]. Leptin is a hormone with a key role in appetite control and body weight homeostasis via actions in the hypothalamus. The main signaling pathway activated by leptin is the melanocortin pathway involving NPY and AgRP neurons that play a crucial role in energy expenditure. The defects of this appetite networks, either insulin or leptin signaling or impaired sensitivity of them, during the gestation as a developmental period, can result in disturbing, long-term body weight set point [40]. In contrast to insulin, leptin presents antilipogenic and lipolytic effects by suppressing expression and activity of lipogenic enzymes. In this field, offspring of food-restricted and low-protein (LP) diet dams show central leptin resistance and an age-related loss of insulin sensitivity in adipocytes, respectively. Further, offspring of LP diet dams are predisposed to adiposity through impaired leptin antilipogenic action [28]. Maternal undernutrition results in higher insulin and leptin and lower adiponectin concentrations in the cord blood. Recent report reveals that imbalance in vitamin B12 and folate associated with deranged 1-carbon metabolism can indeed have an effect on the epigenome, leading to insulin resistance in the offspring [41]. Also, offspring born to overfed mothers show central leptin resistance. Besides increased orexigenic pathways, high suppressor of cytokine signaling 3 (SOCS3) mRNA expression levels with blunted leptin-induced phospho-signal transducer and activator of transcription 3 (pSTAT3) are possible causes of the persistent central leptin resistance observed in the overfed mother's offspring, which leads to impaired leptin performance [28]. Intrauterine exposure to germinated brown rice (GBR) and GBR-derived gamma (γ) aminobutyric acid (GABA) extract increased adiponectin levels and reduced insulin and leptinlevels in rat offspring. Additionally, GBR and GABA extract can increase mRNA levels of glucose transporter 2 (GLUT2) and insulin promoter factor-1 (IPF1) and reduce global DNA methylation, and modulate H3 and H4 acetylation levels [42].

Decreased hepatic mRNA expression of insulin-like growth factor–binding protein 1 (IGFBP1) and 2 (IGFBP2) and reduced IGF-1 and IGFBP3 levels which lead to metabolic disorders later in life can explain metabolic derangements in offspring with maternal undernutrition and over nutrition [43].

With regard to epigenetics, some findings suggest that prenatal LP diet among animals via the modified expression in the IGF2 gene and DNA methylation within adipocytes results in adipose tissue catch-up growth [44].

15.2.3 The role of maternal diet on white adipose tissue and programmed obesity

Enhanced white adipose tissue (WAT) mRNA expression levels in the offspring are modified by maternal LP diet [28]. WAT has been established as a dynamic tissue that is actively involved in metabolic reactions and produces hormonal factors. This role can become dysregulated following excess adiposity. In contrast, brown adipose tissue (BAT) is only present in comparatively small amounts in the body but it is the main site of thermogenesis, and thus could prevent excess white adiposity. Maternal calorie restriction during gestation has been associated with WAT dysfunction in offspring [45]. It has been suggested that maternal nutrient restriction is an important predisposing factor for functional impairment of the sympathetic innervations of WAT as an inhibitor of fat cell proliferation and/or activator of lipolysis and increased adiposity in adult offspring [28]. Also, adverse nutritional effects on sympathetic outflow activity to offspring's adipose tissue and reduced noradrenergic innervations and thermogenesis may contribute indirectly to programmed obesity in intrauterine [24]. BAT thermogenic capacity of offspring involving impaired BAT sympathetic innervation and thyroid hormone signaling is diminished when calorie restriction during pregnancy is applied to mothers. Reduced protein levels of uncoupling protein 1 (UCP1), tyrosine hydroxylase (TyrOH), triiodothyronine (T3) plasma levels, lipoprotein lipase, and mRNA levels of carnitine palmitoyl transferase 1 (CPT1) contribute to metabolic alterations and obesity [46].

15.2.4 The role of maternal diet on fetal growth and programmed obesity

It has been proposed that maternal malnutrition is associated with fetal growth and small for gestational age (SGA) [47]. Therefore, it seems logical that SGA has an inverse programming effect on neuroprogenitor cell proliferation/differentiation such as adipose tissue cells. Also, it causes enhanced cellular orexigenic responses and expression of NPY versus satiety neurons such as POMC, resulting in increase appetite and decrease satiety. Finally, these differences lead to early catch-up growth and developing adult obesity [29,48,49]. Also, intrauterine growth restriction (IUGR) offspring are prone to developing adiposity in adulthood [28].

Besides the adverse effects of low birth weight (LBW) on obesity, a positive association between high levels of birth weight and increased risk of obesity was observed among children in 12 countries [50], which may tend to be stable till adulthood [51]. Low or high birth weights, as some of the most identifiable markers of a suboptimal prenatal environment, were associated with more rapid weight gainand increased risk of obesity [52,53]. As considerable observational literature describes that changes in maternal diet during pregnancy can reduce the risk of high infant birth weight, dietary intervention may be a significant strategy to tackle the increasing problem of adulthood obesity [54].

Prenatal nutrition, linked to regulation of gene expression that can depend on the epigeneticchanges such as methylation, was shown to mediate some of the effects of maternal diet on offspring adult obesity [55].

DNA methylation is characterized by the addition of a methyl group to the cytosine residue of DNA. DNMTs catalyze methylation of a wide variety of proteins and DNA substrates by utilizing S-adenosylmethionine (SAM) as methyl donor. As it was mentioned previously, micronutrients such as folate, choline, and methionine play key roles in provision of methyl donors for DNA and protein methylation [5]. Also, some amino acids (e.g., glycine, histidine, methionine, and serine) are methyl-group donors and contribute to the production of SAM [56]. On the other contrary, dietary maternal supplementations (i.e., taurine, glycine, vitamin D, and n-3 fatty acids) may alleviate adverse consequences of perinatal programming [24].

One of the studies suggests that chronic disorders in offspring caused by maternal HFD can be reduced by supplementation of methyl donors during pregnancy. Analysis of DNA methylation of obesogenic-related genes including PPAR γ, fatty acid synthase, leptin, and adiponectin in visceral fat of offspring showed that dietary supplementation with methyl donors can prevent the adverse effects of maternal HFD on female mice offspring [57]. In contrast, methyl vitamins (HMethyl, tenfold folate, and vitamins B12 and B6) in gestational diets contained high multivitamin which increased food intake and obesity in the rat offspring. These obesogenic effects of methyl vitamins, specifically folate, were consistent with their epigenetic alterations in the hypothalamic feeding pathways [58].

So, variation in SAM levels as a universal methyl donor for DNMTs following dietary factors changes can influence DNA methylation and histone modifications and may impact the epigenetic alterations in the key metabolic genes in developing tissues.

Although evidence from human and animal studies indicates that epigenetic inheritance via both maternal and paternal lineages involves in transgenerational effects of obesity, however, there is evidence that these epigenetic modifications are reversible and there are possibilities that intervention strategies could decrease the risk of obesity [5].

Taken together, as observed in maternal nutrition models, these programmed mechanisms might contribute directly or indirectly to long-term higher energy intake and impaired fat storage in adipocytes.

Exposure to an HFD in utero might affect glucose and lipid metabolism of female offspring through epigeneticmodifications to adiponectin and leptin genes for multiple generations. Obesogenic and diabetogenic traits were abolished after a maternalnormal diet for three generations [59].

15.3 Prenatal nutrition exposure and diabetes in adults

Diabetes mellitus is one of the most common metabolic disorders with prevalence rates reaching epidemic proportions. Because of the significant social and economic burden of diabetes,one of the global targets for this noncommunicable diseases is to halt by 2025 [60]. The underlying cause of the problem has been only partially identified, but impact of early environmental exposures has recently emerged as an important responsible factor for the development of adult-onset diabetes. Substantial evidence supports the role of the intrauterine nutrition in development of offspring diabetes by developmental programming [61]. The consequence of fetal programming as a result of suboptimal maternal diet, excess or an insufficiency of nutrients, can apply as diabetes prevention approaches.

The first epidemiologic observations by Hales and Barker in 1992 led to the proposal of the "thrifty phenotype" hypothesis, which posited that malnutrition during pregnancy resulted in fetal malnutrition and LBW that "set in train mechanisms of fetal nutritional thrift," including underdevelopment of pancreatic beta cells, increased insulin resistance, and hyperglycemia, resulting in increased risk for T2DM [62,63].

The evolved thrifty phenotype theory called "developmental plasticity," explains the association between increased risk for T2DM and poor intrauterine environment that causes reduction of skeletal muscle development, insulin insensitivity, and enhancement of fat deposition as a survival mechanism in an abnormal postnatal environment [63]. It has been widely accepted that the epigenetic mechanism, such as DNA methylation, is the essence of this hypothesis and some organs related to glucose metabolism, including liver, pancreas, adipose tissue and skeletal muscle can involve [8].

15.3.1 The role of maternal diet on insulin-like growth factor 2 and development of diabetes

The retrospective cohort study analyses confirmed the dose-response relation between restricted nutrition in early gestation and odds of type 2 diabetes in later life [64]. After 60 years of early gestational exposure, the Dutch famine individuals exhibited a lower methylation level of insulin-like growth factor

2 (IGF2)-H19 locus, compared with those who were unexposed [65]. IGF-axis Insulin is closely related to the maintenance of normal glucose and pathogenesis of type 2 diabetes [66]. Also, these subjects had an increased risk of some metabolic disorder such as insulin resistance in later life [67].

Some interesting research clarified that periconceptional folic acid use of the mother is also associated with an increased methylation of the IGF2 gene differentially methylation region (IGF2 DMR) in the child that may decrease birth weight and affect the development of metabolic disorder throughout life [68].

Also, maternal undernutrition or over nutrition can regulate the IGF-IGFBP axis in adult male rat offspring [43].

15.3.2 The role of maternal diet on some nuclear receptors, signaling molecules, and transcription factors and development of diabetes

A complex network of transcription factors and signals influences on the pancreatic beta cells differentiation and function. Low-protein (LP) stress in the early stages of development can modify transcription factor hepatocyte nuclear factor 4a (Hnf4a), a transcription factor which has a central role in B-cell differentiation and glucose homeostasis [69]. LP diet can induce differentiation at the expense of proliferation through up-regulation of some transcription factors such as Hnf4a that decreased β-cell reserve, resulting in susceptibility to type 2 diabetes[70].Also, exposure to a LP diet during pregnancy decreases mechanistic target of rapamycin (mTOR) signaling in neonatal and adult that participates in β-cell programming during fetal development [71,72].

The PPARs are nuclear receptors that contribute to the placenta development through regulation of lipogenesis, steroidogenesis, glucose transporters, and placental signaling pathways. One of the PPAR subfamily, PPARγ is the main modulator of mammalian placentation. Some nutrients such as fatty acids act as a PPAR ligand. Also, maternal nutrition during gestation impacts on epigenetic regulation, methylation pattern, of PPAR. So, placenta metabolism of fetus being exposed tounbalance maternal diet can disrupt [73].

The recognized impact of maternal HFD on increased serum insulin, tumor necrosis factor α, and interleukin 1β has been reported in rat model. Also, c-Jun N-terminal kinases (JNK), I kappa B kinase phosphorylation, and PEPCK expression were increased and basal ACC phosphorylation and insulin signaling were decreased in the liver of adult offspring that were consistent with the development of liver damage and insulin resistance [74]. Also, decreased gene expression of insulin, glucokinase, the glucose transporter (Glut2), and transcription factors such as PDX-1 (pancreatic and duodenal homeobox-1) [75,76] and increased risk of insulin resistance in the adult stage via decreases in mRNA expression of adiponectin receptor 1 and glucose transporter 4 in the skeletal muscle have been shown after the mentioned diet [77]. Further, lower

PDX-1 mRNA levels following the HF maternal diet induces insulin resistance and deterioration of pancreatic β-cell function in adult male offspring [78].

Moreover, the epigenome sensitivity to maternal diet in periconceptional period in animal model was shown. Dietary restriction can reduce the hepatic insulin-signaling molecules including insulin receptor substrate 1 (IRS-1), 3-phosphoinositide-dependent protein kinase 1 (*PDK1*) and atypical protein kinase C (aPKCζ), and phosphoenolpyruvate carboxykinase-c (PEPCK-c) and glucose-6-phosphatase (G6Pase) expression [79].

Some miRNAs influence the regulation of gene expression of pancreas and play an important role in inhabitation of insulin secretion (miR-375 is an). The miR-375 locus has binding sites for PDX-1 in at least two regions. Protein restriction during pregnancy programmed higher expression of miR-375 that caused reduced levels of the PDK1 protein (3-phosphoinositide-dependent protein kinase-1) and phosphatidylinositol-3-kinase (PI3K)-signaling of pancreatic β cells [80].

15.3.3 The role of maternal diet on intrauterine growth restriction and development of diabetes

Impairments in maternal nutrient supply to the fetus lead to IUGR and LBW, which in combination with rapid postnatal growth may subsequently lead to the development of diabetes and insulin resistance [81,82]. Animal studies have documented that this postnatal catch-up growth can cause liver dysfunction in later life, which is associated with higher levels of hyperinsulinemia [83]. Also, development of LBW following exposure to a LP diet in utero can lead to programmed reduction in insulin receptor substrate-1 and p110-β. However, expressions of these protein mRNAs have not been changed that suggested that posttranscriptional regulation have occurred [84].

IUGR followed by maternal gestational nutritional restriction possibly through the increase in the DNA methylation of specific CpG sites of PPARγ coactivator-1α (PGC-1α), as a key orchestrator in energy homeostasis, decrease in the transcriptional activity of PGC-1α, mitochondrial content, phosphatidylinositide 3-kinases (PI3K), and phosphorylated-Akt2 levels in liver and muscle tissues can program an insulin-resistant phenotype [85].

Additionally, loss of USF-1 binding site at the proximal promoter of PDX-1 transcription factor by epigenetic modifications may play a role in the development of adult diabetes following IUGR. These modifications recruit the HDAC1 and the corepressor Sin3A, and deacetylation of histones H3 and H4 (H3K4). Following birth, demethylation of H3K4 and methylation of histone 3 lysine 9 (H3K9) were seen. Although these epigenetic changes and the reduction in PDX-1 expression could be reversed by HDAC inhibition in the neonatal period, after the onset of diabetes, permanent silencing of the PDX-1 locus following the methylation of CpG island in the proximal promoter was illustrated [86].

Histone covalent modifications have also been implicated in mediating the effect of caloric restriction and IUGR during the pregnancy on the programmed repress skeletal muscle *glut4* transcription in the rat offspring. These deacetylations of histone inactivate postnatal and adult IUGR glut4 gene transcription. Furthermore, modifications in transcriptional factors including increased MEF2D (inhibitor) and decreased MEF2A (activator) and MyoD (coactivator) binding to the glut4 promoter affect reduction of glut4 expression [87].

15.3.4 The role of maternal diet on pancreatic β cell and development of diabetes

Chronic nutritional stress is associated with alterations of epigenetic indices, factors controlling β-cell development, and gene regulation during pancreatic development and function. These alterations can lead to dysfunctional states in pancreatic β cells, which in the long run are responsible for the onset of metabolic diseases like type 2 diabetes [88].

Many studies with experimental animal models have demonstrated that a maternal proteins deficiency during critical periods of development decreases the size and number of cells of pancreatic islets of Langerhans, and premature aging of the secretory function of pancreatic β cells, and alters tissue sensitivity to the action of insulin in offspring [75,89–92]. Also, increased duration of the cell cycle of pancreatic β cell in offspring was shown [88]. Further, increased consumption of sucrose and decreased intake of copper induce type 2 diabetes in rats via alterations in epigenetic steady states, pancreatic oxidative stress, and apoptotic rate in fetal pancreas [93]. In addition, high saturated fat diet resulting in increase in maternal obesity can modify the ability of maintaining fetal β-cell mass that may be an important contributor to the high susceptibility to develop diabetes [94]. Interestingly, hypomethylation of the IL13-RA2 gene (interleukin 13 receptor, alpha 2) and consequently with apoptosis and β cell dysfunction in rat offspring has been associated with high-fat paternal diet [95].

Loss of methylation at the *ZAC1/PLAGL1* differentially methylated region (DMR) and misexpression of this gene that may play roles in pancreas development involve in the transient neonatal DM. It might cause adolescent relapse with type 2 diabetes in half of the patients. Maternal dietary intake of alcohol and vitamin B2 were positively associated with regulation of ZAC1 methylation [96–98].

High maternal folate level, vitamin B12 deficiency, and high circulating level of homocysteine during pregnancy can predict insulin resistance among children and suggest an important role of maternal 1-carbon metabolism in synthesis of nucleic acids, genomic stability, and the epigenetic regulation of gene function and finally fetal programming of diabetes risk [99]. It should be mentioned that childhood elevated fasting insulin concentrations are associated with elevated risk for type 2 DM in early and mid-adult life [100].

15.3.5 The role of maternal diet on insulin receptor and development of diabetes

Maternal LP diet reduced the insulin receptor substrate 2 and phosphatidylinositol 3'-kinase p85α phosphorylation in the hypothalami of fetuses [101]. Reductions in the insulin-signaling proteins p110-β and insulin receptor substrate-1 in adipose tissue are also associated with mentioned diet in male rats [84]. Moreover, modest caloric restriction coupled with changes in insulin receptor gene expression in multiple organs contributes to the development of insulin resistance [102].

15.3.6 The role of maternal diet on mitochondrial function and development of diabetes

Besides genetic and non-genetic modifications, recently mitochondrial function programming has been proposed to explain how abnormal nutrition results in a phenotype observed in the progeny. Mitochondrial alterations have been observed in diabeticpatients. Nutritional restrictions such as anti-oxidant nutrients contribute to increased oxidative stress leading to alterations in mitochondrial DNA transcription that suggests a nutrition-mitochondrial regulation-insulin signaling axis. Also, nutrients can affect membrane fluidity, following which the gene products function are changed [103–105]. SIRT3 protein belongs to HDACs family that is rich in mitochondria and plays a key regulatory role in this organelle. Reduced expression of SIRT3 that leads to impaired fatty acid oxidation was reported in offspring of high-fat-fed dams. Reduced hepatic fatty acid oxidation resulted in developed insulin resistance and onset of T2D [106].

Also, severe caloric restriction in rodent models during pregnancy causes significant placental mitochondrial defects and abnormal placental metabolism that were associated with increased β-cell apoptosis [106,107].

However, dysregulation of mentioned pathways is heavily implicated. Inconsistent, animal offspring of suboptimal maternal nutrition and lower body condition score did not have glucose intolerance in adult life that may be associated with postnatal nutrient environment [108]. Although some evidence has suggested that prenatal and postnatal high-fat/fructose diet is able to cause hyperglycemia and severe insulin resistance, offspring with normal diet partially compensated the adverse effects of prenatal high-fat/fructose diet [109].

It has been hypothesized that induced permanent changes in metabolism and chronic disease susceptibility following unbalanced nutrition in early life are dependent on the presence of later risk factors such as physical inactivity, malnutrition, and aging [63].

However, the needs for maternal dietary interventions that maximize metabolic benefits and minimize metabolic cost for the next generation [79].

15.4 Prenatal nutrition exposure and hypertension in adults

Hypertension continues to be a major contributor to metabolic diseases such as coronary heart disease, stroke, and heart failure despite the multitude of pharmacological options available [110]. Also, it is a complex condition with many contributing risk factors including environmental exposure and genetic susceptibility [111]. The developmental originof hypertension based on the human evidence showed that the perinatal nutrition can significantly impact on the risk for hypertension [112,113]. As more information is discovered, epigenomic factors during pregnancy play a significant role in adult-onset hypertension [114].

Phenotypic plasticity, different phenotypes from one genome following environmental stimulation, of cardiovascular, renal, neural, and endocrine systems in response to malnourished conditions during early phases of development can affect the high prevalence of hypertension among adult [115]. DNA methylation, histone acetylation, and microRNA expression as the epigenetic alterations are the molecular mechanisms of phenotypic plasticity [115].

15.4.1 The role of maternal diet on renin–angiotensin system, structure and function of glomeruli, and programmed hypertension

The renin–angiotensin system (RAS) is considered to be an important pathway in the development of programmed hypertension. The RAS comprises different angiotensin peptides with diverse biological actions mediated by distinct receptor subtypes. Renin cleaves angiotensinogen to angiotensin I (ANG I), which is further processed to the active peptides angiotensin II (ANG II) by angiotensin-converting enzyme (ACE). The predominant effecter peptide of the RAS, ANG II, causes arterioles to constrict and activates its type-1 receptor to mediate both peripheral and central mechanisms in the regulation of blood pressure [116]. Moreover, deregulation in the nephrogenesis could impact on the development of hypertension [117].

A substantial literature highlights the importance of maternal diet during pregnancy in the programming of hypertension via RAS and glomerular system in later life.

Some of these studies suggested that in pregnant dams fed with a LP diet, adultmice hypertension through suppressed expression of RAS was developed [118]. Moreover, perinatal malnutrition environment can not only significantly destroy function of the renin- angiotensin-aldosterone system but also reduce glomerular filtration rate [113]. Consistent with these, results of other studies also demonstrated that perinatal protein restriction in the rat leads to a reduced number of glomeruli, glomerular enlargement, and hypertension in the adult due to the suppressed RAS [119]. Also, maternal protein-reduced diet can contribute to the programming of hypertension risk by mechanisms including reduced nephron number, greater pressor response to angiotensin I, and lower renal expression of the angiotensin II type 2 receptor [120].

Most interestingly, hypomethylation of angiotensin receptor gene AT(1b) in the adrenal gland of the offspring was seen in maternal LP diet rat models. As the AT(1b) gene expression is highly dependent on promoter methylation, this alteration can result in the development of hypertensionin adult life [121].

The association between programmed reduced renal Na+, K+-ATPase and renin activity, and exposure to maternal HFDs is consistent with previous observations [122].

In addition, in offspring of a maternal high-salt (HS) diets, general reduction in antioxidant capacity and excessive reactive oxygen species (ROS) were associated with increased ANG II in renal and coronary arteries [114]. However, other studies could not associate prenatally programmed hypertension with unfavorable effects of HS diet in adult offspring rats [123].

Other well-studied mechanisms suggested decreased large calcium-activated potassium channels (BKCa) expression and activity and increased vessel tone, induced by angiotensin II and involvement of the AT1 receptor in ANG II-mediated vasoconstriction in mesenteric arteries following maternal exposure to high-sucrose diet in offspring rats [124].

Another consequence of maternal protein malnutrition during pregnancy is increased mRNA expression of ACE-1 with a decrease in mRNA levels of angiotensin II type-2 (AT2) receptors. Also, altered miRNA may be involved in regulating the RAS pathway in animal models of programmed hypertension. In fetal brains from mentioned model, mir27a and mir27b levels were significantly increased, which are regulators of ACE translation, while mir330, which regulates the AT2 receptor, was significantly decreased [125]. Other miRNAs have been found to be altered in renal tissue from offspring of maternal low-protein rats, including mir200a, mir141, and mir429, which may contribute to glomerular dysfunction, fibrosis, and ultimately programmed hypertension [126].

However, some controversy exists in the researches regarding alterations in the various components of the RAS which might be due to gender of the offspring [114].

15.4.2 The role of maternal diet on vascular changes and programmed hypertension

Vascular structural alternations, in particular increased arterial stiffness, reduced density of arterioles and capillaries, and vascular functional changes that include impaired vasodilation and endothelial cells dysfunctions, are considered as mechanisms that may be associated with unbalanced prenatal nutrition, causing IUGR and later hypertension [127].

Although a human study has suggested that severe undernutrition during gestation had no effect on arterial stiffness in the offspring [128], in this field, a clear correlation has been obtained with animal models.

Increased aortic stiffness, smooth muscle cell number, and reduced endothelium-dependent relaxation following a maternal HFD were illustrated in Sprague–Dawley rat offspring [122]. Offspring of the animal receiving HFD and high-sucrose diet–induced programming during pregnancy had carotid artery and aorta contractility dysfunction and arterial abnormality, respectively [114]. Further, some studies provided evidence that a protein-restricted diet [129], high-salt diet [130], or a zinc-restricted diet [131] during pregnancy reduces endothelial nitric oxide synthase expression in vascular tissues in offspring, which might have consequences for hypertension risk. However, in the smooth muscle, the association between sensitivity to nitric oxide (NO) and poor in utero nutrition has not been reported [132,133].

15.4.3 The role of maternal diet on respiratory system and sympathetic function and programmed hypertension

Other hypotheses considering the role of respiratory function that contribute to the development of arterial hypertension have been highlighted.

Sympathetic respiratory over-activity and enhanced peripheral chemoreceptor responses were associated with respiratory dysfunction and hypertension among rats exposed to protein undernutrition during gestation and lactation. It is particularly important to note that some of the mediators such as high levels of hypoxia-inducible factor 1α (HIF-1α) expression in carotid bodies peripheral chemoreceptor might be involved in this impact [134]. Some studies provide evidence that maternal nutrient restriction induces the histone acetylation and HIF-1α binding levels in ET-1 gene promoter of pulmonary vascular endothelial cells in offspring rats. These epigenetic changes can cause pulmonary vascular remodelingand pulmonary arterial hypertension, following being highly sensitive to hypoxia later in life [135]. In addition, feeding a LP diet during gestation can increase the risk of adult arterial hypertension in male rat offspring, which follows alterations in the respiratory rhythm and O_2/CO_2 chemo-sensitivity at early ages [136]. Furthermore, the potential impact of an increase in the cardiovascular sympathetic tone as a predisposing factor for increased arterial pressure in animals subjected to maternal protein restriction was presented [137].

15.4.4 The role of maternal diet on low birth weight and programmed hypertension

Rate of weight gain, consequently LBW, as one of the most identifiable markers of a suboptimal prenatal environment,seems to have an increased risk to developing hypertension [52,53].

After rapid catch-up growth following LBW, rats exhibit some accelerated stress-induced senescence markers and mitochondrial stress indices in kidneys which are the important contributor to the progression of hypertension [138].

Given that no new nephrons are formed in human kidneys after gestation of approximately 36 weeks, LBW influences renal development, nephrogenesis and hypertension, and renal disease [139,140]. In this field, kidney undevelopment, decreased glomerular number, and renal dysfunction followed by LBW and maternal LP diet cause a long-term hypertension risk inrat offspring [141].

Long non-coding RNAs (lncRNAs), which are longer than 200 nucleotides in length, are crucial regulators involved in normal development and a variety of biological processes. A number of lncRNAs were aberrantly expressed in the kidneys of LBW rats and might have an important role in low nephron number induced by the restriction of maternal protein intake. Low nephron numbers at the beginning of life can lead to hypertension in adult life [142].

In the IUGR kidney following deprivation in utero and utero-placental insufficiency, decreased CpG methylation of the renal p53 BstU I site promoter was shown that may be significantly affected on increased renal apoptosis, and decreased nephron number [143].

Fetal growth restriction is also associated with altered autonomic regulation and increased sympatho-adrenal activity in childhood, which possibly develops hypertension in adulthood [144]. Other studied mechanisms that might be associated with SGA and hypertension development include elevatedcirculating noradrenalin levels and increased angiotensin II and ACE activity [145].

Moreover, during only the pre-implantation period, maternal LP diet can induce programming of hypertension by a reduction of cellular proliferation rate, first within the inner cell mass (ICM; early blastocyst), and later within both ICM and trophectoderm lineages (mid/late blastocyst) [146].

Overall, although, LBW influences renal development and hypertension [139, 140], it was reported that these effects may not be sufficient to induce long-lasting vascular disorders and renal disease, and postnatal overfeeding should act as a "second hit" [147].

15.4.5 The role of maternal diet on glucocorticoids and programmed hypertension

Programmed hypertension is also mediated by excess exposure to glucocorticoids and increased renal glucocorticoid sensitivity, with consequent stimulatory effects on Na/K-ATPase-alpha1 and intra-renal RAS [148]. Also, prenatal excess of glucocorticoids can permanently program the HPA axis that may contribute to hypertension in adulthood [149].

The glucocorticoid-inactivating enzyme, 11β-hydroxysteroid dehydrogenase type 2 (HSD2), which highly expresses within the placenta, limits excess exposure of the fetus to glucocorticoids. Down-regulation of placental 11β-HSD2 is also associated with some adverse intrauterine environment such as low-protein maternal diet as well as low fetal growth and birth weight [149,150].

Some literatures exist investigating the key mechanisms underlying maternal diet during gestation and glucocorticoid pathways predisposing to hypertension in later life.

In the Mother Well cohort study, the link between unbalanced diet in pregnancy and increased risk of offspring hypertension in adulthood has been shown. This elevated blood pressure was due to increased CpGs methylation in the HSD2 and glucocorticoid receptor and IGF2 differentially methylated regions (H19 ICR) [16].

A clear correlation between a Ca-deficient diet for a dam during gestation and a reduction in methylation of 11β-hydroxysteroid dehydrogenase type 1 (11β-HSD1) gene, GR (Nr3c1) expression, and high glucocorticoid and corticosterone concentrations has been obtained in female and male offspring, respectively [151]. It should be mentioned that the relation of 11β-HSD1 hypomethylation with high blood pressure may be explained by 11β-HSD1-related effects on an increase in conversion of cortisone to active cortisol [152].

In addition, increased intake of folic acid during pregnancy promotes methylation of GR promoter in rats. Evidently, these epigenetic changes will increase blood pressure in offspring [152].

So, a balanced prenatal diet might have an antihypertensive effect by protecting from genomic and non-genomic dysregulation and reducing the future burden of hypertension. However, the offspring hypertension following imbalanced diet of dams can be normalized by improving the postnatal environment [153]. These data highlight the complexities of fetal programming of hypertension, which is highly sensitive to both the type and timing of the insult [114].

Overall, the role of maternal dietary factors during pregnancy in disease etiology could be confounded by demographic, life style, and psychological characteristics. Furthermore, between and within individual variability, genetic factors and gene–environment interactions for susceptibility to diet-induced disease should be considered in interpreting these results.

In future, more longitudinal and well-designed studies are needed to decipher the impact of maternal diet on long-lasting programming of chronic disease. They will help us to understand the possible link between epigenetic alterations and its role in health and disease. However, it should be considered a personalized diet intervention that not only account for the nutritional needs but also include the genotype ofpregnant women which might impart far-reaching benefits to the health of their children.

References

1. Abente EJ, Subramanian M, Ramachandran V, Najafi-Shoushtari SH. MicroRNAs in obesity-associated disorders. *Archives of Biochemistry and Biophysics*. 2016;589:108–19.
2. Irazola VE, Gutierrez L, Bloomfield G, Carrillo-Larco RM, Dorairaj P, Gaziano T, et al. Hypertension prevalence, awareness, treatment, and control in selected LMIC communities: Results from the NHLBI/UHG network of centers of excellence for chronic diseases. *Global Heart*. 2016;11(1):47–59.
3. Dyer JS, Rosenfeld CR. Metabolic imprinting by prenatal, perinatal, and postnatal overnutrition: A review. *Seminars in Reproductive Medicine*. 2011;29(3):266–76.
4. Vickers MH. Early life nutrition, epigenetics and programming of later life disease. *Nutrients*. 2014;6(6):2165–78.
5. Gali Ramamoorthy T, Begum G, Harno E, White A. Developmental programming of hypothalamic neuronal circuits: Impact on energy balance control. *Frontiers in Neuroscience*. 2015;9:126.
6. Chango A, Pogribny IP. Considering maternal dietary modulators for epigenetic regulation and programming of the fetal epigenome. *Nutrients*. 2015;7(4):2748–70.
7. Canani RB, Costanzo MD, Leone L, Bedogni G, Brambilla P, Cianfarani S, et al. Epigenetic mechanisms elicited by nutrition in early life. *Nutrition Research Reviews*. 2011;24(2):198–205.
8. Zheng J, Xiao X, Zhang Q, Yu M. DNA methylation: The pivotal interaction between early-life nutrition and glucose metabolism in later life. *The British Journal of Nutrition*. 2014;112(11):1850–7.
9. Vanhees K, Vonhogen IG, van Schooten FJ, Godschalk RW. You are what you eat, and so are your children: The impact of micronutrients on the epigenetic programming of offspring. *Cellular and Molecular Life Sciences: CMLS*. 2014;71(2):271–85.
10. Kabasakal Cetin A, Dasgin H, Gulec A, Onbasilar I, Akyol A. Maternal low quality protein diet alters plasma amino acid concentrations of weaning rats. *Nutrients*. 2015;7(12):9847–59.
11. Lanham S, Cagampang FR, Oreffo RO. Maternal high fat diet affects offspring's vitamin K-dependent proteins expression levels. *PLoS One*. 2015;10(9):e0138730.
12. Sebert S, Sharkey D, Budge H, Symonds ME. The early programming of metabolic health: Is epigenetic setting the missing link? *The American Journal of Clinical Nutrition*. 2011;94(6 Suppl):1953S–8S.
13. Soubry A. Epigenetic inheritance and evolution: A paternal perspective on dietary influences. *Progress in Biophysics and Molecular Biology*. 2015;118(1–2):79–85.
14. Delage B, Dashwood RH. Dietary manipulation of histone structure and function. *Annual Review of Nutrition*. 2008;28:347–66.
15. Bultman SJ. Interplay between diet, gut microbiota, epigenetic events, and colorectal cancer. *Molecular Nutrition & Food Research*. 2017;61(1):1500902.
16. Drake AJ, McPherson RC, Godfrey KM, Cooper C, Lillycrop KA, Hanson MA, et al. An unbalanced maternal diet in pregnancy associates with offspring epigenetic changes in genes controlling glucocorticoid action and foetal growth. *Clinical Endocrinology*. 2012;77(6):808–15.
17. McMillen IC, Edwards LJ, Duffield J, Muhlhausler BS. Regulation of leptin synthesis and secretion before birth: Implications for the early programming of adult obesity. *Reproduction (Cambridge, England)*. 2006;131(3):415–27.
18. Granado M, Fuente-Martin E, Garcia-Caceres C, Argente J, Chowen JA. Leptin in early life: A key factor for the development of the adult metabolic profile. *Obesity Facts*. 2012;5(1):138–50.
19. Jansson T, Powell TL. Role of placental nutrient sensing in developmental programming. *Clinical Obstetrics and Gynecology*. 2013;56(3):591–601.

20. Jansson T, Powell TL. Role of the placenta in fetal programming: Underlying mechanisms and potential interventional approaches. *Clinical Science (London, England: 1979).* 2007;113(1):1–13.

21. Liotto N, Miozzo M, Gianni ML, Taroni F, Morlacchi L, Piemontese P, et al. [Early nutrition: The role of genetics and epigenetics]. La Pediatria medica e chirurgica. *Medical and Surgical Pediatrics.* 2009;31(2):65–71. Nutrizione nelle prime epoche della vita: ruolo della genetica e dell' epigenetica.

22. Symonds ME, Budge H, Stephenson T, Gardner DS. Experimental evidence for long-term programming effects of early diet. *Advances in Experimental Medicine and Biology.* 2005;569:24–32.

23. Tobi EW, Lumey LH, Talens RP, Kremer D, Putter H, Stein AD, et al. DNA methylation differences after exposure to prenatal famine are common and timing- and sex-specific. *Human Molecular Genetics.* 2009;18(21):4046–53.

24. Lukaszewski MA, Eberle D, Vieau D, Breton C. Nutritional manipulations in the perinatal period program adipose tissue in offspring. *American Journal of Physiology Endocrinology And Metabolism.* 2013;305(10):E1195–207.

25. Correia-Branco A, Keating E, Martel F. Maternal undernutrition and fetal developmental programming of obesity: The glucocorticoid connection. *Reproductive Sciences.* 2015;22(2):138–45.

26. Grissom NM, George R, Reyes TM. The hypothalamic transcriptional response to stress is severely impaired in offspring exposed to adverse nutrition during gestation. *Neuroscience.* 2017;342:200–11.

27. Desai M, Han G, Ross MG. Programmed hyperphagia in offspring of obese dams: Altered expression of hypothalamic nutrient sensors, neurogenic factors and epigenetic modulators. *Appetite.* 2016;99:193–9.

28. Breton C. The hypothalamus-adipose axis is a key target of developmental programming by maternal nutritional manipulation. *The Journal of Endocrinology.* 2013;216(2):R19–31.

29. Ross MG, Desai M. Developmental programming of appetite/satiety. *Annals of Nutrition & Metabolism.* 2014;64 Suppl 1:36–44.

30. Fraser M, Dhaliwal CK, Vickers MH, Krechowec SO, Breier BH. Diet-induced obesity and prenatal undernutrition lead to differential neuroendocrine gene expression in the hypothalamic arcuate nuclei. *Endocrine.* 2016;53(3):839–47.

31. Plagemann A, Harder T, Brunn M, Harder A, Roepke K, Wittrock-Staar M, et al. Hypothalamic proopiomelanocortin promoter methylation becomes altered by early overfeeding: an epigenetic model of obesity and the metabolic syndrome. *The Journal of Physiology.* 2009;587(Pt 20):4963–76.

32. Stevens A, Begum G, White A. Epigenetic changes in the hypothalamic pro-opiomelanocortin gene: A mechanism linking maternal undernutrition to obesity in the offspring? *European Journal of Pharmacology.* 2011;660(1):194–201.

33. Vucetic Z, Kimmel J, Totoki K, Hollenbeck E, Reyes TM. Maternal high-fat diet alters methylation and gene expression of dopamine and opioid-related genes. *Endocrinology.* 2010;151(10):4756–64.

34. Jiang X, Yan J, West AA, Perry CA, Malysheva OV, Devapatla S, et al. Maternal choline intake alters the epigenetic state of fetal cortisol-regulating genes in humans. *FASEB Journal.* 2012;26(8):3563–74.

35. Lillycrop KA, Phillips ES, Jackson AA, Hanson MA, Burdge GC. Dietary protein restriction of pregnant rats induces and folic acid supplementation prevents epigenetic modification of hepatic gene expression in the offspring. *The Journal of Nutrition.* 2005;135(6):1382–6.

36. Begum G, Stevens A, Smith EB, Connor K, Challis JR, Bloomfield F, et al. Epigenetic changes in fetal hypothalamic energy regulating pathways are associated with maternal undernutrition and twinning. *FASEB Journal.* 2012;26(4):1694–703.

37. Budge H, Gnanalingham MG, Gardner DS, Mostyn A, Stephenson T, Symonds ME. Maternal nutritional programming of fetal adipose tissue development: Long-term consequences for later obesity. *Birth Defects Research Part C, Embryo Today: Reviews.* 2005;75(3):193–9.

38. Cannon MV, Buchner DA, Hester J, Miller H, Sehayek E, Nadeau JH, et al. Maternal nutrition induces pervasive gene expression changes but no detectable DNA methylation differences in the liver of adult offspring. *PLoS One.* 2014;9(3):e90335.

39. Zhang ZY, Dodd GT, Tiganis T. Protein tyrosine phosphatases in hypothalamic insulin and leptin signaling. *Trends in Pharmacological Sciences.* 2015;36(10):661–74.

40. Gardner DS, Rhodes P. Developmental origins of obesity: Programming of food intake or physical activity? *Advances in Experimental Medicine and Biology.* 2009;646:83–93.

41. Yajnik CS. Transmission of obesity-adiposity and related disorders from the mother to the baby. *Annals of Nutrition & Metabolism.* 2014;64 Suppl 1:8–17.

42. Adamu HA, Imam MU, Ooi DJ, Esa NM, Rosli R, Ismail M. Perinatal exposure to germinated brown rice and its gamma amino-butyric acid-rich extract prevents high fat diet-induced insulin resistance in first generation rat offspring. *Food & Nutrition Research.* 2016;60:30209.

43. Smith T, Sloboda DM, Saffery R, Joo E, Vickers MH. Maternal nutritional history modulates the hepatic IGF-IGFBP axis in adult male rat offspring. *Endocrine.* 2014;46(1):70–82.

44. Claycombe KJ, Uthus EO, Roemmich JN, Johnson LK, Johnson WT. Prenatal low-protein and postnatal high-fat diets induce rapid adipose tissue growth by inducing Igf2 expression in Sprague Dawley rat offspring. *The Journal of Nutrition.* 2013;143(10):1533–9.

45. Konieczna J, Palou M, Sanchez J, Pico C, Palou A. Leptin intake in suckling rats restores altered T3 levels and markers of adipose tissue sympathetic drive and function caused by gestational calorie restriction. *International Journal of Obesity (2005).* 2015;39(6):959–66.

46. Palou M, Priego T, Romero M, Szostaczuk N, Konieczna J, Cabrer C, et al. Moderate calorie restriction during gestation programs offspring for lower BAT thermogenic capacity driven by thyroid and sympathetic signaling. *International Journal of Obesity (2005).* 2015;39(2):339–45.

47. Murphy MM, Stettler N, Smith KM, Reiss R. Associations of consumption of fruits and vegetables during pregnancy with infant birth weight or small for gestational age births: a systematic review of the literature. *International Journal of Women's Health.* 2014;6:899–912.

48. Saggese G, Fanos M, Simi F. SGA children: auxological and metabolic outcomes—The role of GH treatment. *The Journal of Maternal-Fetal & Neonatal Medicine.* 2013;26 Suppl 2:64–7.

49. Cho WK, Suh BK. Catch-up growth and catch-up fat in children born small for gestational age. *Korean Journal of Pediatrics.* 2016;59(1):1–7.

50. Qiao Y, Ma J, Wang Y, Li W, Katzmarzyk PT, Chaput JP, et al. Birth weight and childhood obesity: A 12-country study. *International Journal of Obesity Supplements.* 2015;5(Suppl 2):S74–9.

51. Evensen E, Wilsgaard T, Furberg AS, Skeie G. Tracking of overweight and obesity from early childhood to adolescence in a population-based cohort—The Tromso Study, fit futures. *BMC Pediatrics.* 2016;16:64.

52. Mhanna MJ, Iqbal AM, Kaelber DC. Weight gain and hypertension at three years of age and older in extremely low birth weight infants. *Journal of Neonatal-Perinatal Medicine.* 2015;8(4):363–9.

53. Bruno RM, Faconti L, Taddei S, Ghiadoni L. Birth weight and arterial hypertension. *Current Opinion in Cardiology.* 2015;30(4):398–402.

54. Dodd JM, O'Brien CM, Grivell RM. Modifying diet and physical activity to support pregnant women who are overweight or obese. *Current Opinion in Clinical Nutrition and Metabolic Care.* 2015;18(3):318–23.
55. Martinez JA, Milagro FI, Claycombe KJ, Schalinske KL. Epigenetics in adipose tissue, obesity, weight loss, and diabetes. *Advances in Nutrition.* 2014;5(1):71–81.
56. Ji Y, Wu Z, Dai Z, Sun K, Wang J, Wu G. Nutritional epigenetics with a focus on amino acids: Implications for the development and treatment of metabolic syndrome. *The Journal of Nutritional Biochemistry.* 2016;27:1–8.
57. Jiao F, Yan X, Yu Y, Zhu X, Ma Y, Yue Z, et al. Protective effects of maternal methyl donor supplementation on adult offspring of high fat diet-fed dams. *The Journal of Nutritional Biochemistry.* 2016;34:42–51.
58. Cho CE, Pannia E, Huot PS, Sanchez-Hernandez D, Kubant R, Dodington DW, et al. Methyl vitamins contribute to obesogenic effects of a high multivitamin gestational diet and epigenetic alterations in hypothalamic feeding pathways in Wistar rat offspring. *Molecular Nutrition & Food Research.* 2015;59(3):476–89.
59. Masuyama H, Mitsui T, Nobumoto E, Hiramatsu Y. The effects of high-fat diet exposure in utero on the obesogenic and diabetogenic traits through epigenetic changes in adiponectin and leptin gene expression for multiple generations in female mice. *Endocrinology.* 2015;156(7):2482–91.
60. Zhou B, Lu Y, Hajifathalian K, Bentham J, Di Cesare M, Danaei G, et al. Worldwide trends in diabetes since 1980: A pooled analysis of 751 population-based studies with 4.4 million participants. *The Lancet.* 2016;387(10027):1513–30.
61. Smith CJ, Ryckman KK. Epigenetic and developmental influences on the risk of obesity, diabetes, and metabolic syndrome. *Diabetes, Metabolic Syndrome and Obesity: Targets and Therapy.* 2015;8:295–302.
62. Hales CN, Barker DJ. Type 2 (non-insulin-dependent) diabetes mellitus: The thrifty phenotype hypothesis. *Diabetologia.* 1992;35(7):595–601.
63. Millar K, Dean HJ. Developmental origins of type 2 diabetes in aboriginal youth in Canada: It is more than diet and exercise. *Journal of Nutrition and Metabolism.* 2012;2012:127452.
64. Lumey LH, Khalangot MD, Vaiserman AM. Association between type 2 diabetes and prenatal exposure to the Ukraine famine of 1932-33: A retrospective cohort study. *The Lancet Diabetes Endocrinology.* 2015;3(10):787–94.
65. El Hajj N, Schneider E, Lehnen H, Haaf T. Epigenetics and life-long consequences of an adverse nutritional and diabetic intrauterine environment. *Reproduction (Cambridge, England).* 2014;148(6):R111–20.
66. Kim MS, Lee DY. Insulin-like growth factor (IGF)-I and IGF binding proteins axis in diabetes mellitus. *Annals of Pediatric Endocrinology & Metabolism.* 2015;20(2):69–73.
67. Painter RC, Roseboom TJ, Bleker OP. Prenatal exposure to the Dutch famine and disease in later life: An overview. *Reproductive Toxicology.* 2005;20(3):345–52.
68. Steegers-Theunissen RP, Obermann-Borst SA, Kremer D, Lindemans J, Siebel C, Steegers EA, et al. Periconceptional maternal folic acid use of 400 mu g per day is related to increased methylation of the IGF2 gene in the very young child. *PLoS One.* 2009;4(11):e7845.
69. Sandovici I, Smith NH, Nitert MD, Ackers-Johnson M, Uribe-Lewis S, Ito Y, et al. Maternal diet and aging alter the epigenetic control of a promoter-enhancer interaction at the Hnf4a gene in rat pancreatic islets. *Proceedings of the National Academy of Sciences of the United States of America.* 2011;108(13):5449–54.
70. Rodriguez-Trejo A, Ortiz-Lopez MG, Zambrano E, Granados-Silvestre Mde L, Mendez C, Blondeau B, et al. Developmental programming of neonatal pancreatic beta-cells by a maternal low-protein diet in rats involves a switch from proliferation to differentiation. *American Journal of Physiology Endocrinology and Metabolism.* 2012;302(11):E1431–9.

71. Alejandro EU, Gregg B, Wallen T, Kumusoglu D, Meister D, Chen A, et al. Maternal diet-induced microRNAs and mTOR underlie beta cell dysfunction in offspring. *Journal of Clinical Investigation.* 2014;124(10):4395–410.

72. Blandino-Rosano M, Chen AY, Scheys JO, Alejandro EU, Gould AP, Taranukha T, et al. mTORC1 signaling and regulation of pancreatic beta-cell mass. *Cell Cycle.* 2012;11(10):1892–902.

73. Lendvai A, Deutsch MJ, Plosch T, Ensenauer R. The peroxisome proliferator-activated receptors under epigenetic control in placental metabolism and fetal development. *American Journal of Physiology Endocrinology and Metabolism.* 2016;310(10):E797–810.

74. Ashino NG, Saito KN, Souza FD, Nakutz FS, Roman EA, Velloso LA, et al. Maternal high-fat feeding through pregnancy and lactation predisposes mouse offspring to molecular insulin resistance and fatty liver. *Journal of Nutritional Biochemistry.* 2012;23(4):341–8.

75. Chamson-Reig A, Thyssen SM, Arany E, Hill DJ. Altered pancreatic morphology in the offspring of pregnant rats given reduced dietary protein is time and gender specific. *Journal of Endocrinology.* 2006;191(1):83–92.

76. Heywood WE, Mian N, Milla PJ, Lindley KJ. Programming of defective rat pancreatic beta-cell function in offspring from mothers fed a low-protein diet during gestation and the suckling periods. *Clinical Science.* 2004;107(1):37–45.

77. Hou M, Chu ZY, Liu T, Lv HT, Sun L, Wang B, et al. A high-fat maternal diet decreases adiponectin receptor-1 expression in offspring. *The Journal of Maternal-Fetal & Neonatal Medicine.* 2015;28(2):216–21.

78. Yokomizo H, Inoguchi T, Sonoda N, Sakaki Y, Maeda Y, Inoue T, et al. Maternal high-fat diet induces insulin resistance and deterioration of pancreatic beta-cell function in adult offspring with sex differences in mice. *American Journal of Physiology Endocrinology and Metabolism.* 2014;306(10):E1163–75.

79. Nicholas LM, Rattanatray L, MacLaughlin SM, Ozanne SE, Kleemann DO, Walker SK, et al. Differential effects of maternal obesity and weight loss in the periconceptional period on the epigenetic regulation of hepatic insulin-signaling pathways in the offspring. *FASEB Journal.* 2013;27(9):3786–96.

80. Dumortier O, Hinault C, Gautier N, Patouraux S, Casamento V, Van Obberghen E. Maternal protein restriction leads to pancreatic failure in offspring: Role of misexpressed microRNA-375. *Diabetes.* 2014;63(10):3416–27.

81. Vaiserman AM. Early-life exposure to substance abuse and risk of type 2 diabetes in adulthood. *Current Diabetes Reports.* 2015;15(8):48.

82. Martin-Gronert MS, Ozanne SE. Mechanisms linking suboptimal early nutrition and increased risk of type 2 diabetes and obesity. *Journal of Nutrition.* 2010;140(3):662–6.

83. Tarry-Adkins JL, Fernandez-Twinn DS, Hargreaves IP, Neergheen V, Aiken CE, Martin-Gronert MS, et al. Coenzyme Q10 prevents hepatic fibrosis, inflammation, and oxidative stress in a male rat model of poor maternal nutrition and accelerated postnatal growth. *The American Journal of Clinical Nutrition.* 2016;103(2):579–88.

84. Tarry-Adkins JL, Fernandez-Twinn DS, Madsen R, Chen JH, Carpenter A, Hargreaves IP, et al. Coenzyme Q10 prevents insulin signaling dysregulation and inflammation prior to development of insulin resistance in male offspring of a rat model of poor maternal nutrition and accelerated postnatal growth. *Endocrinology.* 2015;156(10):3528–37.

85. Xie XM, Lin TL, Zhang MH, Liao LH, Yuan GD, Gao HJ, et al. IUGR with infantile overnutrition programs an insulin-resistant phenotype through DNA methylation of peroxisome proliferator-activated receptor-gamma coactivator-1 alpha in rats. *Pediatric Research.* 2015;77(5):625–32.

86. Park JH, Stoffers DA, Nicholls RD, Simmons RA. Development of type 2 diabetes following intrauterine growth retardation in rats is associated with progressive epigenetic silencing of Pdx1. *Journal of Clinical Investigation.* 2008;118(6):2316–24.

87. Raychaudhuri N, Raychaudhuri S, Thamotharan M, Devaskar SU. Histone code modifications repress glucose transporter 4 expression in the intrauterine growth-restricted offspring. *Journal of Biological Chemistry.* 2008;283(20):13611–26.
88. Sosa-Larios TC, Cerbon MA, Morimoto S. Epigenetic alterations caused by nutritional stress during fetal programming of the endocrine pancreas. *Archives of Medical Research.* 2015;46(2):93–100.
89. Reusens B, Theys N, Dumortier O, Goosse K, Remacle C. Maternal malnutrition programs the endocrine pancreas in progeny. *The American Journal of Clinical Nutrition.* 2011;94(6 Suppl):1824S–9S.
90. Guan HY, Arany E, van Beek JP, Chamson-Reig A, Thyssen S, Hill DJ, et al. Adipose tissue gene expression profiling reveals distinct molecular pathways that define visceral adiposity in offspring of maternal protein-restricted rats. *American Journal of Physiology. Endocrinology and Metabolism.* 2005;288(4):E663–E73.
91. Morimoto S, Calzada L, Sosa TC, Reyes-Castro LA, Rodriguez-Gonzalez GL, Morales A, et al. Emergence of ageing-related changes in insulin secretion by pancreatic islets of male rat offspring of mothers fed a low-protein diet. *British Journal of Nutrition.* 2012;107(11):1562–5.
92. Morimoto S, Sosa TC, Calzada L, Reyes-Castro LA, Diaz-Diaz E, Morales A, et al. Developmental programming of aging of isolated pancreatic islet glucose-stimulated insulin secretion in female offspring of mothers fed low-protein diets in pregnancy and/or lactation. *Journal of Developmental Origins of Health and Disease.* 2012;3(6):483–8.
93. Ergaz Z, Neeman-Azulay M, Weinstein-Fudim L, Weksler-Zangen S, Shoshani-Dror D, Szyf M, et al. Diabetes in the Cohen rat intensifies the fetal pancreatic damage induced by the diabetogenic high sucrose low copper diet. *Birth Defects Research Part B, Developmental and Reproductive Toxicology.* 2016;107(1):21–31.
94. O'Dowd JF, Stocker CJ. Endocrine pancreatic development: Impact of obesity and diet. *Frontiers in Physiology.* 2013;4:170.
95. Ng SF, Lin RCY, Laybutt DR, Barres R, Owens JA, Morris MJ. Chronic high-fat diet in fathers programs beta-cell dysfunction in female rat offspring. *Nature.* 2010;467(7318):963–U103.
96. Azzi S, Sas TCJ, Koudou Y, Le Bouc Y, Souberbielle JC, Dargent-Molina P, et al. Degree of methylation of ZAC1 (PLAGL1) is associated with prenatal and post-natal growth in healthy infants of the EDEN mother child cohort. *Epigenetics.* 2014;9(3):338–45.
97. Du X, Rousseau M, Ounissi-Benkalha H, Marchand L, Jetha A, Paraskevas S, et al. Differential expression pattern of ZAC in developing mouse and human pancreas. *Journal of Molecular Histology.* 2011;42(2):129–36.
98. Hoffmann A, Spengler D. Role of ZAC1 in transient neonatal diabetes mellitus and glucose metabolism. *World Journal of Biological Chemistry.* 2015;6(3):95–109.
99. Yajnik CS, Deshmukh US. Fetal programming: Maternal nutrition and role of one-carbon metabolism. *Reviews in Endocrine & Metabolic Disorders.* 2012;13(2):121–7.
100. Sabin MA, Magnussen CG, Juonala M, Shield JPH, Kahonen M, Lehtimaki T, et al. Insulin and BMI as predictors of adult type 2 diabetes mellitus. *Pediatrics.* 2015;135(1):E144–E51.
101. Liu X, Qi Y, Gao H, Jiao Y, Gu H, Miao J, et al. Maternal protein restriction induces alterations in insulin signaling and ATP sensitive potassium channel protein in hypothalami of intrauterine growth restriction fetal rats. *Journal of Clinical Biochemistry and Nutrition.* 2013;52(1):43–8.
102. Palou M, Konieczna J, Torrens JM, Sanchez J, Priego T, Fernandes ML, et al. Impaired insulin and leptin sensitivity in the offspring of moderate caloric-restricted dams during gestation is early programmed. *The Journal of Nutritional Biochemistry.* 2012;23(12):1627–39.
103. Reusens B, Theys N, Remacle C. Alteration of mitochondrial function in adult rat offspring of malnourished dams. *World Journal of Diabetes.* 2011;2(9):149–57.

104. Berdanier CD. Mitochondrial gene expression in diabetes mellitus: Effect of nutrition. *Nutrition Reviews*. 2001;59(3 Pt 1):61–70.
105. Zheng LD, Linarelli LE, Liu L, Wall SS, Greenawald MH, Seidel RW, et al. Insulin resistance is associated with epigenetic and genetic regulation of mitochondrial DNA in obese humans. *Clinical Epigenetics*. 2015;7:60.
106. Bruce KD. Maternal and in utero determinants of type 2 diabetes risk in the young. *Current Diabetes Reports*. 2014;14(1):446.
107. Mayeur S, Lancel S, Theys N, Lukaszewski MA, Duban-Deweer S, Bastide B, et al. Maternal calorie restriction modulates placental mitochondrial biogenesis and bioenergetic efficiency: Putative involvement in fetoplacental growth defects in rats. *American Journal of Physiology. Endocrinology and Metabolism*. 2013;304(1):E14–22.
108. Costello PM, Hollis LJ, Cripps RL, Bearpark N, Patel HP, Sayer AA, et al. Lower maternal body condition during pregnancy affects skeletal muscle structure and glut-4 protein levels but not glucose tolerance in mature adult sheep. *Reproductive Sciences*. 2013;20(10):1144–55.
109. Li L, Xue J, Li HY, Ding J, Wang YY, Wang XT. Over-nutrient environment during both prenatal and postnatal development increases severity of islet injury, hyperglycemia, and metabolic disorders in the offspring. *Journal of Physiology and Biochemistry*. 2015;71(3):391–403.
110. Landsberg L, Aronne LJ, Beilin LJ, Burke V, Igel LI, Lloyd-Jones D, et al. Obesity-related hypertension: Pathogenesis, cardiovascular risk, and treatment—A position paper of the The Obesity Society and The American Society of Hypertension. *Obesity*. 2013;21(1):8–24.
111. Ewald DR, Haldeman Ph DL. Risk factors in adolescent hypertension. *Global Pediatric Health*. 2016;3:2333794X15625159.
112. Simeoni U, Ligi I, Grandvuillemin I, Boubred F. [Early origins of arterial hypertension and cardiovascular diseases]. *Bulletin de l'Academie nationale de medecine*. 2011;195(3):499–508; discussion—10. Les origines precoces de l'hypertension arterielle et des maladies cardio-vasculaires.
113. Nuyt AM, Alexander BT. Developmental programming and hypertension. *Current Opinion in Nephrology and Hypertension*. 2009;18(2):144–52.
114. Morton JS, Cooke CL, Davidge ST. In utero origins of hypertension: Mechanisms and targets for therapy. *Physiological Reviews*. 2016;96(2):549–603.
115. Costa-Silva JH, de Brito-Alves JL, Barros MA, Nogueira VO, Paulino-Silva KM, de Oliveira-Lira A, et al. New insights on the maternal diet induced-hypertension: Potential role of the phenotypic plasticity and sympathetic-respiratory overactivity. *Frontiers in Physiology*. 2015;6:345.
116. Chappell MC. Biochemical evaluation of the renin-angiotensin system: The good, bad, and absolute? *American Journal of Physiology Heart and Circulatory Physiology*. 2016;310(2):H137–52.
117. Mazzei L, Garcia M, Calvo JP, Casarotto M, Fornes M, Abud MA, et al. Changes in renal WT-1 expression preceding hypertension development. *BMC Nephrology*. 2016;17:34.
118. Tsukuda K, Mogi M, Iwanami J, Min LJ, Jing F, Ohshima K, et al. Influence of angiotensin II type 1 receptor-associated protein on prenatal development and adult hypertension after maternal dietary protein restriction during pregnancy. *Journal of the American Society of Hypertension: JASH*. 2012;6(5):324–30.
119. Woods LL, Ingelfinger JR, Nyengaard JR, Rasch R. Maternal protein restriction suppresses the newborn renin-angiotensin system and programs adult hypertension in rats. *Pediatric Research*. 2001;49(4):460–7.
120. McMullen S, Gardner DS, Langley-Evans SC. Prenatal programming of angiotensin II type 2 receptor expression in the rat. *The British Journal of Nutrition*. 2004;91(1):133–40.

402 Nutrigenomics and Nutraceuticals

121. Bogdarina I, Welham S, King PJ, Burns SP, Clark AJ. Epigenetic modification of the renin-angiotensin system in the fetal programming of hypertension. *Circulation Research*. 2007;100(4):520–6.

122. Armitage JA, Lakasing L, Taylor PD, Balachandran AA, Jensen RI, Dekou V, et al. Developmental programming of aortic and renal structure in offspring of rats fed fat-rich diets in pregnancy. *The Journal of Physiology*. 2005;565(Pt 1):171–84.

123. Porter JP, King SH, Honeycutt AD. Prenatal high-salt diet in the Sprague-Dawley rat programs blood pressure and heart rate hyperresponsiveness to stress in adult female offspring. *American Journal of Physiology. Regulatory, Integrative and Comparative Physiology*. 2007;293(1):R334–42.

124. Li S, Fang Q, Zhou A, Wu L, Shi A, Cao L, et al. Intake of high sucrose during pregnancy altered large-conductance Ca^{2+}-activated K^+ channels and vessel tone in offspring's mesenteric arteries. *Hypertension Research*. 2013;36(2):158–65.

125. Goyal R, Goyal D, Leitzke A, Gheorghe CP, Longo LD. Brain renin-angiotensin system: Fetal epigenetic programming by maternal protein restriction during pregnancy. *Reproductive Sciences*. 2010;17(3):227–38.

126. Sene Lde B, Mesquita FF, de Moraes LN, Santos DC, Carvalho R, Gontijo JA, et al. Involvement of renal corpuscle microRNA expression on epithelial-to-mesenchymal transition in maternal low protein diet in adult programmed rats. *PLoS One*. 2013;8(8):e71310.

127. Ligi I, Grandvuillemin I, Andres V, Dignat-George F, Simeoni U. Low birth weight infants and the developmental programming of hypertension: A focus on vascular factors. *Seminars in Perinatology*. 2010;34(3):188–92.

128. Painter RC, de Rooij SR, Bossuyt PM, de Groot E, Stok WJ, Osmond C, et al. Maternal nutrition during gestation and carotid arterial compliance in the adult offspring: The Dutch famine birth cohort. *Journal of Hypertension*. 2007;25(3):533–40.

129. Torrens C, Brawley L, Anthony FW, Dance CS, Dunn R, Jackson AA, et al. Folate supplementation during pregnancy improves offspring cardiovascular dysfunction induced by protein restriction. *Hypertension*. 2006;47(5):982–7.

130. Piecha G, Koleganova N, Ritz E, Muller A, Fedorova OV, Bagrov AY, et al. High salt intake causes adverse fetal programming—Vascular effects beyond blood pressure. *Nephrology, Dialysis, Transplantation*. 2012;27(9):3464–76.

131. Tomat A, Elesgaray R, Zago V, Fasoli H, Fellet A, Balaszczuk AM, et al. Exposure to zinc deficiency in fetal and postnatal life determines nitric oxide system activity and arterial blood pressure levels in adult rats. *The British Journal of Nutrition*. 2010;104(3):382–9.

132. Samuelsson AM, Matthews PA, Argenton M, Christie MR, McConnell JM, Jansen EH, et al. Diet-induced obesity in female mice leads to offspring hyperphagia, adiposity, hypertension, and insulin resistance: A novel murine model of developmental programming. *Hypertension*. 2008;51(2):383–92.

133. Musha Y, Itoh S, Hanson MA, Kinoshita K. Does estrogen affect the development of abnormal vascular function in offspring of rats fed a low-protein diet in pregnancy? *Pediatric Research*. 2006;59(6):784–9.

134. de Brito Alves JL, Nogueira VO, Cavalcanti Neto MP, Leopoldino AM, Curti C, Colombari DS, et al. Maternal protein restriction increases respiratory and sympathetic activities and sensitizes peripheral chemoreflex in male rat offspring. *The Journal of Nutrition*. 2015;145(5):907–14.

135. Xu XF, Lv Y, Gu WZ, Tang LL, Wei JK, Zhang LY, et al. Epigenetics of hypoxic pulmonary arterial hypertension following intrauterine growth retardation rat: Epigenetics in PAH following IUGR. *Respiratory Research*. 2013;14:20.

136. de Brito Alves JL, Nogueira VO, de Oliveira GB, da Silva GS, Wanderley AG, Leandro CG, et al. Short- and long-term effects of a maternal low-protein diet on ventilation, O(2)/CO(2) chemoreception and arterial blood pressure in male rat offspring. *The British Journal of Nutrition*. 2014;111(4):606–15.

137. Barros MA, De Brito Alves JL, Nogueira VO, Wanderley AG, Costa-Silva JH. Maternal low-protein diet induces changes in the cardiovascular autonomic modulation in male rat offspring. *Nutrition, Metabolism, and Cardiovascular Diseases: NMCD.* 2015;25(1):123–30.

138. Luyckx VA, Compston CA, Simmen T, Mueller TF. Accelerated senescence in kidneys of low-birth-weight rats after catch-up growth. *American Journal of Physiology. Renal Physiology.* 2009;297(6):F1697–705.

139. Bertram JF, Douglas-Denton RN, Diouf B, Hughson MD, Hoy WE. Human nephron number: Implications for health and disease. *Pediatric Nephrology.* 2011;26(9):1529–33.

140. Fanni D, Gerosa C, Nemolato S, Mocci C, Pichiri G, Coni P, et al. "Physiological" renal regenerating medicine in VLBW preterm infants: Could a dream come true? *The Journal of Maternal-Fetal & Neonatal Medicine.* 2012;25 Suppl 3:41–8.

141. Xie Z, Dong Q, Ge J, Chen P, Li W, Hu J. Effect of low birth weight on impaired renal development and function and hypertension in rat model. *Renal Failure.* 2012;34(6):754–9.

142. Li Y, Wang X, Li M, Pan J, Jin M, Wang J, et al. Long non-coding RNA expression profile in the kidneys of male, low birth weight rats exposed to maternal protein restriction at postnatal day 1 and day 10. *PLoS One.* 2015;10(3):e0121587.

143. Pham TD, MacLennan NK, Chiu CT, Laksana GS, Hsu JL, Lane RH. Uteroplacental insufficiency increases apoptosis and alters p53 gene methylation in the full-term IUGR rat kidney. *American Journal of Physiology. Regulatory, Integrative and Comparative Physiology.* 2003;285(5):R962–70.

144. Johansson S, Norman M, Legnevall L, Dalmaz Y, Lagercrantz H, Vanpee M. Increased catecholamines and heart rate in children with low birth weight: Perinatal contributions to sympathoadrenal overactivity. *Journal of Internal Medicine.* 2007;261(5):480–7.

145. Franco MC, Casarini DE, Carneiro-Ramos MS, Sawaya AL, Barreto-Chaves ML, Sesso R. Circulating renin-angiotensin system and catecholamines in childhood: Is there a role for birthweight? *Clinical Science (London, England: 1979).* 2008;114(5):375–80.

146. Kwong WY, Wild AE, Roberts P, Willis AC, Fleming TP. Maternal undernutrition during the preimplantation period of rat development causes blastocyst abnormalities and programming of postnatal hypertension. *Development.* 2000;127(19):4195–202.

147. Boubred F, Daniel L, Buffat C, Feuerstein JM, Tsimaratos M, Oliver C, et al. Early postnatal overfeeding induces early chronic renal dysfunction in adult male rats. *American Journal of Physiology. Renal Physiology.* 2009;297(4):F943–51.

148. Wyrwoll CS, Mark PJ, Waddell BJ. Developmental programming of renal glucocorticoid sensitivity and the renin-angiotensin system. *Hypertension.* 2007;50(3):579–84.

149. Nuyt AM. Mechanisms underlying developmental programming of elevated blood pressure and vascular dysfunction: Evidence from human studies and experimental animal models. *Clinical Science (London, England: 1979).* 2008;114(1):1–17.

150. Cottrell EC, Seckl JR, Holmes MC, Wyrwoll CS. Foetal and placental 11beta-HSD2: A hub for developmental programming. *Acta Physiologica (Oxford, England).* 2014;210(2):288–95.

151. Takaya J, Iharada A, Okihana H, Kaneko K. A calcium-deficient diet in pregnant, nursing rats induces hypomethylation of specific cytosines in the 11beta-hydroxysteroid dehydrogenase-1 promoter in pup liver. *Nutrition Research.* 2013;33(11):961–70.

152. Anwar MA, Saleh AI, Al Olabi R, Al Shehabi TS, Eid AH. Glucocorticoid-induced fetal origins of adult hypertension: Association with epigenetic events. *Vascular Pharmacology.* 2016;82:41–50.

153. Siddique K, Guzman GL, Gattineni J, Baum M. Effect of postnatal maternal protein intake on prenatal programming of hypertension. *Reproductive Sciences.* 2014;21(12):1499–507.SS

16

Microbiome, Diet, and Health

Himaja Nallagatla, Hemalatha Rajkumar, and Kamala Krishnaswamy
Indian Council of Medical Research
Hyderabad, India

Contents

16.1 Introduction..405
16.2 Gut microbiota and infections 406
16.3 Gut microbiota regulates immune response and inflammation 407
16.4 Gut microbiota and obesity 408
16.5 Gut microbiota and noncommunicable diseases 408
16.6 Gut microbiota and brain function..409
16.7 Diet and gut microbiota: An interrelated pair 409
    16.7.1 Fermented products affect health and gut microbiota.......... 410
    16.7.2 Effect of macronutrients and some diets on the gut microbiome 411
    16.7.3 Effect of polyphenols and flavonoids on the gut microbiota..413
    16.7.4 Effect of vitamins on gut microbiota....................................413
    16.7.5 Effect of minerals and micronutrients on gut microbiota 414
    16.7.6 Impact of malnutrition on gut flora and its implications on health 414
    16.7.7 Rebalancing the gut microbiota 415
References..416

16.1 Introduction

The interactions between microorganisms and humans have coexisted for billions of years. It is estimated through HMP metagenomic sequencing and analysis that human beings harbor 10 times more bacteria than cells in their bodies [1]. The largest number of bacteria exists in the colon, making it the largest bacterial ecosystem of the body [2]. Some bacteria do not interact much with their host and live as commensals, but most bacteria exhibit a symbiotic relationship with the host. The role of gut microbiota in overall health and disease was known long before bacteria were actually discovered and cultured in the laboratory. In 400 BC, Hippocrates proposed that bad digestion was the root cause for all diseases and stated that "death sits in bowels." In the early 1900s, Elie Metchnikoff correlated the longevity of people in the Balkans to their increased intake of fermented milk rich in "Bulgarian bacillus," now commonly known as *Lactobacillus bulgaricus*. He designed a recipe with certain amount of milk, sugar, and *L. bulgaricus* and found that consuming the drink helped bring down the sulfo-conjugate ethers in his urine [3]. Elie Metchnikoff tried to put forth the concept of replacing the bad bacteria or harmful bacteria with beneficial bacteria through diet. This marked the era of shaping or balancing the gut microbiota using dietary components.

In normal conditions, the gastrointestinal tract of the fetus remains sterile and devoid of microbes. The colonization of the gut microbiota in infants begins during childbirth when the child passes through the birth canal. This is followed by breastfeeding; breastmilk contains live microbes, metabolites, immune cells, and cytokines. In contrast, infants born by cesarean section are known to have less microbial diversity in addition to less abundance of the phylum Bacteroidetes compared to infants born vaginally [4]. Bacteroidetes carry out polysaccharide degradation and fermentation and produce short-chain fatty acids like acetate, butyrate, and propionate, which are important in the metabolic reactions of the body [5]. The microflora of pregnant women changes dramatically over the course of pregnancy to provide vaginally delivered babies with the bacteria needed to break down certain complex carbohydrates, such as oligosaccharides, found in breastmilk. These earliest exposures to the microbial world are also paramount for educating the newborn immune system and also potentially programming their metabolic function.

The general functions carried out by gut microbiota include maintenance of self-tolerance, regulation of immune responses, and prevention of allergy and autoimmune reactions. In addition, it decreases the endotoxin load and improves intestinal integrity and thereby prevents inflammatory effects in the host [6]. Gut microbiota is also known to improve satiety and regulates appetite by influencing hormones like ghrelin and peptide YY [7]. Furthermore, recent studies have put forth the concept of the gut–brain axis, which proposes the effect of the gut microbiome in influencing behavior and stress levels in the host [8].

16.2 Gut microbiota and infections

Early research on the microbiota focused mostly upon prevention and treatment of diarrhea, but today the gut microbiota has been linked to many infections such as urinary tract infections (UTIs), reproductive tract infections (RTIs), and pancreatitis, apart from antibiotic-associated diarrhea, traveler's diarrhea, and rotavirus diarrhea. Gut microbiome imbalance impairs immune response and thereby increases the frequency and severity of infections. Other major mechanisms involved in the prevention of infections include the competition for space and nutrition between normal flora and pathogenic bacteria. The gut microbiome disturbances often occurring with chronic drug/ antibiotic usage results in efficient binding and colonization of pathogenic bacteria and establishment of colonic infections. Similarly, marked reduction in the numbers of Firmicutes and Bacteroidetes in the gut was demonstrated to increase susceptibility to *Vibrio cholerae* infection; and *Ruminococcus obeum* was found to prevent *V. cholerae* infection in Bangladeshi children, by a mechanism involving quorum sensing and repression of pathogen colonizing factors [9,10]. However, the role of gut microbiota on various other distant infections like vaginal infections was unclear. The concept of recommending probiotics for vaginal infections orally began in 2001 and the bacteria thus supplemented could be recovered from the rectum [11,12]. The last few decades has seen extensive research on probiotics, which are extensively used as a cost-effective, alternative means of treatment for many infections such as UTIs, RTIs, and hospital-acquired infections apart from diarrheal diseases [13]. Most notably, species of lactobacilli, bifidobacteria, and the yeast *Saccharomyces boulardii* have potential for use in clinical practice due to their anti-infective properties.

16.3 Gut microbiota regulates immune response and inflammation

The intestine is the body's largest immune organ. The gut microbiome is in constant crosstalk with the host immune system and plays a paramount role in immune system development, immune regulation, and immune responses. That the germ-free animal models have immature immune systems and are susceptible to infections is evidence enough to confirm the role of a beneficial gut microbiome on maintaining a healthy immune system [14]. The early colonization of microorganisms in the gut helps in protection of the intestinal barrier through an increase in the duodenal IgA immunoglobulin population and also in the number of enteroendocrine cells in the epithelium of the jejunum and colon. Intestinal microflora that are found to be present throughout the intestinal tract affect the transportation of luminal antigens to Peyer's patches and stimulate the activity of specific and nonspecific immune cells. The gut microbiota not only aids in preventing infections but also in modulating the immune responses and counteracting allergic reactions and autoimmune disorders [15,16]. Studies have shown that prenatal exposure to *Acinetobacter lwoffii* and *Lactococcus lactis* results in reduced allergic responses in murine models, suggesting that prenatal exposure to probiotics can impact immune development in offspring and disease susceptibility in adult life [17,18].

Inflammation is the natural immune reaction in the body against any environmental stimuli and plays a major role in the healing process. Inflammation is tightly regulated by many mechanisms, one of which is microbe and immune cell interaction at the intestinal epithelium interphase [19]. Microbes in the gastrointestinal tract impact the development and functioning of the gut-associated lymphoid tissue (GALT) and the mucosa-associated lymphoid tissue (MALT), both of which regulate the inflammatory responses against pathogens, toxins, etc. [20–23]. In addition, the endotoxin present in the cell wall component of gram-negative bacteria and some gram-positive pathogenic bacteria directly trigger inflammation [24,25]. Colonization of beneficial microbiota in the gut might prevent undesirable local and systemic inflammation by three mechanisms: (1) through production of anti-inflammatory compounds such as cytokines; (2) through gut mucosa repair and enhanced intestinal integrity and thereby prevention of transfer of inflammation-inducing compounds into the circulation; and (3) by discouraging the growth of inflammation-inducing bacteria in the gut. Bacterial genera that are usually anti-inflammatory belong to the groups *Lactobacillus* and *Bifidobacterium* and are extensively studied for their anti-inflammatory properties. It was observed that 9% of differences in the fecal microbiota were associated with an increase in pro-inflammatory cytokines, IL-6, and IL-8 [26].

16.4 Gut microbiota and obesity

Accumulating evidence suggests that the gut microbiota plays an important role in the harvest, storage, and expenditure of energy obtained from the diet. The Firmicutes group of bacteria cause fermentation of the indigestible carbohydrates and higher acetate production that results in higher energy absorption [27]. Likewise, conventionalization of germfree mice with cecal bacteria from wild animals showed increased adiposity and body weight despite reduced consumption of chow diet [28]. The composition of the gut microbiota has been shown to differ between lean and obese mice [29]. Fewer Bacteroidetes and more Firmicutes were observed in obese humans compared with lean controls [30]. Transplantation of the gut microbiome from obese and lean mice to germ-free mice resulted in higher acetate and butyrate production in obese microbiome recipients [31]. Similarly, propionate was increased in fecal samples of obese adults [32]. Short chain fatty acids (SCFA) produced by the intestinal bacteria have a role in appetite, intestinal transit time, and energy absorption and harvest [33,34]. Paradoxically, gut bacteria are also associated with prevention of obesity and complications associated with high calorie intake by reducing the exogenous cholesterol absorption; in particular, bifidobacteria produce conjugated linoleic acid, which modulates the fatty acid composition in the liver and adipose tissue in mice [35]. In general, studies suggest that lean people have more densely populated and diverse types of bacteria and have higher levels of three types of bacteria—Firmicutes, bifidobacteria, and *Clostridium leptum.*

16.5 Gut microbiota and noncommunicable diseases

Diet has a major role to play in the occurrence of noncommunicable diseases. Metabolic syndrome is defined as a combination of physiological, biochemical, clinical, and metabolic factors that are linked to an increased risk of noncommunicable diseases like type 2 diabetes (T2D), hypertension, and cardiovascular diseases (CVDs) [36]. Metabolic syndrome (MS) is one of the most potent causes of insulin resistance and T2D [24]. It was observed in animal models that broad-spectrum antibiotic treatment modulated the gut microbiota, led to a reduced glucose tolerance, and influenced the inflammatory and metabolic status of the obese mice that were insulin resistant [37]. Similarly, gut microbiota also has an impact on hypertension, as demonstrated by meta-analysis data that showed that daily consumption of probiotics reduced the systolic and diastolic pressure among patients suffering from hypertension [38]. It has also been reported that microbial richness, such as diversity and little alteration over time, has been associated with reduced hypertension among spontaneously hypertensive rats [39]. Likewise, depletion in the numbers of bifidobacteria and Actinobacteria was observed among the spontaneously hypertensive rat models [39]. Emerging metabolomic studies have demonstrated that harmful products produced as a result of microbial metabolism are responsible for promoting atherosclerosis. Phosphatidylcholine, which is an important component of high fat diets such as those containing red meat, is metabolized into trimethylamine N-oxide (TMAO) by various bacterial genera like *Clostridium*, *Proteus*, *Shigella*, and *Aerobacter* [40]. Shotgun sequencing of the gut metagenome in atherosclerotic patients showed an increased numbers of *Collinsella*, whereas *Roseburia* and *Eubacterium* were higher among the healthier controls [41].

16.6 Gut microbiota and brain function

The role of the gut microbiome in brain functions like cognition and behavior is being increasingly appreciated and has been suggested to begin during the fetal stage [42–46]. The mechanism of the action of gut microbiota on brain function has been proposed to be either through the inhibition of stress-causing hormones like corticosterone or through a reduction in substance P, which has been highly associated with anxiety, aggression, and depression [46–48]. However, gaps exist in the knowledge regarding the mechanism of signaling between the microbiome and the brain. Most studies have been carried out in animal models and it is therefore difficult to extrapolate the results to humans. The components of bacteria that are responsible for the effect on brain need to be identified and tested further for their application as therapeutic drugs or formulations to be used in treatment of various psychological disorders (Figure 16.1).

16.7 Diet and gut microbiota: An interrelated pair

Diet is a strong trigger, which is known to influence the colonization within 24 hours after its consumption by the host [49]. However, it has been suggested that early priming of the gut microbiota using diet leads to prolonged colonization of the desired microbiota in the gut. Different components of the

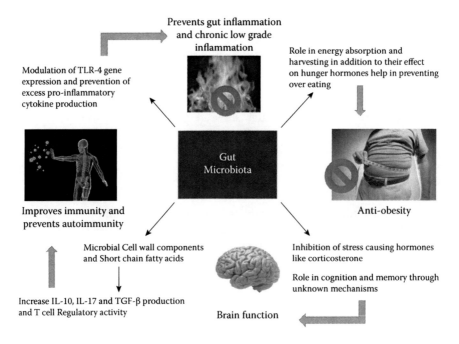

Figure 16.1 *Pictorial representation of the role of gut microbiome in overall body functions.*

diet, especially macronutrients like carbohydrates, lipids, and micronutrients, are known to influence the type of the bacteria in the gut.

16.7.1 Fermented products affect health and gut microbiota

Fermentation, which is achieved by using microorganisms, especially lactic acid bacteria (LAB) and yeast, is an ancient food preservation technology. Fermented foods and drinks like yogurt or curd, kefir, cheese, and sour cream are rich sources of probiotic bacteria. Among these, yogurt or curd is considered as the probiotic carrier food. However, though Indian cuisine comprises various fermented foods like idli, dosa, and dhokla, their benefits are limited only to improved digestion and absorption due to the proteolytic activity during fermentation and lack live bacteria at the time of consumption. Therefore, though foods cooked after fermentation offer limited advantages, uncooked fermented food products such as curd, buttermilk, etc. are important sources of probiotic bacteria.

Curd, prepared by fermenting milk with an inoculum of previously made curd, is used in most households in India. Homemade curd has been found to contain a spectrum of lactic acid bacteria (LAB—*Lactobacillus, Lactococcus, Leuconostoc, Bifidobacterium*, etc.) with potential to exert probiotic effects. These microbes have probiotic properties such as the ability to survive the upper gut, epithelial cell adherence, anti-inflammation, and enhancement of the mucosal innate immune response [50]. LAB from homemade curd could also prevent colonization of pathogenic *Vibrio cholerae* and *Salmonella typhimurium* growth [50]. Other investigators showed reduction in antibiotic-associated diarrhea and improved oral health when children were supplemented with yogurt [51,52]. Augmented linear growth was also observed in female children consuming curd [53]. Some studies have demonstrated improved lipid profile with curd supplementation, and recently a meta-analysis concluded that probiotic or fermented milk consumption may prevent hypercholesterolemia and thereby reduce cardiovascular disease risk [54–56]. Among diabetic patients, supplementation of yogurt containing probiotics like *Lactobacillus acidophilus* La5 and *Bifidobacterium lactis* Bb12 improved fasting blood glucose [57]. In pregnant women, oral probiotic yogurt reduced the vaginal pH, and complete symptomatic cure of bacterial vaginosis was observed, besides reduction in preterm births [58]. Although fermented foods such as curd or yogurt are beneficial and can deliver probiotics directly to the gut, the whole process of household curd preparation need to be standardized to ensure appropriate bacterial strains and sufficient inoculum to achieve maximum benefits from curd consumption.

16.7.2 Effect of macronutrients and some diets on the gut microbiome

All macronutrients, including complex carbohydrates and soluble dietary fiber, play a pivotal role in shaping the gut microbiota [59]. Even as nondigestible carbohydrates such as soluble fiber promote the growth of beneficial commensals in the gut, diets high in fats, carbohydrates, and proteins also impact the intestinal microbiota greatly. Diets rich in fiber are healthier than those containing high quantities of protein and fats, such as in the case of red meats, which discourage the proliferation of beneficial microbes in the gut. A high fat diet is also associated with increased endotoxemia and chronic inflammation [60]. Western diets rich in saturated fats and proteins encourage the growth of *Bacteroides*, which are known to be higher in numbers among patients suffering from colorectal cancer [61]. Likewise, high fat diets are known to decrease the *Bacteroides*/Firmicutes ratio, whereas fat-restricted diets with high carbohydrates increase both *Bacteroides* and Firmicutes and also bifidobacteria [62,63]. A high sucrose diet increases *Clostridium* and *Bacteroides* numbers, and these disturbances in the gut microbiota were associated with poorer cognitive flexibility, especially long-term and short-term memory, in animal models fed a high sucrose diet versus animals fed a normal diet [64]. The effects of different types of diets on gut microbiota and health consequences are given in Table 16.1.

Fermentation of protein results in beneficial compounds, whereas putrefactive action leads to the production of harmful byproducts like indole and *p*-cresol [65,66]. High protein diets are known to favor the *Bacteroides* group [49]. Similarly, excess red meat consumption has been associated with increased production of trimethylamine (TMA) and trimethylamine N-oxide (TMNO). These metabolites, which result from the activity of the microbes in the gut,

Table 16.1 Effect of Various Diets on Gut Bacterial Profile and Its Impact on Health

S.No	Type of Diet	Effect on Gut Bacteria	Effect on Health
1	Mediterranean diet (35% fat and 22% monounsaturated)	↓ *Prevotella* spp. ↑ *Roseburia* spp. ↑ *Oscillospira* ↑ *Parabacteroides distasonis*	Protective effect against development of type 2 diabetes [116]
2	Low fat, high complex carbohydrate diet (28% fat and 12% monounsaturated)	↑ *Prevotella* spp. ↓ *Roseburia* spp. ↑ *Faecalibacterium prausnitzii* ↑ *Parabacteroides distasonis*	Protective effect against development of type 2 diabetes [116]
3	Omnivore diet (both plant- and animal-based diets)	↑ *C. coccoides* ↑ *E. rectale* ↑ *Roseburia*	Improved butyryl-CoA CoA-transferase gene resulting in increased butyrate production and better colonic health [117]
4	Vegetarian diet (only plant-based diet)	↑ *Clostridium* species belonging to clusters XIVa and IV ↓ *Enterobacteriaceae* [117]	Amelioration of gut inflammation Reduced intestinal lipocalin-2, a marker for colitis and colorectal cancer [118]
5	Western diet (high fat and high carbohydrate)	↑ *Rikenellaceae* [119] ↓ *Ruminococcaceae* [119]	Associated with type 2 diabetes in humans [120]

are responsible for atherosclerotic plaque formation and thereby might contribute to cardiovascular diseases [67,68]. Moreover, feeding excessively on red meat and the resulting alteration in gut microbiota may lead to low bowel movements and production of carcinogens that may predispose an individual to development of colorectal cancer [69,70]. However, interestingly, high protein diets (nearly 22% of the total diet) associated with high physical activity, as in the case of athletes, was proven to improve the microbial diversity in the gut and mucosal immunity among rugby players [71]. The athletes were also found to be at a lower risk of obesity and systemic inflammation due to the presence of Akkermansiaceae members in their gut compared to nonathletes, suggesting that the accompanying physical activity also impacts gut microbiome modulation [71]. Dairy is another important source of high protein, and consumption of fermented dairy products is known to impact the gut microbiota by improving beneficial bacteria like *Lactobacillus* and *Bifidobacterium*; moreover, lactose present in the milk is capable of acting as a prebiotic [72].

With the Mediterranean diet, which includes plenty of plant-based foods like whole grains, fruits and vegetables, and lean meat like fish, the gut microbiome is modulated favorably. Moreover, the Mediterranean diet is also rich in polyphenols, which encourage the dominance of *Prevotella*, *Enterococcus*, *Bifidobacterium*, and *Lactobacillus* and discourage *Clostridium* growth significantly, and therefore has been suggested to patients suffering from obesity and high serum cholesterol [73]. Similarly, consumption of "ancestral diets" or the "paleolithic diet," which includes natural foods like fruits and tubers and lesser amount of grains, are known to have more influence on satiety and improve the microbial diversity in the gut compared to modern day diets [61,74–76].

16.7.3 Effect of polyphenols and flavonoids on the gut microbiota

In addition to the major components of diet, such as carbohydrates, proteins, and fats, minor components like vitamins, minerals, polyphenols, flavonoids, isoflavones, tannins, etc. also play a major role in gut microbial colonization. Polyphenols are compounds that are not readily assimilated by human beings but are known to have a role in modulating the gut flora. However, interestingly, the extent of absorption of polyphenols by each individual is different and depends on the type of bacteria lodged in the gut. Polyphenols, in turn, also help in preventing infections by reducing the population of pathogenic bacteria and sometimes when consumed in excess might inhibit beneficial microbiota existing in the gut. Foods like fruits and soy and beverages like wine, tea, and cocoa are well-known sources of polyphenols. Phenolic compounds are known to especially alter the Bacteroides–Firmicutes ratio [77,78]. *In vitro* studies have demonstrated the effect of catechin (the breakdown product of phenols) on the control of pathogenic bacteria like *Clostridium histolyticum* and enhancement of the growth of *Escherichia coli* and members of the *Clostridium coccoides–Eubacterium rectale* group. However, *Lactobacillus* and *Bifidobacterium* remained unaffected [79]. Similarly, animal models fed with red wine extract that was rich in proanthocyanidin showed a shift in the bacterial populations, with increased numbers of *Bacteroides*, *Lactobacillus*, and *Bifidobacterium* [80]. Also, phenolics derived from tea discouraged the growth of *Clostridium perfringens*, *Clostridium difficile*, and *Bacteroides* spp., whereas bifidobacteria and lactobacilli concentrations remained unaltered [77].

Cocoa-derived flavanols are known to have an identical effect on *Lactobacillus* and *Bifidobacterium* concentrations in addition to their detrimental effect on *Clostridium* spp. Supplementation also reduces plasma triglyceride and CRP levels among the subjects, indicating that minor nutrients also modulate the overall health of the host through modulation of gut flora [81]. This might be the mechanism behind the antidepressive effect of dark chocolate that is rich in cocoa, through the modification of gut flora.

16.7.4 Effect of vitamins on gut microbiota

Among the vitamins, fat-soluble vitamins like A and D are known to influence the composition of the gut microbiome. It has been observed that deficiency of retinoic acid leads to a decrease in the numbers of both aerobic and anaerobic bacteria, especially Firmicutes like enterococci, *Clostridium difficile*, and lactobacilli. This effect has also been observed in Proteobacteria and segmented filamentous bacteria in the small intestine [82]. Similarly, vitamin D is also known to impact the gut microbiota composition and gut health. It was observed in a mouse model that could not produce active Vitamin D and another model without Vitamin D receptors that susceptibility to dextran sodium sulfate (DSS) induced colitis corresponded with increased levels of Proteobacteria and lower numbers of the phyla Firmicutes and Deferribacteres [83]. Similarly, an *in vitro* study demonstrated the impact of vitamin D on the tight junction architecture and intestinal epithelial barrier homeostasis, thereby preventing the invasion of adherent-invasive *E. coli* [84]. Likewise, vitamin K, which is highly essential for blood clotting, is also synthesized by the gut microbiota in addition to water-soluble B vitamins like biotin, cobalamin, folate, nicotinic acid, pantothenic acid, pyridoxine, riboflavin, and thiamine [85,86].

16.7.5 Effect of minerals and micronutrients on gut microbiota

Studies on microbiota and nutrients show that deficiency of magnesium, zinc, and copper and supplementation of iron may adversely affect the gut microbiome balance. Magnesium has recently been associated with gut bacteria–associated mood swings. Magnesium deficiency led to decreased *Bifidobacterium* with no effect on *Lactobacillus* and *Bacteroides* [87]. Bifidobacteria are the group of bacteria that prevent inflammation in the host. Depression is associated with inflammation, and amelioration of inflammation may be one of the mechanisms by which gut bacteria might affect mood swings [88]. As for zinc deficiency, it was associated with decreased bacterial diversity in the gut of chickens [89]. A major influence of zinc deficiency was observed on Phylum Proteobacteria and Genera like, *Enterococcus*, *Enterobacter*, and *Ruminococcus* predominated, whereas Firmicutes were significantly diminished among the zinc-deficient group. These disturbances in the balance of Proteobacteria and Firmicutes have an inverse relationship on the body weight of the host, leading to decreased lean body mass and body weight [89]. Selenium also has significant influence on shaping the gut microbiota. Selenium increased the microbial diversity in the mice; an especially remarkable effect was observed on the Bacteroidia class and Parabacteroides genera, where the former showed an increase in numbers and the latter decreased with Se supplementation [90]. In contrast, iron supplementation in humans led to an increase in the Enterobacteriaceae and *Bacteroides* members and a decrease in the Lactobacilli and *Bifidobacteria* groups of bacteria, indicating an increase in the inflammation-promoting microbiome [91–97]. This influence on the gut microbiota was also associated with decreased production of butyrate and propionate and increased production of lactate and formate [98,99]. Butyrate is the energy substrate for colonic epithelial cells and promotes glucose homeostasis, while propionate is a substrate for lipogenesis and gluconeogenesis in the liver. Propionate is also known to reduce serum lipids and therefore reduces the risk of CVDs [100].

16.7.6 Impact of malnutrition on gut flora and its implications on health

It has been observed that malnourished children have disrupted gut flora compared to their healthier counterparts; the disruption is usually permanent and replenishing the diet with wholesome nutrition does not rejuvenate the balance or the balance that has been achieved is short lived, thus suggesting the importance of early nutrition [61,101,102]. A study conducted by Monira et al. has shown that in Bangladeshi children with undernutrition there were low concentrations of the three major phyla, Bacteroidetes, Actinobacteria, and Firmicutes, while the concentration of Proteobacteria was significantly higher compared to healthy children [103]. The study also showed that pathogenic bacteria like *Klebsiella, Enterobacteria*, and *Neisseria* were higher among the undernourished children compared to their healthier counterparts. Notably, the above bacteria are capable of causing gastrointestinal illnesses such as diarrhea and thereby contribute to further malnourishment by impaired absorption of the essential nutrients due to intestinal inflammation. This interrelation between malnutrition and disturbances in the gut microbiota is a vicious circle and each problem tends to contribute to the other, making the host vulnerable to many other illnesses. Similarly, a study conducted in India by Ghosh et al. in 2014 showed a significant difference in the gut bacterial taxonomic groups between chronically undernourished and acutely undernourished groups of children [104]. It was observed that bacteria like *Shigella, Veillonella, Streptococcus, Escherichia*, and *Enterobacter* were negatively correlated with improved nutrition. This suggests the importance of nutrition on the prevention of infections in children.

Diet consumed during gestation and lactation is known to further influence the gut flora in the mother and the offspring born to them. In a study where mothers were fed a high fat diet during lactation and weaning, the pups showed higher adiposity and gut microbiota alterations compared to the control pups, whose mothers were fed a normal diet. The high fat diet increased Firmicutes population and also caused dwindling of *Bacteroides* numbers in the cecum, thereby causing disturbances in energy homeostasis, leading to adiposity in the pups [105].

16.7.7 Rebalancing the gut microbiota

In modern times, in addition to diet, multiple external factors like stress, pollution, alcoholism, and indiscriminate use of antibiotics are responsible for imbalances in the gut microbiota, leading to dysbiosis [106–108]. Dysbiosis is a condition where the balance between beneficial microbes and pathogenic organisms is disturbed. However, very few human studies have shown how exactly the disturbances in the gut flora can be rebalanced, though wholesome diet is known to improve gut bacteria balance. However, in some cases of chronic dysbiosis where the gastrointestinal tract has already suffered damage and where the gut flora imbalance is permanent, alternate methods of regaining the lost flora are proposed.

Some of the commonly employed methods include long-term supplementation of probiotics or prebiotics to patients suffering from various gastrointestinal disturbances. According to the World Health Organization, probiotics are defined as "live microorganisms which when administered in adequate amounts, confer a health benefits on the host." However, loss of colonization after discontinuation of supplementation is a major drawback of probiotics use [109–112]. In recent times, the dietary compounds that encourage the growth of probiotics termed *prebiotics* have gained popularity. A prebiotic is a selectively fermented ingredient that allows specific changes, both in the composition and activity of the gastrointestinal microflora, that confers benefits upon host well-being and health [113]. Dietary fiber or prebiotics might have a long-term impact on the microbiota of the host, as they provide the substrate for the existing beneficial flora in the gut [114]. Recently, fecal transplants have been considered as an alternative for rebalancing the gut flora in various clinical conditions like autoimmunity, inflammatory bowel disease, multiple sclerosis, and obesity [115]. Though fecal transplants are considered for rebiosis of the gut, disadvantages like difficulty in performing the procedures and remote chance of the presence of the desirable bacteria in the donor and their effective colonization in the gut are the limiting factors. Supplementation of prebiotics alone or in combination with probiotics might be useful in rebalancing the gut flora. In conclusion, a fiber-rich, calorie-restricted diet that includes fermented milk such as curd or yogurt is the key to healthy living.

References

1. McFall-Ngai M, Hadfield MG, Bosch TCG, Carey HV, Domazet-Lošo T, Douglas AE, et al. Animals in a bacterial world, a new imperative for the life sciences. *Proc Natl Acad Sci USA.* 2013;110(9):3229–3236. doi: 10.1073/pnas.1218525110
2. Willey J, Sherwood L, Woolverton C. 2011. *Prescott's Microbiology.* 8th ed. New York: McGraw Hill. pp. 731–737. ISBN 978-0-07-017259-3. LCCN 2009033823. OCLC 434613235.
3. Mackowiak PA. Recycling Metchnikoff: Probiotics, the intestinal microbiome and the quest for long life. *Front Publ Health* 2013;1:52. doi: 10.3389/fpubh.2013.00052
4. Jakobsson HE, Abrahamsson TR, Jenmalm MC, Harris K, Quince C, Jernberg C, et al. Decreased gut microbiota diversity, delayed *Bacteroidetes* colonisation and reduced Th1 responses in infants delivered by caesarean section. *Gut* 2014;63(4):559–566.
5. Thomas F, Hehemann J-H, Rebuffet E, Czjzek M, Michel G. Environmental and gut *bacteroidetes*: The food connection. *Front Microbiol.* 2011;2:93. doi: 10.3389/fmicb.2011.00093
6. Ignacio A, Morales CI, Câmara NOS, Almeida RR. Innate sensing of the gut microbiota: Modulation of inflammatory and autoimmune diseases. *Front Immunol.* 2016;7:54. doi: 10.3389/fimmu.2016.00054
7. Parekh PJ, Arusi E, Vinik AI, Johnson DA. The role and influence of gut microbiota in pathogenesis and management of obesity and metabolic syndrome. *Front Endocrinol.* 2014;5:47. doi: 10.3389/fendo.2014.00047
8. Foster JA, Lyte M, Meyer E, Cryan JF. Gut microbiota and brain function: An evolving field in neuroscience. *Int J Neuropsychopharmacol.* 2016;19(5):pyv114.
9. Monira S, Nakamura S, Gotoh K, Izutsu K, Watanabe H, Alam NH, et al. Metagenomic profile of gut microbiota in children during cholera and recovery. *Gut Pathog.* 2013;5:1.
10. Hsiao A, Ahmed AM, Subramanian S, Griffin NW, Drewry LL, Petri WA, et al. Members of the human gut microbiota involved in recovery from *Vibrio cholerae* infection. *Nature* 2014;515:423–426.
11. Reid G, Bruce AW, Fraser N, Heinemann C, Owen J, Henning B. Oral probiotics can resolve urogenital infections. *FEMS Immunol Med Microbiol.* 2001;30(1):49–52.

12. Gardiner GE, Heinemann C, Baroja ML, Bruce AW, Beuerman D, Madrenas J, et al. Oral administration of the probiotic combination *Lactobacillus rhamnosus* GR-1 and *L. fermentum* RC-14 for human intestinal applications. *Int Dairy J.* 2002;12(2–3):191–196.
13. Plowman R, Graves N, Griffin MA, Roberts JA, Swan AV, Cookson B, et al. The rate and cost of hospital-acquired infections occurring in patients admitted to selected specialties of a district general hospital in England and the national burden imposed. *J Hosp Infect.* 2001;47(3):198–209.
14. Round JL, Mazmanian SK. The gut microbiome shapes intestinal immune responses during health and disease. *Nat Rev Immunol.* 2009;9(5):313–323. doi: 10.1038/nri2515
15. Purchiaroni F, Tortora A, Gabrielli M, Bertucci F, Gigante G, Ianiro G, et al. The role of intestinal microbiota and the immune system. *Eur Rev Med Pharmacol Sci.* 2013;17:323–333.
16. Wu H-J, Wu E. The role of gut microbiota in immune homeostasis and autoimmunity. *Gut Microbes.* 2012;3(1):4–14. doi: 10.4161/gmic.19320
17. Debarry J, Garn H, Hanuszkiewicz A, Dickgreber N, Blümer N, von Mutius E, et al. *Acinetobacter lwoffii* and *Lactococcus lactis* strains isolated from farm cowsheds possess strong allergy-protective properties. *J Allergy Clin Immunol.* 2007; 119(6):1514–1521.
18. Penders J, Thijs C, van den Brandt PA, Kummeling I, Snijders B, Stelma F, et al. Gut microbiota composition and development of atopic manifestations in infancy: The KOALA Birth Cohort Study. *Gut* 2007;56(5):661–667. Infant gut microbial colonization events at 1 month are associated with the subsequent development of atopic diseases in childhood.
19. Hakansson A, Molin G. Gut Microbiota and inflammation. *Nutrients* 2011;3(6):637–682. doi: 10.3390/nu3060637
20. Umesaki Y, Setoyama H, Matsumoto S, Okada Y. Expansion of alpha beta T cell receptor- bearing intestinal intraepithelial lymphocytes after microbial colonization in germ-free mice and its independence from thymus. *Immunology* 1993;79:32–37.
21. Helgeland L, Vaage JT, Rolstad B, Midtvedt T, Brandtzaeg P. Microbial colonization influences composition and T cell receptor V beta repertoire of intraepithelial lymphocytes in rat intestine. *Immunology* 1996;89:494–501.
22. Cebra JJ, Periwal SB, Lee G, Lee F, Shroff KE. Development and maintenance of the gut-associated lymphoid tissue (GALT): The roles of enteric bacteria and viruses. *Dev Immunol.* 1998;6:13–18.
23. Butler JE, Sun J, Weber P, Navarro P, Francis D. Antibody repertoire development in fetal and newborn piglets, III. Colonization of the gastrointestinal tract selectively diversifies the preimmune repertoire in mucosal lymphoid tissues. *Immunology* 2000;100:119–130.
24. Cani PD, Amar J, Iglesias MA, Poggi M, Knauf C, Bastelica D, et al. Metabolic endotoxemia initiates obesity and insulin resistance. *Diabetes* 2007;56:1761–1772.
25. González-Navajas JM, Bellot P, Francés R, Zapater P, Munoz C, García-Pagán JC, et al. Presence of bacterial-DNA in cirrhosis identifies a subgroup of patients with marked inflammatory response not related to endotoxin. *J Hepatol.* 2008;48:61–67.
26. Biagi B, Nylund L, Candela M, Ostan R, Bucci L, Pini E, et al. Through ageing, and beyond: Gut microbiota and inflammatory status in seniors and centenarians. *PLoS One* 2010;5:e10667.
27. Zhang H, DiBaise JK, Zuccolo A, Kudrna D, Braidotti M, Yu Y, et al. Human gut microbiota in obesity and after gastric bypass. *Proc Natl Acad Sci USA.* 2009;106(7):2365–2370.
28. Kallus SJ, Brandt LJ. The intestinal microbiota and obesity. *J Clin Gastroenterol.* 2011;46:16–24.
29. Backhed F, Ding H, Wang T, Hooper LV, Koh GY, Nagy A, et al. The gut microbiota as an environmental factor that regulates fat storage. *Proc Natl Acad Sci USA.* 2004;101:15718–15723.

30. Kotzampassi K, Giamarellos-Bourboulis EJ, Stavrou G. Obesity as a consequence of gut bacteria and diet interactions. *ISRN Obes.* 2014;2014:651895.
31. Turnbaugh PJ, Ley RE, Mahowald MA, Magrini V, Mardis ER, Gordon JI. An obesity-associated gut microbiome with increased capacity for energy harvest. *Nature* 2006;444(7122):1027–1031.
32. Schwiertz A, Taras D, Schafer K, Beijer S, Bos NA, Donus C, et al. Microbiota and SCFA in lean and overweight healthy subjects. *Obesity* 2009;18(1):190–195.
33. Samuel BS, Shaito A, Motoike T, Rey FE, Backhed F, Manchester JK, et al. Effects of the gut microbiota on host adiposity are modulated by the short-chain fatty-acid binding G protein-coupled receptor, Gpr41. *Proc Natl Acad Sci USA.* 2008;105(43):16767–16772.
34. Tolhurst G, Heffron H, Lam YŞ, Parker HE, Habib AM, Diakogiannaki E, et al. Short-chain fatty acids stimulate glucagon-like peptide-1 secretion via the G-protein-coupled receptor FFAR2. *Diabetes* 2012;61(2):364–371.
35. Gorissen L, Raes K, Weckx S, Dannenberger D, Leroy F, De Vuyst, et al. Production of conjugated linoleic acid and conjugated linolenic acid isomers by Bifidobacterium species. *Appl Microbiol Biotechnol.* 2010;87:2257–2266.
36. Kaur J. A comprehensive review on metabolic syndrome. *Cardiol Res Pract.* 2014; 2014:943162.
37. Membrez M, Blancher F, Jaquet M, Bibiloni R, Cani PD, Burcelin RG, et al. Gut microbiota modulation with norfloxacin and ampicillin enhances glucose tolerance in mice. *FASEB J.* 2008;22(7):2416–2426.
38. Khalesi S, Sun J, Buys N, Jayasinghe R. Effect of probiotics on blood pressure: A systematic review and meta-analysis of randomized, controlled trials. *Hypertension* 2014;64(4):897–903.
39. Yang T, Santisteban MM, Rodriguez V, Li E, Ahmari N, Carvajal JM, et al. Gut microbiota dysbiosis is linked to hypertension. *Hypertension* 2015;65(6):1331–1340. doi: 10.1161/HYPERTENSIONAHA.115.05315
40. Zeisel SH, Wishnok JS, Blusztajn JK. Formation of methylamines form ingested choline and lecithin. *J Pharmacol Exp Ther.* 1983;225:320–324.
41. Karlsson FH, Fåk F, Nookaew I, Tremaroli V, Fagerberg B, Petranovic D, et al. Symptomatic atherosclerosis is associated with an altered gut metagenome. *Nat Commun.* 2012;3:1245. doi: 10.1038/ncomms2266
42. Cryan JF, Dinan TG. Mind-altering microorganisms: The impact of the gut microbiota on brain and behavior. *Nat Rev Neurosci.* 2012;13:701–712.
43. Collins SM, Kassam Z, Bercik P. The adoptive transfer of behavioral phenotype via the intestinal microbiota: Experimental evidence and clinical implications. *Curr Opin Microbiol.* 2013;16:240–245.
44. Foster JA, McVey Neufeld KA. Gut-brain axis: How the microbiome influences anxiety and depression. *Trends Neurosci.* 2013;36:305–312.
45. Lyte M. Microbial endocrinology in the microbiome-gut-brain axis: How bacterial production and utilization of neurochemicals influence behavior. *PLoS Pathog.* 2013;9:e1003726.
46. Douglas-Escobar M, Elliott E, Neu J. Effect of intestinal microbial ecology on the developing brain. *JAMA Pediatr.* 2013;167:374–379.
47. Bravo J, Forsythe P, Chew M, Escaravage E, Savignac H, Dinan T, et al. Ingestion of *Lactobacillus* strain regulates emotional behavior and central GABA receptor expression in a mouse via the vagus nerve. *Proc Natl Acad Sci USA.* 2011;108: 16050–16055.
48. Bested AC, Logan AC, Selhub EM. Intestinal microbiota, probiotics and mental health: From Metchnikoff to modern advances: Part III—convergence toward clinical trials. *Gut Pathog.* 2013;5:4. doi: 10.1186/1757-4749-5-4
49. Wu GD, Chen J, Hoffmann C, Bittinger K, Chen YY, Keilbaugh SA, et al. Linking long-term dietary patterns with gut microbial enterotypes. *Science* 2011;334:105–108.

50. Balamurugan R, Chandragunasekaran AS, Chellappan G, Rajaram K, Ramamoorthi G, Ramakrishna BS. Probiotic potential of lactic acid bacteria present in home made curd in southern India. *Indian J Med Res.* 2014;140(3):345–355.
51. Fox MJ, Ahuja KD, Robertson IK, Ball MJ, Eri RD. Can probiotic yogurt prevent diarrhoea in children on antibiotics? A double-blind, randomised, placebo-controlled study. *BMJ Open* 2015;5(1):e006474. doi: 10.1136/bmjopen-2014-006474
52. Karuppaiah RM, Shankar S, Raj SK, Ramesh K, Prakash R, Kruthika M. Evaluation of the efficacy of probiotics in plaque reduction and gingival health maintenance among school children—A randomized control trial. *J Int Oral Health.* 2013;5(5):33–37.
53. Berkey CS, Colditz GA, Rockett HRH, Frazier AL, Willett WC. Dairy consumption and female height growth: Prospective cohort study. *Cancer Epidemiol Biomarkers Prev.* 2009;18(6):1881–1887. doi: 10.1158/1055-9965.EPI-08-1163
54. Shiva Prakash M, Madhavi G, Hemalatha R. Effect of supplementation of probiotic curd on lipid profile in obese subjects. *Int J Food Nutr Sci.* 2014;3(4),148–152.
55. Shimizu M, Hashiguchi M, Shiga T, Tamura H-O, Mochizuki M. Meta-Analysis: Effects of probiotic supplementation on lipid profiles in normal to mildly hypercholesterolemic individuals. *PLoS One* 2015;10(10):e0139795. doi: 10.1371/journal.pone.0139795
56. Astrup A. Yogurt and dairy product consumption to prevent cardiometabolic diseases: Epidemiologic and experimental studies. *Am J Clin Nutr.* 2014;99(Suppl):1235 S–1242S. doi: 10.3945/ajcn.113.073015
57. Ejtahed HS, Mohtadi-Nia J, Homayouni-Rad A, Niafar M, Asghari-Jafarabadi M, Mofid V. Probiotic yogurt improves antioxidant status in type 2 diabetic patients. *Nutrition* 2012;28(5):539–543.
58. Hantoushzadeh S, Golshahi F, Javadian P, Khazardoost S, Aram S, Hashemi S, et al. Comparative efficacy of probiotic yoghurt and clindamycin in treatment of bacterial vaginosis in pregnant women: A randomized clinical trial. *J Matern Fetal Neonatal Med.* 2012;25(7):1021–1024.
59. Slavin J. Fiber and prebiotics: Mechanisms and health benefits. *Nutrients* 2013;5(4): 1417–1435. doi: 10.3390/nu5041417
60. Clemente-Postigo M, Queipo-Ortuno MI, Murri M, Boto-Ordonez M, Perez-Martinez P, Andres-Lacueva C, et al. Endotoxin increase after fat overload is related to postprandial hypertriglyceridemia in morbidly obese patients. *J Lipid Res.* 2012;53:973–978. doi: 10.1194/jlr.P020909
61. Yatsunenko T, Rey FE, Manary MJ, Trehan I, Dominguez-Bello MG, Contreras M, et al. Human gut microbiome viewed across age and geography. *Nature* 2012;486:222–227.
62. Furet JP, Kong LC, Tap J, Poitou C, Basdevant A, Bouillot JL, et al. Differential adaptation of human gut microbiota to bariatric surgery-induced weight loss; links with metabolic and low-grade inflammation markers. *Diabetes* 2010;59:3049–3057. doi: 10.2337/db10-0253
63. Fava F, Gitau R, Griffin BA, Gibson GR, Tuohy KM, Lovegrove JA. The type and quantity of dietary fat and carbohydrate alter faecal microbiome and short-chain fatty acid excretion in a metabolic syndrome "at-risk" population. *Int J Obes (Lond.).* 2013;37:216–223. doi: 10.1038/ijo.2012.33
64. Magnusson KR, Hauck L, Jeffrey BM, Elias V, Humphrey A, Nath R, et al. Relationships between diet-related changes in the gut microbiome and cognitive flexibility. *Neuroscience* 2015;300:128–140.
65. Alemany M. The problem of nitrogen disposal in the obese. *Nutr Res Rev.* 2012;25(1):18–28.
66. Geypens B, Claus D, Evenepoel P, Hiele M, Maes B, Peeters M, et al. Influence of dietary protein supplements on the formation of bacterial metabolites in the colon. *Gut* 1997;41:70–76.
67. Shen W, Gaskins HR, McIntosh MK. Influence of dietary fat on intestinal microbes, inflammation, barrier function and metabolic outcomes. *J Nutr Biochem.* 2014;25:270–280.

Microbiome, Diet, and Health   419

68. Tang WH, Wang Z, Levison BS, Koeth RA, Britt EB, Fu X, et al. Intestinal microbial metabolism of phosphatidylcholine and cardiovascular risk. *N Engl J Med.* 2013;368:1575–1584.
69. Chao A, Thun MJ, Connell CJ, McCullough ML, Jacobs EJ, Flanders WD, et al. Meat consumption and risk of colorectal cancer. *JAMA* 2005;293(2):172–182.
70. Norat T, Bingham S, Ferrari P, Slimani N, Jenab M, Mazuir M, et al. Meat, fish, and colorectal cancer risk: The European Prospective Investigation into cancer and nutrition. *J Natl Cancer Inst.* 2005;97:906–916.
71. Clarke SF, Murphy EF, O'Sullivan O, Lucey AJ, Humphreys M, Hogan A, et al. Exercise and associated dietary extremes impact on gut microbial diversity. *Gut* 2014;63(12):1913–1920. doi: 10.1136/gutjnl-2013-306541
72. Barile D, Rastall RA. Human milk and related oligosaccharides as prebiotics. *Curr Opin Biotechnol.* 2013;24(2):214–219.
73. Lopez-Legarrea P, Fuller NR, Zulet MA, Martinez JA, Caterson ID. The influence of Mediterranean, carbohydrate and high protein diets on gut microbiota composition in the treatment of obesity and associated inflammatory state. *Asia Pac J Clin Nutr.* 2014;23(3):360–368. doi: 10.6133/apjcn.2014.23.3.16
74. Schnorr SL, Candela M, Rampelli S, Centanni M, Consolandi C, Basaglia G, et al. Gut microbiome of the Hadza hunter-gatherers. *Nat Commun.* 2014;5:3654.
75. De Filippo C, Cavalieri D, Di Paola M, Ramazzotti M, Poullet JB, Massart S, et al. Impact of diet in shaping gut microbiota revealed by a comparative study in children from Europe and rural Africa. *Proc Natl AcadSci U S A.* 2010;107:14691–14696.
76. Tyakht AV, Kostryukova ES, Popenko AS, Belenikin MS, Pavlenko AV, Larin AK, et al. Human gut microbiota community structures in urban and rural populations in Russia. *Nat Commun.* 2013;4:2469.
77. Lee HC, Jenner AM, Low CS, Lee YK. Effect of tea phenolics and their aromatic fecal bacterial metabolites on intestinal microbiota. *Res Microbiol.* 2006;157(9):876–884.
78. Hervert-Hernandez D, Pintado C, Rotger R, Goni I. Stimulatory role of grape pomace polyphenols on *Lactobacillus acidophilus* growth. *Int J Food Microbiol.* 2009;136(1):119–122.
79. Tzonuis X, Vulevic J, Kuhnle GG, George T, Leonczak J, Gibson GR, et al. Flavanol monomer-induced changes to the human faecal microflora. *Br J Nutr.* 2008;99(4):782–792.
80. Dolara P, Luceri C, De Filippo C, Femia AP, Giovannelli L, Caderni G, et al. Red wine polyphenols influence carcinogenesis, intestinal microflora, oxidative damage and gene expression profiles of colonic mucosa in F344 rats. *Mutat Res.* 2005;591(1–2):237–246.
81. Tzounis X, Rodriguez-Mateos A, Vulevic J, Gibson GR, Kwik-Uribe C, Spencer JP. Prebiotic evaluation of cocoa-derived flavanols in healthy humans by using a randomized, controlled, double-blind, crossover intervention study. *Am J Clin Nutr.* 2011;93(1):62–72.
82. Cha HR, Chang SY, Chang JH, Kim JO, Yang JY, Kim CH, et al. Downregulation of Th17 cells in the small intestine by disruption of gut flora in the absence of retinoic acid. *J Immunol.* 2010;184:6799–6806.
83. Ooi JH, Li Y, Rogers CJ, Cantorna MT. Vitamin D regulates the gut microbiome and protects mice from dextran sodium sulfate-induced colitis. *J Nutr.* 2013;143(10):1679–1686.
84. Assa A, Vong L, Pinnell LJ, Rautava J, Avitzur N, Johnson-Henry KC, et al. Vitamin D deficiency predisposes to adherent-invasive *Escherichia coli*-induced barrier dysfunction and experimental colonic injury. *Inflamm Bowel Dis.* 2015;21(2):297–306.
85. Conly JM, Stein K. The production of menaquinones (vitamin-K2) by intestinal bacteria and their role in maintaining coagulation homeostasis. *Progr Food Nutr Sci.* 1992;16:307–343.

86. Leblanc JG, Milani C, de Giori GS, Sesma F, van Sinderen D, Ventura M. Bacteria as vitamin suppliers to their host: A gut microbiota perspective. *Curr Opin Biotechnol.* 2013;24(2):160–168.
87. Pachikian BD, Neyrinck AM, Deldicque L, De Backer FC, Catry E, Dewulf EM, et al. Changes in intestinal bifidobacteria levels are associated with the inflammatory response in magnesium-deficient mice. *J Nutr.* 2010;140:509–514.
88. Moya-Pérez A, Neef A, Sanz Y. *Bifidobacterium pseudocatenulatum* CECT 7765 reduces obesity-associated inflammation by restoring the lymphocyte-macrophage balance and gut microbiota structure in high-fat diet-fed mice. *PLoS One.* 2015;10(7):e0126976. doi: 10.1371/journal.pone.0126976
89. Reed S, Neuman H, Moscovich S, Glahn RP, Koren O, Tako E. Chronic zinc deficiency alters chick gut microbiota composition and function. *Nutrients* 2015;7(12):9768–9784.
90. Kasaikina MV, Kravtsova MA, Lee BC, Seravalli J, Peterson DA, Walter J, et al. Dietary selenium affects host selenoproteome expression by influencing the gut microbiota. *FASEB J.* 2011;25(7):2492–2499. doi: 10.1096/fj.11-181990. 63
91. Zimmermann MB, Chassard C, Rohner F, N'goran EK, Nindjin C, Dostal A, et al. The effects of iron fortification on the gut microbiota in African children: A randomized controlled trial in Cote d'Ivoire. *Am J Clin Nutr.* 2010;92(6):1406–1415.
92. Jaeggi T, Kortman GA, Moretti D, Chassard C, Holding P, Dostal A, et al. Iron fortification adversely affects the gut microbiome, increases pathogen abundance and induces intestinal inflammation in Kenyan infants. *Gut* 2015;64(5):731–742.
93. Mevissen-Verhage EA, Marcelis JH, Harmsen-Van Amerongen WC, de Vos NM, Verhoef J. Effect of iron on neonatal gut flora during the first three months of life. *Eur J Clin Microbiol.* 1985;4(3):273–278.
94. Tompkins GR, O'Dell NL, Bryson IT, Pennington CB. The effects of dietary ferric iron and iron deprivation on the bacterial composition of the mouse intestine. *Curr Microbiol.* 2001;43:38–42. doi: 10.1007/s002840010257
95. Lee SH, Shinde P, Choi J, Park M, Ohh S, Kwon IK, et al. Effects of dietary iron levels on growth performance, hematological status, liver mineral concentration, fecal microflora, and diarrhea incidence in weanling pigs. *Biol Trace Elem Res.* 2008;126(Suppl 1):S57–S68. doi: 10.1007/s12011-008-8209-5
96. Werner T, Wagner SJ, Martinez I, Walter J, Chang JS, Clavel T, et al. Depletion of luminal iron alters the gut microbiota and prevents Crohn's disease-like ileitis. *Gut* 2011;60:325–333. doi: 10.1136/gut.2010.216929
97. Krebs NF, Sherlock LG, Westcott J, Culbertson D, Hambidge KM, Feazel LM, et al. Effects of different complementary feeding regimens on iron status and enteric microbiota in breastfed infants. *J Pediatr.* 2013;163:416–423. doi: 10.1016/j.jpeds.2013.01.024
98. Dostal A, Fehlbaum S, Chassard C, Zimmermann MB, Lacroix C. Low iron availability in continuous in vitro colonic fermentations induces strong dysbiosis of the child gut microbial consortium and a decrease in main metabolites. *FEMS Microbiol Ecol.* 2013;83(1):161–175.
99. Dostal A, Lacroix C, Bircher L, Pham VT, Follador R, Zimmermann MB, et al. Iron modulates butyrate production by a child gut microbiota *in vitro.* mBio. 2015;6(6):e01453–e01415. doi: 10.1128/mBio.01453-15
100. Wong JM, de Souza R, Kendall CW, Emam A, Jenkins DJ. Colonic health: Fermentation and short chain fatty acids. *J Clin Gastroenterol.* 2006;40(3):235–243.
101. Subramanian S, Huq S, Yatsunenko T, Haque R, Mahfuz M, Alam MA, et al. Persistent gut microbiota immaturity in malnourished Bangladeshi children. *Nature* 2014;510:417–421. doi: 10.1038/nature13421
102. Gordon JI, Dewey KG, Mills DA, Medzhitov RM. The human gut microbiota and undernutrition. *Sci Transl Med.* 2012;4:137ps112.

103. Monira S, Nakamura S, Gotoh K, Izutsu K, Watanabe H, Alam NH, et al. Gut microbiota of healthy and malnourished children in Bangladesh. *Front Microbiol.* 2011;2:228.

104. Ghosh TS, Sen Gupta S, Bhattacharya T, Yadav D, Barik A, Chowdhury A, et al. Gut microbiomes of Indian children of varying nutritional status. *PLoS One* 2014;9(4):e95547. doi: 10.1371/journal.pone.0095547

105. Mozes S, Bujnáková D, Sefcíková Z, Kmet V. Developmental changes of gut microflora and enzyme activity in rat pups exposed to fat-rich diet. *Obesity (Silver Spring).* 2008;16(12):2610–2615. doi: 10.1038/oby.2008.435

106. Hawrelak JA, Myers SP. The causes of intestinal dysbiosis: A review. *Altern Med Rev.* 2004;9(2):180–197.

107. Bailey MT, Coe CL. Maternal separation disrupts the integrity of the intestinal microflora in infant rhesus monkeys. *Dev Psychobiol.* 1999;35:146–155.

108. Lizko NN. Stress and intestinal microflora. *Nahrung* 1987;31:443–447.

109. Alander M, Satokari R, Korpela R, Saxelin M, Salmela VM, Sandholm TM, et al. Persistence of colonization of human colonic mucosa by a probiotic strain, *Lactobacillus rhamnosus* GG, after oral consumption. *Appl Environ Microbiol.* 1999;65:351–354.

110. Himaja N, Hemalatha R, Narendrababu K, Shujauddin M. *Lactobacillus rhamnosus* GG supplementation during critical windows of gestation influences immune phenotype in Swiss albino mice offspring. *Benef Microbes.* 2016;7(2):195–204.

111. Tannock GW, Munro K, Harmsen HJ, Welling GW, Smart J, Gopal PK. Analysis of the fecal microflora of human subjects consuming a probiotic product containing *Lactobacillus rhamnosus* DR20. *Appl Environ Microbiol.* 2000;66:2578–2588.

112. Sanders ME. Impact of probiotics on colonizing microbiota of the gut. *J Clin Gastroenterol.* 2011;l45:115–119.

113. Roberfroid MB. Prebiotics: The concept revisited. *J Nutr.* 2007;137(3 Suppl 2):830S–837S.

114. Shen Q, Zhao L, Tuohy KM. High-level dietary fibre up-regulates colonic fermentation and relative abundance of saccharolytic bacteria within the human faecal microbiota *in vitro. Eur J Nutr.* 2012;51(6):693–705. doi: 10.1007/s00394-011-0248-6

115. Borody TJ, Khoruts A. Fecal microbiota transplantation and emerging applications. *Nat Rev Gastroenterol Hepatol.* 2012;9:88–96.

116. Haro C, Montes-Borrego M, Rangel-Zúñiga OA, Alcalá-Díaz JF, Gómez-Delgado F, Pérez-Martínez P, et al. Two Healthy Diets Modulate Gut Microbial Community Improving Insulin Sensitivity in a Human Obese Population. *J Clin Endocrinol Metab.* 2016; 101(1):233–242. doi: 10.1210/jc.2015-3351.

117. Kabeerdoss J, Devi RS, Mary RR, Ramakrishna BS. Faecal microbiota composition in vegetarians: comparison with omnivores in a cohort of young women in southern India. *Br J Nutr.* 2012; 28;108(6):953–957. doi: 10.1017/S0007114511006362.

118. Kim MS, Hwang SS, Park EJ, Bae JW. Strict vegetarian diet improves the risk factors associated with metabolic diseases by modulating gut microbiota and reducing intestinal inflammation. *Environ Microbiol Rep.* 2013;5(5):765–775. doi: 10.1111/1758-2229.12079.

119. Daniel H, Moghaddas Gholami A, Berry D, Desmarchelier C, Hahne H, Loh G, Mondot S, Lepage P, Rothballer M, Walker A, Böhm C, Wenning M, Wagner M, Blaut M, Schmitt-Kopplin P, Kuster B, Haller D, Clavel T. High-fat diet alters gut microbiota physiology in mice. *ISME J.* 2014;8(2):295–308. doi: 10.1038/ismej.2013.155.

120. Qin J, Li Y, Cai Z, Li S, Zhu J, Zhang F et al . A metagenome-wide association study of gut microbiota in type 2 diabetes. *Nature* 2012; 490: 55–60.

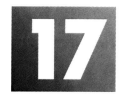

Genetic Susceptibility to Common Diseases and Diet Intakes

Jayvadan Patel and Anita Patel
Sankalchand Patel University
Visnagar, Gujarat, India

Contents

17.1 Genetic susceptibility 424
17.2 Approaches to demonstrate genetic susceptibility to common diseases 424
17.3 An interface between the nutritional environment and genetic processes 426
17.4 Alteration of gene expression or structure by common dietary chemicals 427
17.5 Diet can be a risk factor for disease 429
    17.5.1 Micronutrients 431
    17.5.2 Macronutrients: Fats 433
    17.5.3 Macronutrients: Carbohydrates 433
    17.5.4 Macronutrients: Protein 434
    17.5.5 Caloric restriction 434
17.6 Some diet-regulated genes can play a role in chronic diseases 435
    17.6.1 Molecular approach 435
    17.6.2 Genetic approach 437
17.7 The balance between health and disease states may depend on an individual's genetic makeup 438
17.8 Dietary intervention based on individualized nutrition 438
    17.8.1 Hypertension 439
    17.8.2 Cardiovascular health 440
    17.8.3 Cancer 440
17.9 Population screening for genetic susceptibility to disease 440
17.10 Commercial interests 441
17.11 Public health perspective 442
17.12 Summary 443
References 443

17.1 Genetic susceptibility

A genetic susceptibility is an increased probability of developing a particular disease rooted in a person's genetic framework. Having a genetic predisposition for a disease does not mean that you will get that disease—in other words, it does not directly cause a disease—but your risk may be higher than that of the general population. Definite genetic variations those are frequently innate from a parent result in genetic susceptibility. These changes in genetics may be responsible for the progress of a disease, although they do not directly cause a disease. A number of people with an inclining genetic variation within the same family will never get the disease at the same time as others will. Therefore, genetic susceptibility is the only one component in the etiology of common diseases such as coronary heart disease. The risk of passing on common diseases to offspring is difficult to predict because of complex interactions between different genes, and between behavioral, environmental, and genetic factors (Carol and Kate 2006). To have a genetic susceptibility to something seem to be vulnerable to it or else to be expected to encounter it attributable to inborn genes. Individuals can be hereditarily disposed to certain diseases or behaviors. Hereditary susceptibility is passed down all the way through family histories. Individuals are more probable to develop the conditions like bad teeth, hairlessness, or diabetes themselves because of the genes that they inherit through family histories. These are biological conditions and also a few believe that people can be genetically inclined to behave in a certain way.

A small proportion of common disease cases have single gene causes. The major proportion of the genetic basis of common diseases can be considered to be the result of an inherited predisposition of genetic susceptibility. Common diseases result from a complex interaction of the effects of multi different genes (polygenic inheritance), with environmental factors and influences (multifactorial inheritance).

17.2 Approaches to demonstrate genetic susceptibility to common diseases

Linkage or association studies are the two major approaches to demonstrate genetic susceptibility to common diseases.

In linkage as well as association studies, contiguous marker diversity is shown in Figure 17.1 (Cardon and Bell 2001). On a particular haplotypic milieu, the functional mutation "m" takes place. The variety of contiguous markers that can be used to track the disease gene region will be large because in linkage studies (also called family studies) there is minute time for recombination to take place. And the resultant disease gene region will be small because in association studies it focuses on populations that have previously undergone random mating over a long period of time. Eventually, the disease gene or mutation becomes separated from genes through its original haplotypic

424　Nutrigenomics and Nutraceuticals

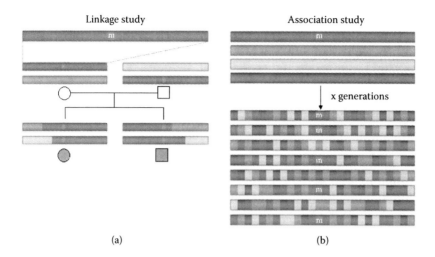

Figure 17.1 (a) Linkage versus (b) association studies.

milieu, even if a few can stay in concert; this type of non-random association of alleles forms the base for linkage disequilibrium (Figure 17.1).

Generally in linkage analysis, a genome-wide set of several hundred or else thousand markers spaced millions of bases separately is typed in families with numerous affected relatives in whom a mannerism has been measured. Markers that separate out with disease in relatives more over and over again than probable are used to localize the genes for disease. This approach has the advantage of being an unbiased, comprehensive search across the genome for susceptibility alleles, and has been successfully applied to find the genes for many single gene disorders. On the contrary, linkage analysis has not been as much victorious for polygenic diseases and quantitative traits (Altmuller et al. 2001; Hirschhorn and Daly 2005), possibly to some extent due to limited control to detect the effect of common alleles with unpretentious effects on disease (Altshuler et al. 2000; Risch and Merikangas 1996).

In association studies, a meticulous marker correlated with disease across a population more willingly than within families. Association studies have much better control to detect the effects of widespread variants (Risch 1990). The insulin VNTR class III allele, which has a frequency of just about 70%, has definitively shown to diffidently have an effect on the risk of type 1 diabetes, with a *p*-value of 10^{-22}, by means of association studies (Barratt et al. 2004). In contrast, the region containing the insulin gene is just scarcely higher than the threshold for statistical significance even after the entire world's linkage data for type 1 diabetes are combined (Cox et al. 2001). In the same way, the common Pro12Ala polymorphism reproducibly influences the risk of type 2 diabetes; however, studies of millions of sib pairs would be requisite to acquire a momentous signal using linkage (Altshuler et al. 2000; Florez et al. 2003).

Nevertheless, association studies necessitate lots of extra markers than linkage analysis. In linkage analysis, the marker as well as the disease allele has to normally be inherited jointly within the one or two generations spanned by a family, and as a result, the markers can be more than a few million bases away from the pertinent gene. In association studies, the marker as well as the disease allele has to normally be inherited jointly all the way through the population. For the reason that segments of linkage disequilibrium are measured in tens of thousands of bases, hundreds of thousands of markers will be necessary to scan the genome for association (Carlson et al. 2004; Gabriel et al. 2002). As well, association studies, even though potentially more commanding than linkage, still need thousands of individual's samples sizes. Therefore, association studies are at present restricted to candidate genes or regions, on account of the expenditure of a genome-wide approach.

17.3 An interface between the nutritional environment and genetic processes

Progression in the fight against human disease along with suffering is being accelerated through the availability of genomic information for humans as well as other organisms. The process of localizing and identifying the genes concerned in the disease has been transformed by the techniques as well as knowledge emerging from genome projects. Up till now, approximately 1,000 human disease genes have been identified plus partially characterized, among 97% of them known to cause monogenic diseases (Jimenez-Sanchez et al. 2001). Nevertheless, the majority cases of obesity, cancer, diabetes, cardiovascular disease (CVD), and other chronic diseases are attributable to complex interactions among environmental factors and a number of genes. It is not surprising, therefore, that the strategies for characterizing as well as identifying monogenic diseases have been ineffective when applied to chronic diseases. Notwithstanding the more than 600 association studies published as of 2002 (Hirschhorn et al. 2002), the molecular basis of chronic diseases remains intangible. Such consequences led to the progress of the "common disease/common variant hypothesis" (i.e., CDCV hypothesis) (Collins et al. 1997; Lander 1996), stating that chronic diseases are typically caused by sets of gene variants that together contribute to initiate and develop disease. Why it has been not easy for molecular epidemiological studies to localize genes associated with chronic diseases explained by means of the complexity of genetic interactions in addition to the numeral and spacing of mapping markers? Further, complete single-nucleotide polymorphism (SNP) as well as haplotype maps (Daly et al. 2001; Gabriel et al. 2002; Johnson et al. 2001; Judson et al. 2002; Zaykin et al. 2002) will generate supplementary resources for identifying genes involved in the diseases. Such type of genome-centric approaches typically is unsuccessful to take into account the most vital variable in expression of genetic information in addition to a chief contributor to disease development, to be precise,

426   Nutrigenomics and Nutraceuticals

nutritional chemicals. And such interface between the nutritional environment and cellular/genetic processes is being referred to as "nutrigenomics" or nutritional genomics. Nutritional genomics looks for to give a genetic considerate of how common nutrition affects the balance between health and disease by altering the gene expression or genetic structure of an individual. The theoretical basis for this new branch of genomic research can best be summarized with the following five tenets.

1. Common nutritional chemicals are active on the human genome to alter gene expression or structure, either directly or indirectly.
2. In some individuals, under certain circumstances, diet can act as a serious risk factor for numerous diseases.
3. A few diet-regulated genes (and their normal, common variants) are expected to play a role in the onset, occurrence, development, and severity of chronic diseases.
4. Individual's genetic framework decides at what degree diet influences the balance between healthy and disease states.
5. Dietary interference derived from the understanding of individual's nutritional requirement, nutritional status, as well as genotype can be used to prevent, mitigate, or treat common disease.

17.4 Alteration of gene expression or structure by common dietary chemicals

Associations between food intakes and the occurrence and severity of chronic diseases are repetitively shown by epidemiological studies (Jenkins et al. 1998; Willett 2002a); however, the fact that food contains bioactive chemicals is not obvious from the design of numerous molecular and genetic association studies or else laboratory animal or cell culture experiments. Consider the complexity of a "simple" food, for example, the constituents of corn oil are fatty acids, triglycerides, sterols, sterol esters, and tocopherols. The diversity and concentrations of fatty acids, triglycerides, sterols, sterol esters, and tocopherols are probable to have lots of as well as varied effects on physiology in view of the fact that dietary chemicals have a number of fates upon entering a cell.

Gene expression can be affected by dietary chemicals directly or indirectly. At the cellular level, nutrients may undergo the following:

I. Act as a ligand for transcription factor receptors (Dauncey et al. 2001; Jacobs and Lewis 2002);
II. Be metabolized by primary or else secondary metabolic pathways, in that way altering concentrations of intermediates or substrates;
III. Affect signal pathways positively or negatively (Clarke 1999; Eastwood 2001).

Gene expression can be affected by dietary chemicals directly or indirectly as shown in Figure 17.2. Fatty acids, for instance, are metabolized by the β-oxidation pathways to produce cellular energy (Figure 17.2, II). Altering intracellular energy balance possibly will indirectly alter gene expression all the way through changes in cellular nicotinamide adenine dinucleotide (NAD) homeostasis (Lin and Guarente 2003). NAD reoxidation is linked with mitochondrial electron transport activity in addition to it being a cofactor for proteins involved in chromatin remodeling (Gasser and Cockell 2001; Moazed 2001). Because of reactions, for instance, histone acetylation or DNA methylation, chromatin remodeling processes have short- and long-term consequences for gene regulation, which alter access to, and consequently regulation of, eukaryotic genes (Edwards et al. 2000).

For nuclear receptors, a number of dietary chemicals act as ligand (Figure 17.2, I). A lot of genes are involved in fatty acid metabolism, which are regulated by means of one of the three members of the peroxisome proliferator-activated receptor (PPARα, PPARδ, and PPARγ) family (Auwerx 1992). The astonishing judgment was that the fatty acids, palmitic (16:0), oleic (18:1 n9), linoleic (18:2 n6), and arachidonic (20:4 n6) acid (Dreyer et al. 1992; Gottlicher et al. 1992; Schmidt et al. 1992), and the eicosanoids, 15-deoxy-Δ12,14prostaglandin J2 and 8-(S) hydroxyeicosatetraenoic acid (Forman et al. 1995; Kliewer et al. 1995) are ligands for PPARs family (Kliewer et al. 2001). Specifically, these nuclear receptors act as sensors for fatty acids. Lipid sensors typically heterodimerize by retinoid X receptor (RXR), whose ligand is derived from different dietary chemical, named retinol (vitamin A) (Dauncey et al. 2001). A number of dietary chemicals, for example, genistein, hyperforin, and vitamin A, bind directly to nuclear receptors and alter gene expression. On

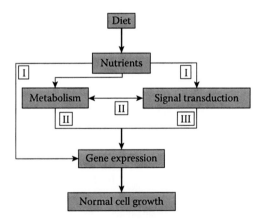

Figure 17.2 Fate and activities of nutrients in the cell. Nutrients may act directly as ligands for transcription factor receptors (pathway I); may be metabolized by primary or secondary metabolic pathways, in that way altering concentrations of intermediates or substrates (pathway II) involved in gene regulation or cell signaling; (pathway III). See text for details.

the contrary, transcription factors are indirectly regulated by dietary chemicals. The sterol regulatory element-binding proteins (SREBPs) are activated as a result of protease cleavage, which is regulated via low levels of oxysterols as well as changes in insulin/glucose and polyunsaturated fatty acids (PUFA) events (Edwards et al. 2000). The carbohydrate-responsive element-binding protein (ChREBP) is activated in response to elevated glucose levels, and an event is regulated by reversible phosphorylation (Uyeda et al. 2002).

For gene expression, metabolic conversion of dietary chemicals moreover serves as a control mechanism (Nobel et al. 2001). The steroid hormone level is eventually derived from cholesterol and is regulated by means of the activities of the combined 10 steps in the steroid biosynthetic pathway. In addition, various intermediates branch into other metabolic pathways. Overall, intracellular concentrations of intermediates along with end products are influenced through degradative pathways (Figure 17.2, II). For this reason, the concentration of any given ligand (Nobel et al. 2001) will be to a great extent influenced by explicit combinations of alleles for the enzymatic steps in these assorted pathways. Specific pair of alleles may be heterozygous and diverge in frequency from one subpopulation to another, which is an essential precept of nutrigenomics.

As shown in Figure 17.2(III), dietary chemicals also can directly have an effect on signal transduction pathways. Green tea contains the polyphenol and 11-epigallocatechin-3-gallate (EGCG). Tyrosine phosphorylation of Her-2/ neu receptor and epidermal growth factor (EGF) receptor are inhibited by EGCG, which sequentially reduces signaling through the phosphatidylinositol 3-kinase (PI-3) 3 Akt kinase 3 NF-κB pathway (Masuda et al. 2001; Pianetti et al. 2002). The NF-κB pathway activation is related to a few virulent forms of breast cancer. EGCG and its derivatives inhibit platelet-derived growth factor receptor phosphorylation (Sachinidis et al. 2002). Inositol hexaphosphate (InsP6) present in grains such as rice inhibits tetradecanoylphorbol-13-acetate (TPA) or EGF-induced cell transformation all the way through its effects on PI-3 kinase (Dong et al. 1999). Genistein, resveratrol, phenethyl isothiocyanate (PEITC), and retinoids (vitamin A and its metabolites) also have an effect on signal transduction pathways (Dong 2000).

Dietary chemicals playing such key roles in regulating gene expression away from their eminent roles of producing energy in addition to affecting insulin levels are reliable with evolutionary hypothesis. It is sensible to conclude that many human genes evolved in response to the plant- and animal-derived dietary chemicals we consume because the human genome is so elegantly receptive to its dietary environment.

17.5 Diet can be a risk factor for disease

The idea that undesirable diet or genome interactions can cause disease is not new-fangled. Discovery of galactosemia by Goppart in 1917 was the first example (http://www.ncbi.nlm.nih.gov/htbin-post/Omim/dispmim?230400).

Galactosemia is an uncommon recessive defect in galactose-1-phosphate uridyltransferase (GALT). The deficiency of GALT results into accumulation of galactose in the blood, causing numerous health problems like mental retardation. Another recessive trait, phenylketonuria was discovered by Asbjorn Folling in 1934 (http://www.ncbi.nlm.nih.gov/htbin-post/Omim/dispmim? 261600). Phenylketonuria is a deficiency in the enzyme phenylalanine hydroxylase that results into accumulation of phenylalanine in the blood. High levels of phenylalanine accumulation can cause neurological damage. Both galactosemia and phenylketonuria can be screened in infants in a moment after birth, and both diseases can be managed with diets low in lactose and phenylalanine, in that order. Galactosemia and phenylketonuria are single gene traits and hence are easy to identify and treat by changes in diet.

The associations of cholesterol with hypercholesterolemia and hypercholesterolemia with atherosclerosis focused much attention on the link between amount of calories (Willett 2002a) and the levels and types of vitamins (Fairfield and Fletcher 2002), fat (Krauss 1994; Willett 2002b), and carbohydrates (Jenkins et al. 2002) with atherosclerosis, cancer, diabetes, obesity, and other chronic diseases. Although some associations have been confirmed by subsequent genetic or biochemical studies in laboratory animals or humans, others remain controversial. The much-debated association between level and type of dietary fat with breast cancer occurrence (Smith-Warner et al. 2001; Willett 2001) illustrates the complexity of epidemiological studies to verify causation.

The restrictions of epidemiological studies might be in design, sample size, measurement errors, dietary assessment tools, statistical methods, and nutritionally irrelevant differences in fat intake amongst study populations (Lee and Lin 2000). Additionally, even though epidemiological methods frequently comprise family histories, individual genotypes are more often than not analyzed. All the same, the fundamental assumption of non-molecular epidemiology studies is that individual genetic difference is inconsequential in addition to that all individual responds in the same way to their environment. There are potentially millions of base pair differences between individuals, and a few of these differences could have an effect on the way one individual responds to their dietary environment relative to another individual demonstrated by the human genome (Lander et al. 2001; Venter et al. 2001) as well as SNP projects (Gabriel et al. 2002; Lee et al. 2003; Sachidanandam et al. 2001; Schork et al. 2000). Assumptions, for that reason, be unsuccessful to take into account that these genetic differences are not likely to make known significant connections between specific nutrients with chronic diseases. Analyzing SNPs or other polymorphisms in multiple genes is now possible with the advent of genomic sequence information and high-throughput technologies as well as reagents. Sophisticated statistical tools and large populations or many family studies are required for analyzing patterns of SNPs with patterns of disease sub-phenotypes.

430   Nutrigenomics and Nutraceuticals

The differences in allele frequencies among human subpopulations are correlated confusing factors. Humans became geographically isolated after the migrations from Africa, limiting genetic exchanges along with fixing distinct alleles and haplotypes (Tishkoff and Williams 2002). Seeing that one case, the gene encoding arylamine *N*-acetyltransferase, NAT2 (Hietanen et al. 1997; Risch et al. 1995), is polymorphic. Fast acetylator alleles as well as quite a few subtypes of slow acetylators are encoded by the variants. Among the populations in different geographic regions, these allele types are represented in a different way: Slow allele subtypes are mostly found in 72% of the Caucasians in the United States but only in 31% of Japanese. Slow acetylator NAT2 allele individuals are more vulnerable to bladder cancer when exposed to procarcinogens (Risch et al. 1995). The NAT2 allele frequencies exemplify the significance of knowing allele distributions in populations as well as contact to environmental influences, in view of the fact that molecular epidemiology studies rely upon statistical associations of convinced haplotypes or SNPs with disease phenotypes, occurrence, and severity. The distribution of alleles in the population is studied more willingly than a true association between an allele and a phenotype or disease, so that false-positive associations of SNPs as well as disease might be found. Determination of allele frequencies requires re-sequencing genes in culturally different individuals ($\geq \sim 90$). In the intervening time, ethnic difference markers (Collins-Schramm et al. 2002; McKeigue et al. 2000; Parra et al. 1998; Shibata and Whittemore 1997) be capable of determining the source of chromosomal regions, which may perhaps encode ethnic-specific alleles and in addition may be used to assess population substructures in epidemiological studies. Even though population substructures stun statistical association studies, analyzing varied admixtures possibly will allow for the recognition of genes causative to certain definite chronic diseases (Collins-Schramm et al. 2002; McKeigue et al. 2000; Parra et al. 1998; Shibata and Whittemore 1997; Tishkoff and Williams 2002), in view of the fact that for chronic diseases certain ethnic populations are at increased risk.

Attributable to population heterogeneity, analyzing genotype as a variable in association studies of disease phenotypes or sub-phenotypes will eradicate perplexing (Willett 2002b). Many times measuring or monitoring dietary intakes must also be done, as epidemiological as well as laboratory animal studies have always demonstrated an effect of diet on disease initiation along with succession. The literature linking diet to disease is too capacious to review in this; however, certain current advances are summarized below.

17.5.1 Micronutrients

The human diet required approximately 40 micronutrients. Suboptimal intakes of specific micronutrients have been associated with cancer (carotenoids, folate), CVD (carotenoids, B vitamins, and vitamin E), bone mass (vitamin D), and neural tube defects (folate) (Fairfield and Fletcher 2002). B6, B12, and folate deficiencies have been associated with increased serum homocysteine levels. For coronary artery disease, hyperhomocysteinemia is considered to be a risk factor as well as marker; however, the mechanism(s) is not implicit at the molecular level (Falk et al. 2001). While to explain its action, several theories have been proposed (Schaefer 2002). A lot of these conclusions are based upon cohort, randomized trials, and meta-analysis in which the origin of the disease cannot be convincingly determined.

Vitamins B6, folic acid, B12, niacin, C, or E, or iron or zinc deficiency appear to imitate radiation in damaging DNA by causing oxidative lesions, single- and double-strand breaks or both (Ames 2001) (Table 17.1). Nutrient deficiencies are orders of magnitude more significant than radiation on account of reliability of exposure to environment promoting DNA damage (Ames 2001; Ames and Gold 2000; Ames and Wakimoto 2002). Owing to substantial incorporation of uracil in human DNA (4 million uracil/cell), folate deficiency breaks chromosomes (Blount et al. 1997). In DNA, single-strand breaks are afterward formed during base excision repair, by means of two nearby single-strand breaks on opposite DNA strands resulting in fragmentation of chromosome. Deficiency of micronutrient can give explanation why the quarter of the US population that consumes a smaller amount than the suggested five portions a day of vegetables as well as fruits has just about double the rate for most types of cancer as compared with the quarter with the maximum intake (Ames 2001).

Table 17.1 Micronutrient Deficiency and DNA Damage

Micronutrient	Percent of US Population	DNA Damage	Health Effects
Folic acid	10%	Chromosome breaks	Colon cancer; heart diseases; brain dysfunction
Vitamin B12	4% (<Half RDA)	Uncharacterized	Same as folic acid; neuronal damage
Vitamin B6	10% (<Half RDA)	Uncharacterized	Same as folic acid
Vitamin C	15% (<Half RDA)	Radiation mimic (DNA oxidation)	Cataracts (4×); cancer
Vitamin E	12% (<Half RDA)	Radiation mimic (DNA oxidation)	Colon cancer (2×); heart disease (1.5×); immune dysfunction
Iron	7% (<Half RDA)	DNA breaks; radiation mimic	Brain and immune dysfunction; cancer
	19% women 12–50years old		
Zinc	18% (<Half RDA)	Chromosome breaks; radiation mimic	Brain and immune dysfunction; cancer
Niacin	2% (<Half RDA)	Disables DNA repair (poly ADP ribose)	Neurological symptoms; memory loss

Source: Adapted from Ames, B.N., and Gold, L.S, *Biotherapy,* 11, 205–220, 1998.
Note: RDA, recommended dietary allowance; number in parentheses for "Health Effects" indicates increased risk for condition/disease.

Many other degenerative diseases of aging are as well associated with low fruit as well as vegetable intake. In determining exact mechanisms for the role of definite minerals (calcium, copper, magnesium, manganese, and selenium) along with vitamins in heart disease as of work done in humans as well as in cell culture systems, advancement is also being made (Witte et al. 2001).

17.5.2 Macronutrients: Fats

The initiation, growth, and severity of chronic diseases might be contributed as a result of unbalanced intake of any of the three most important macronutrients, carbohydrates, fat, or protein. Intake of saturated fatty acids (SFA) is linked with elevated levels of low-density lipoprotein (LDL) cholesterol, which is the principal target of interference for the reduction of coronary disease risk (Krauss 2001). Besides CVDs, SFA possibly will add to diabetes as well as obesity (NCEP 2001). A lots of human and laboratory animal experiments support the associations predicted from epidemiological studies.

Also, human studies showing associations between the amount along with the type of fat and breast (Lee and Lin 2000), colorectal (Gatof and Ahnen 2002), and prostate (Bairati et al. 1998; Powell and Meyskens 2001; Veierod et al. 1997) cancers are conflicting (Skibola et al. 1999; Willett 2002a). Laboratory animal studies wherein genotype as well as environment can be more meticulously controlled every time demonstrate that the type in addition to the level of dietary fat is associated with occurrence and is powerfully associated with promotion (Lee and Lin 2000) of definite cancers.

17.5.3 Macronutrients: Carbohydrates

For minimizing the risk of obesity and its related comorbidities, CVDs and diabetes (Krauss 2001), nutritional guidelines carry on to put emphasis on diets low in saturated as well as total fat. Spurred by the increase in diabetes and obesity at the same time as fat intake scarcely decreased (36.4% to 34.1% of total calories) stuck between 1970 and 1990 (Ernst et al. 1997), an innovative focus of numerous epidemiological studies is carbohydrates. Metabolisms of the simple as well as complex carbohydrates are at different rates and for that reason have discrepancy effects on blood glucose concentrations. The glycemic index (GI) is a quantitative measure of foods based upon postprandial blood glucose response (Jenkins et al. 1981), which is expressed as a percentage of the response to an equivalent carbohydrate portion of glucose or white bread (Wolever et al. 1991). The glycemic load (GL) is a product of the average dietary GI and total carbohydrate intake, and is a measure of total insulin demand (Salmeron et al. 1997). For example, if glucose has a GI of 100, potatoes have a GI of 87, and tomatoes have a GI of 9. Several polysaccharides or refined simple sugars that are cleaved quickly to glucose produce elevated blood glucose levels as well as a larger demand for insulin (Augustin et al. 2002). High levels of GI would add to insulin production and, simultaneously, diminish synthesis of insulin receptors.

Virtually one cohort study of type 2 diabetes and GI (Augustin et al. 2002) showed a connection between GI and type 2 diabetes or breast cancer and GI or coronary artery disease and colon in case control studies. After multiple adjustments, these type of associations were observed (e.g., for fiber or other dietary variables) and typically for the 5th quintile of GI (Augustin et al. 2002). For the determination of the biochemical effects of GI on physiology, molecular epidemiological analysis of the links of candidate genes and dietary variables is desirable.

17.5.4 Macronutrients: Protein

As fat and micronutrients are important variable components of meat, analyzing the consequence of protein intake on health is not easy. The chemical composition of meat as well as other foods can be altered by baking, broiling, and frying differentially, (Ames and Gold 1997), and sometimes it creates nitrosamines along with other carcinogens (Sachse et al. 2002). Diverse amounts and types of natural or heat-generated nutritional chemicals may be produced by preparing foods in a different way, in that way introducing confounding into epidemiological analyses. Through these cautions, meat consumption appears to be linked with increased chronic disease risk (Ames and Gold 1998; Kolonel 2001) together with bowel (Bingham 1997) in addition to colorectal (Freedman et al. 1996) cancers and type 2 diabetes (van Dam et al. 2002). Certain genes, such as epoxide hydrolase (Ulrich et al. 2001), glutathione-S-transferase (Cortessis et al. 2001), and other detoxifying enzymes (Sachse 2002), may alter the effect of meat on disease risk suggested by molecular epidemiology.

The production of urea may be increased by increased metabolism of protein, through the corresponding increase in membrane permeable ammonia (NH_3) as well as its ionized form NH_4^+. Microbial enzymes released ammonia in the alimentary tract of animals, which is capable of modifying the gastrointestinal mucosa (Figura 1997), interrupting metabolic pathways (Visek 1972), changing brain function (Felipo and Butterworth 2002), inhibiting growth rates in animals (Wamberg et al. 1979), and promoting cancer (Clinton et al. 1988).

17.5.5 Caloric restriction

Early epidemiological studies neglected to give an explanation for the differences in energy content between carbohydrates and proteins (each at ~4 kcal/g) and lipids (~9 kcal/g). Through increased energy intake, almost every association studies show an increased risk for common diseases (Kant 2000). Reducing caloric intake is the most effectual means to reduce the occurrence as well as the severity of chronic diseases, slow down the effects of aging, and increase genetic reliability demonstrated by laboratory animal studies (Turturro et al. 1994; Weindruch et al. 2001). Experiments performed in *Saccharomyces cerevisiae* put forward that caloric restraint may produce its main effects by increasing respiration by the concomitant increase in the NAD: NADH (Lin and Guarente 2003). By changes in reducing equivalents, energy balance may possibly be monitored. NAD as well is a cofactor for Sir2, a histone deacetylase involved in chromatin silencing of nucleolar rDNA, telomere, and mating type locus (Gasser and Cockell 2001; Moazed 2001). In mammals, other cellular targets, for example, uncoupling proteins, as well as neuroendocrine peptides of the central nervous system (CNS), are probable targets of regulation by caloric restriction.

17.6 Some diet-regulated genes can play a role in chronic diseases

Changes in gene expression or by differences in activities of proteins and enzymes lead to the progression from a healthy phenotype to a chronic disease phenotype. A subset of genes regulated by diet must be involved in disease initiation, progression, and severity since dietary chemicals are regularly ingested and participate indirectly and directly in regulating gene expression (Kaput et al. 1994; Park et al. 1997), the example of which may be chronic disease like type 2 diabetes, a condition that frequently occurs in sedentary, obese individuals, and certain minority groups which is of genotype–diet interactions pathophysiology (Black 2002; Boden 2001). Some patients can control symptoms by increasing physical activities and by reducing caloric (and specific fat) intake (Nathan 2002), and by changing environmental (i.e., dietary) variables, expression of genomic information is changed. However, other patients are refractory to such environmental interventions and thus require drug treatments. There are many chronic diseases which do not show the phenotypic plasticity like some type 2 diabetics and thus symptoms are not reversible after some initiating event; the reason may be chromatin remodeling and changes in DNA methylation induced by unbalanced diets, which contributes to irreversible gene expression changes. On the contrary, genotype × diet interactions lead to the incidence and severity of obesity, atherosclerosis, many cancers, asthma, and other chronic conditions (Mucci et al. 2001; Reifsnyder et al. 2000; Sunde 2001; Willett 2002b).

17.6.1 Molecular approach

Identification of diet-regulated genes that cause or contribute to disease process can be one approach to understand the molecular mechanisms whereby diet alters health and can be done by examining the expression of a candidate gene or groups of genes (Spindler et al. 1990) in response to diets as per an approach pioneered by Goodridge and coworkers (Morris et al. 1982; Goodridge 1990). The expression of candidate genes in a variety of tissues in laboratory animals has been characterized in many laboratories in response to dietary variables (Fafournoux et al. 2000; Goodridge 1987) and caloric restriction (Cao et al. 2001; Lee et al. 1999). This approach has been extended by DNA and oligo-array technologies to multiple genes within a pathway (Dhahbi et al. 1999) or all genes on an array (Hirschi et al. 2001; Song et al. 2001). Genetic variants in nuclear receptors, *cis*-acting elements in promoters, or differences in metabolism that produce altered concentrations of transcriptional ligands can explain changes in gene expression, which are then associated with phenotype.

The limitations of assessing regulation of individual or multiple genes by diet are as follows:

1. Determining the cause from effect for each gene and the subset of causative genes responsible for a given phenotype?
2. Gene expression patterns in one strain (or genotype) may be unique to that genotype.

The study conducted in inbred mouse strains suggests that individual humans (Yan et al. 2002) may have unique patterns of gene expression depending upon their genotype and diet, and such individual qualitative and quantitative differences may complicate attempts to find patterns in gene expression results for dietary intake. Moreover, identifying these complex interactions is challenging since diet recall is imprecise and controlling diets is difficult in large population studies.

The health of the subject (laboratory animal or human) defines a separate confounding influence on analyses of diet-induced changes in gene expression patterns. The presence of a disease can be considered an additional environmental influence affecting gene expression patterns. For example, the presence of obesity unmasks additional type 2 diabetes loci in C57BL/6 and BTBR mice (Stoehr et al. 2000). Particularly, phenotypic expression of two interacting loci affecting fasting glucose and insulin levels were observed only in obese mice, and the alleles from the two parental strains (C57BL/6 and BTBR) having different effects on the diabetic subphenotypes suggest that there might be changes in gene expression based upon the presence or absence of disease processes and changes caused by dietary differences, and separating these variables will be an important component of future experimental designs for determining the effect of diet on susceptibility and disease progression.

Examination of diet–disease interactions at the molecular level has been possibly useful by employing inbred strains of laboratory animals because of the fact that (1) each individual member of a strain is genetically identical; (2) their environment can be rigorously controlled; (3) statistics can be applied to molecular, physiological, and genetic measurements; and (4) experiments can be repeated (Frankel 1995; Linder 2001) and thus the limitation of a unique genotype can be overcome by examining multiple strains of mice (Wade et al. 2002). A study conducted by researchers (Kaput et al. 1994; Park et al. 1997) introduced a comparative method for laboratory animals identifying genes regulated differently by dietary variables between two or more genotypes, and the genotypes (or inbred strains) of mice were selected on the basis of their susceptibility to disease caused by diet. It was found that certain genes were differentially regulated based upon genotype (in this case, Avy/A obese yellow versus A/a agouti mice) and/or on caloric intake (100% versus 70% calories) or by the interaction between diet and genotype. The criteria for identifying a candidate disease gene of are (1) differential regulation of gene by diet, (2) differential regulation by genotype, and (3) mapping to chromosomal regions [e.g., quantitative trait loci (QTL)] associated with the disease (Kaput et al. 1994; Park et al. 1997). This approach identifies candidate genes in an unbiased manner; however, additional testing in humans or animal models is necessary for validation of this hypothesis.

17.6.2 Genetic approach

The successes in identifying genes causing monogenic diseases have greatly influenced strategies for identifying genes that cause chronic diseases in humans (Jimenez-Sanchez et al. 2001). The difficulty in identifying chronic disease genes (Hirschhorn et al. 2002) has been attributed to factors such as small sample size, poorly matched control groups, population stratification, and over interpreting data (Lander and Kruglyak 1995; Tabor et al. 2002). But these methods and approaches are being improved for eliminating such errors and reliably identifying genes involved in chronic diseases (McKeigue et al. 2000; Reich and Goldstein 2001).

However, the effects of environmental variables such as diet have been noticeably missing from discussions of the limitations of genetic mapping techniques and gene association studies. A research conducted by Patterson et al. (1991) observed the importance of environment on expression of phenotypic traits in F2 and F3 generation tomato plants grown in Davis or Gilroy, California, and compared them with plants grown near Rehovot, Israel, to which it was observed that only 4 of a total of 29 quantitative trait loci (QTL) were found at all three sites, and 10 QTL were found in only two sites. QTL identify multiple regions within all chromosomes that collectively contribute to a complex phenotype (Risch et al. 1993) and encode many genes; thus, identifying the causative genes within the QTL is quite challenging (Tabor et al. 2002). Moreover, QTL mapping that accounts for differences in diet has not been done till date largely because controlling for diet in large population association studies is often not possible.

The factors that affect molecular (gene expression) analyses, epigenetic interactions between genes (Stoehr et al. 2000), in utero effects, diet–gene interactions, the lifelong exposure to changing diets, have compounded the complexities of gene–environment interactions and are postulated to alter expression of genetic information later in life (Sing et al. 2003). Maternal nutrition during pregnancy has also been linked to altered phenotypes in laboratory and farm animals (Cooney et al. 2002; Da Silva et al. 2002), and such epigenetic phenomena might affect gene–disease association studies.

Different health outcomes can be produced by maternal exposure to different nutrients and an organism's exposure during its lifetime to changing diets because the exposure to food and xenobiotics acts upon the genome to alter gene expression. Sing et al. (2003) presented an excellent discussion of the complexity of genotype x environmental history.

17.7 The balance between health and disease states may depend on an individual's genetic makeup

All humans are 99.9% identical at the gene sequence level, and the 0.1% variation in sequence produces the differences in phenotypes (hair and skin color, height, weight, etc.) and an individual's susceptibility to disease or health. Differences in gene expression or altered macromolecular activities can lead to alterations in phenotype. For example: (1) SNP is a polymorphism that alters gene expression and tolerance to dietary lactose (milk). Adult mammals are typically lactose intolerant, and a mutation that occurred ~9,000 years ago in Northern Europeans allowed expression of the lactase-phlorizin hydrolase gene (LCH locus) to continue into adulthood. Although there are 11 polymorphisms in this gene clustered into 4 (A, B, C, and U) prevalent haplotypes (0.05%), a C13910T SNP located 14 kb upstream of the LCH (Enattah et al. 2002) is said to be highly associated with lactase persistence (lactose tolerance), and this polymorphism is thought to alter regulatory protein–DNA interactions controlling the expression of the gene (Hollox et al. 1999). (2) SNPs alter splicing, for example, two insulin receptor splice variants differ in the presence (type B) or absence (type A) of exon 11 (Huang et al. 1996; Sugimoto et al. 2000). Genome-wide analyses of human have been identified over 30,000 alternative splice sites (Lee et al. 2003). (3) A subset of coding SNPs (cSNPs) alters the biochemical activities of enzymes, proteins, and cellular processes. For example, steroid 5 α-reductase (designated SRD5A2), a key enzyme in androgen metabolism in the prostate, has 13 naturally occurring variants in the human population, 9 of which reduce SRD5A2 activity by 20% or more and 3 increase activity by more than 15% and one results in essentially unaltered kinetic properties suggesting that it is a truly neutral ('polymorphic') amino acid substitution. Since SRD5A produces dihydrotestosterone (DHT) and DHT regulates genes in the prostate, variants in steroid 5α-reductase may affect incidence or severity of prostate cancer (Reichardt 1999). Polymorphisms in 5′ or 3′ regulatory regions or splice sites may also alter the level of expression of a gene or the variant produced (Kuokkanen et al. 2003; Yan et al. 2002).

17.8 Dietary intervention based on individualized nutrition

Dietary intervention based on knowledge of nutritional requirement, nutritional status, and genotype (i.e., "individualized nutrition") can be used for prevention, mitigation, or cure of chronic disease. Nonetheless, this assertion is obvious for nutritional deficiencies such as scurvy and beriberi or phenylketonurics, and it is still less obvious for ~50 genetic diseases in humans caused by variants in enzymes (Ames et al. 2002). As many as one-third of enzyme variants are due to increased K_m (a measure of binding affinity of an enzyme for its ligand substrate or coenzyme) for a coenzyme, resulting in a lower rate of reaction (Ames et al. 2002). The Michaelis-Menten constant, K_m, is defined as the concentration of ligand required to fill half of the ligand-binding sites. Work by Ames et al. (2002) proposed the "K_m hypothesis" for describing the effects of polymorphisms on enzymatic activity. High doses of the corresponding vitamin may increase intracellular concentrations of coenzyme which would partially restore enzymatic activity and potentially ameliorate the phenotype. Changing substrate concentrations may circumvent decreased coenzyme binding or decreased enzymatic activities caused by a given cSNP. Some examples that can explain the phenomenon are as follows (Ames et al. 2002):

1. Defects in glucose-6-phosphate dehydrogenase A44G (DNA: C131GP) with NADP as cofactor are involved in favism and hemolytic anemia. Increased dietary intake of nicotinic acid or nicotinamide might increase NADPH coenzyme concentrations and alter the equilibrium of GPDH $\leftrightarrow$ GPDH + NADPH.
2. NAD is a cofactor for aldehyde dehydrogenase (ALDH), an enzyme involved in alcohol intolerance and linked to Alzheimer's and cancer. A cSNP causes E487K, which increases the K_m 150-fold, and this variant could not be treated with diet because the NAD substrate concentration could not be increased sufficiently to overcome the increased K_m.

A web site entitled "K_m Mutants" (http://www.kmmutants.org/), which summarizes nutritional information for a large number of enzymes requiring coenzymes, has also been established by Ames and coworkers (Elson-Schwab et al. 2002).

Prevention or treatment of chronic diseases in an individual by directed dietary intervention is inherently more challenging because multiple genes interacting with each other and with environmental variables contribute to disease etiology. But identification of genes contributing to the most to chronic disease initiation or progression and understanding their regulation by dietary variables is definitely the first step in this process.

17.8.1 Hypertension

An SNP, AA, at nucleotide position 6 of the angiotensinogen (ANG) gene is linked with the level of circulating ANG protein. Individuals with the AA genotype who eat the Dietary Approaches to Stop Hypertension (DASH) diet show reduced blood pressure, but the same diet with a GG genotype was less effective in reducing blood pressure in individuals (Svetkey et al. 2001).

17.8.2 Cardiovascular health

The G-to-A transition in the promoter of APOA1 gene is associated with increased HDL cholesterol concentrations, and thus, Apo-A1 plays a central role in lipid metabolism and coronary heart disease. The A allele (or variant) is associated with decreased serum HDL levels (Ordovas et al. 2002). For example, women eating more PUFA relative to saturated fats (SF) and mono-unsaturated fats (MUFA) have increased serum HDL levels. This type-of-fat effect is significant in men when alcohol consumption and tobacco smoking were considered in the analyses.

Individuals with small, dense LDL particles (phenotype B) have an increased risk of coronary artery disease relative to those individuals exhibiting large, less dense LDL particles (phenotype A) (Krauss 2001). Dreon et al. (1999) in a classic crossover experiment showed that the LDL patterns are influenced by low-fat diets. Thirty-eight men exhibiting phenotype A LDL were switched from a 32% fat diet to a diet containing 10% fat, and the results showed that 12 of these 38 exhibited phenotype B LDL after 10 days on the low-fat diet (Dreon et al. 1999), suggesting that for these 12, low-fat diets were not benefi-cial. Thus, the results suggest three distinct genotypes although not directly analyzed. Two genotypes produce either the A or B phenotype. A third geno-type produces the A phenotype when these individuals eat a diet containing 32% fat, but a B phenotype when fed 10% fat, a result that can be explained by a genotype x environment interaction.

17.8.3 Cancer

A key gene in one-carbon metabolism and, indirectly, in all methylation reac-tions is methylenetetrahydrofolate reductase (MTHFR). Several studies have found that the C667T polymorphism (Ala to Val), which reduces enzymatic activity, is inversely associated with occurrence of colorectal cancer (Chen et al. 1999; Slattery et al. 1999; Ulrich et al. 1999) and acute lymphocyte leu-kemia (Skibola et al. 1999). There is an increased risk for cancer among those with the MTHFR TT genotype in patients with low intake of folate, vitamin B12, vitamin B6, or methionine (Kostulas et al. 1998).

The effects of dietary chemicals on these polymorphisms raise the possibility that candidate gene or SNP association studies may be more accurate if diets and nutritional status are included as variables in the analyses but dietary histories are notoriously inaccurate, and nutritional status is difficult to assess and that environmental factors are likely to alter results of association studies.

17.9 Population screening for genetic susceptibility to disease

The genes responsible for numerous single gene (Mendelian) disorders have been identified in recent time, but the elucidation of the genetic basis of multifactorial disorders has proceeded more slowly. Mendelian diseases are thought to arise from the interaction in an individual of multiple genes, "polygenes," each having a minor effect, with the modifying influence of environmental factors. The process of elucidating the contribution of particular genetic loci to multifactorial disorders is in initial phase. In insulin-dependent diabetes mellitus, genetic susceptibility is influenced by one locus within the major histocompatibility complex on chromosome 6p21, which contributes 42% of the familial clustering, and at least four minor loci (Davies et al. 1994; Hashimoto et al. 1994).

Studies by Baird (1990) have suggested that the dissection of the genetic factors predisposing to the common, multifactorial disorders will lead to a paradigm shift in health care, allowing people at increased risk of these diseases to be identified, and lead to health benefits because those at high risk will be able, and motivated, to alter their lifestyles appropriately. Weber (1994) suggested the immediate banking of DNA from all newborn infants and elderly and sick people so that their DNA can be typed with over 250 markers from across the genome: "global screening of polymorphisms enables the entire genome to be examined in one step." However, benefits of this testing are not clear except to increase the work of genetics laboratories. Like Holtzmann (1992), one can take a more cautious view.

17.10 Commercial interests

The prospect of the application of molecular genetic technology to the general (healthy) population in programs to measure genetic susceptibility to disease is one of the main reasons for conducting human genome research in a commercial climate. Screening tests applicable to the general population hold out promise of enormous profits for corporations that can develop and patent tests and techniques ahead of their competitors.

The control of susceptibility tests by private corporations will have important consequences, and the need to recoup investment makes tests will be introduced into private health care systems before properly evaluated and introduced into state insurance schemes such as the British NHS. The tests will be introduced inequitably if there are health benefits even if they may not yield the promised benefits, because access will be restricted to those who can pay (whether directly or through insurance companies).

The commercial control of susceptibility screening will inevitably lead to the active promotion of such screening. Thus, those who respond to the marketing will be helped to feel in control of their biological destiny and those who do not choose, or cannot afford, to participate may be portrayed as irresponsible and feckless. The notion that genetic endowment and chosen lifestyle together determine future health, while the importance of material circumstances (especially poverty) in creating ill health will be glossed over will be promoted by this commercialization (Phillimore et al. 1994; Townsend 1990; Townsend et al. 1988).

Screening programs for hypertension and high serum cholesterol concentrations (Brett 1991; Lefebvre et al. 1988) indicate that psychological problems are likely to arise in those identified as being susceptible. However, the question is how will the counseling issues be addressed in a commercial environment? Next provision of full information before the test would be expensive and could deter many potential customers, so will counseling before the test be confused with sales talk? Will support through the distress produced by positive results be provided, or will it be left to the NHS and voluntary agencies? All these questions are putative and need conclusive data for support.

17.11 Public health perspective

Predictive testing within known families is beneficial in identifying those at high risk in few uncommon genetic disorders because useful treatments are available or health surveillance improves outcomes. However, there may be no public health benefit in screening the general population for genetic susceptibility for the common multifactorial disorders. Susceptibility screening for multifactorial disorders will be justified only once careful evaluation has shown clear benefits with the help of improved methods of treatment or surveillance for complications. Until then adoption of the privatized screening approach to produce individualized indicators of susceptibility is not worth. As health benefits can be gained by altering lifestyles, the benefits of a healthy lifestyle will apply to everyone and not just those with an increased risk (Chen et al. 1991; Law et al. 1994a, 1994b). Few benefits that could not be achieved by simpler, population-based measures may be caused by individualizing genetic risks that will be inefficient and expensive (Wald et al. 1994).

Population-based measures could achieve a more substantial and more equitable improvement in public health than the individualized approach but would require political action (Mant 1994). Population screening to identify those at high risk may lead to adverse outcomes for the population as a whole, as those not at high risk may feel a sense of invulnerability and modify their lifestyles inappropriately increasing their risk of disease (Kinlay and Heller 1990).

In the future, prevention of the development of disease in those identified as being at increased risk will be able to be prevented by specific interventions that may be devised. Careful research into the risk factors and preventive measures relevant to each disease should be encouraged, which may lead to evidence for justification of trials of screening, but evaluation must include the outcomes of those identified as being at low risk.

Screening programs for the identification of those at high risk need to be clearly presented to potential participants as research studies until the net

442   Nutrigenomics and Nutraceuticals

benefits of specific interventions are established. Subjects may be recruited and labeled as high risk if the labeling of a research-driven susceptibility screening program as a research exercise is not clear and such subjects may feel coerced to participate in subsequent trials of possible interventions. The finding that those at risk of inherited cancers may volunteer to participate in research as they anticipate that this will give them access to better care (Green et al. 1993) makes it important that those entering a research screening program have no such misunderstandings.

17.12 Summary

It is to be expected that nutritional imbalances, starting from micronutrient deficiencies to overconsumption of macronutrients or else nutritional supplements, are the modifiers of metabolism in addition to potentiators of chronic disease. Even though the intricacy of food with genotypic variations appears discouraging, genetic as well as molecular technologies may present the means for identifying causative genes and the nutrients that control them. Understanding the genetic basis of complex traits and common disease is a central goal, since the pathways that affect the risk of disease in patients are also potentially good drug targets. Knowledge of the relevant variants may also aid in prediction and prognosis and in designing optimal therapies and intervention. Identifying the underlying genetic variants will likely require a number of different approaches, but association studies are likely to be a significant tool in the near future. Nevertheless, care must be taken in performing and interpreting these studies, so as to avoid generating false leads and also to correctly identify the *bona fide* genetic risk factors for disease. In the near future, quick, low-cost, point-of-care tests will be available to assist patients and physicians to achieve, manage, and prolong health through dietary invention. The desired outcome of nutrigenomics is the use of personalized diets to delay the onset of disease and optimize and maintain human health.

References

Altmuller J, Palmer LJ, Fischer G, Scherb H, Wjst M. Genomewide scans of complex human diseases: true linkage is hard to find. *Am J Hum Genet.* 2001;69:936–50.

Altshuler D, Hirschhorn JN, Klannemark M, Lindgren CM, Vohl MC, Nemesh J, et al. The common PPARgamma Pro12Ala polymorphism is associated with decreased risk of type 2 diabetes. *Nat Genet.* 2000;26:76–80.

Ames BN. Micronutrients prevent cancer and delay aging. *Toxicol Lett.* 1998;102–103:5–18.

Ames BN. DNA damage from micronutrient deficiencies is likely to be a major cause of cancer. *Mutat Res.* 2001;475:7–20.

Ames BN, Elson-Schwab I, Silver EA. High-dose vitamin therapy stimulates variant enzymes with decreased coenzyme binding affinity (increased Km): relevance to genetic disease and polymorphisms. *Am J Clin Nutr.* 2002;75:616–58.

Ames BN, Gold LS. The causes and prevention of cancer: gaining perspective. *Environ Health Perspect.* 1997;105(4):865–73.

Ames BN, Gold LS. The causes and prevention of cancer: the role of environment. *Biotherapy.* 1998;11:205–20.

Ames BN, Gold LS. Paracelsus to parascience: the environmental cancer distraction. *Mutat Res.* 2000;447:3–13.

Ames BN, Wakimoto P. Are vitamin and mineral deficiencies a major cancer risk? *Nat Rev Cancer.* 2002;2:694–704.

Augustin LS, Franceschi S, Jenkins DJ, Kendall CW, La Vecchia C. Glycemic index in chronic disease: a review. *Eur J Clin Nutr.* 2002;56:1049–71.

Auwerx J. Regulation of gene expression by fatty acids and fibric acid derivatives: an integrative role for peroxisome proliferator activated receptors. The Belgian Endocrine Society Lecture 1992. *Horm Res.* 1992;38:269–77.

Bairati I, Meyer F, Fradet Y, Moore L. Dietary fat and advanced prostate cancer. *J Urol.* 1998;159:1271–5.

Baird PA. Genetics and health care. *Perspect Biol Med.* 1990;33:203–13.

Barratt BJ, Payne F, Lowe CE, Hermann R, Healy BC, Harold D, et al. Remapping the insulin gene/IDDM2 locus in type 1 diabetes. *Diabetes.* 2004;53:1884–9.

Bingham S. Meat, starch and non-starch polysaccharides, are epidemiological and experimental findings consistent with acquired genetic alterations in sporadic colorectal cancer? *Cancer Lett.* 1997;114:25–34.

Black SA. Diabetes, diversity, and disparity: what do we do with the evidence? *Am J Public Health.* 2002;92:543–8.

Blount BC, Mack MM, Wehr CM, Macgregor JT, Hiatt RA, Wang G, et al. Folate deficiency causes uracil misincorporation into human DNA and chromosome breakage: implications for cancer and neuronal damage. *Proc Natl Acad Sci USA.* 1997;94:3290–5.

Boden G. Pathogenesis of type 2 diabetes. Insulin resistance. *Endocrinol Metab Clin North Am.* 2001;30:801–15.

Brett AS. Psychologic effects of the diagnosis and treatment of hypercholesterolemia: lessons from case studies. *Am J Med.* 1991;91:642–7.

Cao SX, Dhahbi JM, Mote PL, Spindler SR. Genomic profiling of short- and long-term caloric restriction effects in the liver of aging mice. *Proc Natl Acad Sci USA.* 2001;98:10630–5.

Cardon LR, Bell JI. Association study designs for complex diseases. *Nat Rev Genet.* 2001;2:91–9.

Carlson CS, Eberle MA, Kruglyak L, Nickerson DA. Mapping complex disease loci in whole-genome association studies. *Nature.* 2004;429:446–52.

Carol E, Kate H. Genetic Susceptibility. In: eLS. John Wiley & Sons Ltd, Chichester, 2006. doi: 10.1002/9780470015902.a0005639

Chen J, Giovannucci EL, Hunter DJ. Mthfr polymorphism, methyl-replete diets and the risk of colorectal carcinoma and adenoma among US men and women: an example of gene-environment interactions in colorectal tumorigenesis. *J Nutr.* 1999;129:560S–4S.

Chen Z, Peto R, Collins R, MacMahon S, Lu J, Li W. Serum cholesterol concentration and coronary heart disease in population with low cholesterol concentrations. *BMJ.* 1991;303:276–82.

Clarke SD. Nutrient regulation of gene and protein expression. *Curr Opin Clin Nutr Metab Care.* 1999;2:287–9.

Clinton SK, Bostwick DG, Olson LM, Mangian HJ, Visek WJ. Effects of ammonium acetate and sodium cholate on N-methyl-N'-nitro- N-nitrosoguanidine-induced colon carcinogenesis of rats. *Cancer Res.* 1988;48:3035–9.

Collins FS, Guyer MS, Charkravarti A. Variations on a theme: cataloging human DNA sequence variation. *Science.* 1997;278:1580–1.

Collins-Schramm HE, Phillips CM, Operario DJ, Lee JS, Weber JL, Hanson RL, et al. Ethnic difference markers for use in mapping by admixture linkage disequilibrium. *Am J Hum Genet.* 2002;70:737–50.

Cooney CA, Dave AA, Wolff GL. Maternal methyl supplements in mice affect epigenetic variation and DNA methylation of offspring. *J Nutr.* 2002;132:2393S–400S.

Cortessis V, Siegmund K, Chen Q, Zhou N, Diep A, Frankl H, et al. A case-control study of microsomal epoxide hydrolase, smoking, meat consumption, glutathione *S*-transferase M3, and risk of colorectal adenomas. *Cancer Res.* 2001;61:2381–5.

Cox NJ, Wapelhorst B, Morrison VA, Johnson L, Pinchuk L, Spielman RS, et al. Seven regions of the genome show evidence of linkage to type 1 diabetes in a consensus analysis of 767 multiplex families. *Am J Hum Genet.* 2001;69:820–30.

Daly MJ, Rioux JD, Schaffner SF, Hudson TJ, Lander ES. High-resolution haplotype structure in the human genome. *Nat Genet.* 2001;29:229–32.

Da Silva P, Aitken RP, Rhind SM, Racey PA, Wallace JM. Impact of maternal nutrition during pregnancy on pituitary gonadotrophin gene expression and ovarian development in growth-restricted and normally grown late gestation sheep fetuses. *Reproduction.* 2002;123:769–77.

Dauncey MJ, White P, Burton KA, Katsumata M. Nutrition hormone receptor-gene interactions: implications for development and disease. *Proc Nutr Soc.* 2001;60:63–72.

Davies IL, Kawaguchi Y, Bennett ST, Copeman JB, Cordell HJ, Pritchard LER, et al. A genomewide search for human type I diabetes susceptibility genes. *Nature.* 1994;371:130–5.

Dhahbi JM, Mote PL, Wingo J, Tillman JB, Walford RL, Spindler SR. Calories and aging alter gene expression for gluconeogenic, glycolytic, and nitrogen-metabolizing enzymes. *Am J Physiol Endocrinol Metab.* 1999;277: E352–60.

Dong Z. Effects of food factors on signal transduction pathways. *Biofactors.* 2000;12:17–28.

Dong Z, Huang C, Ma WY. PI-3 kinase in signal transduction, cell transformation, and as a target for chemoprevention of cancer. *Anticancer Res.* 1999;19:3743–7.

Dreon DM, Fernstrom HA, Williams PT, Krauss RM. A very low- fat diet is not associated with improved lipoprotein profiles in men with a predominance of large, low-density lipoproteins. *Am J Clin Nutr.* 1999;69:411–18.

Dreyer C, Krey G, Keller H, Givel F, Helftenbein G, Wahli W. Control of the peroxisomal beta-oxidation pathway by a novel family of nuclear hormone receptors. *Cell.* 1992;68:879–87.

Eastwood MA. A molecular biological basis for the nutritional and pharmacological benefits of dietary plants. *QJM.* 2001;94:45–8.

Edwards PA, Tabor D, Kast HR, Venkateswaran A. Regulation of gene expression by SREBP and SCAP. *Biochim Biophys Acta.* 2000;1529:103–13.

Elson-Schwab I, Poedjosoedarmo K, Ames BN. *KmMutants.org [Online].* Children's Hospital Oakland Research Institute. http://www. kmmutants.org (updated 19 August 2002).

Enattah NS, Sahi T, Savilahti E, Terwilliger JD, Peltonen L, Jarvela I. Identification of a variant associated with adult-type hypolactasia. *Nat Genet.* 2002;30:233–7.

Ernst ND, Sempos CT, Briefel RR, Clark MB. Consistency between US dietary fat intake and serum total cholesterol concentrations: the National Health and Nutrition Examination Surveys. *Am J Clin Nutr.* 1997;66:965S–72S.

Fafournoux P, Bruhat A, Jousse C. Amino acid regulation of gene expression. *Biochem J.* 2000;351:1–12.

Fairfield KM, Fletcher RH. Vitamins for chronic disease prevention in adults: scientific review. *JAMA.* 2002;287:3116–26.

Falk E, Zhou J, Moller J. Homocysteine and atherothrombosis. *Lipids.* 2001;36:S3–11.

Felipo V, Butterworth RF. Neurobiology of ammonia. *Prog Neurobiol.* 2002;67:259–79.

Figura N. *Helicobacter pylori* factors involved in the development of gastroduodenal mucosal damage and ulceration. *J Clin Gastroenterol.* 1997;25(1): S149–63.

Florez JC, Hirschhorn J, Altshuler D. The inherited basis of diabetes mellitus: implications for the genetic analysis of complex traits. *Annu Rev Genomics Hum Genet.* 2003;4:257–91.

Forman BM, Tontonoz P, Chen J, Brun RP, Spiegelman BM, Evans RM. 15-Deoxy-delta 12,14-prostaglandin J2 is a ligand for the adipocyte determination factor PPAR gamma. *Cell.* 1995;83:803–12.

Frankel WN. Taking stock of complex trait genetics in mice. *Trends Genet.* 1995;11:471–7.

Freedman AN, Michalek AM, Marshall JR, Mettlin CJ, Petrelli NJ, Black JD, et al. Familial and nutritional risk factors for p53 overexpression in colorectal cancer. *Cancer Epidemiol Biomarkers Prev.* 1996;5:285–91.

Gabriel SB, Schaffner SF, Nguyen H, Moore JM, Roy J, Blumenstiel B, et al. The structure of haplotype blocks in the human genome. *Science.* 2002;296:2225–9.

Gasser SM, Cockell MM. The molecular biology of the SIR proteins. *Gene.* 2001;279:1–16.

Gatof D, Ahnen D. Primary prevention of colorectal cancer: diet and drugs. *Gastroenterol Clin North Am.* 2002;31:587–623.

Goodridge AG. Dietary regulation of gene expression: enzymes involved in carbohydrate and lipid metabolism. *Annu Rev Nutr.* 1987;7:157–85.

Goodridge AG. The role of nutrients in gene expression. *World Rev Nutr Diet.* 1990;63:183–93.

Gottlicher M, Widmark E, Li Q, Gustafsson JA. Fatty acids activate a chimera of the clofibric acid-activated receptor and the glucocorticoid receptor. *Proc Natl Acad Sci USA.* 1992;89:4653–7.

Green J, Murton F, Statham H. Psychosocial issues raised by a familial ovarian cancer register. *J Med Genet.* 1993;30:575–9.

Hashimoto L, Habits C, Beressi JP, Delepine M, Besse C, Cambon-Thomsen A, et al. Genetic mapping of a susceptibility locus for insulin-dependent diabetes mellitus on chromosome 1 lq. *Nature.* 1994;371:161–4.

Hietanen E, Husgafvel-Pursiainen K, Vainio H. Interaction between dose and susceptibility to environmental cancer: a short review. *Environ Health Perspect.* 1997;105(4):749–54.

Hirschhorn JN, Daly MJ. Genome-wide association studies for common diseases and complex traits. *Nat Rev Genet.* 2005;6:95–108.

Hirschhorn JN, Lohmueller K, Byrne E, Hirschhorn K. A comprehensive review of genetic association studies. *Genet Med.* 2002;4:45–61.

Hirschi KD, Kreps JA, Hirschi KK. Molecular approaches to studying nutrient metabolism and function: an array of possibilities. *J Nutr.* 2001;131:1605S–9S.

Hollox EJ, Poulter M, Wang Y, Krause A, Swallow DM. Common polymorphism in a highly variable region upstream of the human lactase gene affects DNA-protein interactions. *Eur J Hum Genet.* 1999;7:791–800.

Holtzmann NA. The diffusion of new genetic tests for predicting disease. *FASEBY.* 1992;6:2806–12.

Huang Z, Bodkin NL, Ortmeyer HK, Zenilman ME, Webster NJ, Hansen BC, et al. Altered insulin receptor messenger ribonucleic acid splicing in liver is associated with deterioration of glucose tolerance in the spontaneously obese and diabetic rhesus monkey: analysis of controversy between monkey and human studies. *J Clin Endocrinol Metab.* 1996;81:1552–6.

Jacobs MN, Lewis DF. Steroid hormone receptors and dietary ligands: a selected review. *Proc Nutr Soc.* 2002;61:105–22.

Jenkins D, Wolever TMS, Taylor RH, Barker H, Fielden H, Baldwin JM, et al. Glycemic index of foods: a physiological basis for carbohydrate exchange. *Am J Clin Nutr.* 1981;34(3):362–6.

Jenkins DJ, Kendall CW, Augustin LS, Franceschi S, Hamidi M, Marchie A, et al. Glycemic index: overview of implications in health and disease. *Am J Clin Nutr.* 2002;76:266S–73S.

Jenkins DJA, Kendall CCW, Ransom TPP. Dietary fiber, the evolution of the human diet and coronary heart disease. *Nutr Res.* 1998;18:633–52.

Jimenez-Sanchez G, Childs B, Valle D. Human disease genes. *Nature.* 2001;409:853–5.

Johnson GC, Esposito L, Barratt BJ, Smith AN, Heward J, Di Genova G, et al. Haplotype tagging for the identification of common disease genes. *Nat Genet.* 2001;29:233–7.

Judson R, Salisbury B, Schneider J, Windemuth A, Stephens JC. How many SNPs does a genome-wide haplotype map require? *Pharmacogenomics.* 2002;3:379–91.

Kant AK. Consumption of energy-dense, nutrient-poor foods by adult Americans: nutritional and health implications. The Third National Health and Nutrition Examination Survey, 1988–1994. *Am J Clin Nutr.* 2000;72:929–36.

Kaput J, Swartz D, Paisley E, Mangian H, Daniel WL, Visek WJ. Diet-disease interactions at the molecular level: an experimental paradigm. *J Nutr.* 1994;124:1296S–305S.

Kinlay S, Heller RF. Effectiveness and hazards of case finding for a high cholesterol concentration. *BMJ.* 1990;300:1545–7.

Kliewer SA, Lenhard JM, Willson TM, Patel I, Morris DC, Lehmann JM. A prostaglandin J2 metabolite binds peroxisome proliferator- activated receptor gamma and promotes adipocyte differentiation. *Cell.* 1995;83:813–19.

Kliewer SA, Xu HE, Lambert MH, Willson TM. Peroxisome proliferator-activated receptors: from genes to physiology. *Recent Prog Horm Res.* 2001;56:239–63.

Kolonel LN. Fat, meat, and prostate cancer. *Epidemiol Rev.* 2001;23:72–81.

Kostulas K, Crisby M, Huang WX, Lannfelt L, Hagenfeldt L, Eggertsen G, et al. A methylenetetrahydrofolate reductase gene polymorphism in ischaemic stroke and in carotid artery stenosis. *Eur J Clin Invest.* 1998;28:285–9.

Krauss RM. Dietary and genetic effects on LDL heterogeneity. *World Rev Nutr Diet.* 2001;89:12–22.

Krauss RM. Heterogeneity of plasma low-density lipoproteins and atherosclerosis risk. *Curr Opin Lipidol;*1994;5:339–49.

NCEP (2001) Executive Summary of the Third Report of The National Cholesterol Education Program (NCEP) Expert Panel on Detection, Evaluation, and Treatment of High Blood Cholesterol in Adults (Adult Treatment Panel III). JAMA, 285, 2486–2497. http://dx.doi.org/10.1001/jama.285.19.2486

Kuokkanen M, Enattah NS, Oksanen A, Savilahti E, Orpana A, Jarvela I. Transcriptional regulation of the lactase-phlorizin hydrolase gene by polymorphisms associated with adult-type hypolactasia. *Gut.* 2003;52:647–52.

Lander E, Kruglyak L. Genetic dissection of complex traits: guidelines for interpreting and reporting linkage results. *Nat Genet.* 1995;11:241–7.

Lander ES, Linton LM, Birren B, Nusbaum C, Zody MC, Baldwin J, et al. (International Human Genome Sequencing Consortium). Initial sequencing and analysis of the human genome. *Nature.* 2001;409:860–921.

Lander ES. The new genomics: global views of biology. *Science.* 1996;274:536–9.

Law MR, Thompson SG, Wald NJ. Assessing possible hazards of reducing serum cholesterol. *BMJ.* 1994a;308:373–9.

Law MR, Wald NJ, Thompson SG. By how much and how quickly does reduction in serum cholesterol concentration lower risk of ischaemic heart disease? BMJ. 1994b;308:367–73.

Lee C, Atanelov L, Modrek B, Xing Y. ASAP: the Alternative Splicing Annotation Project. *Nucleic Acids Res.* 2003;31:101–5.

Lee CK, Klopp RG, Weindruch R, Prolla TA. Gene expression profile of aging and its retardation by caloric restriction. *Science.* 1999;285:1390–3.

Lee MM, Lin SS. Dietary fat and breast cancer. *Annu Rev Nutr.* 2000;20:221–48.

Lefebvre RC, Hursey KG, Carleton RA. Labeling of participants in high blood pressure screening programs. Implications for blood cholesterol screenings. *Arch Intern Med.* 1988;148:1993–7.

Lin SJ, Guarente L. Nicotinamide adenine dinucleotide, a metabolic regulator of transcription, longevity and disease. *Curr Opin Cell Biol.* 2003;15:241–6.

Linder CC. The influence of genetic background on spontaneous and genetically engineered mouse models of complex diseases. *Lab Anim (NY).* 2001;30:34–9.

Mant D. Prevention. *The Lancet.* 1994;344:1343–6.

Masuda M, Suzui M, Weinstein IB. Effects of epigallocatechin- 3-gallate on growth, epidermal growth factor receptor signaling pathways, gene expression, and chemosensitivity in human head and neck squamous cell carcinoma cell lines. *Clin Cancer Res.* 2001;7:4220–9.

McKeigue PM, Carpenter JR, Parra EJ, Shriver MD. Estimation of admixture and detection of linkage in admixed populations by a Bayesian approach: application to African-American populations. *Ann Hum Genet.* 2000;64:171–86.

Moazed D. Enzymatic activities of Sir2 and chromatin silencing. *Curr Opin Cell Biol.* 2001;13:232–8.

Morris SM, Jr, Nilson JH, Jenik RA, Winberry LK, McDevitt MA, Goodridge AG. Molecular cloning of gene sequences for avian fatty acid synthase and evidence for nutritional regulation of fatty acid synthase mRNA concentration. *J Biol Chem.* 1982;257:3225–9.

Mucci LA, Wedren S, Tamimi RM, Trichopoulos D, Adami HO. The role of gene-environment interaction in the aetiology of human cancer: examples from cancers of the large bowel, lung and breast. *J Intern Med.* 2001;249:477–93.

Nathan DM. Clinical practice. Initial management of glycemia in type 2 diabetes mellitus. *N Engl J Med.* 2002;347:1342–9.

Nobel S, Abrahmsen L, Oppermann U. Metabolic conversion as a pre-receptor control mechanism for lipophilic hormones. *Eur J Biochem.* 2001;268:4113–25.

Ordovas JM, Corella D, Cupples LA, Demissie S, Kelleher A, Coltell O, et al. Polyunsaturated fatty acids modulate the effects of the APOA1 G-A polymorphism on HDL cholesterol concentrations in a sex-specific manner: the Framingham Study. *Am J Clin Nutr.* 2002;75:38–46.

Park EI, Paisley EA, Mangian HJ, Swartz DA, Wu MX, O'Morchoe PJ, et al. Lipid level and type alter stearoyl CoA desaturase mRNA abundance differently in mice with distinct susceptibilities to diet-influenced diseases. *J Nutr.* 1997;127:566–73.

Parra EJ, Marcini A, Akey J, Martinson J, Batzer MA, Cooper R, et al. Estimating African American admixture proportions by use of population-specific alleles. *Am J Hum Genet.* 1998;63:1839–51.

Patterson AH, Damon S, Hewitt JD, Zamir D, Rabinowitch HD, Lincoln SE, et al. Mendelian factors underlying quantitative traits in tomato: comparison across species, generations, and environments. *Genetics.* 1991;127:181–97.

Phillimore P, Beattie A, Townsend P. Widening inequality of health in northern England, 1981–91. *BMJ.* 1994;308:1125–8.

Pianetti S, Guo S, Kavanagh KT, Sonenshein GE. Green tea polyphenol epigallocatechin-3 gallate inhibits Her-2/neu signaling, proliferation, and transformed phenotype of breast cancer cells. *Cancer Res.* 2002;62:652–5.

Powell IJ, Meyskens FL, Jr. African American men and hereditary/familial prostate cancer: intermediate-risk populations for chemoprevention trials. *Urology.* 2001;57:178–81.

Reich DE, Goldstein DB. Detecting association in a case-control study while correcting for population stratification. *Genet Epidemiol.* 2001;20:4–16.

Reichardt JK. GEN GEN: the genomic genetic analysis of androgen metabolic genes and prostate cancer as a paradigm for the dissection of complex phenotypes. *Front Biosci.* 1999;4:D596–600.

Reifsnyder PC, Churchill G, Leiter EH. Maternal environment and genotype interact to establish diabesity in mice. *Genome Res.* 2000;10:1568–78.

Risch A, Wallace DM, Bathers S, Sim E. Slow *n*-acetylation genotype is a susceptibility factor in occupational and smoking related bladder cancer. *Hum Mol Genet.* 1995;4:231–6.

Risch N. Linkage strategies for genetically complex traits. I. Multilocus models. *Am J Hum Genet.* 1990;46:222–8.

Risch N, Ghosh S, Todd JA. Statistical evaluation of multiple-locus linkage data in experimental species and its relevance to human studies: application to nonobese diabetic (NOD) mouse and human insulin dependent diabetes mellitus (IDDM). *Am J Hum Genet.* 1993;53:702–14.

Risch N, Merikangas K. The future of genetic studies of complex human diseases. *Science.* 1996;273:1516–17.

Sachidanandam R, Weissman D, Schmidt SC, Kakol JM, Stein LD, Marth G, et al. A map of human genome sequence variation containing 1.42 million single nucleotide polymorphisms. *Nature.* 2001;409:928–33.

Sachinidis A, Skach RA, Seul C, Ko Y, Hescheler J, Ahn HY, et al. Inhibition of the PDGF beta-receptor tyrosine phosphorylation and its downstream intracellular signal transduction pathway in rat and human vascular smooth muscle cells by different catechins. *FASEB J.* 2002;16:893–5.

Sachse C, Smith G, Wilkie MJ, Barrett JH, Waxman R, Sullivan F, et al. A pharmacogenetic study to investigate the role of dietary carcinogens in the etiology of colorectal cancer. *Carcinogenesis.* 2002;23:1839–49.

Salmeron JM, Ascherio A, Rimm EB, Colditz GA, Spiegelman D, Jenkins DJ, et al. Dietary fiber, glycemic load, and risk of NIDDM in men. *Diabetes Care.* 1997;20:545–50.

Schaefer EJ. Lipoproteins, nutrition, and heart disease. *Am J Clin Nutr.* 2002;75:191–212.

Schmidt A, Endo N, Rutledge SJ, Vogel R, Shinar D, Rodan GA. Identification of a new member of the steroid hormone receptor superfamily that is activated by a peroxisome proliferator and fatty acids. *Mol Endocrinol.* 1992;6:1634–41.

Schork NJ, Fallin D, Lanchbury JS. Single nucleotide polymorphisms and the future of genetic epidemiology. *Clin Genet.* 2000;58:250–64.

Shibata A, Whittemore AS. Genetic predisposition to prostate cancer: possible explanations for ethnic differences in risk. *Prostate.* 1997;32:65–72.

Sing CF, Stengard JH, Kardia SL. Genes, environment, cardiovascular disease. *Arterioscler Thromb Vasc Biol.* 2003;23:1190–6.

Skibola CF, Smith MT, Kane E, Roman E, Rollinson S, Cartwright RA, et al. Polymorphisms in the methylenetetrahydrofolate reductase gene are associated with susceptibility to acute leukemia in adults. *Proc Natl Acad Sci USA.* 1999;96:12810–15.

Slattery ML, Potter JD, Samowitz W, Schaffer D, Leppert M. Methylenetetrahydrofolate reductase, diet, and risk of colon cancer. *Cancer Epidemiol Biomarkers Prev.* 1999;8:513–18.

Smith-Warner SA, Spiegelman D, Adami HO, Beeson WL, van den Brandt PA, Folsom AR, et al. Types of dietary fat and breast cancer: a pooled analysis of cohort studies. *Int J Cancer.* 2001;92:767–74.

Song F, Srinivasan M, Aalinkeel R, Patel MS. Use of a cDNA array for the identification of genes induced in islets of suckling rats by a high carbohydrate nutritional intervention. *Diabetes.* 2001;50:2053–60.

Spindler SR, Crew MD, Mote PL, Grizzle JM, Walford RL. Dietary energy restriction in mice reduces hepatic expression of glucose regulated protein 78 (BiP) and 94 mRNA. *J Nutr.* 1990;120:1412–17.

Stoehr JP, Nadler ST, Schueler KL, Rabaglia ME, Yandell BS, Metz SA, et al. Genetic obesity unmasks nonlinear interactions between murine type 2 diabetes susceptibility loci. *Diabetes.* 2000;49:1946–54.

Sugimoto K, Murakawa Y, Zhang W, Xu G, Sima AA. Insulin receptor in rat peripheral nerve: its localization and alternatively spliced isoforms. *Diabetes Metab Res Rev.* 2000;16:354–63.

Sunde RA. Research needs for human nutrition in the post-genome sequencing era. *J Nutr.* 2001;131:3319–23.

Svetkey LP, Moore TJ, Simons-Morton DG, Appel LJ, Bray GA, Sacks FM, et al. Angiotensinogen genotype and blood pressure response in the Dietary Approaches to Stop Hypertension (DASH) study. *J Hypertens.* 2001;19:1949–56.

Tabor HK, Risch NJ, Myers RM. Candidate-gene approaches for studying complex genetic traits: practical considerations. *Nat Rev Genet.* 2002;3:391–7.

Tishkoff SA, Williams SM. Genetic analysis of African populations: human evolution and complex disease. *Nat Rev Genet.* 2002;3:611–21.

Townsend P. Individual or social responsibility for premature death? Current controversies in the British debate about health. *Int J Health Serv.* 1990;20:373–92.

Townsend P, Davidson N, Whitehead M, eds. *Inequalities in Health the Black Report and the Health Divide.* 2nd ed. Harmondsworth: Penguin, 1988.

Turturro A, Blank K, Murasko D, Hart R. Mechanisms of caloric restriction affecting aging and disease. *Ann NY Acad Sci.* 1994;719:159–70.

Ulrich CM, Bigler J, Whitton JA, Bostick R, Fosdick L, Potter JD. Epoxide hydrolase Tyr113His polymorphism is associated with elevated risk of colorectal polyps in the presence of smoking and high meat intake. *Cancer Epidemiol Biomarkers Prev.* 2001;10:875–82.

Ulrich CM, Kampman E, Bigler J, Schwartz SM, Chen C, Bostick R, et al. Colorectal adenomas and the C677T MTHFR polymorphism: evidence for gene-environment interaction? *Cancer Epidemiol Biomarkers Prev.* 1999;8:659–68.

Uyeda K, Yamashita H, Kawaguchi T. Carbohydrate responsive element-binding protein (ChREBP): a key regulator of glucose metabolism and fat storage. *Biochem Pharmacol.* 2002;63:2075–80.

van Dam RM, Willett WC, Rimm EB, Stampfer MJ, Hu FB. Dietary fat and meat intake in relation to risk of type 2 diabetes in men. *Diabetes Care.* 2002;25:417–24.

Veierod MB, Laake P, Thelle DS. Dietary fat intake and risk of prostate cancer: a prospective study of 25,708 Norwegian men. *Int J Cancer.* 1997;73:634–8.

Venter JC, Adams MD, Myers EW, Li PW, Mural RJ, Sutton GG, et al. (Celera Genomics). The sequence of the human genome. *Science.* 2001;291:1304–51.

Visek WJ. Effects of urea hydrolysis on cell life-span and metabolism. *Fed Proc.* 1972;31:1178–93.

Wade CM, Kulbokas EJ, III, Kirby AW, Zody MC, Mullikin JC, Lander ES, et al. The mosaic structure of variation in the laboratory mouse genome. *Nature.* 2002;420:574–8.

Wald NJ, Law M, Watt HC, Wu T, Bailey A, Johnson AM, et al. Apolipoproteins and ischaemic heart disease: implications for screening. *The Lancet.* 1994;343:75–9.

Wamberg S, Engel K, Kildeberg P. Balance of net base in the rat. V. Effects of oral ammonium chloride loading. *Biol Neonate.* 1979;36:99–108.

Weber JL. Know thy genome. *Nat Genet.* 1994;7:343–4.

Weindruch R, Keenan KP, Carney JM, Fernandes G, Feuers RJ, Floyd RA, et al. Caloric restriction mimetics: metabolic interventions. *J Gerontol A Biol Sci Med Sci.* 2001;56:20–33.

Willett W. Isocaloric diets are of primary interest in experimental and epidemiological studies. *Int J Epidemiol.* 2002a;31:694–5.

Willett WC. Balancing life-style and genomics research for disease prevention. *Science.* 2002b;296:695–8.

Willett WC. Diet and breast cancer. *J Intern Med.* 2001;249:395–411.

Witte KK, Clark AL, Cleland JG. Chronic heart failure and micronutrients. *J Am Coll Cardiol.* 2001;37:1765–74.

Wolever TMS, Jenkins DJA, Jenkins AL, Josse RG. The glycemic index: methodology and clinical implications. *Am J Clin Nutr.* 1991;54:846–54.

Yan H, Yuan W, Velculescu VE, Vogelstein B, Kinzler KW. Allelic variation in human gene expression. *Science.* 2002;297:1143.

Zaykin DV, Westfall PH, Young SS, Karnoub MA, Wagner MJ, Ehm MG. Testing association of statistically inferred haplotypes with discrete and continuous traits in samples of unrelated individuals. *Hum Hered.* 2002;53:79–91.

18

Nutrition and Healthy Aging

Manjir Sarma Kataki, Ananya Rajkumari, and Bhaskar Mazumder
Dibrugarh University,
Dibrugarh, India

Contents

18.1 Introduction 452
18.2 Healthy nutrition...453
18.3 Healthy aging and nutrition issues 454
     18.3.1 Malnutrition and older persons..457
18.4 Disease concerns in older populations..457
18.5 Key nutrients to help combat age-related disease and disability 459
     18.5.1 Calcium and vitamin D 459
     18.5.2 Antioxidants 463
     18.5.3 Plant polyphenols and catechins—Curcumin, green tea,
            and grape seed 464
     18.5.4 Carotenoids—Lutein, zeaxanthin, and lycopene 465
     18.5.5 Plant stanols/sterols 465
     18.5.6 B vitamins 465
     18.5.7 Omega-3 fatty acids 466
     18.5.8 Glucosamine, chondroitin quercetin, and collagen..............468
     18.5.9 Dietary fibers 468
     18.5.10 Prebiotics and probiotics 469
     18.5.11 Potassium 470
     18.5.12 Whey protein..471
     18.5.13 Zinc..471
     18.5.14 Coenzyme Q10 473
18.6 Formulation challenges 474
18.7 Future opportunities..475
18.8 Conclusion...475
References..475

18.1 Introduction

Aging can be defined as a natural phenomenon of growing matured, manifested by physiological and psychological alteration with time. The process of aging in humans is spontaneous and alters moderately with time. However, it is an ineludible process owing to continuous and unrepairable loss of physiological state causing disability to physical activity as well as increasing the risk of death. Growing old does not necessarily cause sureness to several diseases. Despite, it certainly increases the susceptibility of the older population to many chronic diseases and is definitely a risk factor. Many of the consequences pertaining to aging can be curbed by maintaining a healthy life style. During the past century, there has been an outbreak in the older population all through the world (López-Otín et al. 2013).

In the year 1950, only 8% of the world's population was over the age of 60 years, whereas the estimated proportion for the same will be over 21% by the year 2050. These data certainly mark the longer life expectancies due to improvement in medical care as well as better perceptive and cognizance for healthy lifestyle habits. A strong relation between healthy life style habits and aging definitely exists as shown by research and clinical outcome extensive data. Healthy eating habits also accounts for healthy aging process (Nations 2013).

Morbidity, mortality, and quality of life are greatly influenced by improper nourishment as it may cause several chronic diseases (Anderson and Anderson 2014). It is essential to maintain a complete nutritious diet to lead a healthy life and healthy aging not only for an individual but also for the entire society as a whole. There is still inconsiderable cognizance associated with this point throughout the world and there must be efforts to turn the awareness into alertness (Anderson and Anderson 2014; USDA, 2016; Kalaiselvi et al. 2016). Moreover, the point that healthy diet assists in healthy aging and prevents non-communicable diseases is neglected and is inadequately inferred among general population as well as policymakers and health professionals. Better understanding of the food habits in individuals and populations as well as knowing the effect of modifying diet on them are still poor (Khandelwal et al. 2013).

Balance nutrient consumption has minimized malnutrition and non-communicable disease occurrence to a large extent, thereby reducing healthcare expenses throughout the world. Malnutrition can be circumvented by improving diets along with implementation of constant nutritional education through simple and cost-effective measures like providing specific food supplement and nutrient supplementation of susceptible populations and food addition of micronutrients in the food for general population (Krishnaswamy and Prasad 2001; Oggioni et al. 2014). The problem of malnutrition should be tackled not only concentrating on dietary factors but also through other factors related to it such as physical, social, and medical factors (Piple et al. 2015). Healthy aging and nutrient adequacy can be achieved through considering socio-economic issues along with nutrition and diet as an essential part of the solution (Popkin 2013; Raiten et al. 2016).

A comprehensive national action plan is required in each country through tackling inadequate nutrient status which will eradicate malnutrition in general as well as specific susceptible population. Indeed, this step of expenditure will give fruitful results. Chronic disease, disability, and death are accompanied with aging. It leads to considerable financial burden to society for caring an aging population. In 2011, the expense for health care, long-term care, and nursing home for people with Alzheimer's disease and other dementias alone was $183 billion, which is expected to increase to $1.1 trillion in 2050 as per Center for Disease Control and Prevention (CDC) report (CDC 2015). Therefore, it is utmost essential to prioritize our attention to find out ways to prevent chronic illnesses associated with aging. Each individual should undertake healthy lifestyle practices inclusive of healthful diet consumption. It is now prerequisite to take smarter and healthier decisions on foodstuff purchasing (Gupta et al. 2016; Tulchinsky and Varavikova 2014). The effect of aging varies individually in different ways, yet, some three factors grant to healthy aging including genetic built up and family history, lifestyle habits, and exercise diet and nutrition. Although genetic built up and family history is perpetual, others can be altered to attain healthy life and aging (Akbulut and Ersoy 2008; Amarya et al. 2015; Sixsmith et al. 2014).

18.2 Healthy nutrition

Status of health, physiological changes, and functional disabilities accounted due to aging are largely affected by nutritional choice and physical activity, which in broader extent affect the familial, social, and economic factors. Healthy nutrition is exercised through individuals as well as from collective efforts. Individual factors include age, sex, education, physiological and health issues, psychological attributes, lifestyle practices, knowledge, attitudes, and beliefs and behaviors including income, social status, and culture. Collective contributions include approachable food labels, adequate food shopping atmosphere, popularizing "healthy eating" idea, proper social support, and providing effective, community-based meal delivery services to facilitate healthy eating and dietary habits. Despite, there is unexpectable insufficiency of research in this field, specifically in Canada. A study involving Canadian seniors to find out the knowledge and research gaps in the field of healthy eating habits showed nutritional insufficiency is higher in individuals with poor health and insufficient resources, whereas dietary self-management exists to a great extent in well, independent seniors without financial constraints irrespective of their living arrangements. To allow the development and evaluation of programs and services framed to inspire and avail healthy eating in older Canadians, further study to confirm the contributors to healthy eating are required (Payette and Shatenstein 2005).

Healthy nutrition is very much essential for an optimum health and is always linked to a healthy diet fortified with all the required nutritional components including protein, carbohydrates, fat, water, vitamins, and minerals. A healthy diet is one which aids in the maintenance or improvement of overall health and also destined to supplement the physiological requirement of the body with essential nutrition such as fluid, adequate essential amino acids from protein, essential fatty acids, vitamins, minerals, and adequate calories (Anonymous 2014). Without a balanced nutrition, malnutrition can occur, leading to various symptoms including fatigue, dizziness, and weight loss. If unnoticed and untreated, malnutrition can also cause physical or mental disability. It can occur at any stage of life. However, at an older age, this can precipitate several serious health-related issues which may ultimately cause higher levels of physical and mental disabilities or even death. Therefore, elderly population is vulnerable to malnutrition accompanied by a range of practical issues in maintaining adequate nutrition in this population. Physiological requirement in older age is very much different due to the decrement of basal metabolic rate and lean body mass (LBM) with aging.

According to the World Health Organization (WHO), malnutrition is the biggest single threat to global public health (Nordqvist 2016). It is also a matter of concern that the nutritional requirement in elderly can be individual-specific, and hence, customization on person basis may enhance the healthy nutrition practice in elderly population.

18.3 Healthy aging and nutrition issues

In almost all countries of the world, the number and proportion of older persons aged 60 years or above are increasing and this progression is not likely to sustain soon. According to a report in 2002, out of the total 605 million older population in the world, almost 400 million inhabits in low-income countries. In the year 2000, around 24% of older population which is considered as highest proportion lived in Greece and Italy. However, by 2025, it is estimated that the number of older population will reach above 1.2 billion out of which 840 million survives in low-income countries. In order to attain the final goal of healthy and active aging, WHO has constructed a policy frame that guides in this field (WHO 2016).

The global scenario depicts that the survival of women are longer than men, so most of the older population approximately in almost all countries include women. In both Asia and Africa, the proportion and number of older women may increase from 107 to 373 million and 13 to 46 million, respectively by 2025. Osteoporosis in older women is one of the major health risks which requires special attention for nutrition, significance, and types of malnutrition. The maintenance of osteoporosis and associated fractures are a costly affair with high morbidity and mortality. By 2050, there may be an increase in the annual number of hip fractures from 1.7 million in 1990 to around 6.3 million over the world. About 80% of hip fractures in older population are suffered by women, and the susceptibility of women for osteoporotic fractures is approximately 30% to 40%, which is only 13% for men in their life span. The susceptibility of women for osteoporosis is more, as by post menopause their bone loss expedites. It can be defended by supplementing hormone therapy at menopause. Some of the primary modes of prevention of osteoporosis include balanced diet, physical activity, and caseation of smoking. The most important goal of preventing fractures can be achieved through increasing bone mass, reducing bone loss, and replenishing bone mineral. Exercising intake of sufficient quantity of calcium along with physical activity at adolescence and young adulthood may assist the prevention process (WHO 2016).

There is a physiological and clinical alteration in old age due to free radical damage build-up. Increasing lipid peroxide levels, enzyme activities alterations, and greater osmotic fragility are some of the age-related modifications due to free radical reactions. Studies to analyze the level of lipid peroxidation product malondialdehyde (MDA) and antioxidants catalase and glutathione have shown increase in lipid peroxidation and decrease in antioxidants in normal, elderly individuals. Elderly individuals when complicated with diabetes and hypertension showed substantial increase in MDA and decrease in antioxidants. Antioxidants supplementation in elderly individuals may avoid further oxidative damage (Akila et al. 2007). Aging may cause progressive deterioration of many physiological functions which is substantially affected by nutrition. Level of energy, LBM, and protein intake also decrease progressively with aging. Recommended dietary allowances of calcium, iron, zinc, copper, thiamin, riboflavin, folate, and vitamins B12 and D along with recommended water intake also reduced in aged population (>55 years old). In coming years, the nutritional requirements of the old population required to perform the daily activities are likely to be increased. In order to avail adequate tissue functioning in old age, the food habit modifications should be implemented at a younger age itself as with increased diminished physical activity and old age disabilities, food habits acquired at younger age are required to be altered. Focus for the research and development in nutritional requirements in elderly should be increased by assessing the effect of nutrition on chronic diseases, adopting improved method to analyze nutritional status. The elderly population should be screened for nutritional risk and nutrient-nutrient and nutrient-drug interactions. Educational strategies to provide better nutrition and eliminate health fraud should be implemented. For its effectiveness, dietary interventions and its monitoring prove to be effective (Ahmed 1992).

Remarkable changes are very likely in elderly in terms of body physiology and composition including LBM and total body fat. In elderly, well-evident changes in body composition occur, which trigger loss of skeletal muscle mass leading to "sarcopenia." This is strictly an age-related disability and accounts for the well-documented age-related changes including decreased metabolic rate and muscle strength. This particular issue can also be held accountable for the less energy requirement in elderly (Evans and Cyr-Campbell 1997). Research in gerontology defined several concepts of aging which focus on various factors including genetic makeup, interplay of genes with the environment, underlying disease conditions, early life activities, behavioral practices, and most importantly nutrition and diet practices. Healthy aging is a multidimensional process influenced by cognitive impairments, physical functionalities, concurrent chronic disease conditions, and social–cultural involvement of the elderly including engagement in productive and creative activities.

Cumulative scientific opinions also indicated the concept of reaching old age in good health as a highly complex process encompassing interplay between environmental and genetic factors. Reaching old age in a healthy manner is no more just a "fate-phenomenon," rather it is considered as a multidimensional process with a plethora of controllable factors. A balanced nutrition along with a plethora of other associated factors including physical activity—fitness, weight control, management of chronic diseases, and prevention of obesity, stress management—can pave a path toward healthy aging. In short, there is nothing like a "quick fix" when aging in good health matters; rather, healthy aging is a "package deal" with an exhaustive list of factors to be considered (Figure 18.1). In this context, nutrition and lifestyle factors are considered as the most important contributors to longevity and healthy aging. However, a balanced and optimum nutrition is not a simple goal and it requires a serious monitoring as well as a person-specific surveillance of the overall health of the elderly.

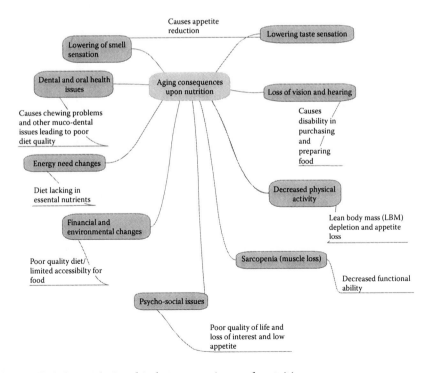

Figure 18.1 Interrelationship between aging and nutrition.

18.3.1 Malnutrition and older persons

Diseases associated with the older population are mostly related to nutritional factors, many of which manifested since childhood. This factor along with degenerative changes with aging accounts for the related diseases. Colon, pancreas, and prostate cancers seem to be precipitated due to consumption of dietary fat. Coronary heart disease is associated with atherogenic risk factors such as increased blood pressure, blood lipids, and glucose intolerance which in turn are linked with diet. Many other common diseases affecting the older populations including cerebrovascular disease, diabetes, osteoporosis and the above mentioned diseases are greatly affected by diet. Micronutrients also play one of the key roles in improving and protecting non-communicable diseases and their importance is increasing day by day. In older population, food consumption decreases along with the lack of varieties in food. As a result, micronutrient deficiencies are observed in this population. Morbidity and mortality in older population also increase due to impaired immune function. The quality of health and life in older population also decreases due to deteriorating vision and depletion of cognitive function. In older population, risks for coronary heart disease due to raised serum cholesterol are usual and the complication lasts till very old age. It is recommended to continue with medicine therapy only if failed to manage through diet modifications, particularly at younger age. As shown by intervention trail, 40% risk of stroke and 15% heart attack can be minimized by minimizing blood pressure by 6 mm Hg and 30% of coronary heart disease can be minimized by 10% reduction in blood cholesterol level. Dietary modifications are key to a better health as they reduce the risks of many diseases and particularly, it has larger influence in old age. Risks of cardiovascular disease can be significantly reduced if intake of saturated fat and salt is generously reduced as it keeps the blood pressure normal. The risk of cardiovascular complications can be reduced by 30% if intake of fruits and vegetables is increased from one to two servings per day (WHO 2016).

18.4 Disease concerns in older populations

Advancement in medications and surgical techniques has increased the life span of individuals but they are often crippled by unfitness. Some of the most common disabilities suffered by old populations are summarized (Chappell and Cooke 2010) in Table 18.1.

CDC states that 80% of older adults suffer from at least one of the diseases mentioned in Table 18.1 and 50% suffer from at least two (CDC 2013). According to them, primary causes of death in older adults in the United States are already predicted. The older population in the United States will increase to 71 million by 2030 (CDC 2003). This colossal change in population will definitely influence healthcare expenditure and hence, extensive preventive measures for diseases will be required (Chappell and Cooke 2010; Robert 2010). One such

Table 18.1 Some Most Common Disabilities in Elderly Population

SN	Name of the Disease
1	Hypertension
2	Congestive heart failure
3	Dementia (Alzheimer's disease)
4	Incontinence Arthritis
5	Osteoporosis
6	Breathing problems Frequent falls/bone fractures
7	Parkinson's disease
8	Vascular disease
9	Coronary heart disease
10	Depression
11	Diabetes
12	Cataracts
13	Glaucoma
14	Cancer
15	Macular degeneration
16	Impaired immunity

step of safeguarding health of older people is by halting of these common chronic disease conditions and other related intricacies (Shneerson et al. 2014; Topp et al. 2004). A healthy lifestyle is maintained by exercising good health practice along with proper diet. When proper diet and good nutrition are consumed, many of the previously mentioned chronic diseases can be prevented. Each year, the estimated deaths are about 50 million worldwide. In 1990, it was estimated that ischemic heart disease (6.3 million), cerebrovascular accidents (4.4 million), lower respiratory infections (4.3 million), diarrheal disease (2.9 million), perinatal disorders (2.4 million), chronic obstructive pulmonary disease (2.2 million), tuberculosis (2.0 million), measles (1.1 million), road-traffic accidents (1.0 million), and lung cancer (0.9 million) are the leading causes of deaths worldwide (Murray and Lopez 1997). A large portion of global deaths in both developing and developed countries of the world are due to lack of nutrition, which is a modifiable disease.

The major area of diseases which are prevalent in aged populations, such as dyslipidemia, heart-related problems like hypertension and stroke, cancer, reduced mobility due to excess body weight, increased risk of developing type 2 diabetes, type 1 diabetes Alzheimer's disease, and other cognitive impairments including depression, physical deterioration of bones and joints associated with osteoporosis and arthritis, vision impairment problems including cataracts and macular degeneration, and an increased risk of pulmonary problems and infectious diseases can be prevented through nutritional modifications (Murray and Lopez 1997; Anderson and Anderson 2014).

18.5 Key nutrients to help combat age-related disease and disability

Some important nutrients and compounds that play a key role in preventing certain age-related chronic diseases and associated disability are listed in Table 18.2 (Everitt et al. 2006).

18.5.1 Calcium and vitamin D

Both calcium and vitamin D are known to play an important role in bone metabolism and prevention of osteoporosis. Recently, the research attention has been shifted to its non-skeletal roles. As investigated, calcium-rich diets have shown its efficacy to reduce the risk of colon cancer and the recurrence of colonic polyps. On the contrary, vitamin D is associated with chronic diseases such as diabetes and various cancers (Garriguet 2011; Rolland et al. 2013).

In EC member states, osteoporosis is a prime public health issue which lowers bone mass and causes high incidence of fragility fractures, especially of hip and vertebrae. The lifestyle in EC states is affected due to increased complications and deaths due to osteoporosis. In 15 countries of EC, the number of hip fractures in 1995 was 382,000 with an expense of 9 billion ECUs for its management. It is important to take public health measures for its prevention due to its significant impact on health sector. Both endogenous (genetic, hormonal) and exogenous (nutritional, physical activity) factors regulate the skeletal bone mass. Bone health is maintained through well-balanced diet or nutrition.

Table 18.2 Some Salient Food Components Linked to Various Disease Conditions in Elderly Population

Food Component	Related Disease or Conditions
Calcium and vitamin D	Osteoporosis, cancer, diabetes
Antioxidants (vitamin E, vitamin, polyphenols)	Cancer, heart disease, neurodegenerative disease
B-Vitamins (folate, vitamin B6, vitamin B12)	Heart disease, cognition
Omega-3 fatty acids (fish oil, DHA, EPA)	Inflammation, heart disease, stroke
Plant stanols/sterols	Elevated blood cholesterol, heart disease
Glucosamine, chondroitin, and collagen	Osteoarthritis
Lutein, zeaxanthin, and lycopene	Macular degeneration
Epigallocatechin-3-gallate (EGCG)	Cancer
Fiber (soluble and insoluble)	Diabetes, constipation
Prebiotics and probiotics	Diarrhea
Potassium	Hypertension
Whey protein	Sarcopenia
Zinc	Immunity and macular degeneration
Coenzyme Q10	Inflammation and endothelial dysfunction.

Calcium and vitamin D are the most essential key nutrients for bone growth and development. Calcium deficiency and significant vitamin deficiency cause osteoporosis, reduced bone mass, and osteomalacia (decreased mineralization of bone). In elderly adults, lack of vitamin D is very common. Lack of vitamin D in physiological system occurs due to reduced renal hydroxylation of vitamin D, insufficient diet, and non-exposure to sunlight and decrease in the production of vitamin D in the skin. In 19 towns of 10 European countries, the average consumption of calcium was evaluated by studying the food habits of the elderly people termed as SENECA study. Dietary calcium consumption was very low in about one-third of the subjects, ranging between 300 and 600 mg/day in women and 350 and 700 mg/day in men. Both bone mass and fracture risk decrease with calcium supplements as reported by some recent studies. In the elderly populations in Europe, the incidence of vitamin D deficiency is rapid as shown by the SENECA study. Several other studies also have shown that the administration of daily doses of 400–800 IU of vitamin D alone or in combination with calcium can replenish the vitamin D deficiency and defend bone loss and ameliorate bone density in the elderly. In the current years, there was controversy regarding consumption of calcium in different age groups and physiological conditions. In the year 1998, the expert committee of the European Community in the Report on Osteoporosis—Action on Prevention has prescribed daily dietary allowances (RDA) for calcium at all stage of life. In the case of elderly population >65 years, the RDA is 700–800 mg/day. The richest origins of calcium in the diet are dairy products such as milk, yoghurts, and cheese; fishes like sardines with bones; few vegetables; and fruits. One of the ideal means to attain adequate calcium levels is through nutrition (Figure 18.2). When nutrition sources are insufficient, extra calcium

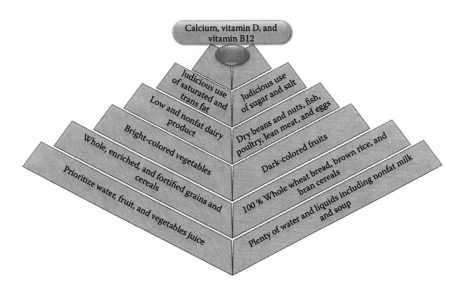

Figure 18.2 An indicative food guide for elderly population.

supplementation is recommended. No side effects are normally associated with calcium. Vitamin D deficiency can be prevented and overcome by sufficient sunlight exposure. Sunlight exposure (ultraviolet irradiation) is avoided in many cases as it may increase the susceptibility to skin cancer. The best way to decrease vitamin D deficiency is through supplementation. For people aged 65 years or above, in Europe, the RDA is 400–800 IU (10–20 µg) daily which is free from side effects and safe. Low calcium consumption and lack of normal vitamin D are very usual in elderly people of Europe. Daily dose of 700–800 mg of calcium and 400–800 IU of vitamin D is recommended on daily basis for these individuals with osteoporosis susceptibility. It can be regarded as the safest, cheapest, and the most effective way to protect osteoporotic fractures (Gennari 2001).

A diet rich in fruits and vegetables (five or more servings/day), sufficient in protein but moderate in animal protein, adequate calcium, and vitamin D intakes with low dairy fat, or calcium-nourished foods can meet the nutritional requirement for healthy bones. The best way of maintaining calcium balance is through foods because many other essential nutrients requirement can be met through calcium-rich food. Additional supplementation of calcium can fulfill the insufficiency of calcium through nutritional sources. For adequate absorption of calcium, the recommended consumption is 500 mg or less per meal extended throughout the day. Vitamin D intakes of at least 600 IU per day (up to 1,000 IU/day) in addition to the calcium requirement of 1200 mg per day are prescribed for all individuals older than 70 years. Vitamin D requirement can be met through foods, supplements, and/or multivitamins. Magnesium may be supplemented to frail elderly individuals who are alcoholics and subjected to malabsorption. To maintain the overall nutrients level, protein supplementation along with multivitamin should be prescribed to elderly individuals indicated with poor nutritional status (low albumin levels) or after hip fracture (Nieves 2003).

Vitamin D deficiency may cause many other complications such as breast, prostate, and colon cancers, type 2 diabetes, and cardiovascular disorders including hypertension in elderly subjects as suggested by epidemiological studies. In randomized intervention studies, causality was not observed for any other complication except hypertension. In elderly women, 800 IU (20 µg) vitamin D per day in combination with calcium decreases systolic blood pressure as shown by studies (Mosekilde 2005).

In postmenopausal women, amount of calcium and vitamin D affects the incidences of their bone loss. Increasing the maximum bone mass and decreasing bone loss can reduce the complications and death associated with osteoporosis. Post menopause, up to first 5 or more years, bone loss in women is very fast. During this tenure, high dose of calcium administration humbly decreases cortical loss from long bones without exerting any effect on more trabecular sites such as the spine. The efficacy of supplemental calcium can be increased by vitamin D. Women who attain late postmenopause are reactive to calcium

Nutrition and Healthy Aging   461

addition and those with least dietary calcium consumption are benefitted the most. Bone loss and fracture frequency decrease in women with adequate calcium levels along with vitamin D administration. Accessible findings confirm that the dose of calcium and vitamin D per day in postmenopausal women should be between 1,000 and 1,500 mg and 400 and 800 IU, respectively (Dawson-Hughes 1996).

The efficacy of dietary calcium and vitamin D in parathyroid hormone serum levels and metabolites of vitamin D in elderly women was analyzed by incorporating 376 free-living women in the age group of 65–77 years. The average consumption of calcium in both groups was in the range of prescribed dietary requirement (800 mg/day). In 245 women without vitamin D supplements, the mean vitamin D intake was 3.53 µg/day (141 IU/d), which was less than the prescribed dietary dose of 5 µg/d (200 IU/day). In order to assess the hypothesis, consumption of vitamin D is essential than calcium in decreasing the parathyroid hormone serum concentration; the origin of dietary calcium intake was further divided into milk-nourished with vitamin D and nonmilk sources. An inverse correlation was observed in serum parathyroid hormone level and calcium consumption derived from milk ($r = -0.20$, $P < 0.01$) which was absent for nonmilk sources ($r = -0.06$). The level of serum calcidiol was also related with milk calcium intake ($r = 0.35$, $P < 0.001$), and the same was found to be significantly lowered for non milk calcium intake ($r = 0.01$). Similarly, level of parathyroid hormone and level of calcidiol in serum are inversely correlated ($r = -0.33$, $P < 0.001$). Regression analysis predicted that average parathyroid hormone level in serum can be decreased in elderly subjects to levels recommended as normal in the young. In serum calcidiol level of 122 nmol/L (49 ng/mL), increase in the dietary intake of vitamin D than normal should be included (Kinyamu et al. 1998).

In recent days, noticeable deficiency in vitamin D characterized by rickets or osteomalacia is unusual. Nevertheless, subclinical vitamin D deficiency is very usual and may account to cause skeletal and non-skeletal complications. Management of this involves administration of mixture of vitamin D and calcium. The advantages of combining calcium with vitamin D are not yet confirmed but may account in decreasing stickiness for its bulky and chalky characteristics. Elderly female patients, age greater than 65 years inhabited in community and long-term care institution, were involved in assessing the response of vitamin D alone or combination of vitamin D and calcium on the levels of vitamin D, parathyroid hormone, and bone health. Post administration of 800 IU of vitamin D3 or combined dose of 800 IU vitamin D3 and 1000 mg calcium were administered in an open-label, observational study. Three months post administration, serum concentrations of 25-hydroxy-vitamin D, parathyroid hormone, calcium, phosphate, and alkaline phosphatase were measured. In patients administered with vitamin D alone, serum 25-hydroxy-vitamin D levels raised from baseline levels of 25 ± 16 to 79 ± 16, whereas in those administered with both vitamin D and calcium increased from 35 ± 24 nmol/L to 70 ± 24 nmol/L. Levels of Parathyroid hormone (PTH)

462 Nutrigenomics and Nutraceuticals

in both the groups decreased up to same level. Study concluded that vitamin D alone is as capable as combined calcium/vitamin D in replenishing serum vitamin D concentration in both older community dwelling and institutionalized patients. However, these findings should be further established by prospective randomized trial (Dinizulu et al. 2011).

18.5.2 Antioxidants

Aging and chronic diseases are related with well-known "free radical theory" according to which free radicals (oxidants) generated in body cause cellular damage owing to an increased risk of disease and disability. Free radicals generation can be inhibited by consumption of diets rich in antioxidants including bioactive polyphenol compounds found in fruits and vegetables along with vitamin E and vitamin C which assist in improving health. The theory has been found to be reliable with positive health outcomes and also implicating protective role in cancer, heart disease, and neurodegenerative diseases (Bonnefoy et al. 2002; Hasnis and Reznick 2003; Gomez-Cabrera et al. 2013). There is a well-balanced equilibrium between oxidants, antioxidants, and biomolecules in normal individuals. Impairment in cellular functional is attributed mainly to excessive production of free radicals which outshines the natural cellular antioxidant protective mechanism. Rates and pathogenesis of disease can be reduced by identifying the free radical reactions promoters and means to prevent it. Supplementation with antioxidant is opted for and has received much attention in Western countries even though favorable declaration is still less and ambiguous. The prime drawbacks in literature are still required to be undertaken to sort out the potential benefits from antioxidant supplementation: a) better understanding of oxidation process on the basis of the aging process, b) to evaluate reliable markers of oxidative damage and antioxidant status, c) Recognition of therapeutic window at which antioxidant dose proves to be beneficial d) to discover further potential of antioxidant molecules which may also prove to be pro-oxidants. Studies should be done to provide better understanding on antioxidants and overcome its limitations (Fusco et al. 2007).

Studies to assess the correlation of consumption of antioxidants (vitamin C, vitamin E, and carotene) on the cognitive function in elderly men and women of Utah in Cache County study showed retardation in cognitive decline. Further, the results were confirmed through systematic review of some prospective review, keeping in view to its methodological quality. Around 3831 residents of 65 years or above were included and interviewed through food frequency questionnaire. Cognitive assessment was measured through modified mini-mental state examination (3MS) at baseline and at three subsequent follow-up interviews up to approximately 7 years. Antioxidant nutrient effects on average 3MS score over time were assessed through multivariable-mixed models. Although the systematic review showed similar results, the results are limited and require additional investigations (Rafnsson et al. 2013; Wengreen et al. 2007).

On aging, free radical damage increases causing physiological and clinical alteration. Complications with aging due to free radical reactions comprise elevation of lipid peroxides levels, modifications in enzymatic activities, and increase in osmotic fragility. Studies on elderly adults to investigate the level of lipid peroxidation product MDA and antioxidants catalase and glutathione showed elevation of lipid peroxidation and depletion of antioxidants. In elderly adults suffering from diabetes and hypertension, further MDA elevation and antioxidants depletion were found. Antioxidants supplementation to elderly people is suggested to inhibit more oxidative damage (Wengreen et al. 2007).

Clinical studies involving 986 Italians aged $\geq$ 65 years (a section of Invecchiare in Chianti) to investigate the relationship of plasma concentrations with everyday dietary consumption of antioxidants on the physical activity and strength of skeletal muscle in those elderly adults showed positive association. Increase in plasma antioxidant concentrations increases the muscle strength and physical activity. Consumption of food rich in antioxidants such as vitamin C increases the skeletal muscle strength. The study incorporated the European Prospective Investigation into Cancer and Nutrition (EPIC) questionnaire to investigate the effect of everyday consumption of vitamin C, vitamin E, beta-carotene, and retinol. Plasma concentration of key compounds like alpha- and gamma-tocopherol concentrations was estimated. Physical activity performance was measured through speed of walk, capacity to rise from chair, and standing balance. Hand-held dynamometer was used to measure the muscle strength through knee extension strength (Cesari et al. 2004).

18.5.3 Plant polyphenols and catechins—Curcumin, green tea, and grape seed

Recently, many of the food supplements are occupied by some identified and isolated plant-based antioxidant components (Cherniack 2016; Khurana et al. 2013). Added benefits of these natural antioxidant components are also revealed by the efforts of researchers (Wang et al. 2014). Potent antioxidant, anti-inflammatory, and anticancer properties are found to be imparted by the curcuminoid polyphenols present in the rhizome (underground stem) of the turmeric plant (*Curcuma longa*) which are also responsible for its yellow color. These studies encouraged to investigate the role of curcumin in combating cognitive decline associated with Alzheimer's disease (Mathew et al. 2012; Mithu et al. 2014; Zhang et al. 2010). During the past decade, a plethora of articles is published due to spectacular increase in research corresponding to the usefulness of these components. Polyphenols found in green tea also possess potential antioxidant, anti-inflammatory, and anticancer properties (Fantini et al. 2015). Epigallocatechin-3-gallate (EGCG) is the most acclaimed polyphenol abundant in green tea (Thakur et al. 2012). Being a member of the catechin family, it has not only antioxidant properties but also other biochemical effects in cells. The most prominent health-stimulating effects of EGCG are due to its potent anticancer activities particularly related to hormone-sensitive cancers (Cimino et al. 2012; Zhu et al. 2011). The second leading cause of death in elderly is cancer (NCHS 2015).

One of the prominent sources of polyphenols is grape seed extract (GSE). Its basic molecular structure is similar to catechins of green tea, with the difference that larger molecular size is attained in the components of GSE. Research on grape seed polyphenols for inflammation and cancer at clinical level is not as facilitated as that for the curcumins and green tea catechins; however, numerous animal and *in vitro* studies have shown positive results revealing GSE as oxidative stress detractor, improving circulation apart from its general anti-inflammatory and anticancer effects (Clifton 2004; Feringa et al. 2011).

18.5.4 Carotenoids—Lutein, zeaxanthin, and lycopene

Lutein and zeaxanthin belong to carotenoid family of compounds which is profuse in green leafy vegetables. It possesses numerous health beneficial properties and is present in the macula of the eye which maintains the central vision (Ahmed et al. 2005). In aged population, macular degeneration is a general complication which also comes under one of the four leading eye diseases prevalent in this population group (Wang et al. 2007). Lutein and zeaxanthin supplementation to patients with early signs of macular degeneration came out to be beneficial (Wang et al. 2007). Recent meta-analysis reported that consumption of diets rich in lutein and zeaxanthin reduces the risk of developing late-stage macular degeneration (Mozaffarieh et al. 2003).

Another carotenoid which imparts red to pink color in tomatoes, watermelons, and some other fruits and vegetables is lycopene. It is a potent antioxidant, and epidemiological studies in animal and cell culture support its role in cancer prevention (Seren et al. 2008; Tanaka et al. 2012). However, activity of lycopene in relation with number of cancers still remains uncertain (Hwang and Bowen 2002).

18.5.5 Plant stanols/sterols

Sterols and stanols are naturally available in small amounts in many plant-based foods. They prevent cholesterol absorption and hence can reduce cholesterol levels (Lichtenstein et al. 2001). This property has made the choice of many manufacturers to use sterols and stanols as food supplements that assist in reducing blood cholesterol and risk of heart disease (Gylling et al. 2014). Plant stanols and sterol-enriched food products should be included as a healthy diet for older people as dyslipidemia is an important risk factor for heart diseases in this group of population (Ras et al. 2013).

18.5.6 B vitamins

A new dawn in interest for B vitamins has arisen due to their possible implications in heart disease and cognitive defects (Mohajeri et al. 2015).

Three important B vitamins that take part in metabolic cycles are vitamin B6, vitamin B12, and folate. They play the crucial role of providing the body with methyl groups (one-carbon metabolites). Metabolism of homocysteine which is otherwise a potential risk factor for heart disease is assisted by them (Fiorito et al. 2014). Vitamins are vital for optimum functioning of human physiological system, which include primarily the B-group vitamins in elderly. It is evident that deficiencies related to vitamin B12, B6, and folate, especially in elderly, have been linked to neuro-psychological dysfunction. Cognitive dysfunction and impairment and dementia have also been found to be related to lack of B vitamins in elderly. B-vitamin status is also linked to rise of plasma homocysteine levels, which indirectly plays a pathophysiological role in neuro-cognitive impairment along with inadequate B-vitamin status (Selhub et al. 2010). As a cardiovascular risk factor, hyperhomocysteinemia has been researched well and also linked to prevalence of dementia and cognitive impairment. Due to the participation of B vitamins in homocysteine metabolism, hyperhomocysteinemia has been indicated as a marker, and therefore it is very much essential to know the effect and interrelationship between homocysteine (tHcy) levels and B-vitamin status, especially in elderly population. In a study involving 218 elderly participants in Spain, high prevalence of hyperhomocysteinemia as well as vitamin B deficiency was reported (Gonzalez-Gross et al. 2007).

18.5.7 Omega-3 fatty acids

Some of the rich sources of omega-3 (n-3) fatty acids include fish oil and flaxseeds. N-3 fatty acids have anti-inflammatory effects (Maroon and Bost 2006), lower blood triglycerides (Goh et al. 1997), and also have protective effect in patients suffering from recent myocardial infarction (heart attack) or heart failure (Zhao et al. 2009). Long-term supplementation of pure eicosapentaenoic acid (EPA) in Japanese patients with hypercholesterolemia was found to have 19% reduction in the risk of coronary heart disease and a significant reduction in recurrent stroke as reported by Japan EPA Lipid Intervention Study (JELIS) (Matsuzaki et al. 2009). A prospective cohort study states that higher circulating long-chain omega-3 fatty acids can reduce risk of congestive heart failure (Mozaffarian et al. 2011). In a recent study, the role of omega-3 intake in halting cancer development was reported, which claimed to decrease breast cancer risk in obese Mexican women (Chajès et al. 2012).

A large randomized, double-blind, placebo-controlled study named as VITAL (Vitamin D and Omega-3 Trial) is currently investigating the activity of this compound for primary cancer and cardiovascular disease prevention (Manson et al. 2012). An entrancing breakthrough related to omega-3 fatty acids was its ability to lower incidence of age-related macular degeneration in female health professionals taking higher amount of EPA and Docosahexaenoic acid (DHA) (Krishnadev et al. 2010; Yashodhara et al. 2009).

The whole world is influenced by the growing aging population. Present scenario forecasts a marked inflation of older population interrogating a pleasant life in the additional years of life to be spent. A fuzz-free life independent of expensive medical requirement should be ensured. One of the flair essential nourishment which is at present perceived to rule out the diseases inevitable with aging is omega-3 fatty acids. Even though studies and reports on the influence of omega-3 fatty acids on the process of normal aging in older adults (≥ 65 years), on its overall health conditions including food intake, perception, muscle strength, and bone quality are observed ambiguously, the amount of studies and procedure incorporated is not enough to draw explicit inference on the role of omega-3 fatty acids in metabolism, pathological state, and overall quality of life in the aging population (Ubeda et al. 2012).

Fish oil along with other sources of omega-3 fatty acids is suggested to be defensive toward age-related debilitated cognition and dementia. Mechanisms depicting the suggested benefits are proposed and experimental studies supporting the claim are well-documented. The defensive role of fish consumption on cognitive function is also supported by observational epidemiological and case control studies in aging population. Cochrane review to investigate the beneficial effect of omega-3 fatty acids' nutritional supplementation in cognitive efficiency in healthy older people with adequate cognition and as well of trials with individuals with prevalent poor cognitive function or dementia has been conducted. It revealed seven relevant trials out of which four included cognitively healthy older people and three persons were already with cognitive retardation or dementia, and concluded that no evidence was observed that showed inhibition or progress of cognitive retardation in older age with daily intake of omega-3 fatty acids. In long-term trials, to see the effect of prevention of dementia and cognitive retardation, where careful consideration, especially in recruitment and retention, is required, numerous challenges are to be faced. The negative correlation as investigated by the review suggests that the consequences may be associated due to disagreement in the results of mechanistic and observational data or intrinsic drawback in the framework of published studies, which is yet to be concluded (Dangour et al. 2012).

One of the most promising mainsprings of healthier aging with reduced risk of disability, adequate physical performance, cognitive capability, and maintaining and confirming a better lifestyle is adequate nutritional consumption. With aging, dietary consumption and nourishment absorption reduce and consequently increase the susceptibility of malnutrition, diseases, and death due to disease. Specific nutritional supplements such as long-chain omega-3 polyunsaturated fatty acids (PUFAs) can reduce and inhibit related diseases in older population. It has the potential to regulate inflammation, hyperlipidemia, platelet aggregation, and hypertension. The possible mechanism by which it can exert the beneficial effect may include conditioning of cell membrane function and composition, production of eicosanoid, and gene expression. The risk of cognitive decline in older population can be significantly reduced through omega-3 fatty acids intake. Numerous complications in old age can be prevented through supplementation of omega-3 PUFAs, although its role for healthy bones and reducing loss of muscle mass is yet to be confirmed (Molfino et al. 2014).

18.5.8 Glucosamine, chondroitin quercetin, and collagen

Arthritis is a joint disorder that causes inflammation of the joints. Osteoarthritis also called "wear and tear" arthritis is the most common type of arthritis characterized by morning stiffness and pain in the hips and knees (Matsuno et al. 2009). Cartilage circumvents the edge of bones in joints which may break down on movement and should be repaired. It is made up of type II collagen. The two main constituents of cartilage are glucosamine and chondroitin (Matsuno et al. 2009). Arthritis pain reduction and bone cartilage can be protected by oral administration of both the components. Even though the efficacy of both the compounds in managing osteoarthritis remains unclear (Kanzaki et al. 2012), recently, 40 Japanese subjects suffering from symptomatic knee osteoarthritis in a randomized, double-blind clinical trial, showed improvements in symptoms when administered with a combination of glucosamine hydrochloride, chondroitin sulphate, and quercetin glycosides than those of the placebo (Kanzaki et al. 2012). Similarly, in Spain, 250 subjects with knee osteoarthritis when treated with collagen hydrolysate showed a significant recovery in knee joint comfort (Benito-Ruiz et al. 2009). In a clinical trial study in Belgium, follow-up of subjects when administered with glucosamine sulfate in knee osteoarthritis for 12 months found that glucosamine treatment group was 57% less likely to require total joint replacement surgery in contrast to the placebo group (Bruyere et al. 2008).

18.5.9 Dietary fibers

There are mainly two types of dietary fiber and are termed as soluble fiber or insoluble fiber. Chemically, as both the fiber differ from each other, their metabolic activity also changes accordingly (Aldoori et al. 1998). Soluble dietary fibers are characterized by its water solubility due to which they produce a gelling effect in the intestine which in turn retards the digestion of carbohydrate and can be confirmed by a flattened out postprandial blood glucose curve when observed (Aldoori et al. 1998). Foods such as peas and soybeans are rich in soluble fiber. Due to this metabolic effect, soluble fibers are beneficial for controlling blood glucose levels in diabetes (Vinik and Jenkins 1988). On the contrary, insoluble dietary fibers help in preventing constipation due to their water insolubility and relative indigestibility, thereby increasing the dry matter content of the stool (Anderson et al. 2009).

Fibers are foods or dietary components that are not absorbed in the upper gastrointestinal tract (GIT) of a healthy human being and reach colon to exert their effect. Recently, the definition of fiber has been modified and termed as any substance other than plant cell wall material can be called as fiber. It can be considered as an extension of the previous definition, expanding it beyond carbohydrates. Evidence suggests it as compounds beyond cell wall polysaccharides that can exert the same physiological effects as those of soluble and insoluble polysaccharides. Dietary intake is fruitful in many aspects. It stimulates lipid and glucose metabolism, acts as prebiotics, helps in treating bowel diseases, and can prevent colonic cancer. In geriatric patients, dietary fiber intake is particularly essential. All national dietary guidelines and food guide pyramid for elderly adult emphasize the importance of increasing consumption of fruits and vegetables which are rich sources of dietary fiber (Donini et al. 2009).

In Essex County Geriatric Center, New Jersey, to combat constipation problem in elderly residents, a fiber-rich dietary plan was implemented. It included bran in the hot breakfast cereal that leads to increase in crude fiber content in diet from 4–6 g to 6–8 g. Due to incorporation of bran in the diet, the total dietary fiber intake raised from 25% to 40%. Sixty per cent of the residents were relieved from constipation, of which many of them were on laxative previously. In case of unresponsive residents to this cereal diet plan or those on nasogastric feedings, extra diet on dietary fiber supplementation was implemented. Laxative administration was basically excluded at the center in that year upon initiation of the diet plan, which in turn recorded a decrease of $44,000 in the cost of laxatives in the institution's pharmacy. In case of patients fed on nasogastric feeding, special diet recipes were enclosed to replace bran-supplemented hot cereal with a special fiber-prune juice supplement and a fiber-rich liquid diet (Hull et al. 1980).

Contrary to the above findings, idiopathic constipation and its related complications can be prevented by eliminating or decreasing dietary fiber intake. A study conducted between May 2008 and May 2010 recorded 63 cases of idiopathic constipation after colonoscopy. A 2-week study without fiber diet and then decreasing it to level acceptable to patients was conducted. Sixteen males and 47 females in the age range of 20–80 years (median age 47 years) were included in the study. A total of 41 patients who restricted fiber completely increased their bowel movement rate from one motion per 3.75 days ($\pm$ 1.59 d) to one motion per 1.0 day ($\pm$ 0.0 d) ($P < 0.001$). For 16 patients on low-fiber diet, movement rate increased from a mean one motion per 4.19 days ($\pm$ 2.09 d) to one motion per 1.9 days ($\pm$ 1.21 d) ($P < 0.001$). Six patients who resumed on high-fiber diet have the least bowel movement rate ranging from one motion per 6.83 days ($\pm$ 1.03 d), same prior to and after deliberation. Bloating rates for all the three groups (without fiber, low fiber, and high-fiber diets) were 0%, 31.3%, and 100% ($P < 0.001$), respectively and constrain to pass stool were 0%, 43.8%, and 100% ($P < 0.001$), respectively (Ho et al. 2012).

18.5.10 Prebiotics and probiotics

Naturally, the large intestine is the store house of large number of different bacteria that helps in maintaining a healthy life. These large inhabitants of friendly bacteria are believed to protect the body from unfriendly pathogenic bacteria and yeast (Chow 2002). Dysbiosis or imbalance in the intestinal bacteria may arise during antibiotic treatment which causes many diseases like that of antibiotic-induced diarrheal disease (Balakrishnan and Floch 2012). Thus, the correct bacterial balance can be regenerated in the body by supplementing with good bacteria (probiotics), such as *Lactobacillis* and *Bifidobacterium* families (Douglas and Sanders 2008).

Prebiotics comprises non-digestible food carbohydrates present in certain food supplements that can stimulate the growth of certain intestinal bacteria in the large intestine. Studies on the beneficial effect of intestinal bacteria in health are hands-on and interesting area in current research, although much is still not known. A recent meta-analysis of the studies conducted revealed unambiguous beneficial effect of probiotics in preventing antibiotic-induced diarrheal disease (Conly and Johnston 2004; Douglas and Sanders 2008; McFarland, 2006).

18.5.11 Potassium

Potassium is one of the essential mineral nutrients that plays a critical role in the physiological system. Fruits and vegetables are abundant in potassium content, hence risk of hypertension (high blood pressure) with these type of diet is less, as dietary potassium has beneficial effects on blood pressure as found in some research studies (Delgado 2004; Houston 2011).

The level of potassium is affected with age and also changes the total body potassium (TBK). Administration of diuretics and cardiac failure have greater significant effect on TBK in older age than in youth or middle age. In a study of 19 elderly patients with diuretics and potassium supplements for cardiac failure, average value of TBK to fat-free mass (TBK:FFM) was significantly less as compared with controlled elderly groups. There was about 13.3% average reduction of potassium in patients group receiving diuretic when compared with the control group, suggesting significant reduction in the TBK:FFM ratio (Ibrahim et al. 1978).

TBK and serum potassium concentration are found to increase in elderly patients with heart failure when administered with potassium supplements. Nine elderly patients with controlled heart failure administered with different diuretic regimens (a potassium-sparing diuretic, frusemide, and furosemide with potassium supplements) for a month were assessed to confirm the findings. The results demonstrated that a 7% increase in TBK levels was found for frusemide with potassium supplements as compared with no supplements ($P < 0.001$) along with increase in serum potassium levels from 4.1 mmol/L to 4.8 mmol/L ($P < 0.01$). This same effect was observed for potassium-sparing diuretic for the TBK levels in six patients. In three cases, the potassium-sparing diuretics did not show increase in TBK when compared with frusemide alone (Potter et al. 1984).

In the United States, elderly population is increasing tremendously and by 2050, the number is expected to be doubled. Aging is accompanied by deleterious health changes affecting many organs including kidney. Post age 40, renal plasma flow and glomerular filtration rate decrease due to increase in the level of cortical glomerulosclerosis. Certain adverse consequences are observed in elderly patients when there is imbalance in electrolyte due to these degenerative changes in kidney. Normally, a perfect water and electrolyte balance is maintained which is likely to be diminished due to a particular illness, depletion in cognition capacity, or on particular medicine regimen. Elderly people suffer from hypernatremia and hyponatremia where electrolyte imbalance in the body occur due to their decline in the efficiency of excreting a concentrated or a dilute urine including ammonium, sodium, or potassium. All these complications lead to higher mortality rates in elderly patients (Schlanger et al. 2010).

Published literature suggests that geriatric patients have the tendency to develop hyperkalemia due to natural imbalance in potassium homeostasis as well as prevalence of diseases that prejudice potassium levels. Elderly people are also likely to be susceptible to hyperkalemia, especially on medications that alert the levels of potassium in the body. Critical diseases such as neuromuscular and cardiac complications can be avoided by proper management of hyperkalemia in them. Management of hyperkalemia is possible by proper awareness such as identifying the risk in physiology, prevention of high-risk medicines, and keeping an eye on plasma potassium concentration and renal function at regular intervals on the medication duration. Once the clinical appearance of hyperkalemia is observed, cellular potassium uptake stimulation, cardiac tissue stabilization, and depletion of potassium from body can manage the complications (Perazella and Mahnensmith 1997).

18.5.12 Whey protein

One of the important protein constituent of milk is whey protein, which is known to show beneficial effect on health. In a recent study on elderly men, it was found that when higher amounts of whey protein (35 g versus 10 g) were fed, it caused increase in amino acid absorption as well increase in muscle protein synthesis (Devries and Phillips 2015). Moreover, whey protein has greater positive impact on muscle synthesis rates than feeding casein to the same group (Wilborn et al. 2013). Studies clearly reveal the beneficial effect of whey protein on building muscle mass in the elderly, as loss of LBM (sarcopenia) is common in aged population, which leads to weakness and disability (Denison et al. 2015; Katsanos et al. 2008).

18.5.13 Zinc

Zinc is one of the essential trace elements which has important biochemical role in a wide variety of reactions as well as DNA synthesis, cell proliferation, and differentiation (Prasad 2008; Tuerk and Fazel 2009). Its deficiency weakens immune system and when administered along with antioxidants, it may involve in defending people from macular degeneration (Rink and Gabriel 2000; Tuerk and Fazel 2009).

Zinc is an important micronutrient which plays a major role in maintaining healthy lifestyle, especially in elderly adults. Zinc insufficiency may cause cell-mediated immune malfunction and increase risk to infections and oxidative stress in elderly adults those above 55 years. It is a potent anti-inflammatory and antioxidative agent. The response of zinc on the frequency of over-all infections as well as cytokines and oxidative stress markers in elderly adults was analyzed through randomized, double-blind, placebo-controlled with zinc supplements clinical trials in elderly adults. The age group of the 50 healthy subjects included in the study ranged between 55 and 87 years, comprising both male and female of all ethnic groups. Zinc gluconate (45 mg elemental Zn/day) was administered orally to the zinc supplement group for 12 months. Frequency of infections and production of inflammatory cytokines was recorded during the zinc intervention period. Plasma concentration of T helper 1 and T helper 2 cytokines and oxidative stress markers was also ana-lyzed after administration. Zinc plasma concentration was significantly higher in younger adults group as that of the elderly adults, whereas ex vivo genera-tion of inflammatory cytokines and interleukin 10, plasma oxidative stress markers, and endothelial cell adhesion molecules was higher in elderly adults. Zinc-intervened group has significantly lower frequency of infections and ex vivo generation of tumor necrosis factor alpha and plasma oxidative stress markers than the placebo group. Moreover, significantly higher level of zinc plasma, phytohemagglutin-induced interleukin 2 mRNA in isolated mono-nuclear cells, was found in zinc-intervened groups than that of the placebo (Prasad et al. 2007).

Zinc (Zn) in elderly subjects is also specifically important for behavioral and mental function. It is the most significant micronutrient for bone metabolism and a proper immune and antioxidant system. Numerous physiological, social, psychological, and economic factors may jeopardize the nutritional status of elderly adults. Absorption and metabolism of nutrition alter with age due to deterioration of physiological function. Food habits and preferences changes with age and are affected by social and economic conditions. Nevertheless, nutrient requirement of the elderly for specific nutrient (such as vitamins, minerals, and proteins) is more than for younger adults (Meunier et al. 2005).

Zinc levels are depleted naturally in elderly adults. It is essential for growth and development including synthesis of DNA, neurosensory functions, and cell-mediated immunity. Lack of zinc and its response on cell-mediated immu-nity in elderly adults are not yet acclaimed. The position of zinc and nutrition on elderly adults was assessed in randomly selected 180 healthy subjects in a study termed as "A Model Health Promotion and Intervention Program for Urban Middle Aged and Elderly Americans." Although the prescribed dietary dose is 15 mg/day, the average dietary consumption of zinc was 9.06 mg/day. As compared to the younger adults of the control group, the level of zinc in granulocytes and lymphocytes was less but plasma zinc concentration was normal. Zinc concentration in both granulocytes and lymphocytes was available in 118 elderly adults but 36 of them lacked the desired level. Production of interleukin 1 (IL-1) was reduced and plasma copper concentration rose. The subjects reduced taste interest and response to the skin-test antigen panel also decreased. Further, 13 elderly zinc-insufficient adults were administered with zinc and different variables were analyzed before and after zinc administration. Along with maintaining the normal level of zinc, its administration maintained the levels of copper. Significant increase in serum thymulin activity, IL-1 production, and lymphocyte ecto-5′-nucleotidase was also observed. Amelioration of all other conditions was observed after zinc supplementation. Thus, slight depletion in the normal levels of zinc may exert serious clinical complications in healthy elderly adults (Prasad et al. 1993).

18.5.14 Coenzyme Q10

Coenzyme Q10 resembles vitamin and plays a prime role in aerobic respiration of the cell in mitochondria, generating ATP to be used as energy by the cells. It is also a potent antioxidant that can prevent oxidative stress (Yamamoto 2016). The inflammatory marker IL-6 is found to be reduced in patients with coronary artery disease when supplemented with coenzyme Q10 (Lee et al. 2012), depicting its anti-inflammatory effect. It is also known to promote endothelial function in patients with heart disease as shown by some studies (Gao et al. 2012; Littarru et al. 2011). A recent study in Chinese women cleared the implication of coenzyme Q10 in cancer prevention as it was found that with decrease in plasma coenzyme Q10 levels, risk of breast cancer was increased (Cooney et al. 2011).

Coenzyme Q10 (CoQ10) is also effective in treating community-acquired pneumonia (CAP), which leads to complications and death in geriatric patients. The efficacy of this adjunctive was assessed in CAP-diagnosed, hospitalized patients administered with oral CoQ10 (200 mg/d) for 14 days with antibiotics. CURB-65 index was utilized to analyze the seriousness of the disease. Out of 150 patients registered in the study, 141 were included in the study, 71 patients in the control, and 70 patients in the trial group. The age groups of the patients in the trial and control group were 67.6 ± 7.2 years and 68.7 ± 7.9 years, respectively. At days 3 and 7, clinical cure were 24 (34.3%) and 62 (88.6%) in the trial group (P value = 0.6745) and 22 (31%) and 52 (73.2%) in the placebo group (P value = 0.0209). Moreover, the trial group has faster defervescence ($P = 0.0206$) and lesser hospital stay ($P = 0.0144$) as that of the placebo group. There were changes in the clinical cure at day 14 when compared with subgroup with severe pneumonia. Although adverse effects were less and similar in both the groups, failure in treatment was less for CoQ10 group than in the placebo group (10% versus 22.5% and $P = 0.0440$) (Farazi et al. 2014).

In males, there are changes in the plasma concentration of antioxidants such as coenzyme Q (10) along with decrease in fat-free body mass (FFM) with aging. One of the major components of FFM is muscle tissue and with aging, metabolic rate decreases; therefore, serum CoQ(10) acts as an indirect index of metabolic activity in the elderly. However, decrease in serum CoQ(10) is not related to aging alone but also to FFM. Serum CoQ(10) concentrations of 73 non-obese, healthy males divided into 4 age groups 20–55 (n = 23), 56–70 (n = 20), 71–90 (n = 8), and 91–100 (n = 22) were analyzed by High-Performance Liquid Chromatography (HPLC). Multi-frequency bioimpedance analysis was utilized to measure the body composition. The group in the age range of 91–100 years revealed lower serum CoQ(10) levels and FFM than the other age groups (p < 0.001). Multi-regression analysis shows that there is correlation between serum CoQ(10) and FFM (p < 0.01), but not for serum CoQ(10) and age (Ravaglia et al. 1996). Selenium and coenzyme Q10 are known to be important antioxidants in the body. Significant reduction in cardiovascular mortality was recorded in healthy elderly group of participants in a 10-year follow-up study administered with selenium and coenzyme Q10 for 4 years. This defensive function was not only restricted to the 4 years intervention period but also lasted in the follow-up period. The mechanism by which this effect is produced is yet to be evaluated and these findings are thus data for generating a hypothesis (Alehagen et al. 2015).

18.6 Formulation challenges

It is essential to consider a number of technical issues to formulate and commercialize a novel fortified food product apart from choosing product components that are suitable with different cultural, ethnic, and medical concerns of aged population during its inception. All these factors encompass the chemical compatibility between the nutrient ingredients, final product approval along with its stability, taste and texture as well as product shelf-life. As many physiological alterations along with loss of taste (ageusia) are associated with aging (Fikentscher et al. 1977; Hoffman et al. 2009), therefore, these issues should also be taken into account for commercialization of new fortified products to strike the aged market. During preformulation studies, addition of flavor enhancers as well their consistency should be carefully addressed and analyzed to get a suitable product. It is utmost essential to consider flavor, masking bad taste and incorporating colorants to the product for its successful launching. An enticing product can be produced by addressing its color intensity, enhancing texture by addition of herbs and spices, and a number of other ingredients during its premix or else in the finished product. One of the prime factors that should be kept in priority is that of investing its possible chemical interaction with common medicines taken in the aged population. As for example, grape fruit juice may have possible interaction with some immunosuppressant drugs (statins) (Bailey et al. 1998) used to lower blood cholesterol, and calcium-channel blockers used to treat high blood pressure (Lim et al. 2003), hence, other fortifying juices, drinks, or health supplements without any possible chemical interactions could be beneficial for the aged population. Moreover, careful reading and surveillance of the labels of supplements as well as foods in packages should be practiced while procuring for elderly population.

18.7 Future opportunities

Mostly, five countries (China, India, United States, Japan, and Russia) of the world are inhabited by 50% of the world's oldest populations. Asia along with rest of the developing world in addition to the United States and Europe is the hub for aged market. Recent demographic studies indicate a total of 901 million older populations (people aged 60 or above) in the world, of which majority of inhabitants are in developing countries. It is estimated that the percent of the world's elderly persons will abode in developing countries by 2020 (UN 2015). More scope for marketing fortified products will be generated for various demographic subgroups within this population in order to hit the aged market.

18.8 Conclusion

Aging is inevitable and universal. The older adult population is growing and is also expected to grow more, which will present potential challenging issues for the individuals and the society. The health care fraternity will be imposed with more responsibilities in terms of caring the elderly as well as managing older adults' health care needs. In future, healthy aging will be encompassed with the careful maintenance of the health of the elderly population. Nutrition science and lifestyle practices will be the major deciding modalities in conceptualizing the process of aging in good health. Moreover, to promote healthy aging and care, it is also very much significant to get an overview of older adults' self-rated health status. The food industry should also be indulged in careful designing of packaged food products, especially for elderly population with proper disclosure of ingredients used in the products. The industry should also focus on the careful selection of food ingredients and additives while targeting the elderly population depending upon solid research evidence. It is a high time to rationalize the lifestyle in terms of healthy nutrition through systematic research on healthy aging and nutrition.

References

Ahmed, F. E. 1992. Effect of nutrition on the health of the elderly. *J Am Diet Assoc*, 92, 1102–8.
Ahmed, S. S., Lott, M. N. & Marcus, D. M. 2005. The macular xanthophylls. *Surv Ophthalmol*, 50, 183–93.
Akbulut, G. Ç. & Ersoy, G. 2008. Assessment of nutrition and life quality scores of individuals aged 65 and over from different socio-economic levels in Turkey. *Arch Gerontol Geriatr*, 47, 241–52.

Akila, V. P., Harishchandra, H., D'souza, V. & D'souza, B. 2007. Age related changes in lipid peroxidation and antioxidants in elderly people. *Indian J Clin Biochem,* 22, 131–4.

Aldoori, W. H., Giovannucci, E. L., Rockett, H. R., Sampson, L., Rimm, E. B. & Willett, W. C. 1998. A prospective study of dietary fiber types and symptomatic diverticular disease in men. *J Nutr,* 128, 714–9.

Alehagen, U., Aaseth, J. & Johansson, P. 2015. Reduced cardiovascular mortality 10 years after supplementation with selenium and coenzyme Q10 for four years: Follow-up results of a prospective randomized double-blind placebo-controlled trial in elderly citizens. *PLoS One,* 10(12), e0141641. doi: 10.1371/journal.pone.0141641.

Amarya, S., Singh, K. & Sabharwal, M. 2015. Changes during aging and their association with malnutrition. *J Clin Gerontol Geriatr,* 6, 78–84.

Anderson, B. D. & Anderson, R. M. 2014. Nutritional Modulation of Aging. *Reference Module in Biomedical Sciences.* Michael Caplan (editor). San Francisco, CA: Elsevier.

Anderson, J. W., Baird, P., Davis, R. H. Jr., Ferreri, S., Knudtson, M., Koraym, A., Waters, V. & Williams, C. L. 2009. Health benefits of dietary fiber. *Nutr Rev,* 67(4), 188–205.

Anonymous. 2014. *What Does Healthy Eating Mean ? [Online].* 120 East Lancaster Avenue, Suite 201 Ardmore, PA 19003: Breastcancer.org Available: http://www.breastcancer.org/tips/nutrition/healthy_eat. Accessed May 02, 2016.

Bailey, D. G., Malcolm, J., Arnold, O. & David Spence, J. 1998. Grapefruit juice–drug interactions. *Br J Clin Pharmacol,* 46, 101–10.

Balakrishnan, M. & Floch, M. H. 2012. Prebiotics, probiotics and digestive health. *Curr Opin Clin Nutr Metab Care,* 15(6), 580–5.

Barkoukis, H. 2016. Nutrition Recommendations in Elderly and Aging. *Medical Clinics of North America,* 100, 1237–1250.

Benito-Ruiz, P., Camacho-Zambrano, M. M., Carrillo-Arcentales, J. N., Mestanza-Peralta, M. A., Vallejo-Flores, C. A., Vargas-Lopez, S. V., Villacis-Tamayo, R. A. & Zurita-Gavilanes, L. A. 2009. A randomized controlled trial on the efficacy and safety of a food ingredient, collagen hydrolysate, for improving joint comfort. *Int J Food Sci Nutr,* 60 Suppl 2, 99–113. doi: 10.1080/09637480802498820.

Bonnefoy, M., Drai, J. & Kostka, T. 2002. Antioxidants to slow aging, facts and perspectives. *Presse Med,* 31, 1174–84.

Bruyere, O., Pavelka, K., Rovati, L. C., Gatterová, J., Giacovelli, G., Olejarová, M., Deroisy, R. & Reginster, J. Y. 2008. Total joint replacement after glucosamine sulphate treatment in knee osteoarthritis: Results of a mean 8-year observation of patients from two previous 3-year, randomised, placebo-controlled trials. *Osteoarthritis Cartilage,* 16, 254–60.

CDC. 2003. *Public Health and Aging: Trends in Aging—United States and Worldwide. Morbidity and Mortality Weekly Report (MMWR) [Online],* 52. Washington, DC: U.S. Government Printing Office (GPO).

CDC. 2013. *Death and Mortality: NCHS FastStats [Online].* Available: http://www.cdc.gov/nchs/fastats/deaths.htm [Accessed 20 December 2015].

CDC. 2015. *2015–2020 Dietary Guidelines—health.gov [Online].* Available: http://health.gov/dietaryguidelines/2015/guidelines/files/56/guidelines.html. Accessed April 04, 2016.

Cesari, M., Pahor, M., Bartali, B., Cherubini, A., Penninx, B. W., Williams, G. R., Atkinson, H., Martin, A., Guralnik, J. M. & Ferrucci, L. 2004. Antioxidants and physical performance in elderly persons: The Invecchiare in Chianti (InCHIANTI) study. *Am J Clin Nutr,* 79, 289–94.

Chajès, V., Torres-Mejía, G., Biessy, C., Ortega-Olvera, C., Angeles-Lleranas, A., Ferrari, P., Lazcano-Ponce, E. & Romieu, I. 2012. ω-3 and ω-6 polyunsaturated fatty acid intakes and the risk of breast cancer in Mexican women: Impact of obesity status. *Cancer Epidemiol Biomarkers Prev,* 21, 319–26.

Chappell, N. L. & Cooke, H. A. 2010. Age Related Disabilities—Aging and Quality of Life. *In:* Stone, J. H. & Blouin, M. (eds.) *International Encyclopedia of Rehabilitation.* New York: University at Buffalo, State University of New York, 1–14.

Cherniack, E. P. 2016. Polyphenols and Aging A2—Malavolta, Marco. *In:* Mocchegiani, E. (ed.), *Molecular Basis of Nutrition and Aging.* San Diego, CA: Academic Press, 649–98.

Chow, J. 2002. Probiotics and prebiotics: A brief overview. *J Ren Nutr,* 12, 76–86.

Cimino, S., Sortino, G., Favilla, V., Castelli, T., Madonia, M., Sansalone, S., Russo, G. I. & Morgia, G. 2012. Polyphenols: Key issues involved in chemoprevention of prostate cancer. *Oxid Med Cell Longev,* 2012, 632959.

Clifton, P. M. 2004. Effect of grape seed extract and quercetin on cardiovascular and endothelial parameters in high-risk subjects. *J Biomed Biotechnol,* 2004, 272–8.

Conly, J. M. & Johnston, L. B. 2004. Coming full circle: From antibiotics to probiotics and prebiotics. *Can J Infect Dis Med Microbiol,* 15, 161–3.

Cooney, R. V., Dai, Q., Gao, Y.-T., Chow, W.-H., Franke, A. A., Shu, X.-O., Li, H., et al. 2011. Low plasma coenzyme Q10 levels and breast cancer risk in Chinese women. *Cancer Epidemiol Biomarkers Prev,* 20, 1124–30.

Dangour, A. D., Andreeva, V. A., Sydenham, E. & Uauy, R. 2012. Omega 3 fatty acids and cognitive health in older people. *Br J Nutr,* 107 Suppl 2, S152–8.

Dawson-Hughes, B. 1996. Calcium and vitamin D nutritional needs of elderly women. *J Nutr,* 126, 1165S–7S.

Delgado, M. C. 2004. Potassium in hypertension. *Curr Hypertens Rep,* 6, 31–5.

Denison, H. J., Cooper, C., Sayer, A. A. & Robinson, S. M. 2015. Prevention and optimal management of sarcopenia: A review of combined exercise and nutrition interventions to improve muscle outcomes in older people. *Clin Interv Aging,* 10, 859–69.

Devries, M. C. & Phillips, S. M. 2015. Supplemental protein in support of muscle mass and health: Advantage whey. *J Food Sci,* 80 Suppl 1, A8–15.

Dinizulu, T., Griffin, D., Carey, J. & Mulkerrin, E. 2011. Vitamin D supplementation versus combined calcium and vitamin D in older female patients—An observational study. *J Nutr Health Aging,* 15, 605–8.

Donini, L. M., Savina, C. & Cannella, C. 2009. Nutrition in the elderly: Role of fiber. *Arch Gerontol Geriatr,* 49 Suppl 1, 61–9.

Douglas, L. C. & Sanders, M. E. 2008. Probiotics and prebiotics in dietetics practice. *J Am Diet Assoc,* 108(3), 510–21.

Evans, W. J. & Cyr-Campbell, D. 1997. Nutrition, exercise, and healthy aging. *J Am Diet Assoc,* 97, 632–8.

Everitt, A. V., Hilmer, S. N., Brand-Miller, J. C., Jamieson, H. A., Truswell, A. S., Sharma, A. P., Mason, R. S., Morris, B. J. & Le Couteur, D. G. 2006. Dietary approaches that delay age-related diseases. *Clin Interv Aging,* 1, 11–31.

Fantini, M., Benvenuto, M., Masuelli, L., Frajese, G. V., Tresoldi, I., Modesti, A. & Bei, R. 2015. In vitro and in vivo antitumoral effects of combinations of polyphenols, or polyphenols and anticancer drugs: Perspectives on cancer treatment. *Int J Mol Sci,* 16, 9236–82.

Farazi, A., Sofian, M., Jabbariasl, M. & Nayebzadeh, B. 2014. Coenzyme q10 administration in community-acquired pneumonia in the elderly. *Iran Red Crescent Med J,* 16(12), e18852. doi: 10.5812/ircmj.18852.

Feringa, H. H., Laskey, D. A., Dickson, J. E. & Coleman, C. I. 2011. The effect of grape seed extract on cardiovascular risk markers: A meta-analysis of randomized controlled trials. *J Am Diet Assoc,* 111(8), 1173–81.

Fikentscher, R., Roseburg, B., Spinar, H. & Bruchmuller, W. 1977. Loss of taste in the elderly: Sex differences. *Clin Otolaryngol Allied Sci,* 2, 183–9.

Fiorito, G., Guarrera, S., Valle, C., Ricceri, F., Russo, A., Grioni, S., Mattiello, A., et al. 2014. B-vitamins intake, DNA-methylation of one carbon metabolism and homocysteine pathway genes and myocardial infarction risk: The EPICOR study. *Nutr Metab Cardiovasc Dis,* 24, 483–8.

Fusco, D., Colloca, G., Monaco, M. R. L. & Cesari, M. 2007. Effects of antioxidant supplementation on the aging process. *Clin Interv Aging,* 2, 377–87.

Gao, L., Mao, Q., Cao, J., Wang, Y., Zhou, X. & Fan, L. 2012. Effects of coenzyme Q10 on vascular endothelial function in humans: A meta-analysis of randomized controlled trials. *Atherosclerosis,* 221(2), 311–6. doi: 10.1016/j.atherosclerosis.2011.10.027.

Garriguet, D. 2011. Bone health: Osteoporosis, calcium and vitamin D. *Health Rep,* 22, 7–14.

Gennari, C. 2001. Calcium and vitamin D nutrition and bone disease of the elderly. *Public Health Nutr,* 4, 547–59.

Goh, Y. K., Jumpsen, J. A., Ryan, E. A. & Clandinin, M. T. 1997. Effect of omega 3 fatty acid on plasma lipids, cholesterol and lipoprotein fatty acid content in NIDDM patients. *Diabetologia,* 40, 45–52.

Gomez-Cabrera, M. C., Ferrando, B., Brioche, T., Sanchis-Gomar, F. & Viña, J. 2013. Exercise and antioxidant supplements in the elderly. *J Sport Health Sci,* 2, 94–100.

Gong, X. and Rubin, L. P. 2015. Role of macular xanthophylls in prevention of common neovascular retinopathies: Retinopathy of prematurity and diabetic retinopathy. *Archives of Biochemistry and Biophysics,* 572, 40–48.

Gonzalez-Gross, M., Sola, R., Albers, U., Barrios, L., Alder, M., Castillo, M. J. & Pietrzik, K. 2007. B-vitamins and homocysteine in Spanish institutionalized elderly. *Int J Vitam Nutr Res,* 77, 22–33.

Gupta, V., Downs, S. M., Ghosh-Jerath, S., Lock, K. & Singh, A. 2016. Unhealthy fat in street and snack foods in low-socioeconomic settings in India: A case study of the food environments of rural villages and an urban slum. *J Nutr Educ Behav,* 48, 269–279.e1.

Gylling, H., Plat, J., Turley, S., Ginsberg, H. N., Ellegård, L., Jessup, W., Jones, P. J., et al. 2014. Plant sterols and plant stanols in the management of dyslipidaemia and prevention of cardiovascular disease. *Atherosclerosis,* 232, 346–60.

Hasnis, E. & Reznick, A. Z. 2003. Antioxidants and healthy aging. *Isr Med Assoc J,* 5, 368–70.

Ho, K.-S., Tan, C. Y. M., Mohd Daud, M. A. & Seow-Choen, F. 2012. Stopping or reducing dietary fiber intake reduces constipation and its associated symptoms. *World J Gastroenterol,* 18, 4593–6.

Hoffman, H. J., Cruickshanks, K. J. & Davis, B. 2009. Perspectives on population-based epidemiological studies of olfactory and taste impairment. *Ann N Y Acad Sci,* 1170, 514–30.

Houston, M. C. 2011. The importance of potassium in managing hypertension. *Curr Hypertens Rep,* 13(4), 309–17.

Hull, C., Greco, R. S. & Brooks, D. L. 1980. Alleviation of constipation in the elderly by dietary fiber supplementation. *J Am Geriatr Soc,* 28, 410–4.

Hwang, E. S. & Bowen, P. E. 2002. Can the consumption of tomatoes or lycopene reduce cancer risk? *Integr Cancer Ther,* 1, 121–32.

Ibrahim, I. K., Ritch, A. E., Maclennan, W. J. & May, T. 1978. Are potassium supplements for the elderly necessary? *Age Ageing,* 7, 165–70.

Kalaiselvi, S., Arjumand, Y., Jayalakshmy, R., Gomathi, R., Pruthu, T. & Palanivel, C. 2016. Prevalence of under-nutrition, associated factors and perceived nutritional status among elderly in a rural area of Puducherry, South India. *Arch Gerontol Geriatr,* 65, 156–70.

Kanzaki, N., Saito, K., Maeda, A., Kitagawa, Y., Kiso, Y., Watanabe, K., Tomonaga, A., Nagaoka, I. & Yamaguchi, H. 2012. Effect of a dietary supplement containing glucosamine hydrochloride, chondroitin sulfate and quercetin glycosides on symptomatic knee osteoarthritis: A randomized, double-blind, placebo-controlled study. *J Sci Food Agric,* 92(4), 862–9. doi: 10.1002/jsfa.4660.

Katsanos, C. S., Chinkes, D. L., Paddon-Jones, D., Zhang, X.-J., Aarsland, A. & Wolfe, R. R. 2008. Whey protein ingestion in elderly results in greater muscle protein accrual than ingestion of its constituent essential amino acid content. *Nutr Res (New York, N.Y.),* 28, 651–8.

Khandelwal, S., Siegel, K. R. & Narayan, K. M. V. 2013. Nutrition research in India: Underweight, stunted, or wasted? *Global Heart,* 8, 131–7.

Khurana, S., Venkataraman, K., Hollingsworth, A., Piche, M. & Tai, T. C. 2013. Polyphenols: Benefits to the cardiovascular system in health and in aging. *Nutrients,* 5, 3779–827.

Kinyamu, H. K., Gallagher, J. C., Rafferty, K. A. & Balhorn, K. E. 1998. Dietary calcium and vitamin D intake in elderly women: Effect on serum parathyroid hormone and vitamin D metabolites. *Am J Clin Nutr,* 67, 342–8.

Krishnadev, N., Meleth, A. D. & Chew, E. Y. 2010. Nutritional supplements for age-related macular degeneration. *Curr Opin Ophthalmol,* 21, 184–9.

Krishnaswamy, K. & Prasad, M. P. R. 2001. The changing epidemiologic scene: malnutrition versus chronic diseases in India. *Nutrition,* 17, 166–7.

Lee, B. J., Huang, Y. C., Chen, S. J. & Lin, P. T. 2012. Effects of coenzyme Q10 supplementation on inflammatory markers (high-sensitivity C-reactive protein, interleukin-6, and homocysteine) in patients with coronary artery disease. *Nutrition,* 28(7–8), 767–72. doi: 10.1016/j.nut.2011.11.008.

Lichtenstein, A. H., Deckelbaum, R. J. & Committee, F. T. A. H. A. N. 2001. Stanol/sterol ester–containing foods and blood cholesterol levels: A statement for healthcare professionals from the nutrition committee of the Council on Nutrition, Physical Activity, and Metabolism of the American Heart Association. *Circulation,* 103, 1177–9.

Lim, G. E., Li, T. & Buttar, H. S. 2003. Interactions of grapefruit juice and cardiovascular medications: A potential risk of toxicity. *Exp & Clin Cardiol,* 8, 99–107.

Littarru, G. P., Tiano, L., Belardinelli, R. & Watts, G. F. 2011. Coenzyme Q(10), endothelial function, and cardiovascular disease. *Biofactors,* 37(5), 366–73. doi: 10.1002/biof.154.

López-Otín, C., Blasco, M. A., Partridge, L., Serrano, M. & Kroemer, G. 2013. The Hallmarks of Aging. *Cell,* 153, 1194-1217.

Manson, J. E., Bassuk, S. S., Lee, I. M., Cook, N. R., Albert, M. A., Gordon, D., Zaharris, E., et al. 2012. The VITamin D and OmegA-3 TriaL (VITAL): Rationale and design of a large randomized controlled trial of vitamin D and marine omega-3 fatty acid supplements for the primary prevention of cancer and cardiovascular disease. *Contemp Clin Trials,* 33, 159–71.

Maroon, J. C. & Bost, J. W. 2006. Omega-3 fatty acids (fish oil) as an anti-inflammatory: An alternative to nonsteroidal anti-inflammatory drugs for discogenic pain. *Surg Neurol,* 65, 326–31.

Mathew, A., Fukuda, T., Nagaoka, Y., Hasumura, T., Morimoto, H., Yoshida, Y., Maekawa, T., Venugopal, K. & Kumar, D. S. 2012. Curcumin loaded-PLGA nanoparticles conjugated with Tet-1 peptide for potential use in Alzheimer's disease. *PLoS One,* 7, e32616.

Matsuno, H., Nakamura, H., Katayama, K., Hayashi, S., Kano, S., Yudoh, K. & Kiso, Y. 2009. Effects of an oral administration of glucosamine-chondroitin-quercetin glucoside on the synovial fluid properties in patients with osteoarthritis and rheumatoid arthritis. *Biosci Biotechnol Biochem* 73, 288–92.

Matsuzaki, M., Yokoyama, M., Saito, Y., Origasa, H., Ishikawa, Y., Oikawa, S., Sasaki, J., et al. 2009. Incremental effects of eicosapentaenoic acid on cardiovascular events in statin-treated patients with coronary artery disease secondary prevention analysis from JELIS. *Circ J,* 73, 1283–90.

Mcfarland, L. V. 2006. Meta-analysis of probiotics for the prevention of antibiotic associated diarrhea and the treatment of *Clostridium difficile* disease. *Am J Gastroenterol,* 101, 812–22.

Meunier, N., O'Connor, J. M., Maiani, G., Cashman, K. D., Secker, D. L., Ferry, M., Roussel, A. M. & Coudray, C. 2005. Importance of zinc in the elderly: The ZENITH study. *Eur J Clin Nutr,* 59, S1–4.

Mithu, V. S., Sarkar, B., Bhowmik, D., Das, A. K., Chandrakesan, M., Maiti, S. & Madhu, P. K. 2014. Curcumin alters the salt bridge-containing turn region in amyloid β(1–42) aggregates. *J Biol Chem,* 289, 11122–31.

Mohajeri, M. H., Troesch, B. & Weber, P. 2015. Inadequate supply of vitamins and DHA in the elderly: Implications for brain aging and Alzheimer-type dementia. *Nutrition,* 31, 261–75.

Molfino, A., Gioia, G., Fanelli, F. R. & Muscaritoli, M. 2014. The role for dietary omega-3 fatty acids supplementation in older adults. *Nutrients*, 6, 4058–72.

Mosekilde, L. 2005. Vitamin D and the elderly. *Clin Endocrinol*, 62, 265-81.

Mozaffarian, D., Lemaitre, R. N., King, I. B., Song, X., Spiegelman, D., Sacks, F. M., Rimm, E. B. & Siscovick, D. S. 2011. Circulating long-chain ω-3 fatty acids and incidence of congestive heart failure in older adults: The cardiovascular health study a cohort study. *Ann Intern Med*, 155, 160–70.

Mozaffarieh, M., Sacu, S. & Wedrich, A. 2003. The role of the carotenoids, lutein and zeaxanthin, in protecting against age-related macular degeneration: A review based on controversial evidence. *Nutr J*, 2, 1–8.

Murray, C. J. & Lopez, A. D. 1997. Mortality by cause for eight regions of the world: Global burden of disease study. *The Lancet*, 349, 1269–76.

NCHS. 2015. *Health, United States, 2014: With Special Feature on Adults Aged 55–64. National Center for Health Statistics [Online]. Available: www.cdc.gov/nchs/hus.htm.* Accessed April 11, 2016.

Nieves, J. W. 2003. Calcium, vitamin D, and nutrition in elderly adults. *Clin Geriatr Med*, 19, 321–35.

Nordqvist, C. 2016. Malnutrition: Causes, symptoms and treatments. *Medical News Today [Online].* Available: <http://www.medicalnewstoday.com/articles/179316.php>. Accessed April 11, 2016.

Oggioni, C., Lara, J., Wells, J. C. K., Soroka, K. & Siervo, M. 2014. Shifts in population dietary patterns and physical inactivity as determinants of global trends in the prevalence of diabetes: An ecological analysis. *Nutr Metab Cardiovasc Dis*, 24, 1105–11.

Payette, H. & Shatenstein, B. 2005. Determinants of healthy eating in community-dwelling elderly people. *Can J Public Health*, 96, S30–5.

Perazella, M. A. & Mahnensmith, R. L. 1997. Hyperkalemia in the elderly: Drugs exacerbate impaired potassium homeostasis. *J Gen Intern Med*, 12, 646–56.

Piple, J., Gora, R., Purbiya, P., Puliyel, A., Chugh, P., Bahl, P. & Puliyel, J. 2015. Food choices and consequences for the nutritional status: Insights into nutrition transition in an hospital community. *PLoS One*, 10(11), e0140807. doi: 10.1371/journal. pone.0140807.

Popkin, B. M. 2013. *Nutrition Transition, Diet Change, and its Implications A2—Caballero, Benjamin. Encyclopedia of Human Nutrition* (3rd ed.). Waltham, MA: Academic Press.

Potter, J. M., Blake, G. M. & Cox, J. R. 1984. Potassium supplements and total body potassium in elderly patients. *Age Ageing*, 13, 238–42.

Prasad, A. S. 2008. Zinc in human health: Effect of zinc on immune cells. *Mol Med*, 14(5–6), 353–7.

Prasad, A. S., Beck, F. W., Bao, B., Fitzgerald, J. T., Snell, D. C., Steinberg, J. D. & Cardozo, L. J. 2007. Zinc supplementation decreases incidence of infections in the elderly: Effect of zinc on generation of cytokines and oxidative stress. *Am J Clin Nutr*, 85, 837–44.

Prasad, A. S., Fitzgerald, J. T., Hess, J. W., Kaplan, J., Pelen, F. & Dardenne, M. 1993. Zinc deficiency in elderly patients. *Nutrition*, 9, 218–24.

Rafnsson, S. B., Dilis, V. & Trichopoulou, A. 2013. Antioxidant nutrients and age-related cognitive decline: A systematic review of population-based cohort studies. *Eur J Nutr*, 52(6), 1553–67. doi: 10.1007/s00394-013-0541-7.

Raiten, D. J., Neufeld, L. M., De-Regil, L. M., Pasricha, S. R., Darnton-Hill, I., Hurrell, R., Murray-Kolb, L. E., et al. 2016. Integration to implementation and the micronutrient forum: A coordinated approach for global nutrition. Case study application: Safety and effectiveness of iron interventions. *Adv Nutr*, 7(1), 135–48. doi: 10.3945/an.115.008581.

Ras, R. T., Hiemstra, H., Lin, Y., Vermeer, M. A., Duchateau, G. S. M. J. E. & Trautwein, E. A. 2013. Consumption of plant sterol-enriched foods and effects on plasma plant sterol concentrations—A meta-analysis of randomized controlled studies. *Atherosclerosis*, 230, 336–46.

Ravaglia, G., Forti, P., Maioli, F., Scali, R. C., Boschi, F., Cicognani, A., Morini, P., Bargossi, A. & Gasbarrini, G. 1996. Coenzyme Q10 plasma levels and body composition in elderly males. *Arch Gerontol Geriatr,* 1, 539–43.

Rink, L. & Gabriel, P. 2000. Zinc and the immune system. *Proc Nutr Soc,* 59, 541–52.

Robert, L. 2010. Aging in the 21st century. *Pathol Biol,* 58, 185–6.

Rolland, Y., De Souto Barreto, P., Abellan Van Kan, G., Annweiler, C., Beauchet, O., Bischoff-Ferrari, H., Berrut, G., et al. 2013. Vitamin D supplementation in older adults: Searching for specific guidelines in nursing homes. *J Nutr Health Aging,* 17(4), 402–12.

Schlanger, L. E., Bailey, J. L. & Sands, J. M. 2010. Electrolytes in the aging. *Adv Chronic Kidney Dis,* 17, 308–19.

Selhub, J., Troen, A. & Rosenberg, I. H. 2010. B vitamins and the aging brain. *Nutr Rev,* 68 Suppl 2, S112–8.

Seren, S., Lieberman, R., Bayraktar, U. D., Heath, E., Sahin, K., Andic, F. & Kucuk, O. 2008. Lycopene in cancer prevention and treatment. *Am J Ther,* 15(1), 66–81.

Shneerson, C., Bartlett, D., Lord, J. & Gale, N. 2014. Supporting healthy ageing: Training multi-disciplinary healthcare students. *Eur J Integr Med,* 6, 104–11.

Sixsmith, J., Sixsmith, A., Fänge, A. M., Naumann, D., Kucsera, C., Tomsone, S., Haak, M., Dahlin-Ivanoff, S. & Woolrych, R. 2014. Healthy ageing and home: The perspectives of very old people in five European countries. *Soc Sci Med,* 106, 1–9.

Swagerty, D. 2017. Integrating Quality Palliative and End-of-Life Care into the Geriatric Assessment. *Clinics in Geriatric Medicine,* 33, 415–429.

Tanaka, T., Shnimizu, M. & Moriwaki, H. 2012. Cancer chemoprevention by carotenoids. *Molecules,* 17(3), 3202–42.

Thakur, V. S., Gupta, K. & Gupta, S. 2012. The chemopreventive and chemotherapeutic potentials of tea polyphenols. *Curr Pharm Biotechnol,* 13, 191–9.

Topp, R., Fahlman, M. & Boardley, D. 2004. Healthy aging: Health promotion and disease prevention. *Nurs Clin North Am,* 39, 411–22.

Tuerk, M. J. & Fazel, N. 2009. Zinc deficiency. *Curr Opin Gastroenterol,* 25(2), 136–43.

Tulchinsky, T. H. & Varavikova, E. A. 2014. Nutrition and Food Safety. *The New Public Health (Third Edition).* San Diego, CA: Academic Press, 419–469.

Ubeda, N., Achon, M. & Varela-Moreiras, G. 2012. Omega 3 fatty acids in the elderly. *Br J Nutr,* 107 Suppl 2, S137–51.

UN. 2015. *World Population Prospects: The 2015 Revision, Key Findings and Advance Tables.* Working Paper No. ESA/P/WP.241. New York: Department of Economic and Social Affairs of the United Nations.

United Nations. 2013. *World Population Ageing 2013.* ST/ESA/SER.A/348. New York: Department of Economic and Social Affairs of the United Nations.

USDA. 2016. Nutrition and Health Are Closely Related—2015–2020 Dietary Guidelines—health. gov [Online]. Available at: http://health.gov/dietaryguidelines/2015/guidelines/introduction/nutrition-and-health-are-closely-related/files/64/nutrition-and-health-are-closelyrelated. html. Accessed on April 2, 2016.

Vinik, A. I. & Jenkins, D. J. 1988. Dietary fiber in management of diabetes. *Diabetes Care,* 11, 160–73.

Wang, S., Moustaid-Moussa, N., Chen, L., Mo, H., Shastri, A., Su, R., Bapat, P., Kwun, I. & Shen, C.-L. 2014. Novel insights of dietary polyphenols and obesity. *J Nutr Biochem,* 25, 1–18.

Wang, W., Connor, S. L., Johnson, E. J., Klein, M. L., Hughes, S. & Connor, W. E. 2007. Effect of dietary lutein and zeaxanthin on plasma carotenoids and their transport in lipoproteins in age-related macular degeneration. *Am J Clin Nutr,* 85, 762–9.

Wengreen, H. J., Munger, R. G., Corcoran, C. D., Zandi, P., Hayden, K. M., Fotuhi, M., Skoog, I., et al. 2007. Antioxidant intake and cognitive function of elderly men and women: The Cache County Study. *J Nutr Health Aging,* 11, 230–7.

WHO 2016. Nutrition for Older Persons. *Nutrition.* Department of Nutrition for Health and Development (NHD). World Health Organization, 1–3.

Wilborn, C. D., Taylor, L. W., Outlaw, J., Williams, L., Campbell, B., Foster, C. A., Smith-Ryan, A., Urbina, S. & Hayward, S. 2013. The effects of pre- and post-exercise whey vs. casein protein consumption on body composition and performance measures in collegiate female athletes. *J Sports Sci Med*, 12(1), 74–9.

Yamamoto, Y. 2016. Coenzyme Q10 redox balance and a free radical scavenger drug. *Arch Biochem Biophys*, 595, 132–5.

Yashodhara, B. M., Umakanth, S., Pappachan, J. M., Bhat, S. K., Kamath, R. & Choo, B. H. 2009. Omega-3 fatty acids: A comprehensive review of their role in health and disease. *Postgrad Med J*, 85, 84–90.

Zhang, C., Browne, A., Child, D. & Tanzi, R. E. 2010. Curcumin decreases amyloid-β peptide levels by attenuating the maturation of amyloid-β precursor protein. *J Biol Chem*, 285, 28472–80.

Zhao, Y. T., Chen, Q., Sun, Y. X., Li, X. B., Zhang, P., Xu, Y. & Guo, J. H. 2009. Prevention of sudden cardiac death with omega-3 fatty acids in patients with coronary heart disease: A meta-analysis of randomized controlled trials. *Ann Med*, 41(4), 301–10.

Zhu, B.-H., Chen, H.-Y., Zhan, W.-H., Wang, C.-Y., Cai, S.-R., Wang, Z., Zhang, C.-H. & He, Y.-L. 2011. (-)-Epigallocatechin-3-gallate inhibits VEGF expression induced by IL-6 via Stat3 in gastric cancer. *World J Gastroenterol*, 17, 2315–25.

19

The Role of Nutritional Factors in Pathogenesis of Diseases

Jayvadan Patel and Anita Patel
Sankalchand Patel University
Gujarat, India

Contents

19.1 The global burden of chronic disease 483
19.2 Nutrition problems in the developing world 486
19.3 Assessment of criteria for the role of nutritional deficiency in causing disease 487
    19.3.1 Evidence of insufficient diet 487
    19.3.2 Evidence of imperfect absorption......................................488
    19.3.3 Evidence of increased utilization..489
19.4 Nutritional mechanism of inflammation.......................................489
19.5 How can diet cause oxidative stress?...492
19.6 How are chronic diseases linked to diet and nutrition?....................492
19.7 Interaction between nutrition and infection....................................493
19.8 The cycle of malnutrition and infection...494
19.9 Diet and nutritional risk factors in diseases 495
    19.9.1 Macronutrients 495
        19.9.1.1 Carbohydrates 496
        19.9.1.2 Protein 497
        19.9.1.3 Fat 499
    19.9.2 Micronutrients..502
        19.9.2.1 Minerals..502
        19.9.2.2 Vitamins..504
        19.9.2.3 Antioxidants 505
19.10 Conclusion...506
References...507

19.1 The global burden of chronic disease

In the promotion and maintenance of good health throughout the human lifespan, diet and nutrition are considered to be vital factors. The role of nutritional factors as determinants of chronic NCDs is well established and so they occupy a prominent position in prevention activities (WHO 2002a). In this chapter, the latest scientific evidence on the nature and strength of the links between diet and chronic diseases is examined as well as discussed in detail. The chronic diseases considered in this chapter, including cancer, cardiovascular diseases, diabetes, obesity, hypertension, and stroke, are related to diet and present the greatest public health burden, either in terms of direct cost to society and government, or in terms of disability-adjusted life years.

The burden of chronic diseases is speedily increasing globally, and it has been calculated that, in 2001, chronic disease contributed to about 60% of the 56.5 million total reported deaths in the world and approximately 46% of the worldwide burden of disease (WHO 2002a). The percentage of the burden of chronic NCDs is likely to increase to 57% by 2020. Approximately half of total chronic disease deaths are due to cardiovascular diseases; obesity and diabetes are also showing disturbing trends, not only because they already affect a large proportion of the population, but also because they have started to appear earlier in life.

The chronic disease problem is far from being limited to the developed regions of the world. Contrary to widely held beliefs, developing countries are suffering from increasingly high levels of public health problems related to chronic diseases (WHO 2002a). While diseases like human immunodeficiency virus/ acquired immunodeficiency syndrome (HIV/AIDS), malaria, tuberculosis, and infectious diseases still predominate in sub-Saharan Africa and will continue to do so for the foreseeable future, 79% of all deaths globally that are caused by chronic diseases are already occurring in developing countries (WHO 2002b).

It is obvious that the previous labeling of chronic diseases as "diseases of affluence" is increasingly a misnomer, as they occur both in poorer countries and in the poorer population groups in richer countries. The alteration in the pattern of disease is taking place at an accelerating rate; also, it is occurring at a more rapid rate in developing countries than it did in the industrialized regions of the earth half a century back (Popkin 2002). This fast rate of change, along with the growing burden of disease, is creating a major public health hazard that demands instant and effectual action.

By 2020, it has been projected that chronic diseases will comprise almost three-quarters of all deaths worldwide and that 71% of deaths due to ischemic heart disease (IHD), 75% of deaths due to stroke, and 70% of deaths due to diabetes will take place in developing countries (WHO 1998). The number of diabetes patients in the developing world will rise by more than 2.5-fold, from 84 million in 1995 to 228 million in 2025 (Aboderin et al. 2001). Indeed, cardiovascular diseases are even now more numerous in India and China than in all the economically developed countries in the world put together (WHO 2002b). For overweight and obesity, not only has the recent prevalence by now reached unprecedented levels but also the rate at which it is yearly growing in the majority of developing regions is considerable (Popkin 2002).

484 Nutrigenomics and Nutraceuticals

The speed of changes in developing countries is such that a double burden of disease may frequently exist. For example, India presently faces a combination of communicable diseases and chronic diseases, with the burden of chronic diseases predicted to soon be greater than that of communicable diseases. On the contrary, projections specify that communicable diseases will still take up a seriously important position up to 2020 (Murray and Lopez 1996). One more expressive example is that of obesity, which is becoming a grave problem throughout Asia, Latin America, and parts of Africa, in spite of the widespread presence of undernutrition.

Chronic diseases are mainly avoidable diseases. Even though additional research is perhaps needed on some aspects of the mechanisms that link diet with health, the presently available scientific evidence provides a satisfactorily strong and reasonable basis to give reason for taking action now. Apart from the suitable medical treatment for those previously affected, the public health approach of primary prevention is considered to be the most lucrative, reasonable, and sustainable course of action to manage the chronic disease outbreak globally. The common risk-factor acceptance approach to chronic disease prevention is a main development in the thinking behind an integrated health policy (Choi et al. 2001).

Recent nutritional as well as physical activity patterns are risk factors that pass through countries and are also transferable from one population to another similar to an infectious disease, affecting disease patterns worldwide. Although age, sex, and genetic susceptibility are nonmodifiable, many of the risks associated with age and sex are modifiable. Such risks comprise behavioral factors (e.g., diet, physical inactivity, tobacco, and alcohol); biological factors (e.g., dyslipidemia, hypertension, hyperinsulinemia, and overweight); and lastly societal factors, which consist of a complex mixture of interacting socioeconomic, cultural, and other environmental parameters.

Diet has been identified for many years as playing a key role as a risk factor for chronic diseases. At the global level, great changes have swept the entire world since the second half of the twentieth century, inducing major modifications in diet, first in industrial regions and in more recent times in developing countries. Customary, mostly plant-based diets have been rapidly replaced by high-fat, energy-dense diets with a considerable content of animal-based foods. However, diet, whilst dangerous to prevention, is presently one risk factor. Physical inactivity, recognized as an important determinant of health, is the result of a progressive shift of lifestyle towards more inactive patterns, in developing countries as much as in industrialized ones. Current data from São Paulo, Brazil, indicate that 70%–80% of the population is amazingly dormant (Matsudo et al. 2002). The combination of these risk factors, along with such factors as tobacco use, is expected to have an additive effect, accelerating the speed at which the chronic disease epidemic is rising in developing countries.

The need to counter the spread of the chronic disease epidemic is at present extensively recognized by a lot of countries, but developing countries are lagging behind in implementing such preventive measures. Positively, on the other hand, efforts to counteract the increase in chronic diseases are gradually being assigned a higher preference. This circumstance is reflected by the increasing curiosity of member states, the concerned international and joint agencies, as well as nongovernmental organizations, in addressing health promotion, food and diet plans, policies for the control and prevention of chronic diseases, promoting healthy aging, and tobacco control. The need to prevent and control the rising public health problem of chronic diseases by promoting proper diets and healthy lifestyles was identified in the International Conference on Nutrition 1992 (WHO 1992a, 1992b, 1992c).

19.2 Nutrition problems in the developing world

The majority of the world's poor and needy people and the health of the world's poorest nations face an overwhelming problem of hunger and malnutrition. Almost 30% of civilization is at present suffering from one or more of the multiple forms of malnutrition (WHO 2000a). The heartbreaking consequences of malnutrition mainly include death, disability, stunted mental and physical growth, and, consequently, retarded nationwide socioeconomic growth. In the developing world, 60% of the 10.9 million deaths every year amongst children aged less than 5 years are linked with malnutrition (WHO 2002c). Worldwide, iodine deficiency is the greatest solitary avoidable cause of brain damage and mental retardation; it is predicted to affect more than 700 million people, the majority of them located in less developed countries (WHO 1999). More than 2,000 million people have iron deficiency anemia (WHO 2001). Vitamin A deficiency remains the single most preventable cause of pointless childhood blindness and higher risk of premature childhood death from infectious diseases, with 250 million children below the age of 5 years suffering from subclinical deficiency (WHO 1995). Birth weight below the 10th percentile of the reference curve for birth weight for gestational age, termed *intrauterine growth retardation*, has an effect on 23.8% or about 30 million newborn babies annually, greatly influencing development, endurance, and physical and mental capacity in the early years (de Onis et al. 1998). Considering the greater risk of developing diet-related chronic diseases later in life, this problem has major public health implications (Barker et al. 1989, 1993; Barker 1995).

Given the rapidity with which traditional diets and lifestyles are changing in many developing countries, it is not surprising that food insecurity and undernutrition persist in the same countries where chronic diseases are emerging as a major epidemic. The outbreak of obesity, with its attendant comorbidities— heart disease, hypertension, diabetes, and stroke—is not a problem restricted to industrialized countries (WHO 2000). Over the past 20 years in developing countries as diverse as India, Mexico, Nigeria, and Tunisia, children have been in a comparable situation: a worrying rise in the incidence of overweight in this group has taken place (de Onis and Blössner 2000).

486 Nutrigenomics and Nutraceuticals

19.3 Assessment of criteria for the role of nutritional deficiency in causing disease

For the development of either recognized disease of previously unidentified etiology or unclear signs and symptoms in an individual, nutritional deficiency may be a responsible factor. Claims are sometimes made that vitamin insufficiency plays a part in the development of renal lithiasis (Higgins 1935) and muscular dystrophies (Bicknell 1940). Yet again, considering a patient with an abnormal form of keratosis of the skin, or edema, which does not effortlessly respond to the usual therapy, or with a tender tongue with few other signs, or with an unusual type of subcutaneous hemorrhage: to what degree are vitamin A, vitamin B, riboflavin, and vitamin C correspondingly concerned in the development of these disorders in the individual?

As Koch's postulates are used in determining the role of specific bacteria in causing disease, accordingly the following criteria have been laid down for assessing the role of nutritional deficiency in causing disease: (1) it should be possible to show the existence of a deficiency of the nutrient; (2) deficiency of the nutrient should result in the development of the disease; and (3) the disease should be cured by replacement of the lacking nutrient. There might be evidence of a deficiency in any part of the pathway between the nutrient and the tissues.

19.3.1 Evidence of insufficient diet

A nutritional history is a necessary first step in diagnosis. The following conditions are particularly appropriate to lead to an insufficient diet.

1. *Low Income Levels* On the whole, foods that are excellent sources of vitamins are more costly; cheaper foods contribute mostly calories (Orr 1936).
2. *War* Wartime measures, such as the introduction of the national loaf and the vitaminization of margarine, jointly with rationing, the cost control of foods, and the supply of cheap or free milk and fruit juices, have decreased the difference between the diets of different classes. However, there are numerous people who still cannot afford to buy their meat or bacon ration or to pay out a lot on vegetables. Furthermore, as war leads to limited imports, to decreased manpower for food production, and to the obliteration of crops and further foodstuffs, it might be a powerful cause in the development of deficiency disease.
3. *Season* A low level of vitamin C is found in foods in the spring and early summer; as a result, at this time the effects of its deficiency are most expected to be seen (Harris 1942).
4. *Geography* Diversity in food production and dietary habits leads to the typical examples of geographically prevalent deficiency disease, for example, beriberi associated with the consumption

of polished rice and pellagra associated with the consumption of maize.

5. *Special Diets* In Britain, the consumption of a too-stiff "gastric" diet by patients with peptic ulcer, devoid of sufficient precautions for assuring the supply of vitamin C, is probably the most common cause of adult scurvy (Harris et al. 1936). Moreover, beriberi has been reported in food cranks that have lived on a diet containing extreme amounts of exceedingly purified carbohydrates. It is also possible that incidence of pellagra in mental hospitals are to a certain extent because of the distorted food habits of the patients.

6. *Institutions* Epidemics of deficiency diseases are habitually reported from institutions; this is surprising in prisons and asylums, where the allowance for food may not be enough to provide even the necessary calories. An insufficiently balanced diet results from the sole nature of institutional feeding, though economic considerations do not limit the option of food. In the first place, the food and its preparation for a large number of people are in the hands of only a few individuals, who may be accountable for a diet of poor quality through unawareness or lack of care. Secondly, the preparation of food on a large scale introduces new problems associated with the preservation of its nutritive value; it necessitates special care, for example, to preserve the vitamin C (King et al. 1942).

19.3.2 Evidence of imperfect absorption

1. *Water-soluble vitamins:* Several affections of the gastrointestinal tract emerge to diminish the absorption of vitamins of the B group. Hyperemesis gravidarum (Strauss and McDonald 1933) as well as alcoholic gastritis (Minot et al. 1933) are frequently connected with deficiency of vitamin B1; in the latter condition there is possibly a second factor in the reduced intake of the vitamin in the diet. Gastrectomy, colitis, and intestinal obstruction frequently lead to a complex deficiency of the vitamin B2 group.

2. *Fat-soluble vitamins*: The absorption of these substances is bound up with the absorption of fat. In obstructive jaundice, absorption of fat is diminished, resulting in decreased absorption of vitamins A (Breese and McCoord 1940) and K; in addition, the complexity of controlling hemorrhage in obstructive jaundice is a result of this "conditioned" deficiency of vitamin K (Brinkhous et al. 1938; Warner et al. 1938). In another example, the effect of large doses of liquid paraffin in delaying the absorption of carotene induced defective absorption of fat-soluble vitamins (Rowntree 1931).

19.3.3 Evidence of increased utilization

1. *Pregnant and lactating women*: Demand for all nutrients increased in pregnancy and lactation, including vitamins. Beriberi and osteomalacia are examples of deficiency that might be precipitated by increased physiological needs.
2. *Heavy manual laborers*: It is to be expected that the required consumption of numerous nutritional factors is larger with increased physical effort. Several Europeans consume diets that possibly contain the same amount of vitamin B as that consumed by several Chinese; the high frequency of beriberi amongst the latter is most likely linked with the extremely heavy work that they perform.
3. *Fever*: During fever there is in fact a greater destruction of vitamin C and probably other vitamins (Abbasy et al. 1936, 1937).

19.4 Nutritional mechanism of inflammation

Acute inflammation is defensive; however, chronic and nonresolving inflammation is destructive and is vital to many chronic diseases. Oxidative stress plays a key role in development of chronic inflammation, resulting in pathogenesis of variety of chronic inflammatory diseases (Hensley et al. 2000) (e.g., type 2 diabetes, cardiovascular disease, and metabolic syndrome) (Figure 19.1) (Milward and Chapple 2013); in fact, it has been proposed as a common association between periodontitis and systemic disease (Chapple 2009; Chapple and Matthews 2007).

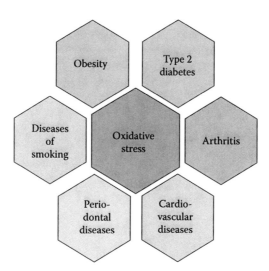

Figure 19.1 Oxidative stress is central to the pathogenesis of numerous systemic diseases and has been proposed as a possible mechanistic link with systemic disease.

In good health, excellent balance exists between oxidants and antioxidants, which are found in all tissues of the body.

Figure 19.2 represents the fine balance that exists at a cellular level in health; diets rich in refined sugars, carbohydrates, and saturated fats will increase oxidative stress and disturb the balance, predisposing susceptible patients to a variety of diseases, while diets rich in antioxidants and micronutrients will help scavenge oxidant species and restore the balance to health (Milward and Chapple 2013).

By surplus production of oxidants and/or diminution of local antioxidants if this excellent balance is disturbed, the resulting surplus oxidant causes oxidative stress and is linked with local tissue damage. An imbalance between oxidants and antioxidants in favor of the oxidants leads to a disturbance of redox signaling and control and/or molecular damage defined as oxidative stress (Sies and Jones 2007). By changing molecules, like proteins, lipids, and deoxyribonucleic acid (DNA), oxidative stress can cause direct tissue damage resulting in cell damage, or else by stimulating redox-sensitive transcription factors within the cell directing to downstream gene expression changes and production of pro-inflammatory molecules (cytokines).

Figure 19.3 shows the complete mechanism of formation of pro-inflammatory molecule cytokines (Milward and Chapple 2013). It shows how bacteria present in the plaque biofilm stimulate a pro-inflammatory cellular response. Bacteria are recognized by cell surface receptors (pattern recognition receptors), which results in activation of pro-inflammatory transcription factors (e.g., nuclear factor kB) in the cytoplasm of the cell. The activated transcription factor migrates into the nucleus, binds to DNA, and causes changes

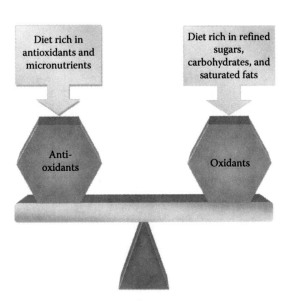

Figure 19.2 In good health, excellent balance exists between oxidants and antioxidants.

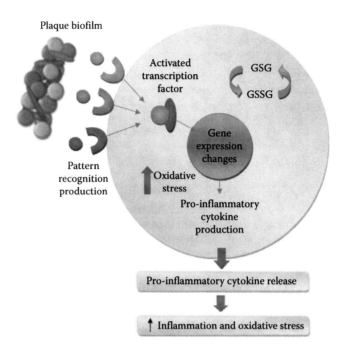

Figure 19.3 Complete mechanism of production and release of pro-inflammatory cytokine.

in gene expression, resulting in pro-inflammatory cytokine production in mitochondria. These cytokines are transported out of the cell and cause an inflammatory response and increases in the local levels of oxidative stress. In vulnerable patients, the body's inflammation-resolving mechanisms do not work competently; a vicious cycle is established, resulting in a shift from acute to chronic inflammatory lesions.

Cellular metabolism can result in elevated levels of oxidative stress, mostly because of leakage of electrons from mitochondria or else through the host's response to a variety of stressful stimuli, for example, periodontal pathogenic bacteria, for example, *Porphyromonas gingivalis*, one of many bacteria strongly associated with periodontitis (Socransky et al. 1998). Receptors present on the cell surface of host cells (pattern recognition receptors, e.g., Toll-like receptors) allow cells to distinguish key bacterial components (e.g., lipopolysaccharide), resulting in stimulation of nuclear factor kappa-B, a pro-inflammatory gene transcription factor, which is as well susceptible to the redox state of the cell, and finally generating downstream pro-inflammatory sequelae (Milward et al. 2007). In sensitive patients, the resultant inflammatory response is unusually elevated and results in collateral tissue damage.

Elevated oxidative stress is antagonized by means of a complex system of antioxidants that comprise antioxidant vitamins; nevertheless, it has been confirmed that the most vital tiny molecule antioxidant species is glutathione

(Sies and Jones 2007). Glutathione presents in both oxidized form glutathione disulfide (GSSG) and reduced form glutathione (GSH), and the proportion of GSH to GSSG usually favors GSH, which preserves a reduced state within the cell. GSH has variety of key distinctions that underpin its significance in antioxidant defense; it is a powerful hunter of free radicals and plays a key role in many other defensive antioxidant systems. GSH has one more important role in cell metabolism and DNA synthesis and repair.

19.5 How can diet cause oxidative stress?

That increased oxidative stress triggers a range of damaging cellular as well as molecular events has already been established, and increases in oxidative stress can be a product of normal cellular metabolism. Oxidative stress levels are additionally enhanced if the nutritional levels of simple sugars are raised through production of mitochondrial superoxide radicals, as a side effect of ATP synthesis, which may be capable of overcoming cellular antioxidant defense mechanisms. Oxidative stress can also be increased by increased dietetic intake of simple sugars or else saturated fat by receptor binding of neutrophils. First, higher glucose in the blood, that is, hyperglycemia, results in the development of advanced glycation end products (AGE), as glucose binds to proteins in tissues in addition to the bloodstream. Neutrophils comprise receptors for AGE, called *RAGE*, and their ligation by AGEs activates NADPH-oxidase enzyme complex (called the "respiratory burst"), generating oxygen radicals. Secondly, metabolism of excess saturated fats generates elevated low density lipoprotein (LDL) cholesterol, which when oxidised forms oxidized LDL; this in turn binds to complementary receptors found on the cell membrane of neutrophils (Toll-like receptors), activating NADPH-oxidase and oxygen radical formation, further adding to the oxidative stress burden (Figure 19.4). Nutritional–cellular interactions are enhanced after eating meals comprised of high levels of simple sugars and saturated fats, producing inflammation, in recent times termed "meal-induced inflammation" (Grant et al. 2010), and are in association with high levels of glucose and lipid in the blood stream and oxidative stress, as well as downstream pro-inflammatory sequelae.

19.6 How are chronic diseases linked to diet and nutrition?

As a consequence of factors such as changes in food availability, food prices, and level of income, diets change over time. Customary, mostly plant-based diets are being replaced by diets high in sugars and animal fats and low in starches, dietary fiber, fruits, and vegetables. This evolution, combined with further inactive lifestyle and a low level of physical activity, is a fundamental factor in the risk of producing chronic diseases. Poverty and inequity are the root causes of malnutrition. Elimination of these causes necessitates political plus social action, of which dietary programs can be

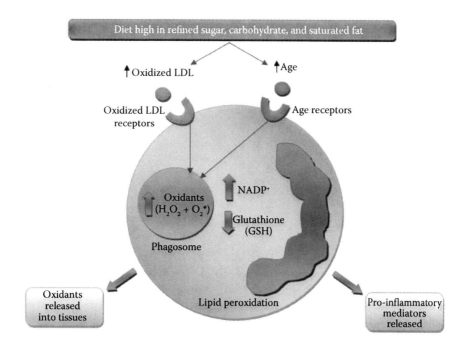

Figure 19.4 Diagrammatic representation of effects of a diet high in refined sugar, carbohydrate, and saturated fat on neutrophil function, which results in production of a "respiratory burst" ultimately leading to release of oxidant species and pro-inflammatory mediators into tissues thereby increasing oxidative stress and causing local tissue damage.

simply solitary aspect. Sufficient, harmless, and wide-ranging food supplies not only avert malnutrition but also lessen the risk of chronic diseases. It is well-known that nutritional deficiency adds to the risk of widespread infectious diseases, notably those of childhood, and vice versa (Scrimshaw et al. 1968; Tompkins and Watson 1989). Diets mainly describe a person's health, growth, and development. Lifestyle factors that have an effect on individuals, for instance, tobacco use and physical inactivity, are progressively more predictable as playing a role in the development of chronic disease. Likewise, the societal, cultural, political, and economic environment can worsen the health of populations, except where healthy lifestyles are energetically promoted (WHO 1990).

19.7 Interaction between nutrition and infection

John Mason and colleagues (Mason et al. 2003) claimed that 32% of the worldwide disease burden could be removed by eliminating malnutrition. Undernutrition is not inevitably developed by a shortage of food, nor is it

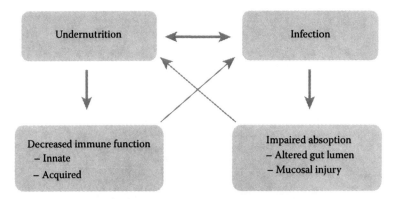

Figure 19.5 Interactions between malnutrition and infection.

unique to poor populations. There are also malnourished people in rich nations. Undernutrition concerns up to 15% of ambulatory outpatients, 25%–60% of patients receiving long-term care, and 35%–65% of hospitalized patients in the United States (Chapman 2006).

Malnutrition is the prime cause of immunodeficiency universally, with infants, children, adolescents, and the elderly nearly all affected. There is a strong relationship between malnutrition and infection and infant mortality; as poor nutrition begins, children become underweight, weaken, and become susceptible to infections, first and foremost owing to epithelial integrity and inflammation (Figure 19.5).

Five infectious diseases including AIDS, diarrhea, malaria, measles, and pneumonia make up more than one-half of all deaths in children aged below 5 years (UNICEF 2006). With this type of interaction between infection and malnutrition, it is vital to keep in mind that a diminished immune function is not a permanently defective one, and numerous indicators of nutritional status are not consistent during infection.

19.8 The cycle of malnutrition and infection

A person suffering from malnutrition becomes more susceptible to infection, and infection as well adds to malnutrition, which causes a vicious cycle (Figure 19.6) (Katona and Katona-Apte 2008). Insufficient nutritional intake leads to weight loss, lowered immunity, mucosal damage, invasion by pathogens, and impaired growth and development in children. An ill person's diet is supplementary motivated by diarrhea, diversion of nutrients to the immune response, loss of appetite, malabsorption, and urinary nitrogen loss, all together leading to loss of nutrients and additional injury to defense mechanisms. These, consequently, cause reduced dietary intake. Additionally, fever raises energy as well as micronutrient requirements.

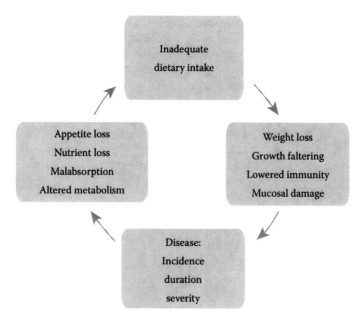

Figure 19.6 The "vicious cycle" of malnutrition and infection.

Malaria and influenza also have mortality rates in proportion to the degree of malnutrition (Müller et al. 2003).

Many a time inadequate or delayed treatment further extends disease occurrence and severity. Several fundamental causes of malnutrition emerge at the national and international levels and relate to the availability and control of food.

19.9 Diet and nutritional risk factors in diseases

Nutrients can be divided into six main classes, that is, fats, carbohydrates, proteins, minerals, vitamins, and water. These can be further subdivided into two broad categories, macronutrients (fats, carbohydrates, and proteins), which are requisite in large quantities from the diet, and micronutrients (minerals, vitamins, trace elements, and amino-acids), which are requisite in small quantities in the diet and which are necessary for a variety of biological processes significant in sustaining optimal health. The role of vitamin deficiency has claimed our attention in current years, and various diseases and syndromes have been treated with a vitamin or combination of vitamins.

19.9.1 Macronutrients

Nutrients are components of foods that a creature utilizes for survival and growth. Macronutrients (e.g., carbohydrates, protein, and fat), desirable in large quantities, provide the bulk of energy needed for an organism's metabolic system to function and can be acquired from the environment (Whitney and Rolfes 2005). Too little or too much of any of these macronutrients may result in poor health and a variety of diseases. A nutrient is considered vital if it must be obtained from an external source, either because the organism cannot synthesize it or because inadequate quantities are produced. The effects of nutrients are dose dependent; shortages are called *deficiencies* (Ensminger 1994). Deficiencies can occur because of numerous causes including insufficiency in nutrient intake, called *dietary deficiency*, or conditions that obstruct the use of a nutrient within an organism. A number of conditions that can hinder nutrient consumption include problems with nutrient absorption, substances that cause a higher-than-usual need for a nutrient, conditions that can cause nutrient destruction, and conditions that can cause greater nutrient excretion. Nutrient toxicity originates when excess of a nutrient does damage to an organism (Ensminger 1994).

19.9.1.1 Carbohydrates

Carbohydrates can be classified into three major groups: monosaccharide and disaccharides (e.g., sugars), oligosaccharides (e.g., fructo-oligosaccharides and maltodextrin), and polysaccharides (e.g., starch and cellulose). They may as well be divided into those that are accessible for metabolism in humans (starch and soluble sugars) and those that remain unavailable (hemicellulose and resistant starch) but are fermented by bacteria in the gastrointestinal tract. The majority of research has focused on available carbohydrates, mostly sugar. Research in rats has revealed that higher sugar intake produces insulin resistance, resulting in chronic inflammation (Cai et al. 2005; Sandu et al. 2005). Whereas insulin resistance and type 2 diabetes in high-fat-fed mice are associated with high glycotoxin intake (Sandu et al. 2005), no mechanism has been recommended to connect starch or sugar intake with higher risk of developing inflammatory bowel disease (IBD). A relationship between sugar intake and IBD is not at present supported by epidemiological research (Sonnenberg 1988).

A research study performed on an experimental gingivitis model revealed high levels of bleeding on probing for participants who were fed a high-carbohydrate diet as compared to those on a low sugar diet (Sidi and Ashley 1984). This was additionally supported by a study performed on volunteers placed on a primitive diet rich in fiber, antioxidants, and fish oils but low in refined sugars and with no oral hygiene measures. It would be expected that plaque levels increased considerably and typical periodontal pathogens emerged within the biofilm; however, unpredictably gingival bleeding notably decreased from 35% to 13% (Baumgartner et al. 2009), supporting a role for nutrition in controlling periodontal inflammation. Nevertheless, the exact mechanisms behind this observed dietary effect have yet to be completely elucidated.

Worldwide, nonalcoholic fatty liver disease (NAFLD) is the most recurrent liver disease and is generally associated with metabolic syndrome. In the occurrence of these diseases, secular trends may be associated with the higher fructose consumption found in the Western diet. NAFLD is mostly described by two steps of liver injury: intrahepatic lipid accumulation and inflammatory succession to nonalcoholic steatohepatitis (NASH) (the "two hit" theory). In the first "hit," hepatic metabolism of fructose encourages *de novo* lipogenesis and intrahepatic lipid, inhibition of mitochondrial β-oxidation of long-chain fatty acids, formation of triglyceride and steatosis, hepatic and skeletal muscle insulin resistance, and hyperglycemia. In the second hit, due to the molecular instability of its five-member furanose ring, fructose promotes protein fructo-sylation and development of reactive oxygen species (ROS), which necessitate quenching by hepatic antioxidants. A lot of patients with NASH also have micronutrient deficiencies, as well as not enough antioxidant capacity to avoid synthesis of ROS, resultant in necro-inflammation. Researchers have claimed that too much dietary fructose consumption might cause the progress of NAFLD and metabolic syndrome and also assumed that NAFLD and alcoholic fatty liver disease contribute to the similar pathogenesis (Jung et al. 2010).

19.9.1.2 Protein

Although a short-term high-protein diet might be essential in some pathologi-cal conditions like malnutrition and sarcopenia, it is obvious that "too much of a good thing" in diet could be ineffective or even injurious for healthy individuals (Kafatos and Hatzis 2008). The main sources of dietary protein are cheese, eggs, fish, meat, milk, and nuts. Diets containing milk, cheese, eggs, and meats, consumed along with cruciferous vegetables and sulfite-preserved foods, present intestinal bacteria with sulfate and sulfite. These are further fermented to generate hydrogen sulfide, which prevents butyrate oxidation and has been linked with mucosal hyperproliferation in ulcerative colitis (Christl et al. 1996).

In epidemiologic investigations, the role of dietary protein in the progress of cancer as well as coronary heart disease (CHD) has not been studied as much as the effects of dietary fats and carbohydrates. In different coun-tries, ecologic data has demonstrated strong positive relationships between the amount of animal protein in the diet and CHD mortality (Carroll 1978), signifying that amount along with type of protein may be significant in the etiology of disease. Comparable results were seen for milk, meat, and overall protein intake with cancer mortality (Tominaga and Kuroishi 1997). Previously, experimental studies established that animal protein diet fed to rabbits was associated with atherosclerosis (Kritchevsky 1995) as well as plaque formation (Katan et al. 1982).

Renal function can also modulated by dietary protein intake (King and Levey 1993). At the center of the disagreement is the concern that routine con-sumption of dietary protein in excess of suggested amounts promotes chronic renal disease by elevated glomerular pressure and hyperfiltration (Brenner et al. 1982; Metges and Barth 2000). Dietary protein intake may be associated with the progression of renal disease confirmed by observational data from epidemiological studies (Lentine and Wrone 2004). Allen and Cope's study showing that increased dietary protein induced renal hypertrophy in dogs (Allen and Cope 1942) led to conjecture that dietary protein intake may possibly have deleterious effects on the kidney.

A large amount of acid in body fluids is generated by a diet high in protein. The kidneys react to this dietary acid challenge with net acid excretion, and at the same time, the skeleton supplies buffer as a result of active resorption of bone, resulting in unnecessary calcium loss (Barzel and Massey 1998). Furthermore, acid loading straight inhibits renal calcium reabsorption, leading to hypercalciuria along with exorbitant bone loss (Goldfarb and Coe 1999; Goldfarb 1988). In another study, the association of animal protein–rich diet with calcium metabolism was studied during a 12-day dietary period. The urinary calcium excretion increased, indicating that the animal protein–induced calciuric response can be a risk factor for the progress of osteoporosis (Breslau et al. 1988). Excessive intake of protein along with low fluid intake are the main risk factors for kidney stones (Goldfarb and Coe 1999). Protein intake increases renal acid excretion, and acid loads, consecutively, can be buffered in part by bone, which releases calcium to be excreted by the kidney. This protein-induced hypercalciuria may well lead to the development of calcium kidney stones (Goldfarb 1988).

Intermittent abdominal pain, transient elevations in transaminases, and hyperalbuminemia were found in persons taking high protein supplements without any identifiable cause. After discontinuation of the high protein intake, the symptoms and abnormalities on the laboratory tests resolved (Mutlu et al. 2006). In one case-control study, individuals (treatment group, TG) were studied for a year using myocardial perfusion imaging (MPI), echocardiography (ECHO), and serial blood work (Fleming 2000). MPI and ECHO were carried out at the beginning as well as the end of the study for every individual. The TG group studied adapted their dietary ingestion as instructed. Additional individuals (high protein group, HPG) selected a different dietary schedule comprised of a high-protein diet (Fleming 2000). TG individuals established a decrease in each of the independent variables studied with regression, in both the extent as well as severity of coronary artery disease (CAD) when quantitatively measured by MPI. Subjects in the HPG showed deterioration of their independent variables. These results suggest that high-protein diets may precipitate development of CAD by increases in lipid deposition in addition to inflammatory and coagulation pathways (Fleming 2000).

Sarcopenia is a multifaceted process facilitated by a combination of factors, counting the acceptance of a more deskbound lifestyle and a less than optimal diet. At present there is a lack of longer-term research with distinct health outcomes to state the best value for protein intake in elderly subjects. In general, fairly rising daily protein ingestion more than 0.8 $g \cdot kg^{-1} \cdot d^{-1}$ may improve muscle protein anabolism and provide a means to decrease the progressive loss of muscle mass with age. The valuable effects of resistance exercise in aging populations are unambiguous. On the contrary, research has not recognized a synergistic result of protein supplementation and resistance exercise in aging populations. There is only modest evidence associating high protein ingestion with higher risk for impaired kidney function in healthy subjects. Conversely, renal function decreases with age, and higher protein ingestion is contraindicated in subjects with renal disease. For older individuals assessment of renal function is suggested prior to adopting a higher-protein diet (Douglas et al. 2008).

In addition to insufficiency, higher amounts of certain nutritional factors like amino acid phenylalanine in the subjects can be damaging, resulting in phenylketonuria (brain damage) as well as mental retardation (Blomquist et al. 1980). Insufficient absorption or malnutrition, like in celiac disease, may lead to anxiety/depressive symptoms, as a gluten-free diet can lead to deficiency of B-complex, iron, zinc, calcium, and vitamin D (Guevara et al. 2014).

Pellagra is a nutritional deficiency disease caused by eating maize, a staple that is poor in tryptophan and in which nicotinic acid occurs in "bound" form. However, pellagra cases found in populations whose staple is "jowar," millet with a tryptophan content near to that of rice, has thrown uncertainty on this theory. Jowar has an unusually high leucine content, like maize. L-leucine was shown to obstruct with tryptophan and nicotinic-acid metabolism, and leucine supplements induced "black tongue" (the canine equivalent of pellagra) in dogs. Leucine acts by distorting the nicotinamide–nucleotide pattern of red blood cells, even if total nucleotide levels are not affected. Thus amino acid supplements appear to aggravate the mental symptoms related to pellagra. As a result, pellagra may be considered as a human nutritional deficiency disease arbitrated by leucine imbalance (Gopalan 1969).

19.9.1.3 Fat

Fat is a macronutrient and is considered to be a main source of calories or energy. Even if some fat in the diet is essential, excess fat can lead to cancers, heart diseases, obesity, and other health-related problems. Red meat is the major dietary source of saturated fat, which has been linked with breast and colorectal cancers (Kafatos and Hatzis 2008). Up to 80% of breast, bowel, and prostate cancers are accredited to dietary practices and optimistic links with high meat diet shown by international comparisons (Bingham 1999). Conversely, the connection between red meat or processed meat with colorectal cancer seems to have been more consistently established (Norat and Riboli 2001). In recent times, studies revealed positive links between the use of well-done red meat and everyday frying, barbecuing, and broiling of meats with the growth of some cancers (Sinha 2002), considered to be explained through augmented exposure to the potent and extremely bioavailable carcinogens heterocyclic aromatic amines (Gooderham et al. 1997; Sugimura 2000). Probable mechanisms comprise the development of heterocyclic amines in meat when it is cooked; the resulting heterocyclic amines need acetylation by P450 enzymes, and subjects with the fast-acetylating genotype who eat elevated amounts of meat might be at increased risk of large-bowel cancer (Bingham 1999).

The relationship among dietary fat consumption and risk of cancer, particularly breast, colon, prostate, and ovarian cancer, has been discussed for several years. For more than 30 years, ecologic studies have confirmed the association of higher dietary fat with greater mortality attributable to various cancers. That greater fat consumption might be linked with higher risk of cancer has also been shown by migrant studies. Definite saturated fatty acids increase blood cholesterol levels and, thus, raise the risk of atherosclerosis. Increased fat ingestion is a major cause of diabetes, gallbladder disease, hypertension, and obesity. The risk of breast cancer may also be intensified by high fat intake directly by raised blood estrogen levels and/or secondarily by increased obesity. Significant experimental studies for determination of the effects of a low-fat diet on disease risk still have not been completed; however, decreasing fat in the US diet has the potential to reduce morbidity and mortality considerably (Kuller 1997).

The pathogenesis of many diseases, including cardiovascular disease, cancer, osteoporosis, and inflammatory and autoimmune diseases, is promoted by a high omega-6/omega-3 ratio, as found in today's Western diets, while higher levels of omega-3 polyunsaturated fatty acids (PUFAs) (a lower omega-6/omega-3 ratio), exert exploitive effects. Greater dietary ingestion of linoleic acid leading to oxidation of low-density lipoprotein (LDL) and platelet aggregation moreover hinders with the incorporation of required fatty acids in cell membrane phospholipids. Gene expression is influenced by both omega-6 and omega-3 fatty acids. Omega-3 fatty acids have anti-inflammatory effects and repress interleukin-1β, tumor necrosis factor-α, and interleukin-6, but omega-6 fatty acids do not. As inflammation is at the base of numerous chronic diseases, dietary ingestion of omega-3 fatty acids plays a key role in the expression of disease, predominantly in persons with genetic variation, as in individuals with genetic variants at the 5-lipoxygenase. Carotid intima media thickness (IMT) used as a marker of atherosclerotic burden is considerably augmented, by 80%, in the variant group as compared to carriers with the regular allele, signifying greater 5-lipoxygenase promoter activity linked with the (variant) allele. Dietary arachidonic acid and linoleic acid raise the risk for cardiovascular disease in individuals with the variants, while dietary ingestion of eicosapentaenoic acid and docosahexaenoic acid reduce the risk (Simopoulos 2006). There is proof that n-3 PUFAs, mainly eicosapentaenoic acid and docosahexaenoic acid, persuade the inflammatory response through antagonizing the generation of inflammatory eicosanoid mediators from arachidonic acid, repress generation of a few inflammatory cytokines, and downregulate the expression of many genes concerned in inflammation (Gil 2002).

Imbalance between omega-6 and omega-3 PUFAs in the peripheral blood causes overproduction of pro-inflammatory cytokines. Moreover, there is proof that alterations in fatty acid composition are concerned in the patho-physiology of major depression. Alterations in serotonin (5-HT) receptor number along with function caused by changes in PUFAs present the hypo-thetical basis linking fatty acids with the existing receptor and neurotransmit-ter theories of depression (Maes et al. 1996, 1997; Peet et al. 1998).

Morris and colleagues observed a sturdy higher risk of Alzheimer's disease with consumption of *trans-unsaturated fat*. Trans-unsaturated fats arise as a result of partial hydrogenation of vegetable oils to make commercially baked prod-ucts and hard-bitten margarine. Researchers observed that an interactive effect between ingestion of trans-unsaturated and polyunsaturated fats and the risk of Alzheimer's disease has also been found for heart disease. The association observed among Alzheimer's patients and ingestion of saturated fat appeared to be limited to black participants; conversely, researchers had restricted data for precise judgment of risks within subgroups (Morris et al. 2003).

Worldwide, breast cancer is the main public health problem amongst women. To find the role of dietary fat and the risk of breast cancer numerous epide-miological studies have been performed. Higher use of total fat and saturated fat were found to be optimistically linked with the progress of breast cancer. Albeit an ambiguous relationship was found between the use of total mono-unsaturated fatty acids (MUFA) and the risk of breast cancer, there exists an opposite relationship in the case of oleic acid, the most copious MUFA. A sensible opposite connection among consumption of n-3 fatty acids and breast cancer risk and a reasonable positive connection between n-6 fatty acids and breast cancer risk were found (Binukumar and Mathew 2005).

Dietary factors play a major role in the pathogenesis of biliary diseases, for example, gallstones and pancreaticobiliary maljunction. Gallstones are prin-cipally classified into cholesterol stone and pigment stone consistent with the main composition. Formation of cholesterol gallstone is to be expected based upon supersaturated bile production, and pigment stones are produced in bile rich in bilirubin. As a result, deficiencies of hepatic metabolism of lipids and organic anions lead to biliary stones. Alternatively, there is one more significant association of biliary lipid degradation to severe biliary disease, that is, pancreaticobiliary maljunction. Lysophosphatidylcholine (lysoPC), derived from phosphatidylcholine hydrolysis by phospholipase A2, is a very plenti-ful bioactive lipid mediator present in the circulation and in bile. Increase in bile of lysoPC and phospholipase A2 have been reported in pancreatico-biliary maljunction and measured to be the main risk factor for biliary tract cancers. Additional, oxidized fatty acids have been recognized as a powerful ligand for G protein coupled receptor 132 (G2A), which arbitrates a varied array of biological processes including cell growth and apoptosis. Therefore, both lysoPC and free fatty acids theoretically play a vital role through G2A in biliary inflammation and carcinogenesis of pancreaticobiliary maljunction. Altogether, dietary factors, particularly lipid compounds, are outwardly criti-cal in the pathogenesis of biliary diseases (Tazuma et al. 2013).

19.9.2 Micronutrients

19.9.2.1 Minerals

Sodium concentrations in the blood are affected by high sodium in the diet, which has an effect on the cells of the blood vessel wall and blood volume, although blood pressure itself does not change. The concluding effects are long-term alterations in vessel wall structure, together with thickening of the vessel wall and altered production of structural proteins, leading to arterial stiffening. A high amount of dietary sodium timely changes in hormonal systems and as well gene expression in endothelial cells of blood vessels. Sequentially, these changes encourage unnecessary growth of vascular smooth muscle cells, which adds to thickening of vessel wall, and distorted manufacture of structural proteins, for example collagen, elastin, and fibronectin, which presents as arterial stiffening. Dietary salt has also been linked with endothelial dysfunction, which is one of the beginning events of atherosclerotic plaque formation (Dickinson et al. 2009; Safar et al. 2000; Sanders 2009; Simon 2003; de Wardener and MacGregor 2002).

In the 1990s, it was established that the association between salt intake and stroke mortality was stronger than the association between blood pressure and stroke mortality, suggesting that salt might have harmful effects on the cardiovascular system that are not correlated to blood pressure (Perry and Beevers 1992). In recent study, increased sodium intake was linked with higher carotid artery IMT, a precise forecaster of future cardiovascular events in persons devoid of high blood pressure. Thickening of vessels is a sign of atherosclerotic plaque development, and as a result indicates greater risk of heart attack or stroke (Lorenz et al. 2007).

Hypertension is the main risk factor for kidney disease; however dietary sodium has additional damaging effects on the kidneys. Excess salt ingestion forces the generation of oxygen radicals, leads to oxidative stress in kidney tissue (de Wardener and MacGregor 2002). Excess salt ingestion is also a risk factor for osteoporosis, as high dietary sodium promotes urinary calcium loss; as a result calcium is lost from bone and so decreases bone density. The daily sodium intake of Americans has been connected with increased bone loss at the hip, and sodium constraint decreases markers of bone breakdown (Devine et al. 1995). Even in the presence of an increased calcium diet, excess salt intake results in net calcium loss from bone (Teucher et al. 2008). In asthmatic patients, excess dietary sodium might increase the severity of the disease (de Wardener and MacGregor 2002).

A high salt diet is associated with gastric cancer; aflatoxin B1, a recurrent food pollutant, with liver cancer; and betel nut chewing with oral cancer (Park et al. 2008). It clearly explains differences in cancer frequency in different countries. For example, gastric cancer is more frequent in Japan with its increased salt diet and colon cancer is more frequent in the United States. Migrants increase the risk of their new country, signifying a considerable connection between diet and cancer (Brenner et al. 2009).

Zinc is a trace mineral that is necessary for all species and is requisite for the activities of 1,300 enzymes, carbohydrate and energy metabolism, protein synthesis and degradation, nucleic acid production, heme biosynthesis, and carbon dioxide transport. It is also a cofactor in the formation of enzymes as well as nucleic acids and takes part in a vital role in the structure of cell membranes and in the functioning of immune cells. Zinc deficiency decreases nonspecific immunity, including neutrophil and natural killer cell function and balance activity; decreases numbers of T and B lymphocytes; and represses delayed hypersensitivity, cytotoxic activity, and antibody production. Insufficient zinc intake stops normal release of vitamin A from the liver; clinically, it is linked with fetal loss, growth retardation, malabsorption syndromes, neonatal death, and congenital abnormalities. Reduced blood zinc concentrations have also been seen in patients with Crohn's disease, diarrheal disease, pneumonia, and tuberculosis. Moreover, zinc deficiency is connected with abnormal pregnancy outcomes (Fawzi and Msamanga 2004) and conditions of relatively compromised immunity, including alcoholism, burns, HIV infection, inflammatory bowel disease and kidney disease.

Iron deficiency is the most widespread trace element deficiency universally, affecting 20%–50% of the world's population, mostly infants, children, and women of childbearing age (Patterson et al. 2001). It is linked with impairments in cell-mediated immunity and declines in neutrophil action, with reduced bacterial and myeloperoxidase activity. It also subordinates the body's defenses against disease and decreases body and brain functions. Regardless of this, iron deficiency has indistinct effects on infectious disease risk. In the treatment of malaria, correcting iron deficiency is significant, as malaria causes hemolysis and anemia. Supplementation in a few cases, conversely, possibly will in fact worsen infection, since the malaria parasite necessitates iron for its multiplication in blood and therefore may be less infective in the iron-deficient person. The mechanism for this might also be connected to the inhibition of zinc absorption (Oppenheimer 2001). Lots of microorganisms have need of trace elements, like iron and zinc, for continued existence and replication in the host and might increase in pathogenicity with supplementation (Shankar 2000).

Selenium is a potent antioxidant that regulates activity of the glutathione peroxidase enzymes, which further catalyze the detoxification of hydrogen peroxide and organic hydroperoxides. Selenium deficiency has been concerned in the etiopathogenesis of Keshan disease (congestive cardiomyopathy), found in China, and in additional cases of congestive cardiomyopathy in individuals on artificial nutrition. Nevertheless, the facts from case-control as well as prospective studies for a relationship among low selenium status and cardiovascular diseases remain contentious (Neve 1996).

Minute changes in magnesium levels may have major effects on cardiac excitability and on vascular tone, contractility as well as reactivity. Hypertension is a multifaceted and quantitative trait under polygenic control. Even if the accurate etiology is unidentified, the basic hemodynamic abnormality in hypertension is raised peripheral resistance, owing mainly to alterations in vascular structure and function. These alterations consist of arterial wall thickening, abnormal vascular tone, and endothelial dysfunction and are due to changes in the biology of the cellular and noncellular constituents of the arterial wall. Many of these processes are influenced by magnesium. In view of this, magnesium may be essential in the physiological regulation of blood pressure, while perturbations in cellular magnesium homeostasis might play a role in pathophysiological processes underlying blood pressure elevation. Nearly all epidemiological and experimental studies have revealed an opposite relationship between magnesium and blood pressure and have supported a role for magnesium in the pathogenesis of hypertension. On the contrary, data from clinical studies have been less believable and the therapeutic value of magnesium in the prevention and management of elementary hypertension remains indistinct (Touyz 2003).

19.9.2.2 Vitamins

Vitamin A preserves the integrity of the epithelium in the respiratory as well as gastrointestinal tracts. The World Health Organization approximates that, universally, 100–140 million children are vitamin A deficient, causing 1.2–3 million deaths per year (Neidecker-Gonzales et al. 2007). The risk of diarrhea, *Plasmodium falciparum* malaria, measles, and overall mortality is increased due to vitamin A deficiency. Vitamin A deficiency along with measles, which is expected to kill 2 million children annually, is directly associated. Measles in a child is to be expected to worsen any existing nutritional deficiency, and children who are already deficient in vitamin A are at much higher risk of mortality from measles. Postmeasles diarrhea is mostly not easy to treat and has an extremely great mortality. Vitamin A deficiency also raises the risk of developing respiratory disease as well as chronic ear infections (Tomkins and Watson 1989). Hypervitaminosis A acute intoxication can lead onto symptoms of increased intracranial tension and individuals can experience extreme headache, drowsiness, irritability, vertigo, and blurred vision (Vallbracht and Gilory 1976).

Dietary factors are integrally associated with Alzheimer's disease. Even if Alzheimer's disease subjects have no alteration in energy metabolism, variations in weight are quite frequent. William and colleagues explored the potential role of vitamin B_{12} and folate, with the production of hyperhomocysteinemia, in the pathophysiology of Alzheimer's disease, as well as the role of free-radical damage in Alzheimer's disease (William et al. 2001).

Researchers tested the assumption that nutritional folate might be able to alter susceptibility of dopaminergic neurons to dysfunction and fatality in a mouse model of Parkinson's disease. Wenzhen and colleagues reported that nutritional folate deficiency sensitized mice to 1-methyl-4-phenyl-1,2,3,6-tetrahydropyridine (MPTP)-induced Parkinson's disease–like pathology and motor dysfunction. Mice kept on a folate-deficient diet showed high levels of plasma homocysteine. While infused straight into either the substantia nigra or striatum, homocysteine aggravates MPTP-induced dopamine depletion, neuronal degeneration, and motor dysfunction. Homocysteine aggravates oxidative stress, mitochondrial dysfunction, and apoptosis in human dopaminergic cells exposed to the pesticide rotenone or the pro-oxidant Fe^{2+} (Wenzhen et al. 2002).

Vitamin E is an antioxidant that scavenges free radicals and its supplementation has been revealed to improve immune function in the elderly, with delayed hypersensitivity skin response and antibody production following vaccination (Meydani et al. 2005). Research has not found any adverse effects from consuming vitamin E in food. Premature babies of very low birth weight (<1,500 grams) may be deficient in vitamin E. Vitamin E supplementation in these infants may decrease the risk of a few complications, such as those affecting the retina, but they can also raise the risk of infections (Brion et al. 2003).

Researchers reported that a single 2.5-mg dose of vitamin D was adequate to improve the immune system's ability to withstand infection. These outcomes came from a study that identified an amazingly elevated incidence of vitamin D deficiency among tuberculosis-vulnerable women in Muslim communities in London (Diamond et al. 2002). It is nowadays accepted that vitamin D deficiency in a pregnant and lactating mother predisposes her breastfed infant to the progress of rickets, and that cultural and social factors are vital in the pathogenesis of the disease for the period of the adolescent growth spurt. Avoidance of rickets is reliant on the alertness of the medical profession and the common public of the need to ensure sufficient ingestion of vitamin D in at-risk populations, and of the significance of increasing nutritional ingestion of calcium using locally obtainable and low-cost foods in communities in which nutritional calcium deficiency rickets is common (John 2013).

19.9.2.3 Antioxidants

A micronutrient is a crucial dietary component present in a trace amount (Witte and Clark 2002). Micronutrients, as opposed to macronutrients, contain minerals and vitamins to ensure normal growth, metabolism, and physical comfort. They are used to build and repair tissues as well as to control bodily processes (Whitney and Rolfes 2005). Globally, ~2 billion people are affected by micronutrient deficiencies, comprising vitamins A, C, and E and the minerals iodine, iron, and zinc. Micronutrient deficiency leads to poor growth, impaired intellect, and increased mortality as well as vulnerability to infection.

Current nutritional alterations comprise lessening ingestion of antioxidants (such as vitamin C, vitamin E, b-carotene, zinc, and selenium). Reduced ingestion of antioxidant-rich foods has been linked with decreased pulmonary function and higher risk of wheeze (Allan et al. 2010). Some evidence has suggested that antioxidant status in pregnancy may influence vulnerability to allergic disease. Decreased maternal consumption of antioxidant-rich foods and vitamin E has been related with a higher risk of developing childhood wheeze (Miyake et al. 2010), asthma, and sensitization (Allan et al. 2010), while dealings between other antioxidants and allergic disease have not been in agreement (Allan et al. 2010). Antioxidant status can change cell processes implicated in immune programming, including T cell regulation (Tan et al. 2005) and induction of interleukin-12 production by antigen presenting cells (Utsugi et al. 2003).

Food insecurity is nowadays related with children's psychological difficulties like anxiety/depression, aggression and hyper-reactivity, and inattention as evidenced from a potential birth cohort study (Melchior et al. 2012). There are now irresistible facts of the importance of diet in a wide range of systemic diseases with diet modification, increasing physical activity and reducing levels of obesity a key public health message. So we require considering dietary intake when managing our dietary deficient patients not only for the potential benefits in terms of their health but also the systemic benefits that it unquestionably provides.

19.10 Conclusion

It is obvious that "too much of a good thing" in diet could be ineffective or even injurious for healthy individuals. The impact of dietary factors on health and longevity is increasingly appreciated. In some cases, there is incontrovertible evidence of a cause-and-effect relationship between a dietary factor and health, while in many other cases the link is inconclusive. Diets are changing rapidly across the world, resulting in a bifurcation of policy challenges. Foods, diets, and nutritional status are important determinants of NCDs. Undernutrition, and its effects on growth, development and maturation has numerous detrimental outcomes, including the potential to increase risk of developing NCDs later in life. Eating red and processed meat increases risk of developing colorectal cancer. Saturated fat and trans-fats increase blood cholesterol and cardiovascular risk. Higher sodium/salt intake is a major risk factor for elevated blood pressure and cardiovascular diseases, and probably stomach cancer. Diets high in meat and dairy also increase blood pressure. Diets high in energy-dense, highly-processed foods and refined starches and/or sugary beverages contribute to overweight and obesity. Infection is inevitably tied to nutrition in both the developing and the developed world. From the available evidence, it is possible to state that unhealthy diets, physical inactivity and smoking are confirmed risk behaviors for chronic diseases; nutrients and physical activity influence gene expression and may define susceptibility; and improving diets and increasing levels of physical activity in adults and older people will reduce chronic disease risks for death and disability.

References

Abbasy MA, Harris LJ, Hill NG. Vitamin C and infection. Excretion of vitamin C in osteomy-elitis. *Ibid.* 1937; 2: 177.

Abbasy MA, Hill NG, Harris LJ. Vitamin C and juvenile rheumatism with some observations on the vitamin C reserves in surgical tuberculosis. *The Lancet.* 1936; 2: 1413.

Aboderin I, Kalache A, Ben-Shlomo Y, Lynch JW, Yajnik CS, Kuh D, Yach D. *Life course perspectives on coronary heart disease, stroke and diabetes: Key issues and implications for policy and research.* Geneva, 2001. (World Health Organization, Document WHO/NMH/NPH/01.4).

Allan K, Kelly FJ, Devereux G. Antioxidants and allergic disease: A case of too little or too much? *Clin Exp Allergy.* 2010; 40: 370–380.

Allen FM, Cope OM. Influence of diet on blood pressure and kidney size in dogs. *J Urol.* 1942; 47: 751.

Al-Rasheed NM, Attia HA, Mohamed RA, Al-Rasheed NM, Al-Amin MA. Preventive effects of selenium yeast, chromium picolinate, zinc sulfate and their combination on oxidative stress, inflammation, impaired angiogenesis and atherogenesis in myocardial infarction in rats. *Journal of Pharmacy & Pharmaceutical Sciences.* A publication of the Canadian Society for Pharmaceutical Sciences, *Societe canadienne des sciences pharmaceutiques.* 2013;16(5):848-67. PubMed PMID: 24393559. Epub 2014/01/08. eng.

Barker DJ. Fetal origins of coronary heart disease. *Br Med J.* 1995; 311: 171–174.

Barker DJ, Martyn CN, Osmond C, Hales CN, Fall CH. Growth in utero and serum cholesterol concentrations in adult life. *Br Med J.* 1993; 307: 1524–1527.

Barker DJ, Winter PD, Osmond C, Margettes B, Simmonds SJ. Weight in infancy and death from ischaemic heart disease. *The Lancet.* 1989; 2: 577–580.

Barzel US, Massey LK. Excess dietary protein may can adversely affect bone. *J Nutr.* 1998; 128(6): 1051–1053.

Baumgartner S, Imfeld T, Schicht O, Rath C, Persson RE, Persson GR. The impact of the stone age diet on gingival conditions in the absence of oral hygiene. *J Periodontol.* 2009; 80: 759–768.

Bicknell F. Vitamin E in the treatment of muscular dystrophies and nervous diseases. *The Lancet.* 1940; 1: 10–13.

Bingham SA. Meat or wheat for the next millennium? Plenary lecture. High-meat diets and cancer risk. *Proc Nutr Soc.* 1999; 58: 243–248.

Binukumar B, Mathew A. Dietary fat and risk of breast cancer. *World J Surg Oncol.* 2005; 3: 45.

Blomquist HK, Gustavson KH, Holmgren G. Severe mental retardation in five siblings due to maternal phynylketonuria. *Neuropediatrics.* 1980; 11: 256–261.

Breese BB, McCoord AB. Vitamin a absorption in catarrhal jaundice. *J Pediatr.* 1940; 16: 139–145.

Brenner BM, Meyer TW, Hostetter TH. Dietary protein intake and the progressive nature of kidney disease: The role of hemodynamically mediated glomerular injury in the pathogenesis of progressive glomerular sclerosis in aging, renal ablation, and intrinsic renal disease. *N Engl J Med.* 1982; 307: 652–659.

Brenner H, Rothenbacher D, Arndt V. Epidemiology of stomach cancer. *Method Mol Biol.* 2009; 472: 467–477.

Breslau NA, Brinkley L, Hill KD, Pak CY. Relationship of animal protein-rich diet to kidney stone formation and calcium metabolism. *J Clin Endocrinol Metab.* 1988; 66(1): 140–146.

Brinkhous KM, Smith HP, Warner ED. Prothrombin deficiency and the bleeding tendency in obstructive jaundice and in biliary fistula. Effect of feeding bile and alfalfa (vitamin K). *Am J Med Sci.* 1938; 196: 50.

Brion LP, Bell EF, Raghuveer TS. Vitamin E supplementation for prevention of morbidity and mortality in preterm infants. *Cochrane Database Syst Rev.* 2003; (4): CD003665.

Bylsma LC, Alexander DD. A review and meta-analysis of prospective studies of red and processed meat, meat cooking methods, heme iron, heterocyclic amines and prostate cancer. *Nutrition Journal*. 2015 Dec 21;14:125. PubMed PMID: 26689289. Pubmed Central PMCID: PMC4687294. Epub 2015/12/23. eng.

Cai D, Yuan M, Frantz DF, Melendez PA, Hansen L, Lee J, Shoelson SE. Local and systemic insulin resistance resulting from hepatic activation of IKK-beta and NF-kappaB. *Nat Med*. 2005; 11: 183–190.

Carroll KK. Dietary protein in relation to plasma cholesterol levels and atherosclerosis. *Nutr Rev*. 1978; 36: 1–5.

Chapman I. Nutritional disorders in the elderly. *Med Clin North Am*. 2006; 90: 887–907.

Chapple ILC. Potential mechanisms underpinning the nutritional modulation of periodontal inflammation. *J Am Dent Assoc*. 2009; 1402: 178–184.

Chapple ILC, Matthews JB. The role of reactive oxygen and antioxidant species in periodontal tissue destruction. *Periodontol 2000*. 2007; 43: 160–232.

Choi BC, Bonita R, McQueen DV. The need for global risk factor surveillance. *J Epidemiol Community Health*. 2001; 55: 370.

Christl SU, Eisner HD, Dusel G, Kasper H, Scheppach W. Antagonistic effects of sulfide and butyrate on proliferation of colonic mucosa: A potential role for these agents in the pathogenesis of ulcerative colitis. *Dig Dis Sci*. 1996; 41: 2477–2481.

Crack JC, Green J, Thomson AJ, Le Brun NE. Iron-sulfur clusters as biological sensors: the chemistry of reactions with molecular oxygen and nitric oxide. *Accounts of Chemical Research*. 2014 Oct 21;47(10):3196-205. PubMed PMID: 25262769. Epub 2014/09/30. eng.

de Onis M, Blössner M. Prevalence and trends of overweight among preschool children in developing countries. *Am J Clin Nutr*. 2000; 72: 1032–1039.

de Onis M, Blössner M, Villar J. Levels and patterns of intrauterine growth retardation in developing countries. *Eur J Clin Nutr*. 1998; 52 (Suppl.1): S5–S15.

de Wardener HE, MacGregor GA. Harmful effects of dietary salt in addition to hypertension. *J Hum Hypertens*. 2002; 16(4): 213–223.

Devine A, Criddle RA, Dick IM, Kerr DA, Prince RL. A longitudinal study of the effect of sodium and calcium intakes on regional bone density in postmenopausal women. *Am J Clin Nutr*. 1995; 62(4): 740–745.

Diamond TH, Levy S, Smith A, Day P. High bone turnover in Muslim women with vitamin D deficiency. *Med J Aust*. 2002; 177: 139–141.

Dickinson KM, Keogh JB, Clifton PM. Effects of a low-salt diet on flow-mediated dilatation in humans. *Am J Clin Nutr*. 2009; 89(2): 485–490.

Douglas PJ, Kevin RS, Wayne WC, Elena V, Robert RW. Role of dietary protein in the sarcopenia of aging. *Am J Clin Nutr*. 2008; 87(5): 1562S–1566S.

Ensminger AH. *Foods & Nutrition Encyclopedia*. vol. 1. Boca Raton, FL: CRC Press, 1994; ISBN 978-0-8493-8980-1. p. 527.

Fawzi W, Msamanga G. Micronutrients and adverse pregnancy outcomes in the context of HIV infection. *Nutr Rev*. 2004; 62: 269–275.

Fleming RM. The effect of high-protein diets on coronary blood flow. *Angiology*. 2000; 51(10): 817–826.

Gil A. Polyunsaturated fatty acids and inflammatory diseases. *Biomed Pharmacother*. 2002; 56: 388–396.

Goldfarb DS, Coe FL. Prevention of recurrent nephrolithiasis. *Am Fam Physician*. 1999; 60(8): 2269–2276.

Goldfarb S. Dietary factors in the pathogenesis and prophylaxis of calcium nephrolithiasis. *Kidney Int*. 1988; 34(4): 544–555.

Gooderham NJ, Murray S, Lynch AM, Yadollahi-Farsani M, Zhao K, Rich K, Boobis AR, Davies DS. Assessing human risk to heterocyclic amines. *Mutat Res*. 1997; 376: 53–60.

Gopalan C. Possible role for dietary leucine in the pathogenesis of pellagra. *The Lancet*. 1969; 293: 197–199. doi:10.1016/S0140-6736(69)91206-9.

Grant MM, Brock GR, Matthews JB, Chapple IL. Crevicular fluid glutathione levels in periodontitis and the effect of non-surgical therapy. *J Clin Periodontol.* 2010; 37: 17–23.

Guevara PG, Chavez CE, Castillo DC. Micronutient deficiencies and celiac disease in pediatrics. *Arch Argent Pediatr.* 2014; 112(5): 457–463.

Hamai A, Caneque T, Muller S, Mai TT, Hienzsch A, Ginestier C, et al. An iron hand over cancer stem cells. *Autophagy.* 2017 Jun 14:1-2. PubMed PMID: 28613094. Epub 2017/06/15. eng.

Hamlat-Khennaf N, Neggazi S, Ayari H, Feugier P, Bricca G, Aouichat-Bouguerra S, et al. [Inflammation in the perivascular adipose tissue and atherosclerosis]. *Comptes rendus biologies.* 2017 Mar;340(3):156-63. PubMed PMID: 28188070. Epub 2017/02/12. Inflammation dans le tissu adipeux peri-arteriel et atherome. fre.

Harris LJ. Critique of the saturation method for determining vitamin C levels. *The Lancet.* 1942; 1: 642–644.

Harris LJ, Abbasy MA, Yudkin J. Vitamins in human nutrition. Vitamin C reserves of subjects of the voluntary hospital class. *The Lancet.* 1936; 1: 1488.

Hashimoto A, Kambe T. Mg, Zn and Cu Transport Proteins: A Brief Overview from Physiological and Molecular Perspectives. *Journal of Nutritional Science and Vitaminology.* 2015;61 Suppl:S116-8. PubMed PMID: 26598820. Epub 2015/11/26. eng.

Hendriks HF. Use of nutrigenomics endpoints in dietary interventions. *The Proceedings of the Nutrition Society.* 2013 Aug;72(3):348-51. PubMed PMID: 23710901. Epub 2013/05/29. eng.

Hensley K, Robinson KA, Gabbita SP, Salaman S, Floyd RA. Reactive oxygen species, cell signaling, and cell injury. *Free Radic Biol Med.* 2000; 28(10): 1456–1462.

Higgins CC. Production and solution of urinary calculi: Experimental and clinical studies. *J Am Med Assoc.* 1935; 104: 1296–1299.

Howard MT, Carlson BA, Anderson CB, Hatfield DL. Translational redefinition of UGA codons is regulated by selenium availability. *The Journal of Biological Chemistry.* 2013;288(27):19401-13. PubMed PMID: 23696641. Pubmed Central PMCID: PMC3707644. Epub 2013/05/23. eng.

John MP. Nutritional rickets: Pathogenesis and prevention. *Pediatr Endocrinol Rev.* 2013; 10(Suppl 2): 7–13.

Jung SL, Michele MS, Annie V, Jean-Marc S, Robert HL. The role of fructose in the pathogenesis of NAFLD and the metabolic syndrome. *Nat Rev Gastroenterol Hepatol.* 2010; 7: 251–264. doi:10.1038/nrgastro.2010.41.

Kafatos A, Hatzis C. *Clinical Nutrition for Medical Students.* Greece: University of Crete, 2008.

Kaniak-Golik A, Skoneczna A. Mitochondria-nucleus network for genome stability. *Free Radical Biology & Medicine.* 2015;82:73-104. PubMed PMID: 25640729. Epub 2015/02/03. eng.

Katan MB, Vroomen LH, Hermus RJ. Reduction of casein-induced hypercholesterolaemia and atherosclerosis in rabbits and rats by dietary glycine, arginine and alanine. *Atherosclerosis.* 1982; 43: 381–391.

Katona P, Katona-Apte J. The interaction between nutrition and infection. *Clin Infect Dis.* 2008; 46: 1582–1588. doi: 10.1086/587658.

King AJ, Levey AS. Dietary protein and renal function. *J Am Soc Nephrol.* 1993; 3: 1723–1737.

King EJ, Haslewood GA, Delbry GE. Beal D. Micro-chemical methods of blood analysis: Revised and extended. *The Lancet.* 1942; 1: 207–209.

Kritchevsky D. Dietary protein, cholesterol and atherosclerosis: A review of the early history. *J Nutr.* 1995; 125: 589S–593S.

Kuller LH. Dietary fat and chronic diseases: Epidemiologic overview. *J Am Diet Assoc.* 1997; 97(7 Suppl): S9–15.

Lee YK, Park SY, Kim YM, Kim DC, Lee WS, Surh YJ, et al. Suppression of mTOR via Akt-dependent and -independent mechanisms in selenium-treated colon cancer cells: involvement of AMPKalpha1. *Carcinogenesis.* 2010;31(6):1092–9.

Lentine K, Wrone EM. New insights into protein intake and progression of renal disease. *Curr Opin Nephrol Hypertens*. 2004; 13: 333–336.

Lorenz MW, Markus HS, Bots ML, Rosvall M, Sitzer M. Prediction of clinical cardiovascular events with carotid intima-media thickness: A systematic review and meta-analysis. *Circulation*. 2007; 115(4): 459–467.

Maes M, Smith R, Christophe A, Cosyns P, Desnyder R, Meltzer H. Fatty acid composition in major depression: Decreased omega 3 fractions in cholesteryl esters and increased C20: 4 omega 6/C20:5 omega 3 ratio in cholesteryl esters and phospholipids. *J Affect Disord*. 1996; 38: 35–46.

Maes M, Smith R, Christophe A, Vandoolaeghe E, Van Gastel A, Neels H, Demedts P, Wauters A, Meltzer HY. Lower serum high-density lipoprotein cholesterol (HDL-C) in major depression and in depressed men with serious suicidal attempts: Relationship with immune-inflammatory markers. *Acta Psychiatr Scand*. 1997; 95: 212–221.

Mason JB, Musgrove P, Habicht JP. *At least one-third of poor countries' burden is due to malnutrition. Working paper no. 1, Disease Control Priorities Project*. Bethesda, MD: Fogarty International Center, National Institutes of Health, 2003.

Matsudo V, Matsudo S, Andrade D, Araujo T, Andrade E, de Oliveira LC, Braggion G. Promotion of physical activity in a developing country: The Agita São Paulo experience. *Public Health Nutr*. 2002; 5: 253–261. doi: 10.1079/PHN2001301.

McCord MC, Aizenman E. The role of intracellular zinc release in aging, oxidative stress, and Alzheimer's disease. Frontiers in aging neuroscience. 2014;6:77. PubMed PMID: 24860495. Pubmed Central PMCID: PMC4028997. Epub 2014/05/27. eng.

Melchior M, Chastang JF, Falissars B, Galéra C, Tremblay RE, Côté SM, Boivin M. Food insecurity and children's mental health: A prospective birth cohort study. *PLoS One*. 2012; 7(12): e52615.

Metges CC, Barth CA. Metabolic consequences of a high dietary-protein intake in adulthood: Assessment of the available evidence. *J Nutr*. 2000; 130: 886–889.

Meydani SN, Han SN, Wu D. Vitamin E and immune response in the aged: Molecular mechanisms and clinical implications. *Immunol Rev*. 2005; 205: 269–284.

Milward MR, Chapple ILC. The role of diet in periodontal disease. *Dental Health* 2013; 52: 18–21.

Milward MR, Chapple ILC, Wright HJ, Millard JL, Matthews JB, Cooper PR. Differential activation of NF-kB and gene expression in oral epithelial cells by periodontal pathogens. *Clin Exp Immunol*. 2007; 148: 307–324.

Minot GR, Strauss MB, Cobb S. "Alcoholic" polyneuritis, dietary deficiency as a factor in its production. *New Engl J Med*. 1933; 208: 1244–1249.

Miyake Y, Sasaki S, Tanaka K, Hirota Y. Consumption of vegetables, fruit, and antioxidants during pregnancy and wheeze and eczema in infants. *Allergy*. 2010; 65: 758–765.

Mocchegiani E, Costarelli L, Basso A, Giacconi R, Piacenza F, Malavolta M. Metallothioneins, ageing and cellular senescence: Current pharmaceutical target. Current pharmaceutical design. 2013;19(9):1753-64. PubMed PMID: 23061732. Epub 2012/10/16. eng.

Morris MC, Evans DA, Bienias JL, Tangney CC, Bennett DA, Aggarwal N, Schneider J, Wilson RS. Dietary fats and the risk of incident alzheimer disease. *Arch Neurol*. 2003; 60(2): 194–200. doi:10.1001/archneur.60.2.194.

Müller O, Garenne M, Kouyaté B, Becher H. The association between protein-energy malnutrition, malaria morbidity and all-cause mortality in West African children. *Trop Med Int Health*. 2003; 8: 507–511.

Murray CJL, Lopez AD. *The global burden of disease: A comprehensive assessment of mortality and disability from diseases, injuries, and risk factors in 1990 and projected to 2020*. Cambridge, Harvard School of Public Health on behalf of the World Health Organization and the World Bank, 1996. (Global Burden of Disease and Injury Series, vol. 1).

Mutlu E, Keshavarzian A, Mutlu GM. Hyperalbuminemia and elevated transaminases associated with high-protein diet. *Scand J Gastroenterol*. 2006; 41(6): 759–760.

Myers SA. Zinc transporters and zinc signaling: new insights into their role in type 2 diabetes. *International Journal of Endocrinology*. 2015;2015:167503. PubMed PMID: 25983752. Pubmed Central PMCID: PMC4423030. Epub 2015/05/20. eng.

Neidecker-Gonzales O, Nestel P, Bouis H. Estimating the global cost of vitamin A capsule supplementation: A review of the literature. *Food Nutr Bull*. 2007; 28: 307–316.

Neve J. Selenium as a risk factor for cardiovascular diseases. *Eur J Cardiovasc Risk*. 1996; 3(1): 42–47.

Neitemeier S, Dolga AM, Honrath B, Karuppagounder SS, Alim I, Ratan RR, et al. Inhibition of HIF-prolyl-4-hydroxylases prevents mitochondrial impairment and cell death in a model of neuronal oxytosis. *Cell Death & Disease*. 2016;7:e2214. PubMed PMID: 27148687. Pubmed Central PMCID: PMC4917646. Epub 2016/05/07. eng.

Neri C, Edlow AG. Effects of Maternal Obesity on Fetal Programming: Molecular Approaches. *Cold Spring Harbor Perspectives in Medicine*. 2015;6(2):a026591. PubMed PMID: 26337113. Epub 2015/09/05. eng.

Norat T, Riboli E. Meat consumption and colorectal cancer: A review of epidemiologic evidence. *Nutr Rev*. 2001; 59: 37–47.

Oppenheimer S. Iron and its relation to immunity and infectious disease. *J Nutr*. 2001; 131: 616S–635S.

Orr JB. *Food, Health and Income: Report on a Survey of Adequacy of Diet in Relation to Income*, London: Macmillan and Co, 1936.

Paglia G, Miedico O, Cristofano A, Vitale M, Angiolillo A, Chiaravalle AE, et al. Distinctive Pattern of Serum Elements During the Progression of Alzheimer's Disease. *Scientific Reports*. 2016;6:22769. PubMed PMID: 26957294. Pubmed Central PMCID: PMC4783774. Epub 2016/03/10. eng.

Park S, Bae J, Nam BH, Yoo KY. Aetiology of cancer in Asia. *Asian Pac J Cancer Prev*. 2008; 9: 371–380.

Patterson AJ, Brown WJ, Roberts DC. Dietary and supplement treatment of iron deficiency results in improvements in general health and fatigue in Australian women of child-bearing age. *J Am Coll Nutr*. 2001; 20: 337–342.

Peet M, Murphy B, Shay J, Horrobin D. Depletion of omega-3 fatty acid levels in red blood cell membranes of depressive patients. *Biol Psychiatry*. 1998; 43: 315–319.

Perry IJ, Beevers DG. Salt intake and stroke: A possible direct effect. *J Hum Hypertens*. 1992; 6(1): 23–25.

Popkin BM. The shift in stages of the nutritional transition in the developing world differs from past experiences! *Public Health Nutr*. 2002; 5: 205–214.

Rowntree JI. The effect of the use of mineral oil upon the absorption of vitamin A. *J Nutr*. 1931; 3: 345.

Safar ME, Thuilliez C, Richard V, Benetos A. Pressure-independent contribution of sodium to large artery structure and function in hypertension. *Cardiovasc Res*. 2000; 46(2): 269–276.

Saha SK, Lee SB, Won J, Choi HY, Kim K, Yang GM, et al. Correlation between Oxidative Stress, Nutrition, and Cancer Initiation. International journal of molecular sciences. 2017 Jul 17;18(7). PubMed PMID: 28714931. Epub 2017/07/18. eng.

Sanders PW. Vascular consequences of dietary salt intake. *Am J Physiol Renal Physiol*. 2009; 297(2): F237–243.

Sandstead HH, Freeland-Graves JH. Dietary phytate, zinc and hidden zinc deficiency. Journal of trace elements in medicine and biology : organ of the Society for Minerals and Trace Elements (GMS). 2014 Oct;28(4):414-7. PubMed PMID: 25439135. Epub 2014/12/03. eng.

Sandu O, Song K, Cai W, Zheng F, Uribarri J, Vlassara H. Insulin resistance and type 2 diabetes in high-fat-fed mice are linked to high glycotoxin intake. *Diabetes*. 2005; 54: 2314–2319.

Sawicki KT, Chang HC, Ardehali H. Role of heme in cardiovascular physiology and disease. Journal of the American Heart Association. 2015 Jan 05;4(1):e001138. PubMed PMID: 25559010. Pubmed Central PMCID: PMC4330050. Epub 2015/01/07. eng.

Scrimshaw NS, Taylor CE, Gordon JE. *Interactions of Nutrition and Infection*. Geneva: World Health Organization, 1968.

Shankar AH. Nutritional modulation of malaria morbidity and mortality. *J Infect Dis.* 2000; 182: S37–S53.

Shetty S, Marsicano JR, Copeland PR. Uptake and Utilization of Selenium from Selenoprotein P. *Biological Trace Element Research.* 2017. PubMed PMID: 28488249. Epub 2017/05/11. eng.

Sidi A, Ashley F. Influence of frequent sugar intakes on experimental gingivitis. *J Periodontol.* 1984; 55: 419–423.

Sies H, Jones DP. Oxidative stress. *Encyclopedia of Stress.* San Diego, CA: Elsevier, 2007.

Simon G. Experimental evidence for blood pressure-independent vascular effects of high sodium diet. *Am J Hypertens.* 2003; 16(12): 1074–1078.

Simopoulos AP. Evolutionary aspects of diet, the omega-6/omega-3 ratio and genetic variation: Nutritional implications for chronic diseases. *Biomed Pharmacother.* 2006; 60: 502–507.

Sinha R. An epidemiologic approach to studying heterocyclic amines. *Mutat Res.* 2002; 506–507: 197–204.

Socransky SS, Haffajee AD, Cugini MA, Smith C, Kent RL Jr. Microbial complexes in subgingival plaque. *J Clin Periodontol.* 1998; 25: 134–144.

Sonnenberg A. Geographic and temporal variations of sugar and margarine consumption in relation to Crohn's disease. *Digestion.* 1988; 41: 161–171.

Strauss MB, McDonald WJ. Polyneuritis of pregnancy: A dietary deficiency disorder. *J Am Med Assoc.* 1933; 100: 1320–1323.

Sugimura T. Nutrition and dietary carcinogens. *Carcinogenesis.* 2000; 21: 387–395.

Tan PH, Sagoo P, Chan C, Yates JB, Campbell J, Beutelspacher SC, Foxwell BM, Lombardi G, George AJ. Inhibition of NF-kappa B and oxidative pathways in human dendritic cells by antioxidative vitamins generates regulatory T cells. *J Immunol.* 2005; 174: 7633–7644.

Tapia G, Valenzuela R, Espinosa A, Romanque P, Dossi C, Gonzalez-Manan D, et al. N-3 long-chain PUFA supplementation prevents high fat diet induced mouse liver steatosis and inflammation in relation to PPAR-alpha upregulation and NF-kappaB DNA binding abrogation. Molecular nutrition & food research. 2014 Jun;58(6):1333-41. PubMed PMID: 24436018. Epub 2014/01/18. eng.

Tazuma S, Kanno K, Sugiyama A, Kishikawa N. Nutritional factors (nutritional aspects) in biliary disorders: Bile acid and lipid metabolism in gallstone diseases and pancreaticobiliary maljunction. *J Gastroenterol Hepatol.* 2013; 28(4): 103–107. doi: 10.1111/jgh.12241.

Teucher B, Dainty JR, Spinks CA, Majsak-Newman G, Berry DJ, Hoogewerff JA, et al. Sodium and bone health: Impact of moderately high and low salt intakes on calcium metabolism in postmenopausal women. *J Bone Miner Res.* 2008; 23: 1477–1485. doi: 10.1359/jbmr.080408.

Tominaga S, Kuroishi T. An ecological study on diet/nutrition and cancer in Japan. *Int J Cancer.* 1997; 10: 2–6.

Tomkins A, Watson F. *Malnutrition and infection—A review. Nutrition policy discussion paper no. 5,* 1989. http://www.unsystem.org/SCN/archives/npp05/ch4.htm. Accessed 31 March 2016.

Tompkins A, Watson F. *Malnutrition and infection: A review.* Geneva, Administrative Committee on Coordination/Subcommittee on Nutrition, 1989. (ACC/SCN State-of-the-art Series Nutrition Policy Discussion Paper, No. 5).

Touyz RM. Role of magnesium in the pathogenesis of hypertension. *Mol Aspects Med.* 2003; 24: 107–136.

UNICEF Statistics. *Progress for children: A child survival report card,* 2006. http://www.cdc.gov/malaria/impact/index.htm. Accessed 31 April 2016.

Utsugi M, Dobashi K, Ishizuka T, Endou K, Hamuro J, Murata Y, Nakazawa T, Mori M. c-Jun N-terminal kinase negatively regulates lipopolysaccharide-induced IL-12 production in human macrophages: Role of mitogen-activated protein kinase in glutathione redox regulation of IL-12 production. *J Immunol.* 2003; 171: 628–635.

Vallbracht R, Gilory J. Vitamin A induced benign intracranial hypertension. *Cac J Neurol Sci.* 1976; 3: 59–61.

Warner ED, Brinkhous KM, Smith HP. Bleeding tendency of obstructive jaundice; prothrombin deficiency and dietary factors. *Proc Soc exp Biol NY.* 1938; 37: 628.

Wenzhen D, Bruce L, Roy GC, Inna IK, Jean LC, Mark PM. Dietary folate deficiency and elevated homocysteine levels endanger dopaminergic neurons in models of Parkinson's disease. *J Neurochem.* 2002; 80: 101–110.

Whitney EN, Rolfes SR. *Understanding nutrition*, 10th edition, p 6. Thomson-Wadsworth. 2005.

WHO. *Diet, nutrition and the prevention of chronic diseases. Report of a WHO Study Group.* Geneva, 1990. (WHO Technical Report Series, No. 797).

WHO. *World declaration and plan of action for nutrition.* Rome, Food and Agriculture Organization of the United Nations and Geneva, 1992a.

WHO. *Nutrition and development: A global assessment.* Rome, Food and Agriculture Organization of the United Nations and Geneva, 1992b.

WHO. Promoting appropriate diets and healthy lifestyles. In: *Major issues for nutrition strategies.* Rome, Food and Agriculture Organization of the United Nations and Geneva, 1992c.

WHO. *WHO/UNICEF. Global prevalence of vitamin A deficiency. MDIS Working Paper No. 2.* Geneva, 1995. (Document WHO/NUT/95.3).

WHO. *Life in the 21st century: A vision for all. The world health report 1998.* Geneva, 1998.

WHO. *WHO/UNICEF/International Council for the Control of Iodine Deficiency Disorders. Progress towards the elimination of iodine deficiency disorders (IDD).* Geneva, 1999. (Document WHO/NHD/99.4).

WHO. *A global agenda for combating malnutrition: Progress report.* Geneva, 2000a. (Document WHO/NHD/00.6).

WHO. *Obesity: Preventing and managing the global epidemic. Report of a WHO Consultation.* Geneva, 2000b. (WHO Technical Report Series, No. 894).

WHO. *WHO/UNICEF/United Nations University. Iron deficiency anemia assessment, prevention and control: A guide for programme managers.* Geneva, 2001. (Document WHO/NHD/01.3).

WHO. *The world health report 2002: Reducing risks, promoting healthy life.* Geneva, 2002a.

WHO. *Diet, physical activity and health.* Geneva, 2002b. (Documents A55/16 and A55/16 Corr.1).

WHO. *Childhood nutrition and progress in implementing the International Code of Marketing of Breast-milk Substitutes.* Geneva, 2002c. (Document A55/14).

Wilkinson N, Pantopoulos K. The IRP/IRE system in vivo: insights from mouse models. Frontiers in pharmacology. 2014;5:176. PubMed PMID: 25120486. Pubmed Central PMCID: PMC4112806. Epub 2014/08/15. eng.

William R, Sandrine A, Fati N, Bruno V. Nutritional factors and alzheimer's disease. *J Gerontol A Biol Sci Med Sci.* 2001; 56: M675–M680. doi: 10.1093/gerona/56.11.M675.

Witte KK, Clark AL. Nutritional abnormalities contributing to cachexia in chronic illness. *Int J Cardiol.* 2002; 85: 23–31.

Yoshida K. [Iron accumulation and neurodegenerative diseases]. Nihon rinsho Japanese journal of clinical medicine. 2016 Jul;74(7):1161–7. PubMed PMID: 27455807. Epub 2016/07/28. jpn.

Yoshikawa S, Shimada A, Shinzawa-Itoh K. Respiratory conservation of energy with dioxygen: cytochrome C oxidase. Metal ions in life sciences. 2015;15:89–130. PubMed PMID: 25707467. Epub 2015/02/25. eng.

Zimmerman MT, Bayse CA, Ramoutar RR, Brumaghim JL. Sulfur and selenium antioxidants: challenging radical scavenging mechanisms and developing structure-activity relationships based on metal binding. Journal of inorganic biochemistry. 2015 Apr;145:30–40. PubMed PMID: 25600984. Epub 2015/01/21. eng.

20

Gene-Based Dietary Advice and Eating Behavior

Aparoop Das
Dibrugarh University
Dibrugarh, India

Manash Pratim Pathak
Dibrugarh University
Dibrugarh, India
and
Defence Research Laboratory
Tezpur, India

Pronobesh Chattopadhyay
Defence Research Laboratory
Tezpur, India

Yashwant V. Pathak
University of South Florida
Tampa, Florida

Contents

20.1 Introduction 516
    20.1.1 Nutrigenomics 517
    20.1.2 Nutrigenetics 517
    20.1.3 Single nucleotide polymorphisms 518
20.2 Impact of dietary habits on prophylactic or therapeutic
    management of some diseases 519
    20.2.1 Cancer 519
    20.2.2 Cardiovascular disease 519
    20.2.3 Diabetes 520
    20.2.4 Other diseases 521
20.3 Gene–diet interaction in management of diseases 521
20.4 Application of nutrigenomics and nutrigenetics: Legal aspects 523
20.5 Conclusion 524
References 524

20.1 Introduction

Worldwide, researchers have been developing numerous strategies for management of noncommunicable chronic disease such as cancer, diabetes, and cardiovascular disease (CVD), but every strategy comes with an adverse effect, directly or indirectly. Food consumption is one of the factors that have both positive as well as negative implications due to the diverse individual response towards food and the bioactive compounds in it. Researcher have gradually started to understand the individual response towards dietary modification and thus have started the process of development of personalized diets for preventing or treating chronic diseases (Table 20.1). Gene-based dietary advice and the field of nutritional genomics have gathered momentum at a fast pace and undergone significant changes and development in the last two decades, due to which two new terms have come into being: *nutrigenetics* and *nutrigenomics*. The ultimate goal for the researchers will be to utilize the available resources for development of a personalized diet that suits the variable genetic makeup of an individual within a population for specific health conditions (Figure 20.1) (Schwartz 2014).

Table 20.1 List of Nutrients/Bio-Active Compounds in Prevention of Some Diseases

Nutrients/Bio-Active Compounds	Presence in Food	Disease	Reference
Resveratrol	Grapes	Coronary artery disease	Carneiro et al. 2013
Oleic acid	Peanut oil	Type-2 diabetes	Vassiliou et al. 2009
Flavonoid	Green vegetables	Cancer, Type-2 diabetes	Kaviarasan and Pugalendi 2009
Eicosapentaenoic acid (EPA) and docosahexaenoic acid (DHA)	Marine products	Type-2 diabetes	Flachs 2006
Naringin		Type-2 diabetes	Jung 2006
Folic acid (Vitamin B9)	Liver, kidney, egg yolk, spinach, beetroot, broccoli, orange	Cancer, heart disease,	Neeha 2013
Fatty acids	Salmon, sardines, herring, mackerel, soyoil, sunflower oil, palm oil	Obesity, CVD, Diabetes	Neeha 2013
Vitamin E (Tocopherols)	Tomato, spinach, broccoli, blueberries, mangoes, kiwi, papaya, almonds,	Colon cancer, heart disease, immune dysfunction	Neeha 2013
Nicotinamide		Type-2 diabetes	Ye 2006
Plant sterol		Hypercholesterolemia	Izer 2011 and Cohen 2006

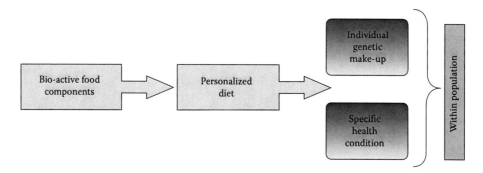

Figure 20.1 *Influence of bioactive food components on specific health condition within a population.*

20.1.1 Nutrigenomics

Nutrigenomics and nutrigenetics are very interrelated terms. Terminologically, nutrigenomics is like other omics technologies, when high-throughput technologies applied to the field of nutrition (Müller et al 2003). An inclusive definition comes into being when nutrigenomics is referred along with nutrigenomics. In such case, nutrigenomics correlates the effects on gene expression and gene regulation by ingested nutrients and other food or dietetic components to identify useful or harmful effects (German 2005; Miggiano 2006). In the postgenomic era, emerging sophisticated research tools have proved to be a boon for geneticists and nutritionists to develop dietary strategies by monitoring the genetic makeup, metabolome, transcriptome, and proteome that are targeted to provide optimum nutrition for single individuals (Neeha 2013). Use of research tools like DNA microarray technology and quantitative real time polymerase chain reaction (PCR) will help determine associations between diet and diseases, which will help researchers understand the etiologic aspect of chronic diseases such as cancer, type 2 diabetes, obesity, and cardiovascular disease (CVS) (Miggiano 2006).

20.1.2 Nutrigenetics

Nutrigenetics deals with the coordination of the genetic makeup of an individual and their response to various dietary nutrients, which paves a way to know the contrasting responses of people to various dietary nutrients (Hawkinson 2007). Nutrigenetics aims to investigate how the phenomena of individual genetic background and underlying genetic polymorphisms specifically determines their response to diet (de Roos 2013). Researchers are on a quest to uncover a treatment strategy for chronic diseases such as diabetes mellitus, cardiovascular disease, hypertension, etc., investigating the genetic variants

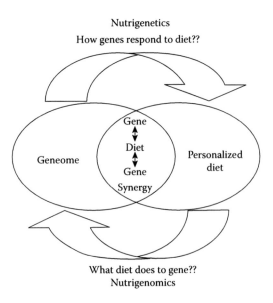

Figure 20.2 *Relationship between nutrigenomics and nutrigenetics.*

that interact with dietary or lifestyle by identifying specific populations classified by specific genotypes with the help of nutrigenetics. In short, nutrigenomics encompasses the effect of nutrients on expressions at the genetic level whereas nutrigenetics deals with the response to the effects of our genetic makeup to nutrients (Figure 20.2).

20.1.3 Single nucleotide polymorphisms

About 99.9% of genomic sequences are identical in every human being and the remaining 0.1% of variations in genomic sequences are responsible for phenotypic differences like height, weight, etc., and an individual's susceptibility to disease conditions and health status (Kaput 2004). Polymorphism is a phenomenon in which genes show small sequence differences in polymorphic sites among the same study population, among which single nucleotide polymorphisms (SNPs) are the most common type of variations (Hawkinson 2007).

SNPs influence dietary absorption and metabolic response, which may lead to onset of chronic diseases in human populations. Study of SNPs provides an integral means to elucidate and prevent numerous chronic diseases such as cardiovascular disease, diabetes mellitus, hypertension, etc. The relationship between folate and the gene for MTHFR (5,10-methylenetetrahydrofolate reductase) is one of the best examples to elucidate the function of SNPs. Folate is a vital component for proper functioning of MTFHR. MTHFR supplies 5-methylenetetrahydrofolate for remethylation of homocysteine to form methionine, which is an important precursor for production of many neurotransmitters and regulation of gene expression.

20.2 Impact of dietary habits on prophylactic or therapeutic management of some diseases

20.2.1 Cancer

Though many literatures have related dietary habits to occurrence of cancer, specific bioactive components found in foods are also reported to provide prophylactic as well as therapeutic treatment to several stages of cancer (World Cancer Research Fund 1997). Approximately 35% of all human cancers considered to be contributed to by dietary habits and, for some specific cancers, the association is as high as 70% (Pet 1981). Absence of genotoxins influences the genome and epigenome, which plays the role of an indicator for deficiency in nutrients that are required as cofactors of DNA repair enzymes as well as in prevention of DNA oxidation, incorporation of uracil into DNA, and for methylation of CpG sequences (Fenech 2005).

Alteration in epigenetics plays an important role in the development and pathogenesis of many forms of cancer. Epigenetic modification suppresses the genes responsible for cell cycle regulation, DNA repair, angiogenesis, and apoptosis in the form of hypermethylation of their specific own CpG islands (Komduur 2011; Panagiotakos et al. 2007). Involvement of SNPs has both positive as well as negative response to a food component. As reported, women that consume <764 g/day of fruits and vegetables, <155 mg/day of ascorbic acid, and <7.5 mg/day of tocopherol on average had a greater risk of developing breast cancer due to polymorphism, which causes a change in valine to alanine change in the 6 position in the signal sequence of superoxide dismutase, which is dependent on the enzyme manganese (Ambrosone 1999). Polymorph of N-acetyl transferase (NAT) is found in two forms: NAT1 and NAT2, which are found in well-cooked red meat. Cooking red meat at high temperature yields heterocyclic aromatic amines (HAA), which binds DNA and lead to the development of cancers by producing reactive metabolites (Garg et al. 2014).

20.2.2 Cardiovascular disease

Nutritional modulation plays an important role in both the progression and prevention of cardiovascular diseases (CVD). CVD morbidity and mortality significantly decreased in different developed countries by recognizing the main dietary risk factors that promote atherogenesis and the effort to reduce the impact of such factors in the study population (Kant 2004; WHO 1997). The public is devoid of clear scientific evidence, which has led to the creation of a certain degree of doubt about which diet to follow to prevent or treat different altered phenotypes involved in CVD (Chahoud 2004). A 7-year longitudinal cohort study showed that a healthy diet rich in fish, raw vegetables, fresh fruit, and poultry, with wine, and low in high-fat dairy products, may modify atherothrombosis and thereby favorably influence the development of CVD.

There have been contrasting opinions on the addition of saturated fatty acids as well as carbohydrates as prophylactic as well as therapeutic strategy for management of CVD. Although epidemiological studies support a beneficial association of ω-3 fatty acids with CVD, this fact has not been confirmed by clinical studies. Dietary patterns consisting of vegetables, fish, nuts, etc., compared to processed grains are the backbone of a heart-healthy diet for CVD. Diets high in omega-3 PUFAs are related with decreased risk of cardiovascular disease (CVD) and prevention of certain types of cancer. Polymorphisms lead to altered response to omega-3 PUFAs in certain enzymes, transcription factors, inflammatory molecules, and lipoproteins (Schwartz 2014). The Framingham Study (Lai 2006) studied the possible modulation of an intermediate phenotype of CVD. Numerous meta-analyses evaluated one or more genetic variant and intermediate phenotypes of CVD. Meta-analysis of the classic APOE and CETP polymorphisms in plasma lipids and CVD risk is one such example (Bennet 2007).

20.2.3 Diabetes

Apart from sedentary lifestyle and environmental factors, diet and its interaction with multiple genes plays a vicious role in the increasing incidence of both types of diabetes mellitus (DM), which is evident from the pathophysiology of the said disorder (Schulze and Hu 2005). Diabetes UK (2011) have published guidelines that have undergone peer review and aim to support self-management, promote healthy lifestyles, and reduce the risk of type 2 diabetes and the comorbidities associated with diabetes (Dyson et al. 2011). A study of food habits suggested the combined effect of fatty fish, bilberries, and wholegrain products to improve endothelial dysfunction and inflammation in overweight and obese individuals at high risk of developing diabetes (De Mello 2011). Another study indicated that diet based on high-heat-treated foods enhances the risk of type 2 diabetes (T2D) as well as CVD, which is evident from the increment of their biological markers in healthy people. Mild cooking techniques in place of high-heat-treatment may help to positively modulate biomarkers associated with an increased risk of DM and CVD (Birlouez 2010).

Ignorance of a disciplined diet–based lifestyle may aggravate the development of DM. Omission of breakfast, which is one of the most important meals of the day to maintain a healthy life, was associated with an increased risk of T2D in men even after adjustment for basal metabolic rate (BMI). Association between snacking between meals and T2D risk is managed by BMI (Mekary et al. 2012). Diets that are high in animal protein are associated with an increased diabetes risk. When protein is consumed as an energy source, replacing carbohydrates or fat, the risk of developing DM increases manifold (Sluijs et al. 2010). The Mediterranean diet (MedDiet) is widely known for use of olive oil. A report suggested that MedDiet without calorie restriction seems to be effective in the prevention of diabetes in subjects at high cardiovascular risk (Salas et al. 2011).

20.2.4 Other diseases

Abdominal pain, diarrhea, and weight loss, etc., are some of the common symptoms of inflammatory bowel diseases (IBD), which includes ulcerative colitis and Crohn's disease. Gene–diet therapy has been implicated in IBD, upon which exclusive enteral nutrition (EEN) therapy with elemental, semi-elemental, or polymeric formula diets has been shown to improve the condition of IBD and is regarded as the first-line therapy (Borrelli 2006; Day et al. 2006; Heuschkel et al. 2000; Sandhu et al. 2010). Phytosterol or plant sterol is recommended as an adjunctive therapy for hypercholesterolemia along with statins that reduce cholesterol absorption at the intestinal lumen through the Niemann-Pick C1 like 1 (NPC1L1) transporter pathway. Plant sterols when prescribed with stains double the efficacy of statins alone by stimulating the expression of NPC1L1 polymorphisms (Cohen 2006; Izar et al. 2011).

20.3 Gene–diet interaction in management of diseases

The diverse response to cancer incidence among and within same study population indicates an individual's outcome to interaction of genetic factors to gene, protein, and metabolite expression patterns (Davis and Milner 2004). Natural products are found to have epigenetic targets in cancer cells and may act in the prevention of cancer. Cruciferous vegetables, herbs, grapes, garlic, tea, and soy products are reported to have compounds that may enhance the defense mechanism against different types of cancer by modulating the epigenetic factors, which thereby impact initiation and progression of oncogenesis (Cheung 2010; Ho et al. 2009; Ravindran et al. 2009; Shu et al. 2010). Apart from the gene–diet interaction, calorie restriction (CR) without malnutrition, and possibly protein restriction, prevents cancer by avoiding accumulation of DNA damage or by potentiating the regression of preneoplastic lesions (Longo and Fontana 2010). CR may promote induction of senescence or apoptosis to prevent accumulation of multiple DNA mutations in critical genes (i.e., oncogenes or tumor suppressor genes), which may lead to transformation of normal healthy human cells to highly malignant tumor cells (Bishop 1996; Lengauer et al. 1998; Sharpless 2002).

Dietary supplements, taken by one class of patients as "natural, safe, and good for you" produce an adverse effect and in the worst-case scenario may increase risk of developing cancer if not properly monitored (Hori et al. 2011). For instance, vitamins generally considered as safe when taken in combination can result in increased risk of aggressive prostate cancer (Lawson et al. 2007;

Neuhouser et al. 2009). Data from the American Association of Poison Control Centers has shown an increase in adverse effects or death due to consumption of dietary supplements. So, patients should be advised of the merits and demerits of dietary supplement before consumption (Figure 20.3). A recent study suggested an "ideal" prostate diet, which comprises high intake of vegetables, tomatoes (both cooked and uncooked), soy, and green tea in addition to a healthy weight and lifestyle through healthy eating and regular exercise (Hori et al. 2011).

For the proper management of CVD, there has been an increasing debate worldwide about the proper selection of fatty acid in the diet for CVD as well as non-CVD patients. A recent study evaluated the effectiveness of replacing dietary saturated fat with omega-6 linoleic acid for effective prevention of coronary heart disease and death, but in contrast substitution of omega-6 linoleic acid increases the risk of death from all causes, coronary heart disease, and cardiovascular disease, which may result in the impact of earlier practice for advising substitution of omega-6 linoleic acid or poly-unsaturated fatty acid (PUFA) for saturated fatty acid (SFA) (Ramsden 2013). CVD is one of the key comorbidities of obesity-related disorders. Regular consumption of fried food aggravates the obese condition, especially in the teenage population. A study was conducted to estimate the potential modification of an individual's genetic makeup. Among many variants, FTO (fat mass and obesity-associated) genotype showed the strongest interaction with fried food consumption on body

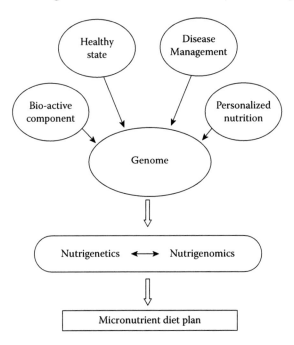

Figure 20.3 *Factors needed to be taken into account while recommending a micronutrient diet plan.*

mass index (BMI). Along with FTO, other variants such as GNPDA2, NEGR1, SEC16B, and MC4R showed potential interactions with fried food consumption on BMI (Qi et al. 2014).

The traditional Mediterranean diet, characterized by a high intake of olive oil, fruit, nuts, vegetables, and cereals; a moderate intake of fish and poultry; a low intake of dairy products, red meat, processed meats, and sweets; and wine in moderation, consumed with meals, is reported to reduce the major risk of CVD among high-risk patients (Estruch et al. 2013). Resveratrol-containing grape supplement was screened for its beneficial effect on patients suffering from coronary artery disease (CAD) for 1 year. After 1 year of administration, the group administered with grape extract showed promising increment of anti-inflammatory serum adiponectin and a decreasing level of thrombogenic plasminogen activator inhibitor type 1 (PAI-1), as compared to the placebo group.

Oleic acid and foods rich in oleic acid such as peanut oil has been shown to reverse the inhibitory effect upon insulin production and can have a beneficial effect in type 2 diabetes (Vassiliou et al. 2009). Flavonoid is reported to augment PPARα expression and stabilize blood triglycerides in high-fat-fed diabetic rats (Kaviarasan and Pugalendi 2009). Association of several single nucleotide polymorphisms (SNPs) with fasting glucose and insulin concentration in diabetes-free individuals has been studied recently by genome-wide association studies (GWAS). The study hinted a possible interaction between variation in (rs780094) GCKR and whole-grain intake in influencing fasting insulin concentrations (Nettleton et al. 2010). The same dietary and lifestyle factors influence individuals differently due to different genetic profiling. Men with a higher genetic risk score (GRS) of type 2 diabetes susceptibility based on certain established single nucleotide polymorphisms were found to have increasing multivariate adjusted odds ratio. Moreover, a significant interaction of diabetes risk with GRS has been found in the Western dietary pattern, comprising processed meat, red meat, and heme iron (Hu 2011).

Adiponectin gene G276T under the APM1 locus has shown a significant association with decreased CVD risk and increased plasma concentration in diabetic men (Qi et al. 2005). As reported by a study, intake of cereal fiber was associated with higher adiponectin concentrations in type 2 diabetic women, whereas dietary glycemic load and glycemic index were inversely associated with plasma adiponectin concentrations (Qi et al. 2006). Intake of diet rich in eicosapentaenoic acid (EPA) and docosahexaenoic acid (DHA) led to stimulation of *Adipoq* (adiponectin gene) expression in mice fed a high-fat diet, which supports the antidiabetic effects of the compounds (Flachs et al. 2006).

20.4 Application of nutrigenomics and nutrigenetics: Legal aspects

Recommendation of the use of nutrigenomics is premature at this juncture, as normalization of altered intermediate CVD phenotypes will be the first application in treatment and prevention of CVD (Corella 2009). Development of gene-targeted products by developers and registered dietitians and nutritional professionals need to consider the legal aspects surrounding nutrigenomics. Owing to the nascent stage of nutrigenomics, proper steps should be undertaken for developing ethical and legal guidelines to protect consumers.

Nutrigenomic tests and associated products and services are sold directly to customers via the Internet; as a result, consumers have more access to genetic information about themselves, but there is always a looming doubt about the authenticity of test results. Bans on direct access to such tests may put a hold on such fraudulent practices. Codes of practice and test registries should be implemented among good players, whereas regulatory guidelines should be passed to check bad players (Ries and Castle 2008). Customers are advised of their personalized nutrition based upon the results of genetic testing via the Internet, but in return they suffer from doubt and protection of consumer's rights added with far-reaching promises and contrasting disclaimers. Therefore, existing rules should be carefully assessed and developed to safeguard fundamental rights and ensure data protection and sufficient guarantees for consumers against potential misuse (Ahlgren 2013).

20.5 Conclusion

The fundamental goal of a gene-based diet is to develop a diet that caters to the health of the individual concerned and thereby makes provision for management of disease progression. Although common foods and other natural products are deemed to be safe for consumption, there are exceptions, too. Adverse effects that may lead to development of oncogenesis is one of the examples generated from the consumption of vitamins as a dietary supplement. At present, implementation of therapeutic strategies developed on the basis of a gene-based diet for prevention of CVD, diabetes, cancer, etc., is premature, owing to the diverse genetic makeup of the target population. Proper utilization of omics technology will help in-depth study of the gene-based dietary regime to check, alleviate, or cure chronic disease. As nutrigenomics and nutrigenetics are a relatively new field, regulatory and legal issues revolving around these fields should be addressed properly, ensuing safety for the individual health of the study population.

References

Ahlgren J, Nordgren A, Perrudin M, Ronteltap A, Savigny J, van Trijp H, Nordström K, Görman U, 2013. Consumers on the Internet: Ethical and legal aspects of commercialization of personalized nutrition. *Genes Nutr.* 8(4), 349–355.

Bennet AM, Di Angelantonio E, Ye Z, Wensley F, Dahlin A, Ahlbom A, Keavney B, Collins R, Wiman B, de Faire U, Danesh J, 2007. Association of apolipoprotein E genotypes with lipid levels and coronary risk. *JAMA.* 298, 1300–1311.

Birlouez-Aragon I, Saavedra G, Tessier FJ, Galinier A, Ait-Ameur L, Lacoste F, Niamba CN, Alt N, Somoza V, Lecerf JM, 2010. A diet based on high-heat-treated foods promotes risk factors for diabetes mellitus and cardiovascular diseases. *Am J Clin Nutr.* 91(5), 1220–1226.

Borrelli O, Cordischi L, Cirulli M, et al., 2006. Polymeric diet alone versus corticosteroids in the treatment of active pediatric Crohn's disease: A randomized controlled open-label trial. *Clin Gastroenterol Hepatol.* 2006; 4: 744–753.

Ambrosone CB, Freudenheim JL, Thompson PA, Bowman E, Vena JE, Marshall JR, Graham S, Laughlin R, Nemoto T, Shields P, 1999. Manganese superoxide dismutase (MnSOD) genetic polymorphisms, *Cancer Res.* 59, 602–606.

Chahoud G, Aude YW, Mehta JL, 2004. Dietary recommendations in the prevention and treatment of coronary heart disease: Do we have the ideal diet yet? *Am J Cardiol.* 94, 1260–1267.

Cheung KL, Khor TO, Huang M-T, Kong A-N, 2010, Differential *in vivo* mechanism of chemoprevention of tumor formation in azoxymethane/dextran sodium sulfate mice by PEITC and DBM. *Carcinogenesis* 31(5), 880–885.

Cohen JC, Pertsemlidis A, Fahmi S, Esmail S, Vega GL, Grundy SM, Hobbs HH, 2006. Multiple rare variants in NPC1L1 associated with reduced sterol absorption and plasma low-density lipoprotein levels. *Proc Natl Acad Sci U S A.* 103, 1810–1815.

Corella D, González JI, Bulló M, et al., 2009. Polymorphisms cyclooxygenase-2–765G_C and interleukin-6 –174G_C are associated with serum inflammation markers in a high cardiovascular risk population and do not modify the response to a Mediterranean diet supplemented with virgin olive oil or nuts. *J Nutr.* 139, 128–134.

Davis CD, Milner J, 2004. Frontiers in nutrigenomics, proteomics, metabolomics and cancer prevention. *Mutat Res.* 551, 51–64.

Day AS, Whitten KE, Lemberg DA, et al., 2006. Exclusive enteral feeding as primary therapy for Crohn's disease in Australian children and adolescents: A feasible and effective approach. *J Gastroenterol Hepatol.* 21: 1609–1614.

De Mello VDF, Schwab U, Kolehmainen M, Koenig W, Siloaho M, Poutanen K, Mykkänen H, Uusitupa M, 2011. A diet high in fatty fish, bilberries and wholegrain products improves markers of endothelial function and inflammation in individuals with impaired glucose metabolism in a randomised controlled trial: The Sysdimet study. *Diabetologia,* 54(11), 2755–2767.

de Roos B, 2013. Personalised nutrition: Ready for practice? *Proc Nutr Soc* 72, 48–52.

Dyson PA, Kelly T, Deakin T, et al., 2011. Diabetes UK evidence-based nutrition guidelines for the prevention and management of diabetes. *Diabetic Med.* 28(11), 1282–1288.

Estruch R, Ros E, Salas-Salvadó J, et al., 2013. Primary prevention of cardiovascular disease with a Mediterranean diet. *N Engl J Med.* 368(14), 1279–1290.

Fenech M, 2005. The genome health clinic and genome health nutrigenomics concepts: Diagnosis and epigenome damage on an individual basis. *Mutagenesis.* 20(4), 255–269.

Flachs P, Mohamed-Ali V, Horakova O, Rossmeisl M, Hosseinzadeh-Attar MJ, Hensler M, Ruzickova J, Kopecky J, 2006. Polyunsaturated fatty acids of marine origin induce adiponectin in mice fed a high-fat diet. *Diabetologia,* 49(2), 394–397.

Garg R, Sharma N, Jain SK, 2014. Nutrigenomics and nutrigenetics: Concepts and applications in Nutrition Research and Practice. *Acta Medica International* 1(2): 124–130.

German JB, 2005. Geetic dietetic: Nutrigenomics ad the future of dietetic practice. *J Am Diet Assoc.* 105, 530–531.

Hawkinson AK, 2007. *Nutrigenomics and nutrigenetics in whole food nutritional medicine. Townsend letters for doctors and patients,* Feb–March, 2007.

Heuschkel RB, Menache CC, Megerian JT, et al., 2000. Enteral nutrition and corticosteroids in the treatment of acute Crohn's disease in children. *J Pediatr Gastroenterol Nutr.* 31, 8–15.

Ho E, Clarke JD, Dashwood RH, 2009. Dietary sulforaphane, a histone deacetylase inhibitor for cancer prevention. *J. Nutr.* 139(12), 2393–2396.

Hori S, Butler E, McLoughlin J, 2011. Prostate cancer and diet: Food for thought?. *BJU Int.* 107(9), 1348–1359.

Hu FB, 2011. Globalization of diabetes: The role of diet, lifestyle, and genes. *Diabetes care.* 34(6), 1249–1257.

Izar MC, Tegani DM, Kasmas SH, Fonseca FA, 2011. Phytosterols and phytosterolemia: Gene–diet interactions. *Genes Nutr.* 6(1), 17–26.

Jung UJ, Lee MK, Park YB, Kang MA, Choi MS, 2006. Effect of citrus flavonoids on lipid metabolism and glucose-regulating enzyme mRNA levels in type-2 diabetic mice. *Int J Biochem Cell Biol.* 38, 1134–1145.

Kant AK, 2004. Dietary patterns and health outcomes. *J Am Diet Assoc* 104, 615–635.

Kaput J, Rodriquez RL, 2004. Nutritional genomics: The next frontier in the postgenomic era. *Physiol Genomics.* 16, 166–177.

Kaviarasan K, Pugalendi KV, 2009. Influence of flavonoid-rich fraction from Spermacoce hispida seed on PPAR-alpha gene expression, antioxidant redox status, protein metabolism and marker enzymes in high-fat-diet fed STZ diabetic rats. *Basic Clin Physiol Pharmacol.* 20, 141–158.

Komduur RH, Korthals M, te Molder H, 2011. The good life: Living for healthand a life without risks? On a prominent script of nutrigenomics. *Br J Nutr.* 101, 307–316.

Lai CQ, Corella D, Demissie S, et al., 2006. Dietary intake of n-6 fatty acids modulates effect of apolipoprotein A5 gene on plasma fasting triglycerides, remnant lipoprotein concentrations, and lipoprotein particle size: The Framingham Heart Study. *Circulation.* 113, 2062–2070.

Lawson KA, Wright ME, Subar A, et al., 2007. Multivitamin use and risk of prostate cancer in the National Institutes of Health-AARP Diet and Health Study. *J Natl Cancer Inst.* 99, 754–764.

Lengauer C, Kinzler KW, Vogelstein B, 1998. Genetic instabilities in human cancers. *Nature* 396, 643–649.

Longo VD, Fontana L, 2010. Calorie restriction and cancer prevention: Metabolic and molecular mechanisms. *Trends Pharmacol Sci.* 31(2), 89–98.

Mekary RA, Giovannucci E, Willett WC, van Dam RM, Hu FB, 2012. Eating patterns and type 2 diabetes risk in men: Breakfast omission, eating frequency, and snacking. *Am J Clin Nutr.* 95(5), 1182–1189.

Miggiano GA, DeSanctis, 2006. Nutritional genomics: Toward a personalized diet US National Library of Medicine, National institutes of health. *Clin Ter.* 157(4), 355–361.

Müller M, Kersten S, 2003. Nutrigenomics: Goals and strategies. *Nat Rev Genet.* 4, 315–322.

Neeha VS, Kinth P, 2013. Nutrigenomics research: A review. *J Food Sci Technol.* 50(3), 415–428.

Nettleton JA, McKeown NM, Kanoni S, et al., 2010. Interactions of dietary whole-grain intake with fasting glucose–and insulin-related genetic loci in individuals of European descent: A meta-analysis of 14 cohort studies. *Diabetes care.* 33(12), 2684–2691.

Neuhouser ML, Barnett MJ, Kristal AR, et al., 2009. Dietary supplement use and prostate cancer risk in the Carotene and Retinol Efficacy Trial. *Cancer Epidemiol Biomarkers Prev.* 18, 2202–2206.

Panagiotakos D, Sitara M, Pitsavos C, Stefanadis C, 2007. Estimating the 10-year risk of cardiovascular disease and its economic consequences, bythe level of adherence to the Mediterranean diet: The ATTICA study. *J Med Food.* 10, 239–243.

Qi L, Li T, Rimm E, Zhang C, Rifai N, Hunter D, Doria A, Hu FB, 2005. The 276 polymorphism of the APM1 gene, plasma adiponectin concentration, and cardiovascular risk in diabetic men. *Diabetes.* 54(5), 1607–1610.

Qi L, Meigs JB, Liu S, Manson JE, Mantzoros C, Hu FB, 2006. Dietary fibers and glycemic load, obesity, and plasma adiponectin levels in women with type 2 diabetes. *Diabetes Care.* 29(7), 1501–1505.

Qi Q, Chu AY, Kang JH, et al. 2014. Fried food consumption, genetic risk, and body mass index: Gene-diet interaction analysis in three US cohort studies. *BMJ.* 348, 1610.

Ramsden CE, Zamora D, Leelarthaepin B, et al., 2013. Use of dietary linoleic acid for secondary prevention of coronary heart disease and death: Evaluation of recovered data from the Sydney Diet Heart Study and updated meta-analysis. *BMJ.* 346, e8707.

Ravindran J, Prasad S, Aggarwal B, 2009. Curcumin and cancer cells: How many ways can curry kill tumor cells selectively? *AAPS J.* 11(3), 495–510.

Ries NM, Castle D, 2008. Nutrigenomics and ethics interface: Direct-to-consumer services and commercial aspects. *OMICS J Integrative Biol.* 12(4), 245–250.

Salas-Salvadó J, Bulló M, Babio N, et al., 2011. Reduction in the incidence of type 2 diabetes with the mediterranean diet results of the PREDIMED-reus nutrition intervention randomized trial. *Diabetes care.* 34(1), 14–19.

Sandhu BK, Fell JM, Beattie RM, et al., 2010. Guidelines for the management of inflammatory bowel disease in children in the United Kingdom. *J Pediatr Gastroenterol Nutr.* 50 Suppl 1, S1–13.

Schulze MB, Hu FB, 2005. Primary prevention of diabetes: What can be done and how much can be prevented? *Ann Rev Public Health.* 26, 445–467.

Schwartz B, 2014. New criteria for supplementation of selected micronutrients in the era of nutrigenetics and nutrigenomics. *Int J Food Sci Nutr.* 65(5), 529–538.

Sharpless NE, DePinho RA, 2002. p53: good cop/bad cop. *Cell* 110, 9–12.

Shu L, Cheung K-L, Khor T, Chen C, Kong A-N, 2010. Phytochemicals: Cancer chemoprevention and suppression of tumor onset and metastasis. *Cancer Metastasis Rev.* 29(3), 483–502.

Sluijs I, Beulens JW, Spijkerman AM, Grobbee DE, Van der Schouw YT, 2010. Dietary intake of total, animal, and vegetable protein and risk of type 2 diabetes in the European Prospective Investigation into Cancer and Nutrition (EPIC)-NL study. *Diabetes care* 33(1), 43–48.

Vassiliou EK, Gonzalez A, Garcia C, Tadros JH, Chakraborty G, Toney JH, 2009. Oleic acid and peanut oil high in oleic acid reverse the inhibitory effect of insulin production of the inflammatory cytokine TNF-alpha both in vitro and in vivo systems. *Lipids Health Dis.* 8, 25–34.

WHO, 1997. *Health for All. Statistical Database 1997.* WHO, Copenhagen.

World Cancer Research Fund, American Institute for Cancer Research, Food, Nutrition and the Prevention of Cancer: A Global Perspective, American Institute for Cancer Research, Washington, DC, 1997.

Ye DZ, Tai MH, Linning KD, Szabo C, Olson LK, 2006. MafA expression and insulin promoter activity are induced by nicotinamide and related compounds in INS-1 pancreatic beta-cells. *Diabetes* 55, 742–750.

21

Dietary Fats and Cancer

Ananya Rajkumari, Manjir Sarma Kataki, and Bhaskar Mazumder
Dibrugarh University
Dibrugarh, India

Contents

21.1 Introduction 530
21.2 The cancer process: A short review 531
21.3 Diet and cancer 533
21.4 Dietary fats: Interventions in cancer 534
    21.4.1 Specific and nonspecific effect of dietary fats on
        carcinogenesis 534
    21.4.2 Polyunsaturated fats 534
    21.4.3 Conjugated linoleic acid and cancer 535
    21.4.4 Monounsaturated fatty acid and cancer 536
    21.4.5 Trans fatty acids and cancer 537
    21.4.6 Saturated fatty acids 537
21.5 Cancers: An overview 538
    21.5.1 Oral cavity, pharynx, and esophagus 538
    21.5.2 Nasopharynx 538
    21.5.3 Lung 539
    21.5.4 Stomach 539
    21.5.5 Pancreas 540
    21.5.6 Liver 540
    21.5.7 Colon and rectum 540
    21.5.8 Breast 542
    21.5.9 Ovary 542
    21.5.10 Endometrium 542
    21.5.11 Cervix 542
    21.5.12 Prostate 543
    21.5.13 Kidney 543
    21.5.14 Bladder 544
21.6 Some cancers and dietary fats: Opinions and outcomes 544
    21.6.1 Breast cancer and fat 544
    21.6.2 Fat and colon cancer 547
21.7 Conclusion 548
References 548

529

21.1 Introduction

Although not in every form of cancer, dietary fats have an explicit consequence on tumor occurrence in numerous experimental studies on animals. Nevertheless, a pivotal concern relevant to this is that if it is related to total energy consumption as restraint of energy typically and significantly limits tumor growth and development (Appleton & Landers 1986; Sonnenschein et al. 1991).

Some animal studies have shown a discrete effect of fat on cancer; however, the results were inadequate and hypothetical for many studies devised separately for this purpose. Therefore, there has been doubt regarding the applicability of these models in human studies (Boissonneault et al. 1986; Freedman et al. 1990; Ip 1990; Welsch 1992). Huge global deviation in the degree of appearance of breast, colon, prostate, and endometrial cancer leads to interpretation of the pertinency between dietary fat intake and cancer rate, as this in turn is connected with possible per capita fat consumption (Carroll et al. 1983; Prentice & Sheppard 1990). Possible per capita fat consumption may not be an etiological factor, as this interrelationship depends only on animal fat and not vegetable fat (Rose et al. 1986). The prime motive for these global comparisons, termed *ecological studies*, is that several other causes apart from fat consumption differ between countries and mix up with that of fat. For instance, the relationship between gross national product and breast cancer occurrence is further convincing than fat consumption and hence several factors linked with national wealth like physical activity, obesity, and reproductive patterns will also be interlinked to breast cancer (Armstrong & Doll 1975).

Fats, also known as *triglycerides*, are esters of three fatty acids and glycerol. Fatty acids are constituted naturally in food stuffs and in the fat repositories of human beings. In cell membranes, fatty acids are in the form of phospholipids and the third fatty acid molecule is substituted by a phosphate ester attached to a hydrophilic moiety like choline, serine, inositol, or ethanolamine. They play an important role in maintaining the sturdiness of the cell membrane along with regulation of enzymatic activities of some membrane enzymes (Kolonel et al. 1999). Most of the inevitable fatty acids for humans are produced naturally, excluding polyunsaturated fatty acids linoleic and linoleic, which are generated through dietary sources like vegetable oils, red meat, and dairy products. The effect on health due to alteration of fatty acid consumption in diet is increasing as there is correlation between cellular functions and the composition of fatty acids on the phospholipids of the cellular membrane (Bougnoux et al. 2010). Polyunsaturated group of fatty acids (PUFAs) are under investigation in the milieu of cancer prevention. They comprise two groups (n-6 and n-3 fatty acids). Precursors of the n-6 series include linoleic acid (LA, 18:2n-6), arachidonic acid (AA, 20:4n-6), and gamma-linolenic acid (GLA, 18:3n-6). Diets of animal origin, vegetables, and oils from sunflower, soybeans, and grape seeds are rich sources of linoleic acid. Arachidonic acid is a substrate of specific lipid oxygenases, which form bioactive inflammatory mediators, and gamma-linolenic acids are bountiful in vegetables. Essential fatty acids like alpha-linolenic acid (ALA, 18:3n-3), highly unsaturated derivatives such as eicosapentaenoic acid (EPA, 20:5n-3) and docosahexaenoic acid (DHA, 22:6n-3) are included in the n-3 series. Alpha-linolenic acids are copious in green vegetables and in several oils (colza, soybean). Eicosapentaenoic acid and docosahexaenoic acid are omnipresent in mammals and plentiful in seafood and marine products. Polyunsaturated fatty acids partake in the biosynthesis of bioactive oxygenated derivatives. The conjugated linoleic acids (CLA) group of fatty acids is also known for cancer prevention. It comprises positional and geometrical isomers of linoleic acid having a conjugated double bond. Dairy products from grass-eating mammals contain high amounts of CLA, produced due to biohydrogenation of polyunsaturated fatty acids (linoleic or alpha-linolenic acids) by the microflora of the ruminants (Turpeinen et al. 2002).

Studies conducted on oncogenic models in animals as well as epidemiological reports from clinical studies indicate a positive relationship between dietary fat intake and development of cancer. This combined experimental and epidemiological report was recommended by the Committee on Diet, Nutrition, and Cancer, held by the US National Academy of Sciences in 1982, for showing a causal relationship between fat intake and occurrence of cancer. They suggest presumable affirmations that increase in consumption of total fat increases the prevalence of cancer in some particular sites like breast and colon. Studies conducted on animals revealed that under special conditions polyunsaturated fats increase tumor development more efficiently than saturated fats. However, clinical studies suggest that there does not exist any solid differentiation in types of fatty acids for exaggerating cancer (Guthrie & Carroll 1999).

Data on studies involving experimental animals and intercountry studies show a positive correlation between dietary fat intake and cancer risk. On the contrary, case-control and cohort studies are wary to impose the possibility of increased cancer risk with intake of high fat diet. However, all these epidemiological studies are associated with one or other methodological problem (McGinnis & Nestle 1989; Fay et al. 1997).

21.2 The cancer process: A short review

The quest for the cause of cancer has been ongoing for centuries. Over 2,000 years ago, Hippocrates made the observation that the long extended veins that expand out from some breast tumors resemble the limbs of a crab [National Institutes of Health (US); Biological Sciences Curriculum Study (NIH 2007)]. Cancers are a vast group of diseases that comprise irregular cell development with the ability to pervade and expand to different segments of the body (WHO 2014). Neoplasms are formed, which grow irregularly and expand gradually (WHO 2013). Every tumor cells exhibits six traits of cancer. Each of these traits is required to generate a malignant tumor. In a cancerous cell, there is deformity in the regulation process that control its division as well as setbacks in homeostasis that supervise these processes. A normal cell grows and divides in a controlled manner. It is responsive to growth factors when innervated. If injured it stops invading as directed by molecular signals until improved. If it is not repaired, the cell dies and the process is termed *apoptosis*. Cell division is a controlled process that is restricted to certain times. The growth of normal cells is confined to their origin and they grow when supplied by a healthy blood flow.

A normal cell forms a cancerous cell only when it can withstand all these mechanisms. The mechanisms involved are controlled by specific proteins that, when malfunctioning, result in the ultimate condition. The process is generated through several stages, which is referred to as the six traits of cancer by Hanahan and Weinberg (2000; Anonymous 2011) (Figure 21.1).

There has been considerable progress over the past 30 years in understanding the molecular base of cancer. It has brought us to the conclusion that cancer is a type of well-defined disease and that deformed genes cause this disease. Deformed genes are a wide subject to know, and it can either cause addition or reduction of its quality. Several inherited disorders linked with increase in the susceptibility to cancer have been recognized. Most cancers (90%–95%) are attributed to environmental factors; 5%–10% are genetically inherited (Anand et al. 2008). The term *environmental factors* does not solely mean pollution but includes factors like lifestyle, economic, and social factors (Kravchenko et al. 2009). Some of the common environmental factors that account for cancer death include tobacco (25%–30%), diet and obesity (30%–35%), infections (15%–20%), radiation (both ionizing and nonionizing, up to 10%), stress, lack of physical activity, and environmental pollutants (Anand et al. 2008).

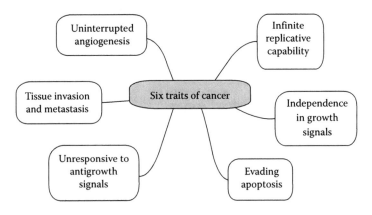

Figure 21.1 Six traits of cancer: A pictorial representation.

21.3 Diet and cancer

During the last considerable decade there has been increasing engrossment on the pertinence of the connection between diet and human cancer. This may be due to differences in occurrence of rates of cancers between countries and noticeable differences among migrating populations; fast changes in the rates within the countries with time reveals that common cancers especially in Western countries may be precipitated by some facet of lifestyle or environment. All these findings unveil the fact that some possibly changeable factors may play key role in the genesis and impediment of cancer. The role of diet has been implied by the possible substantial interrelationship between cancer rates and national per capita consumption of characteristic supplements. In an extensive review by Americans Doll and Peto in 1981 on the veritable causes of cancer mortality, the authors recommended that approximately 35% of cancer deaths may be precipitated due to dietary factors that resemble the impingement of smoking (Sonnenschein et al. 1991). Nevertheless, assessment of risk from diet was erratic and it was assumed that this may fluctuate from as low as 10% to as high as 70%. Although detailed analysis of prospective studies do not support the contribution of dietary fat in cancer, it has been presumed as a prime cause, as consumption at the national level is related with differences at the international level. Alternatively, an important causal factor for breast and colon cancers is positive energy balance observed during menarche at an early age and weight gain as an adult, supported by several animal studies. Physical inactivity is another key factor for cancer, as it is also a bestower to positive energy balance along with other possible mechanism that may partially contribute to international differences. Possible contributors other than fat per se are considerable, as percentage of calories from fat in the diet does not show any connection to its risk for colon cancer, as higher intake of red meat has shown greater risk. Recent prospective studies have claimed the hypothesis of many case-control studies associating high intake of fruits and vegetables with reduced risks of numerous cancers as being exaggerated. Risks of colon and breast cancers can be reduced by higher folic acid intake, as analyzed by factors in fruits and vegetables that have been studied in connection to cancer risk. A relationship between colon cancer occurrence and polymorphism in the gene for methylene tetrahydrofolate reductase, which takes part in folic acid metabolism, reinforced these findings. Individuals who regularly consume alcohol experience the beneficial effects of folic acid the most, as they are more prone to the risk of cancer (Ferlay et al. 2000).

Thus the effects of diet on the occurrence of cancer have been confirmed by several studies. If public health policies are to be furnished for nutrition based on cancer patients, it should be on the prime and extensive research study databases. Certain inclusive and exclusive criteria primely affect the risks of occurrence. Reducing weight or obesity along with low alcohol consumption will minimize the risk. In a population group where there is consumption of Chinese-style salted fish and exposure to aflatoxin, limiting them decreases the risk. The probability of reducing the risk of cancer increases when average consumption of fruits and vegetables is low. Alternatively, minimizing intake of red meat as well as meat in preserved form, salted preserved foods, and too-hot drinks and food can decrease the risk. It is of utmost importance to extricate the influence of diet on cancer risk, which can greatly support public health management, but unfortunately some areas of research are still left with scant findings (Willett 2000).

21.4 Dietary fats: Interventions in cancer

21.4.1 Specific and nonspecific effect of dietary fats on carcinogenesis

A possible mechanism through which cancer occurs is postulated on the fact that as the growth and development of cancer requires energy, a greater amount of energy from diet can induce the process, whereas lack of energy will retard the process of growth and development. Fatty diets have high energy density as compared to carbohydrates and proteins. Moreover, a fatty diet requires less energy for metabolism along with faster deposition in the body. This consequently leads to obesity, which is known to cause cancer at different sites. Hence, excess fat in diets can induce the process of carcinogenesis as compared to a low-fat diet (Willett 2000).

21.4.2 Polyunsaturated fats

Polyunsaturated fats are reported to promote the growth of tumors in breast cancer in rats induced by 7,12-dimethylbenz[a]anthracene (DMBA). Saturated fats alone are not capable of increasing tumor growth, but a mixture of polyunsaturated fat and saturated fat in the diet increases the growth of tumors as shown by experiments (Carroll et al. 1981). In a more systematic study in a rat mammary cancer model, inclusion of a mixture of polyunsaturated fat (corn oil) with a saturated fat (coconut oil) in the ratio of 18:2 as linoleic acid (n-6) in diet caused a cumulative increase in tumor yield up to a level of 4% ± 5%. Increase in tumor beyond this was not observed and n-6 polyunsaturated fat is also reported to increase carcinogenesis in pancreatic cancer and colon cancer induced by carcinogens (Ip 1987; Bull et al. 1989; Appel et al. 1994; Heber & Kritchevsky 2012). Again, studies in mammary cancer, pancreatic cancer, and colon cancer showed that n-6 polyunsaturated fat promotes growth, whereas n-3 polyunsaturated fat inhibits its growth (Reddy 1992).

Another study in xenografts of human breast cancer cells in nude mice confirmed that eicosanoids in n-6 polyunsaturated fatty acid promotes the growth of cancer. Linoleic acid stimulates the extracellular matrix for local invasion of tumor cells through metastasis. This process is triggered due to induction of type IV collagen by 12-hydroxy eicosapentaenoic acid. On the other hand, separate eicosanoids derived from n-3 fatty acids inhibited the growth of cancer derived from human xenograft model breast cancer in nude mice. However, studies have also confirmed the obstruction of growth is also associated with peroxidized lipids obtained from unsaturated fatty acids (Gonzalez et al. 1993; Liu et al. 1996).

The growth-promoting effect of polyunsaturated fatty acids in breast cancer has been observed and reported only in animal studies; epidemiological data in humans decline to demonstrate a positive correlation between consumption of linoleic acid and death due to breast cancer. An underlying reason behind this may be due to the lesser quantity of fats required, which can also be obtained from other sources of normal diet. However, an extensive review on epidemiological and experimental data presenting the relationship of consumption of linoleic acid and cancer risk revealed that high intake of linoleic acid does not increase the chance of breast, colorectal, or prostate cancer in humans (Carroll et al. 1986; Zock & Katan 1998). Expansion of tumor cells did not depend upon the type of fatty acids incorporated in diet when the necessity of a n-6 fatty acid was fulfilled. Merely increasing the amount of fat enhanced tumor cell proliferation irrespective of the type of dietary fats, which may also include saturated or monounsaturated fatty acids (Carroll et al. 1986; Ip 1987).

21.4.3 Conjugated linoleic acid and cancer

Conjugated linoleic acid, popularly known as *CLA*, is composed of blend of positional and geometric isomers of n-6 (polyunsaturated fatty acids) in the ratio of 18:2. Although available in different types of nourishment in small amounts, milk products and meat from ruminants are the richest sources. Linoleic acid and CLA are two of a kind but the latter is reported to obstruct mammary carcinogenesis in an animal model at a concentration as low as 1% of the diet.

Concentration and variety of dietary fat have a negligible effect on the action of CLA, as mammary carcinogenesis was prohibited by different varieties of either corn oil or lard included in diet. Interestingly, when the concentration of CLA was increased over 1%, extra inhibition was not observed. This propounded prevalence of a limiting step in transforming CLA to a compound that veritably produces the desired protective effect (Ip et al. 1991; Ip et al. 1994; Ip 1997).

New research has shown that CLA prompts apoptosis in mammary epithelial cells. Moreover, it was also found that N-methylurea (NMU)-induced mammary gland tumor in rats can be inhibited when supplemented with CLA administered intravenously throughout the experiment. Other research has proved that immunodeficient mice induced with breast or prostate cancer formed tumors of smaller sizes as well as prevented its further spread. Supplementation of CLA in the range of 1% and 1.5% also inhibits skin tumors caused by phorbol esters generated through the combined effect of both synthesis of eicosanoids and metabolism of linoleic acid. Another group of researchers in experiments conducted on rat carcinogenic models found that inhibition of cancer by CLA was not associated with synthesis of eicosanoids and metabolism of linoleic acid. They also observed that inhibitory effect of CLA was not predominantly affected by the amount of fat in the diet. It was able to exert the desired effect when given as a free acid or as part of triacylglycerol molecule (Ip et al. 1995; Ip et al. 1996; Belury et al. 1996; Visonneau et al. 1997).

21.4.4 Monounsaturated fatty acid and cancer

Among all the monounsaturated fatty acids, oleic acid (18:1) is the most bountiful. It is the primary ingredient of several fats and oils like olive oil, high-oleic safflower oil, canola oil, and palm oil. Reports on studies involving the consequences of high-oleic oil intake in mammary carcinogenesis are inconsistent. A considerable increase in tumor equivalent with those when fed with linoleic oils in rats induced through DMBA was observed for experiments when fed with olive oil and high oleic safflower oil. Mammary tumors promoted by NMU are least affected by olive oil. Inconsistencies in the report may be due to a difference in the amount of linoleic acid in different oils. When the effects of safflower oil containing 17% linoleic acid (LA, 18.2) and olive oil containing 5% linoleic acid (LA, 18.2) were compared in a rat model treated with DMBA, high tumor yield was observed for safflower oil. Apparently when linoleic acid (LA, 18.2) content of the olive oil was increased to 17%, the difference vanished. However, studies on intercountry comparisons revealed a substantial relationship between dietary monounsaturated fatty acid and breast cancer mortality rate (Cohen et al. 1986). Therefore it can be concluded that the effect produced is due to total dietary far rather than oleic acid alone.

Recent studies on oleic acid for its effect on intake and breast cancer growth failed to show a positive relationship only in Spanish centre. The study was conducted and compared between postmenopausal breast cancer patients and a matched control from five European centers.

It can be concluded from this that the defensive action of olive oil is associated with ingredients of olive oil other than that of oleic acid as well as lifestyle modification and high consumption of olive oil. Studies conducted with palmitoleic acid (16:1) and myristoleic acid (14:1) in those five centers proved to be positively associated in some centers and negatively in other. However, the results obtained from this study are not particularly relevant as these fatty acids are a comparatively minor component of diet. Rather than consumption of fatty acids through diet, their concentration in tissues is more significant for disease condition. Polyunsaturated fatty acids are not produced endogenously in the body, so their concentration in the blood depends upon the consumption of fatty acids in the diet. In the case of monounsaturated fatty acids, which are synthesized by desaturation of the corresponding saturated fatty acids, the scenario differs (Lasekan et al. 1990; Simonsen et al. 1998).

21.4.5 Trans fatty acids and cancer

Trans fatty acids are abundant in margarine and the milk and flesh of ruminant animals. They are synthesized through partial hydrogenation of unsaturated fats like by bacterial microflora in the rumen of ruminant animals. In hydrogenation, the double bonds of the unsaturated fatty acids are converted from cis to trans configuration along with a change in position of the carbon chain. Mostly, 18-carbon monoenestrans fatty acids are produced by this process. Elaidic acid (18:1 Δ9) is the principal byproduct, but the double bond may take up a different position along the chain (Beare-Rogers 1983).

Interest in the function of trans fatty acids in carcinogenesis was reignited by a report on epidemiological data that revealed a connection between increased consumption of trans fatty acids and high risk of breast cancer. Some earlier studies did not provide any confirmation of the difference in the effect on mammary cancer by cis and trans fatty acids. Studies in a rat mammary cancer model induced by DMBA, reported fewer mammary tumors when fed with trans fats. However, the report of the study was not statistically significant when compared between partially hydrogenated fat, comprising 22.5% cis monoene and 35% transmonoene, and nonhydrogenated fat, containing approximately 55% cis monoene. Another study in the same animal model showed that rats supplemented with hydrogenated soybean oil have a relatively lower occurrence and development of mammary tumors than those fed unhydrogenated soybean oil (Selenskas et al. 1984; Watanabe et al. 1985). Various studies on animals in a colon cancer model induced by azoxymethane or by dimethylhydrazine failed to exhibit any distinction between rats fed diets containing either cis or trans fats (Erickson et al. 1984).

Some comparison studies of cis-fat diet with trans-fat diet revealed that trans fats promote growth and expand the tumor cells that are generated from a tumor in BALBc±fC3H breeding mouse mammary tumor when cells were embedded subcutaneously into female BALBc mice; no difference in dormancy period and final tumor size was studied in mice fed with cis and trans fat (Erickson et al. 1984).

21.4.6 Saturated fatty acids

Saturated fats have a negligible effect on the growth and development of mammary cancer, except when they are mixed with a small amount of polyunsaturated fatty acids, as reported by studies (Carroll & Khor 1971; Carroll et al. 1981). An epidemiological study report obtained from different countries showed that dietary saturated fatty acids impart a significant relationship with breast cancer lethality equivalent to that observed for dietary monounsaturated fatty acids. Mostly, the composition of saturated fatty acids of varying chain length in diet is small, and palmitic acid (16:0) is the most ample dietary saturated fatty acid. Reports on the effects of mammary cancer by specific fatty acids are scant. However, one of the studies on medium-chain fatty acids

(C10 ± C14) available in coconut oil provided little confirmation of its stimulating effect on mammary cancer (Carroll et al. 1986; Cohen et al. 1986).

21.5 Cancers: An overview

21.5.1 Oral cavity, pharynx, and esophagus

The rates at which cancers of the oral cavity, pharynx, and esophagus occur differ greatly depending upon the origin of the population. In Europe, North America, and West Africa, the occurrence of esophageal cancer is much lower than in parts of Central Asia, China, and southern Africa. In fact, the possibility of occurrence is a hundred times higher in the latter countries (IARC 1990).

Two lifestyle factors that increase the risk of cancer are alcohol and tobacco in developed countries and up to 75% of these cancers are affected (IARC 1988). The possible mechanism by which alcohol induces these cancers is not clear but it may be due to some direct effect on the epithelium (Brown et al. 1995). One of the most important confirmed risk factors of adenocarcinoma (but not squamous cell carcinoma) of the esophagus is overweight or obesity (AICR 1997b; Cheng et al. 2000; IARC 2002). Micronutrient deficiencies, having inadequate diet that is low in fruits and vegetables and animal products, are thought to be the principal cause of 60% of cancers of the oral cavity, pharynx, and esophagus in developing countries (WHO 1990; AICR 1997a). Confirmation of the defensive effect of fruits and vegetables is mainly based on case-control studies as well as prospective studies. The reliant activities of different micronutrients are unclear, but lack of riboflavin, folate, vitamin C, and zinc may prove to bring complications (WHO 1990; Sharp et al. 2001). Intake of drinks and foods at high temperature increases the incidence of these cancers, as shown by persistent evidence (Blot et al. 1993). Although encouraging results of reducing esophageal cancer rates with micronutrient supplements were observed in trials in Linxian, China, the results were not definite (Li et al. 1993; Parkin et al. 2001). However, in 2000, there were approximately 582,000 deaths for 867,000 cases of cancer of the oral cavity, pharynx, and esophagus (Glade 1999).

21.5.2 Nasopharynx

Nasopharyngeal cancer is specifically typical in Southeast Asia (Armstrong & Doll 1975). This particular cancer has been known to be linked with an increase in consumption of Chinese-style salted fish during adolescence (IARC 1995; Doll & Peto 1996). Infection with Epstein–Barr virus (Bjelke 1975) may also precipitate the disease. Association of Chinese-style salted fish with this cancer may be associated with its tendency to get softened by partial decomposition before or during salting (IARC 1995). However, other varieties of salted fish are not associated with increased risk of nasopharyngeal cancer.

21.5.3 Lung

Lung cancer is the most prevalent cancer in the world, resulting in approximately 1,239,000 cases and 1,103,000 deaths in 2000 (Glade 1999). In Western countries, more than 80% of lung cancers are due to smoking, as it increases the risk by 30 times (Hennekens et al. 1996). An observation made in the 1970s contributed to discovering the possibility that diet might influence lung cancer risk (Blot et al. 1993). It was observed that low dietary intake of vitamin A followed by smoking increases the risk of lung cancer. Many observational studies since 1970 have revealed that, as compared to controls, lung cancer patients consume a smaller amount of fruits, vegetables, and related nutrients (such as β-carotene). Despite this, controlled trial studies were unsuccessful in observing any beneficial effect of β-carotene when administered as a supplement for 12 years (Clark et al. 1998; Heinonen et al. 1998; Correa et al. 2000). The potential effect of diet on lung cancer is still unclear. Even though some current observational studies have shown an inverse relation with increase intake of fruits and vegetables, prospective studies have failed to show the same (Armstrong & Doll 1975; Welsch 1992). Again, smoking may intervene the effect and smokers are known to consume fewer fruits and vegetables than nonsmokers. Reduction of smoking will prove to be beneficial for public health.

21.5.4 Stomach

It was estimated around 20 years ago that stomach cancer was the most common cancer in the world. Since then, however, there has been a downturn in mortality rates, especially in Western countries, and now stomach cancer dominates in Asia rather than Europe or North America (Bergstrom et al. 2001b). In the year 2000, approximately 876,000 cases and 647,000 deaths due to stomach cancer were recorded worldwide (Kolonel et al. 1999). *Helicobacter pylori* is a well-known probable factor but not an adequate component for inducing cancer (Bergstrom et al. 2001b). The role of diet in the etiology of this disease is an important factor to be considered, and recent studies have claimed the responsibility of diet in its occurrence and deaths in many countries. Reports from case-control studies demonstrate that probability increases with increased consumption of a few customarily stored salted foods, especially meats and pickles, and decreases with increased consumption of fruits and vegetables (WHO 2016), which may be due to their high vitamin content. However, prospective studies do not agree with the preventive effect of fruits and vegetables (Palli 2000; Helicobacter 2001). One of the factors that supports the changing scenario is the advent of refrigeration, which facilitates preservation of fruits and vegetables year-round, which in turn has decreased the intake of salted and preserved foods. In developing countries, some encouraging results were obtained with supplementation of micronutrients in certain trials, but the results were not conclusive. In trials involving combined supplementation of β-carotene, selenium, and α-tocopherol, a considerable decline in stomach cancer mortality was observed, which failed with vitamin C supplementation in Linxian, China (McCullough et al. 2001). However, some newer studies in Colombia found an increased lapse of precancerous gastric dysplasia when β-carotene and vitamin C were administered (Botterweck et al. 1998). More prospective studies clarifying the role of diet as well as its implications along with *H. pylori* are required.

21.5.5 Pancreas

Pancreatic cancer is more prevalent in Western countries as compared to developing countries. There were 216,000 cases and 214,000 deaths in 2000 due to pancreatic cancer (Armstrong & Doll 1975; Glade 1999). In most parts of the world, the incidence and rates of mortality due to pancreas cancer are increasing daily, which may be associated with advancements in diagnostic methods (Hennekens et al. 1996). Health factors like obesity or overweight may increase susceptibility (IARC 1994; Saracco 1995). Case-control studies have reported increased risk with high intake of meat and low intake of vegetables with inconsistent data (Zeegers et al. 2001). The precise relationship between diet and pancreatic cancer can be predicted in the next few years through considerable data from prospective studies.

21.5.6 Liver

The incidence of liver cancer varies by 20 times among different countries of the world; it is higher in sub-Saharan Africa and Southeast Asia than in Europe and North America (Armstrong & Doll 1975). Seventy-five percent of liver cancers occur in developing countries; 564,000 cases and 549,000 deaths from liver cancer were recorded in 2000 (Glade 1999). The main form of liver cancer is hepatocellular carcinoma, which is mainly due to chronic infection with hepatitis B and to a minor extent by the hepatitis C virus (Sesink et al. 2001). Active hepatitis virus infection in developing countries occurs due to intake of foods infected with the mycotoxin aflatoxin (IARC 1995; Baron et al. 1999). The major diet-related risk factor for liver cancer in Western countries is excessive intake of alcohol, which occurs through liver cirrhosis and alcoholic hepatitis (IARC 1988). Much less information has been acquired regarding the possible role of nutritional cofactors in viral carcinogenesis and this is now an emerging area of research (Zeegers et al. 2001).

21.5.7 Colon and rectum

The incidence of colon cancer is tenfold higher in developed countries than developing countries (Carroll et al. 1983). It is the third most common cancer of the world and 945,000 cases and 492,000 deaths were recorded in 2000 (Kolonel et al. 1999). Up to 80% of the intercountry differences are due to diet-related factors (Ip et al. 1994). Overweight or obesity is the best confirmed factor related to risk through diet (McGinnis & Nestle 1989). Alcohol consumption may also partially increase the risk (Welsch 1992). Nutrition supplemented during childhood and adolescence, which determines adult height, is weakly related with the increase in risk, whereas increased physical activity can reduce the risk as supported by consistent data (McGinnis & Nestle 1989; Ip et al. 1996). The large differences in incidences among different population cannot be attributed solely to these factors, and diet especially in Western countries is suspected to play a crucial role. Different mechanisms have been proposed suggesting an increase in cancer rate with increased intake of meat. It is suspected to produce carcinogenic N-nitroso compounds in the colon due to consumption of meat cooked at high temperatures, which leads to production of mutagenic heterocyclic amines and polycyclic aromatic hydrocarbons during the process (Ip et al. 1995; Visonneau et al. 1997). Nitrites and their related compounds found in smoked, salted, and some processed meat also produce the same compounds in the colon (Belury et al. 1996). Fat may also increase the risk, as it causes an increase in the levels of cytotoxic free fatty acids or secondary bile acids in the lumen of the large intestine. However, observational study reports are controversial (Beare-Rogers 1983; Welsch 1992).

Fiber increases stool bulk and speeds the transit of food through the colon, thus diluting the gut contents and perhaps reducing the absorption of carcinogens by the colonic mucosa (Watanabe et al. 1985). Fermentation of fiber (and resistant starch) in the large intestine produces short chain fatty acids such as butyrate, which may protect against colorectal cancer through the ability to promote differentiation, induce apoptosis, and/or inhibit the production of secondary bile acids by reducing luminal pH (Erickson et al. 1984).

Some recent prospective studies have suggested that a methyl-depleted diet (i.e., a diet low in folate and methionine and high in alcohol) is associated with an increased risk of colon cancer (Wynder et al. 1997; Willet and Lenart 1998). Diminished folate status may contribute to carcinogenesis by alteration of gene expression and increased DNA damage (Hunter et al. 1998; Holmes et al. 1999), as well as chromosome breakage (Hu et al. 1997).

The finding that a common polymorphism in the methylenetetrahydrofolate reductase gene involved in folic acid metabolism may also be associated with colorectal cancer (Toniolo et al. 1995) strengthens the hypothesis that dietary folate may be an important factor in colorectal carcinogenesis.

Calcium. Another promising hypothesis is that relatively high intakes of calcium may reduce the risk for colorectal cancer, perhaps by forming complexes with secondary bile acids in the intestinal lumen (Welsch 1992) or by inhibiting the hyperproliferative effects of dietary heme (Hankinson et al. 1995). Several observational studies have supported this hypothesis (Freedman et al. 1990; Welsch 1992), and two trials have suggested that supplemental calcium may have a modest protective effect on the recurrence of colorectal adenomas (Lubin et al. 1981; Goldin et al. 1982; Ip 1990). More data are needed to evaluate this hypothesis.

21.5.8 Breast

Breast cancer is known to be the second most common cancer in the world, though it is the most common one in women. About 1,105,000 cases and 373,000 deaths in women occurred due to this disease in 2000 (Goldin et al. 1982). Western countries are five times more susceptible to it than less developed countries and Japan (Goldin et al. 1982). These differences in the international level may be accounted for by well-known reproductive risk factors such as age at puberty, parity, and age at births, as well as breastfeeding along with dietary habits and physical activity variation (Goldin et al. 1982). Diet plays an important role in onset of puberty, as inadequate dietary consumption during childhood and adolescence delays it. Moreover, adult height is weakly positively associated with susceptibility, which in turn is partially linked with dietary habits in childhood and adolescence (Goldin et al. 1982). The etiology of breast cancer is primarily mediated by estradiol and related hormones and any additional effect of diet on its risk may be governed by hormonal mechanisms (Goldin et al. 1982).

21.5.9 Ovary

Ovarian cancer is found to be highest in Western countries, with 192,000 cases and 114,000 deaths in women reported in the year 2000 (Goldin et al. 1982). Long-term use of combined oral contraceptives and parity is associated with reduced risk (Goldin et al. 1982). Susceptibility to this cancer increases with higher consumption of fat or dairy products and reduction in intake of vegetables. More prospective studies on the possible correlation is further required, as available data are inconsistent (Goldin et al. 1982).

21.5.10 Endometrium

The maximum incidence of endometrial cancer is recorded in Western countries, with 189,000 cases and 45,000 deaths in women in 2000 (Goldin et al. 1982). This cancer is three times more likely to occur in obese women than lean ones (Goldin et al. 1982; Banks et al. 1997). The mechanism by which obese women are more prone to endometrial cancer is same as that of breast cancer, and it is likely to manifest as an elevation in serum concentrations of estradiol and depletion in serum concentrations of sex hormone–binding globulin. In premenopausal women, anovulation increases, which in turn leads to increased susceptibility to estradiol unobstructed by progesterone (Banks et al. 1997). Although data are limited, some case-control studies have revealed a reduction in risk with high intake of fruits and vegetables and an increase in risk with diets high in saturated or total fat (Zeegers et al. 2001).

21.5.11 Cervix

Cervical cancers are predominant in sub-Saharan Africa, Central and South America, and Southeast Asia (Zeegers et al. 2001). There were approximately

471,000 and 233,000 cervical cancer cases and deaths in women, respectively, in 2000. The prime causal factor for cervical cancer is infection with certain subtypes of the human papillomavirus (Zeegers et al. 2001). Smoking and other factors along with papillomavirus infections may intervene with the protective activity from consuming fruits, vegetables, and related nutrients such as carotenoids and folate (Zeegers et al. 2001). Nevertheless, further studies are required, particularly on folate deficiency (Zeegers et al. 2001).

21.5.12 Prostate

The rates of mortality due to prostate cancer are about tenfold higher in North America and Europe than in Asia (Zeegers et al. 2001). The rate is strongly influenced by diagnostic practices and hence difficult to predict. Ecological studies suggest a positive association of prostate cancer with Western-style diet, although little is known about the etiology of prostate cancer (Schuurman et al. 1999). The total cases and deaths due to prostate cancer in 2000 were 543,000 and 204,000, respectively (Schuurman et al. 1999). Prospective studies have not shown any causal or protective correlation for specific nutrients or diets (Chan et al. 2001; Zeegers et al. 2001). Although data are not completely homogeneous, excessive consumption of red meat, dairy products, and animal fat is often found to be connected with prostate cancer development (Hennekens et al. 1996; Omenn et al. 1996; Michaud et al. 2001; Zeegers et al. 2001). Beta-carotene supplements (Clark et al. 1998; Heinonen et al. 1998; Kristal & Cohen 2000) do not have any effect on prostate cancer risk, as supported by randomized controlled trials, whereas vitamin E (Kristal & Cohen 2000) and selenium (Eaton et al. 1999) might have a protective effect. The results of a few observational studies have correlated a reduced risk of prostate cancer with intake of lycopene from tomatoes, but the results are not consistent (Gann et al. 1996). Medications that can reduce the levels of androgen are mildly successful for managing this disease, and hormones are known to control the growth of the prostate. Even though there are inadequate data showing a correlation between concentrations of hormone on serum and prostate cancer risk, prospective studies have shown increased risk with increased levels of bioavailable androgens (Chan et al. 1998; Stattin et al. 2000) and of insulin-like growth factor-I (IGF-I) (Heaney et al. 1999; Allen et al. 2000). Prostate cancer may be indirectly affected by diet, as it can affect the hormonal level of the body. Moreover, certain recent studies have revealed that animal protein may increase levels of IGF-I (Yu 1991; IARC 1993).

21.5.13 Kidney

There were approximately 189,000 cases and 91,000 deaths due to kidney cancer in 2000 (Glade 1999). Differences in incidences due to geographic variation are average and highest in Scandinavia and among the members of northern Canada and parts of Greenland and Alaska (Bergstrom et al. 2001a).

One of the confirmed risk factors for kidney cancer is overweight or obesity, and 30% of kidney cancers in both men and women are due to this (COMA 1998). The role of diet in the etiology of kidney cancer is supported by little data. However, studies conducted have suggested an increase in risk with higher consumption of meat and dairy products and a reduced risk with higher consumption of vegetables (Zeegers et al. 2001).

21.5.14 Bladder

Findings on bladder cancer suggest that increased consumption of fruits and vegetables might decrease risk, although for solid confirmation further prospective data are required (IARC 1990a; Michaud et al. 1999; Zeegers et al. 2001). Large variations in incidences of cancer of up to tenfold, with comparatively higher rates in Western countries, are observed for bladder cancer (Bergstrom et al. 2001a). Moreover, smoking accelerates the chances of bladder cancer (Armstrong & Doll 1975). In the year 2000, there were approximately 336,000 cases and 132,000 deaths due to bladder cancer (Glade 1999).

21.6 Some cancers and dietary fats: Opinions and outcomes

21.6.1 Breast cancer and fat

Contrary to the hypothesis regarding a global relationship between fat consumption and national breast cancer mortality, a study conducted in 65 Chinese countries claimed an inadequate positive relationship between fat consumption and breast cancer mortality when per capita fat intake varied from 6% to 25% of energy (Marshall et al. 1992). In China the differences in wealth and industrialization are less common than other countries around the globe. When comparison was done in five countries where 25% of energy was consumed through fat, the frequency of breast cancer was much lower than for US women consuming the same amount of fat. This support the fact that factors apart from fat consumption account for the large global differences (Willett et al. 1992). During the present century, based upon per capita fat consumption and food disappearance data, the frequency of breast cancer has increased considerably in the United States. Only two case-control studies showing a positive relationship between dietary fat and breast cancer were reported in 1982 by the National Academy of Sciences review of diet and cancer. However, it was also reported elsewhere that confirmed data did not show any positive correlation conducted by their dietary assessment method. Some studies failed to show a strong dietary assessment and inclusion of several interviewers for cases and control created bias (Miller et al. 1978; Lubin et al. 1981). There are now an adequate number of case-control studies with relation to dietary fat intake and breast cancer risk. However, animal fat and total fat intake have not shown any association with breast cancer in the most extensive study conducted to date (Graham et al. 1982). A review of 12 smaller case-control studies in a meta-analysis reported 4,312 cases

544 Nutrigenomics and Nutraceuticals

and 5,978 controls. Results revealed that the pooled relative risk was 1.35 ($p < 0.0001$) when total daily fat intake was increased to 100 grams, while the relative risk was greater for postmenopausal women (relative risk = 1.48; $p < 0.001$). The extent of this comparative risk could be confusing as change to fat intake of 100 grams may not be possible for a wide category of women, since approximately only 70 grams per day average intake was observed. In addition the positive association could be linked with change in diet and inclusion of controls (Giovannucci et al. 1993).

Cohort studies conducted in developed countries have significant data to evaluate the correlation of dietary fat intake and breast cancer. When total energy from fat intake was in the range of <20% to >45%, pooled analysis data of some prospective studies in more than 200 cases of breast cancer did not reveal any connection. Positive correlation with particular type of fats was not observed even in postmenopausal women. In some studies involving a smaller number of women and intake of less than 15% of energy from fat showed a strong association, which can be regarded as a twofold increase in risk. Hence, dissimilarities were observed in the findings of case-control and cohort studies that could be due to elusive methodological biases.

Due to lack of effective correlation between dietary fat intake and breast cancer in huge prospective studies and differences in extensive dietary consumption, as well as strong belief in a causal relationship, these types of studies have come under abnormal inspection and appraisal (Prentice & Sheppard 1990; Wynder et al. 1997).

A prime issue related to this is that dietary connections are not adequate to figure out the possible connections; in addition, there exist some insufficient differences in fat within the study population, and differences would exist due to consumption of fat by obese women. These issues have been undertaken by different measures. At first, the study was validated by comparison of consumption of fat analyzed through a standard questionnaire incorporated in prospective studies through illustrative investigation of meal-by-meal intake conducted for many weeks over more than a year. As a result, a correlation of approximately 0.5–0.7 was found due to modification of energy consumption and revision for weekly differences in dietary consumption record (Willet and Lenart 1998).

Secondly, statistical techniques should be developed in order to consider the extent of analysis error when estimating relative risk and confidence interval (Rosner et al. 1992). These measures exclude the degree of relationship of fat intake and breast cancer risk evaluated by international correlations, as the confidence interval becomes wider by including uncertainty due to measurement error (Rosner et al. 1992; Hunter et al. 1998).

Thirdly, international pooling of prospective data was conducted to evaluate the risk of breast cancer over a broad extent of fat intake as it enabled analysis of further extreme groups and the addition of several countries allowed a wide range of fat consumption. Consequently, a large range of fat intake was provided as for ecological studies, which also showed that a positive relation was found only in women who consumed 15% of energy from fat; as well, low risk was not observed in women who consumed less fat.

Fourthly, none of the reported prospective studies noted the fact that absence of positive connection may be due to underreporting of fat intake is not based on experimental data as well as serious inference is required to claim that fat consumption is firmly inversely associated with body fat (Hunter et al. 1998).

Fifthly, in the Nurses' Health Study, methods have been chosen to minimize errors by repeated dietary measurements. A poor but statistically significant inverse association was observed with total fat intake for about 3,000 breast cancer cases in a 14-year follow-up study up to four measurements (Holmes et al. 1999). Finally, metabolic studies of blood lipids have reported risk of coronary heart diseases correlated with specific types of fat in the same study populations with the same dietary assessment method (Hu et al. 1997). Astonishingly, the strong outlook with relation to dietary fat intake and breast cancer does not have any solid proof related to the biological mechanism of action. However, there is experimental evidence that increase in the level of estrogen in the body increases the risk of breast cancer (Hankinson et al. 1995; Toniolo et al. 1995). Therefore, the effects of fats as well as other dietary components on the level of estrogens are of possible importance. Women (vegetarians) with higher fiber intake and lower fat intake were found to have low blood levels and lower urinary excretion of estrogens related to increased fecal excretion (Goldin et al. 1982). Studies without simultaneous controls have shown that women consuming diets high in fiber and low in fat had decreased levels of estrone sulfate but not other estrogens, whereas postmenopausal women had decreased estradiol but not estrone sulfate. Interpretation of this type of study is difficult as there are no concurrent groups (Prentice & Sheppard 1990). In premenopausal women, a relatively significant decrease was found in estrogen level with low fat diet compared to controls; however women eating a low fat diet had a slightly negative energy balance (Ingram et al. 1987). Positive association of fat intake and breast cancer is known to be highest in postmenopausal women but crossover studies have shown no prominent effect of fat on plasma estrogen levels (Hopkins & Carroll 1979). There was a decrease in the level of serum estradiol in women with higher baseline serum estradiol levels. This may be due to regression analysis, as adequate comparison with control groups again showed no effect of dietary fat (Willet & Lenart 1998).

Therefore, it can be concluded that specifically in postmenopausal women dietary fat has negligible or minimum effect on endogenous estrogen levels in properly controlled studies.

Prospective epidemiologic studies have shown that total fat intake is not related to breast cancer risk; however, there has been some confirmation that type of fat may be an important consideration. In an animal model of mammary carcinoma, this positive effect for tumor growth was observed

546 Nutrigenomics and Nutraceuticals

for polyunsaturated fat when administered with high fat diets comprising approximately 45% of energy (Howe et al. 1990). A meta-analysis of case-control studies revealed that risk of breast cancer was least for polyunsaturated fat (relative risk 1.25 for 45 g/day), followed by monounsaturated fats (relative risk 1.41 for 45 g/day), and highest for saturated fats (relative risk 1.46 for 45 g/day) (Howe et al. 1990). A detailed food frequency questionnaire data by the Nurses' Health Study in 1984 claimed a negative association of monounsaturated fat intake and breast cancer risk (Martin-Moreno et al. 1994). An interesting observation was also found where a very low risk of breast cancer was found in Southern European countries, where there is higher intake of monounsaturated fat consisting of olive oil as the primary fat. In Spain and Greece, case-control studies have reported lower risks of breast cancer in women who consumed olive oil (Welsch 1992; Trichopoulou et al. 1995). Moreover; olive oil has preventive activity as compared to other kind of fats, observed in some animal studies (Armstrong & Doll 1975).

21.6.2 Fat and colon cancer

The frequency at which colon cancer occurs when compared among several countries was found to be significantly related with national per capita consumption of animal fat and meat, with correlation coefficients in the range of 0.8 and 0.9 (Rose et al. 1986; Giovannucci et al. 1992). A hypothesis has been postulated based upon these community health report and animal studies stating that, with the increased intake of dietary fat, excretion of bile acids increases, which in turn can be transformed into carcinogens or promoters of cancer in the colon (Macquart-Moulin et al. 1986). However, fat intake alongside inactive lifestyle and habits also contributes to the same. The results of case-control studies have shown a positive relation between the risk of colon cancer and intake of fat or red meat with few exceptions (Jain et al. 1980; Willett et al. 1990; Peters et al. 1992; Meyer & White 1993).

Positive association observed between total energy intake and risk of colon cancer seems to create confusion regarding the underlying etiological factors, whether excess intake of food or fat increases the risk of cancer. Moreover, a meta-analysis report of 13 case-control studies also showed that type of fat is independent from total energy intake that increases the risk of colon cancer.

Some differences can be observed in the reports of prospective and case-control studies, where positive association of colon cancer with total energy intake was confirmed only in case-control studies; this may be related to bias. However, the Nurses' Health Study also confirmed a twofold increase in colon cancer for women who consumed higher amounts of animal fat compared to those with lower intake (Thun et al. 1992; Goldbohm et al. 1994).

When these data are subjected to multivariate analysis, which comprises red meat and animal fat in the same model, only red meat emerged as indicative of colon cancer and animal fat was excluded from the same. This was supported by a cohort study from Netherlands, where positive association was found for processed meat intake, independent of fresh meat or overall fat intake (Bostick et al. 1994).

Another cohort study in Iowa also claimed a direct positive relation with processed meats, though statistically insignificant (Giovannucci et al. 1992). In spite of a considerable range of fat intake, the study did not show an overall relationship between total or saturated fat and colon cancer risk (Doll & Peto 1981).

The large American Cancer Society Cohort study claimed that there is very little association of either meat or fat intake with colon cancer mortality rate. However, the interview questionnaire was concise and also of unknown authenticity (Goldbohm et al. 1994).

21.7 Conclusion

There is no skepticism about that fact that nutritional status of an individual impacts the overall health status. A healthy diet can defend the body by building a strong immune system and consequently many diseases can be prevented. On the contrary, diet, which has the tendency to exert negative impact, like increasing serum cholesterol level, may precipitate many life-threatening diseases. Cancer is a deadly disease affecting the life of individuals through its manifestations and outcomes. Therapy, management, and prevention of cancer are a complex set of tasks associated with several facts. However, diet intake may have a substantial impact on its prevention and management. Maintaining healthy eating habits from a young age can protect the body from the same. It is always recommendable to avoid excessive energy intake from all sources in general and animal sources in particular, like red meat. Moreover, increasing the intake of a variety of whole grains, vegetables, and fruits and physical activity can reduce the susceptibility to numerous cancers, viz. breast, colorectal, and prostate cancer. At times disputes over the need to reduce overall fat intake and its role in cancer prevention and manifestation have arisen. Studies are in process for its validation, and more evidence-based research is the need of the hour. It is advisable to focus and conduct trials with and without dietary fat intervention in order to get a firm affirmation.

References

AICR 1997a. Food, nutrition, and the prevention of cancer: A global perspective. In: *Food, Nutrition, and the Prevention of Cancer: A Global Perspective,* Fund, W. C. R. (ed.). Washington, DC: American Institute for Cancer Research, p. 233–357.

AICR. 1997b. *World Cancer Research Fund: Food, Nutrition, and the Prevention of Cancer: A Global Perspective.* Washington, DC: AICR.

Allen, N. E., Appleby, P. N., Davey, G. K. & Key, T. J. 2000. Hormones and diet: Low insulin-like growth factor-I but normal bioavailable androgens in vegan men. *Br J Cancer,* 83, 95–7.

Anand, P., Kunnumakkara, A. B., Kunnumakara, A. B., Sundaram, C., Harikumar, K. B., Tharakan, S. T., Lai, O. S., Sung, B. & Aggarwal, B. B. 2008a. Cancer is a preventable disease that requires major lifestyle changes. *Pharm Res,* 25, 2097–116.

Anonymous. 2011. 'Scientists Revisit "Hallmarks of Cancer"'. *Science Daily [Online].* https://www.sciencedaily.com/releases/2011/03/110316113057.htm. Acessed March 16, 2011.

Appel, M. J., Garderen-Hoetmer, A. V. & Woutersen, R. A. 1994. Effects of dietary linoleic acid on pancreatic carcinogenesis in rats and hamsters. *Cancer Res,* 54, 2113–2120.

Appleton, B. S. & Landers, R. E. 1986. Oil gavage effects on tumor incidence in the National Toxicology Program's 2-year carcinogenesis bioassay. *Adv Exp Med Biol,* 206, 99–104.

Arends, J., Bachmann, P., Baracos, V., Barthelemy, N., Bertz, H., et al. 2017. ESPEN guidelines on nutrition in cancer patients. *Clinical Nutrition,* 36, 11–48.

Armstrong, B. & Doll, R. 1975. Environmental factors and cancer incidence and mortality in different countries, with special reference to dietary practices. *Int J Cancer,* 15, 617–31.

Banks, E., Beral, V. & Reeves, G. 1997. The epidemiology of epithelial ovarian cancer: A review. *Int J Gynecol Canc,* 7, 425–38.

Baron, J. A., Beach, M., Mandel, J. S., Van Stolk, R. U., Haile, R. W., Sandler, R. S., Rothstein, R., Summers, R. W., Snover, D. C., Beck, G. J. et al. 1999. Calcium supplements and colorectal adenomas. Polyp Prevention Study Group. *Ann N Y Acad Sci,* 889, 138–45.

Beare-Rogers, J. L. 1983. Trans- and postional isomers of common fatty acids. *Adv Nutr Res,* 5, 171–200.

Belury, M. A., Nickel, K. P., Bird, C. E. & Wu, Y. 1996. Dietary conjugated Linoleic acid modulation of phorbol ester skin tumor promotion. *Nutr Canc,* 26, 149–57.

Bergstrom, A., Hsieh, C. C., Lindblad, P., Lu, C. M., Cook, N. R. & Wolk, A. 2001a. Obesity and renal cell cancer–a quantitative review. *Br J Cancer,* 85, 984–90.

Bergstrom, A., Pisani, P., Tenet, V., Wolk, A. & Adami, H. O. 2001b. Overweight as an avoidable cause of cancer in Europe. *Int J Cancer,* 91, 421–30.

Bjelke, E. 1975. Dietary vitamin a and human lung cancer. *Int J Canc,* 15, 561–5.

Blot, W. J., Li, J. Y., Taylor, P. R., Guo, W., Dawsey, S., Wang, G. Q., Yang, C. S., Zheng, S. F., Gail, M., Li, G. Y. et al. 1993. Nutrition intervention trials in Linxian, China: Supplementation with specific vitamin/mineral combinations, cancer incidence, and disease-specific mortality in the general population. *J Natl Cancer Inst,* 85, 1483–92.

Boissonneault, G. A., Elson, C. E. & Pariza, M. W. 1986. Net energy effects of dietary fat on chemically induced Mammary Carcinogenesis in F344 Rats. *J Natl Canc Inst,* 76, 335–8.

Bostick, R. M., Potter, J. D., Kushi, L. H., Sellers, T. A., Steinmetz, K. A., Mckenzie, D. R., Gapstur, S. M. & Folsom, A. R. 1994. Sugar, meat, and fat intake, and non-dietary risk factors for colon cancer incidence in Iowa women (United States). *Canc Causes Contr,* 5, 38–52.

Botterweck, A. A. M., Van Den Brandt, P. A. & Goldbohm, R. A. 1998. A prospective cohort study on vegetable and fruit consumption and stomach cancer risk in the Netherlands. *Am J Epidemiol,* 148, 842–53.

Bougnoux, P., Hajjaji, N., Maheo, K., Couet, C. & Chevalier, S. 2010. Fatty acids and breast cancer: Sensitization to treatments and prevention of metastatic re-growth. *Prog Lipid Res,* 2010;49(1):76–86. doi:10.1016/j.plipres.2009.08.003.

Brown, L. M., Swanson, C. A., Gridley, G., Swanson, G. M., Schoenberg, J. B., Greenberg, R. S., Silverman, D. T., Pottern, L. M., Hayes, R. B., Schwartz, A. G. et al. 1995. Adenocarcinoma of the esophagus: Role of obesity and diet. *J Natl Cancer Inst,* 87, 104–9.

Bull, A. W., Bronstein, J. C. & Nigro, N. D. 1989. The essential fatty acid requirement for azoxymethane induced intestinal carcinogenesis in rats. *Lipids,* 24, 340–6.

Campbell, T. C. 2017. Nutrition and Cancer: An Historical Perspective-The Past, Present, and Future of Nutrition and Cancer. Part 2. Misunderstanding and Ignoring Nutrition. *Nutr Cancer,* 1–7.

Carroll, K. K., Braden, L. M., Bell, J. A. & Kalamegham, R. 1986. Fat and cancer. *Cancer,* 58, 1818–25.

Carroll, K. K., Hopkins, G. J., Kennedy, T. G. & Davidson, M. B. 1981. Essential fatty acids in relation to mammary carcinogenesis. *Prog Lipid Res,* 20, 685–90.

Carroll, K. K. & Khor, H. T. 1971. Effects of level and type of dietary fat on incidence of mammary tumors induced in female Sprague-Dawley rats by 7, 12-dimethylbenz(α) anthracene. *Lipids,* 6, 415–20.

Carroll, M. D., Abraham, S. & Dresser, C. M. 1983. Dietary intake source data: United States, 1976–80. *Vital Health Stat*, 11, 1–483.

Chan, J. M., Stampfer, M. J., Giovannucci, E., Gann, P. H., Ma, J., Wilkinson, P., Hennekens, C. H. & Pollak, M. 1998. Plasma insulin-like growth factor-I and prostate cancer risk: A prospective study. *Science*, 279, 563–6.

Chan, J. M., Stampfer, M. J., Ma, J., Gann, P. H., Gaziano, J. M. & Giovannucci, E. L. 2001. Dairy products, calcium, and prostate cancer risk in the Physicians' Health Study. *Am J Clin Nutr*, 74, 549–54.

Cheng, K. K., Sharp, L., Mckinney, P. A., Logan, R. F. A., Chilvers, C. E. D., Cook-Mozaffari, P., Ahmed, A. & Day, N. E. 2000. A case-control study of oesophageal adenocarcinoma in women: A preventable disease. *Br J Canc*, 83, 127–132.

Clark, L. C., Dalkin, B., Krongrad, A., Combs, G. F., JR., Turnbull, B. W., Slate, E. H., Witherington, R., Herlong, J. H., Janosko, E., Carpenter, D., Borosso, C., Falk, S. & Rounder, J. 1998. Decreased incidence of prostate cancer with selenium supplementation: results of a double-blind cancer prevention trial. *Br J Urol*, 81, 730–4.

Cohen, L. A., Thompson, D. O., Maeura, Y., Choi, K., Blank, M. E. & Rose, D. P. 1986. Dietary fat and mammary cancer. I. Promoting effects of different dietary fats on N-nitrosomethylurea-induced rat mammary tumorigenesis. *J Natl Cancer Inst*, 77, 33–42.

COMA. 1998. *Nutritional Aspects of the Development of Cancer (Report of the Working Group on Diet and Cancer of the Committee on Medical Aspects of Food and Nutrition Policy)*.

Correa, P., Fontham, E. T., Bravo, J. C., Bravo, L. E., Ruiz, B., Zarama, G., Realpe, J. L., Malcom, G. T., Li, D., Johnson, W. D. & Mera, R. 2000. Chemoprevention of gastric dysplasia: Randomized trial of antioxidant supplements and anti-helicobacter pylori therapy. *J Natl Cancer Inst*, 92, 1881–8.

Doll, R. & Peto, R. 1981. The causes of cancer: Quantitative estimates of avoidable risks of cancer in the United States today. *J Natl Cancer Inst*, 66, 1191–308.

Doll, R. & Peto, R. 1996. Epidemiology of cancer. *In*: Weatherall, D. J., Ledingham, J. G. G. & Warrell, D. A. (eds.) *Oxford Textbook of Medicine*. Oxford: Oxford University Press, p. 197–221.

Eaton, N. E., Reeves, G. K., Appleby, P. N. & Key, T. J. 1999. Endogenous sex hormones and prostate cancer: A quantitative review of prospective studies. *Br J Cancer*, 80, 930–4.

Erickson, K. L., Schlanger, D. S., Adams, D. A., Fregeau, D. R. & Stern, J. S. 1984. Influence of dietary fatty acid concentration and geometric configuration on murine mammary tumorigenesis and experimental metastasis. *J Nutr*, 114, 1834–42.

Fay, M. P., Freedman, L. S., Clifford, C. K. & Midthune, D. N. 1997. Effect of different types and amounts of fat on the development of mammary tumors in rodents: A review. *Cancer Res*, 57, 3979–88.

Ferlay, J. B. F., Pisani, P. & Parkin, D.M. 2000. *GLOBOCAN 2000: Cancer incidence, mortality, and prevalence worldwide, Version 1.0. 2001 International Agency for Research on Cancer CancerBase No. 5*. Available: [http://www-dep.iarc.fr].

Freedman, L. S., Clifford, C. & Messina, M. 1990. Analysis of dietary fat, calories, body weight, and the development of mammary tumors in rats and mice: A review. *Cancer Res*, 50, 5710–9.

Gann, P. H., Hennekens, C. H., Ma, J., Longcope, C. & Stampfer, M. J. 1996. Prospective study of sex hormone levels and risk of prostate cancer. *J Natl Canc Inst*, 88, 1118–26.

Giovannucci, E., Stampfer, M. J., Colditz, G., Rimm, E. B. & Willett, W. C. 1992. Relationship of diet to risk of colorectal adenoma in men. *J Natl Cancer Inst*, 84, 91–8.

Giovannucci, E., Stampfer, M. J., Colditz, G. A., Manson, J. E., Rosner, B. A., Longnecker, M., Speizer, F. E. & Willett, W. C. 1993. A comparison of prospective and retrospective assessments of diet in the study of breast cancer. *Am J Epidemiol*, 137, 502–11.

Glade, M. J. 1999. Food, nutrition, and the prevention of cancer: A global perspective. American Institute for Cancer Research/World Cancer Research Fund, American Institute for Cancer Research, 1997. *Nutrition*, 15, 523–6.

Goldbohm, R. A., Van Den Brandt, P. A., Van 'T Veer, P., Brants, H. A., Dorant, E., Sturmans, F. & Hermus, R. J. 1994. A prospective cohort study on the relation between meat consumption and the risk of colon cancer. *Cancer Res,* 54, 718–23.

Goldin, B. R., Adlercreutz, H., Gorbach, S. L., Warram, J. H., Dwyer, J. T., Swenson, L. & Woods, M. N. 1982. Estrogen excretion patterns and plasma levels in vegetarian and omnivorous women. *N Engl J Med,* 307, 1542–7.

Gonzalez, M. J., Schemmel, R. A., Dugan, L., Jr., Gray, J. I. & Welsch, C. W. 1993. Dietary fish oil inhibits human breast carcinoma growth: A function of increased lipid peroxidation. *Lipids,* 28, 827–32.

Graham, S., Marshall, J., Mettlin, C., Rzepka, T., Nemoto, T. & Byers, T. 1982. Diet in the epidemiology of breast cancer. *Am J Epidemiol,* 116, 68–75.

Guthrie, N. & Carroll, K. K. 1999. Specific versus non-specific effects of dietary fat on carcinogenesis. *Prog Lipid Res,* 38, 261–71.

Hanahan, D. & Weinberg, R. A. 2000. The hallmarks of cancer. *Cell,* 100, 57–70.

Hankinson, S. E., Willett, W. C., Manson, J. E., Hunter, D. J., Colditz, G. A., Stampfer, M. J., Longcope, C. & Speizer, F. E. 1995. Alcohol, height, and adiposity in relation to estrogen and prolactin levels in postmenopausal women. *J Natl Cancer Inst,* 87, 1297–302.

Heaney, R. P., Mccarron, D. A., Dawson-Hughes, B., Oparil, S., Berga, S. L., Stern, J. S., Barr, S. I. & Rosen, C. J. 1999. Dietary changes favorably affect bone remodeling in older adults. *J Am Diet Assoc,* 99, 1228–33.

Heber, D. & kritchevsky, D. 2012. *Dietary Fats, Lipids, Hormones, and Tumorigenesis: New Horizons in Basic Research,* New York: Springer.

Heinonen, O. P., Albanes, D., Virtamo, J., Taylor, P. R., Huttunen, J. K., Hartman, A. M., Haapakoski, J., Malila, N., Rautalahti, M., Ripatti, S. et al. 1998. Prostate cancer and supplementation with alpha-tocopherol and beta-carotene: Incidence and mortality in a controlled trial. *J Natl Canc Inst,* 90, 440–6.

Helicobacter, A. 2001. Gastric cancer and Helicobacter pylori: A combined analysis of 12 case control studies nested within prospective cohorts. *Gut,* 49, 347–53.

Hennekens, C. H., Buring, J. E., Manson, J. E., Stampfer, M., Rosner, B., Cook, N. R., Belanger, C., Lamotte, F., Gaziano, J. M., Ridker, P. M. et al. 1996. Lack of effect of longterm supplementation with beta carotene on the incidence of malignant neoplasms and cardiovascular disease. *N Engl J Med,* 334, 1145–9.

Holmes, M. D., Hunter, D. J., Colditz, G. A., Stampfer, M. J., Hankinson, S. E., Speizer, F. E., Rosner, B. & Willett, W. C. 1999. Association of dietary intake of fat and fatty acids with risk of breast cancer. *Jama,* 281, 914–20.

Hopkins, G. J. & Carroll, K. K. 1979. Relationship between amount and type of dietary fat in promotion of mammary carcinogenesis induced by 7,12-dimethylbenz[a]anthracene. *J Natl Cancer Inst,* 62, 1009–12.

Howe, G. R., Hirohata, T., Hislop, T. G., Iscovich, J. M., Yuan, J. M., Katsouyanni, K., Lubin, F., Marubini, E., Modan, B., Rohan, T. et al. 1990. Dietary factors and risk of breast cancer: Combined analysis of 12 case-control studies. *J Natl Cancer Inst,* 82, 561–9.

Hu, F. B., Stampfer, M. J., Manson, J. E., Rimm, E., Colditz, G. A., Rosner, B. A., Hennekens, C. H. & Willett, W. C. 1997. Dietary fat intake and the risk of coronary heart disease in women. *N Engl J Med,* 337, 1491–9.

Hunter, D. J., Spiegelman, D. & Willett, W. 1998. Dietary fat and breast cancer. *J Natl Cancer Inst,* 90, 1303–6.

IARC. 1988. IARC Monographs on the Evaluation of Carcinogenic Risks to Humans. *Alcohol Drinking.* Vol. 44. Lyon, France: IARC.

IARC. 1990. *Cancer: Causes, Occurrence and Control.* IARC Scientific Publications No. 100.

IARC. 1993. *IARC Monographs on the Evaluation of Carcinogenic Risks to Humans. Some Naturally Occurring Substances: Food Items and Constituents, Heterocyclic Aromatic Amines and Mycotoxins.* Vol. 56. Lyon, France: IARC.

IARC. 1994. *IARC monographs on the evaluation of carcinogenic risks to humans. Hepatitis Viruses.* Vol. 59. Lyon: IARC.

IARC. 1995. *IARC Monographs on the Evaluation of Carcinogenic Risks to Humans. Human Papillomaviruses.* Vol. 64. Lyon: IARC.

IARC. 2002. Overweight and lack of exercise linked to increased cancer risk. *IARC Handbooks of Cancer Prevention [Online],* April 21, 2016, 6, 41–51.

Ingram, D. M., Bennett, F. C., Willcox, D. & De Klerk, N. 1987. Effect of low-fat diet on female sex hormone levels. *J Natl Cancer Inst,* 79, 1225–9.

Ip, C. 1987. Fat and essential fatty acid in mammary carcinogenesis. *Am J Clin Nutr,* 45, 218–24.

Ip, C. 1990. Quantitative assessment of fat and calorie as risk factors in mammary carcinogenesis in an experimental model. *Prog Clin Biol Res,* 346, 107–17.

Ip, C. 1997. Review of the effects of trans fatty acids, oleic acid, n-3 polyunsaturated fatty acids, and conjugated linoleic acid on mammary carcinogenesis in animals. *Am J Clin Nutr,* 66, 1523S–9S.

Ip, C., Briggs, S. P., Haegele, A. D., Thompson, H. J., Storkson, J. & Scimeca, J. A. 1996. The efficacy of conjugated linoleic acid in mammary cancer prevention is independent of the level or type of fat in the diet. *Carcinogenesis,* 17, 1045–50.

Ip, C., Chin, S. F., Scimeca, J. A. & Pariza, M. W. 1991. Mammary cancer prevention by conjugated dienoic derivative of linoleic acid. *Cancer Res,* 51, 6118–24.

Ip, C., Scimeca, J. A. & Thompson, H. 1995. Effect of timing and duration of dietary conjugated linoleic acid on mammary cancer prevention. *Nutr Cancer,* 24, 241–7.

Ip, C., Singh, M., Thompson, H. J. & Scimeca, J. A. 1994. Conjugated linoleic acid suppresses mammary carcinogenesis and proliferative activity of the mammary gland in the rat. *Cancer Res,* 54, 1212–5.

Jain, M., Cook, G. M., Davis, F. G., Grace, M. G., Howe, G. R. & Miller, A. B. 1980. A case-control study of diet and colo-rectal cancer. *Int J Canc,* 26, 757–68.

Kolonel, L. N., Nomura, A. M. & Cooney, R. V. 1999. Dietary fat and prostate cancer: Current status. *J Natl Cancer Inst,* 91, 414–28.

Kravchenko, J., Akushevich, I. & Manton, K. G. 2009. *Cancer Mortality and Morbidity Patterns in the U. S. Population: An Interdisciplinary Approach,* Berlin, Springer.

Kristal, A. R. & Cohen, J. H. 2000. Invited commentary: Tomatoes, lycopene, and prostate cancer. How strong is the evidence?. *Am J Epidemiol,* 151, 124–7.

Lasekan, J. B., Clayton, M. K., Gendron-Fitzpatrick, A. & Ney, D. M. 1990. Dietary olive and safflower oils in promotion of DMBA-induced mammary tumorigenesis in rats. *Nutr Canc,* 13, 153–63.

Li, J. Y., Taylor, P. R., Li, B., Dawsey, S., Wang, G. Q., Ershow, A. G., Guo, W., Liu, S. F., Yang, C. S., Shen, Q. et al. 1993. Nutrition intervention trials in Linxian, China: Multiple vitamin/mineral supplementation, cancer incidence, and disease-specific mortality among adults with esophageal dysplasia. *J Natl Cancer Inst,* 85, 1492–8.

Liu, X. H., Connolly, J. M. & Rose, D. P. 1996. Eicosanoids as mediators of linoleic acid-stimulated invasion and type IV collagenase production by a metastatic human breast cancer cell line. *Clin Exp Metastasis,* 14, 145–52.

Lubin, J. H., Burns, P. E., Blot, W. J., Ziegler, R. G., Lees, A. W. & Fraumeni, J. F., Jr. 1981. Dietary factors and breast cancer risk. *Int J Cancer,* 28, 685–9.

Macquart-Moulin, G., Riboli, E., Cornee, J., Charnay, B., Berthezene, P. & Day, N. 1986. Case-control study on colorectal cancer and diet in Marseilles. *Int J Cancer,* 38, 183–91.

Marshall, J. R., Qu, Y., Chen, J., Parpia, B. & Campbell, T. C. 1992. Additional ecological evidence: Lipids and breast cancer mortality among women aged 55 and over in China. *Eur J Cancer,* 28a, 1720–7.

Martin-Moreno, J. M., Willett, W. C., Gorgojo, L., Banegas, J. R., Rodriguez-Artalejo, F., Fernandez-Rodriguez, J. C., Maisonneuve, P. & Boyle, P. 1994. Dietary fat, olive oil intake and breast cancer risk. *Int J Cancer,* 58, 774–80.

Mccullough, M. L., Robertson, A. S., Jacobs, E. J., Chao, A., Calle, E. E. & Thun, M. J. 2001. A prospective study of diet and stomach cancer mortality in United States men and women. *Cancer Epidemiol Biomarkers Prev,* 10, 1201–5.

Mcginnis, J. M. & Nestle, M. 1989. The surgeon general's report on nutrition and health: Policy implications and implementation strategies. *Am J Clin Nutr,* 49, 23–8.

Meyer, F. & White, E. 1993. Alcohol and nutrients in relation to colon cancer in middle-aged adults. *Am J Epidemiol,* 138, 225–36.

Michaud, D. S., Augustsson, K., Rimm, E. B., Stampfer, M. J., Willet, W. C. & Giovannucci, E. 2001. A prospective study on intake of animal products and risk of prostate cancer. *Canc Causes Contr,* 12, 557–67.

Michaud, D. S., Spiegelman, D., Clinton, S. K., Rimm, E. B., Willett, W. C. & Giovannucci, E. L. 1999. Fruit and vegetable intake and incidence of bladder cancer in a male prospective cohort. *J Natl Canc Inst,* 91, 605–13.

Miller, A. B., Kelly, A., Choi, N. W., Matthews, V., Morgan, R. W., Munan, L., Burch, J. D., Feather, J., Howe, G. R. & Jain, M. 1978. A study of diet and breast cancer. *Am J Epidemiol,* 107, 499–509.

NIH. 2007. NIH Curriculum Supplement Series [Internet]. *A service of the National Library of Medicine, National Institutes of Health [Online].* https://www.ncbi.nlm.nih.gov/books/NBK20364/. Accessed April, 26, 2016.

Omenn, G. S., Goodman, G. E., Thornquist, M. D., Balmes, J., Cullen, M. R., Glass, A., Keogh, J. P., Meyskens, F. L., Valanis, B., Williams, J. H. et al. 1996. Effects of a combination of beta carotene and vitamin A on lung cancer and cardiovascular disease. *N Engl J Med,* 334, 1150–5.

Palli, D. 2000. Epidemiology of gastric cancer: An evaluation of available evidence. *J Gastroenterol,* 12, 84–9.

Parkin, D. M., Bray, F., Ferlay, J. & Pisani, P. 2001. Estimating the world cancer burden: Globocan 2000. *Int J Canc,* 94, 153–6.

Peters, R. K., Pike, M. C., Garabrant, D. & Mack, T. M. 1992. Diet and colon cancer in Los Angeles County, California. *Canc Causes Contr,* 3, 457–73.

Prentice, R. L. & Sheppard, L. 1990. Dietary fat and cancer: Consistency of the epidemiologic data, and disease prevention that may follow from a practical reduction in fat consumption. *Canc Causes Contr,* 1, 81–97; discussion 99–109.

Reddy, B. S. 1992. Dietary fat and colon cancer: Animal model studies. *Lipids,* 27, 807–13.

Rose, D. P., Boyar, A. P. & Wynder, E. L. 1986. International comparisons of mortality rates for cancer of the breast, ovary, prostate, and colon, and per capita food consumption. *Cancer,* 58, 2363–71.

Rosner, B., Spiegelman, D. & Willett, W. C. 1992. Correction of logistic regression relative risk estimates and confidence intervals for random within-person measurement error. *Am J Epidemiol,* 136, 1400–13.

Saracco, G. 1995. Primary liver cancer is of multifactorial origin: Importance of hepatitis B virus infection and dietary aflatoxin. *J Gastroenterol Hepatol,* 10, 604–8.

Schuurman, A. G., Brandt, P. A. V. D., Dorant, E. & Goldbohm, R. A. 1999. Animal products, calcium and protein and prostate cancer risk in the Netherlands Cohort Study. *Br J Canc,* 80, 1107–13.

Selenskas, S. L., Margot, M. I. & Clement, I. 1984. Similarity between frans fat and saturated fat in the modification of Rat Mammary Carcinogenesis. *Canc Res,* 44, 1321–6.

Sesink, A. L., Termont, D. S., Kleibeuker, J. H. & Van Der Meer, R. 2001. Red meat and colon cancer: Dietary haem-induced colonic cytotoxicity and epithelial hyperproliferation are inhibited by calcium. *Carcinogenesis,* 22, 1653–9.

Sharp, L., Chilvers, C. E., Cheng, K. K., Mckinney, P. A., Logan, R. F., Cook-Mozaffari, P., Ahmed, A. & Day, N. E. 2001. Risk factors for squamous cell carcinoma of the oesophagus in women: A case-control study. *Br J Cancer,* 85, 1667–70.

Simonsen, N. R., Fernandez-Crehuet Navajas, J., Martin-Moreno, J. M., Strain, J. J., Huttunen, J. K., Martin, B. C., Thamm, M., Kardinaal, A. F., Van't Veer, P., Kok, F. J. & Kohlmeier, L. 1998. Tissue stores of individual monounsaturated fatty acids and breast cancer: The EURAMIC study. European Community Multicenter Study on Antioxidants, Myocardial Infarction, and Breast Cancer. *Am J Clin Nutr,* 68, 134–41.

Sonnenschein, E. G., Glickman, L. T., Goldschmidt, M. H. & Mckee, L. J. 1991. Body conformation, diet, and risk of breast cancer in pet dogs: A case-control study. *Am J Epidemiol,* 133, 694–703.

Stattin, P., Bylund, A., Rinaldi, S., Biessy, C., Déchaud, H., Stenman, U.-H., Egevad, L., Riboli, E., Hallmans, G. & Kaaks, R. 2000. Plasma insulin-like growth Factor-I, Insulin-Like growth factor-binding proteins, and prostate cancer risk: A prospective study. *J Natl Canc Inst,* 92, 1910–7.

Thun, M. J., Calle, E. E., Namboodiri, M. M., Flanders, W. D., Coates, R. J., Byers, T., Boffetta, P., Garfinkel, L. & Heath, C. W. 1992. Risk factors for fatal colon cancer in a large prospective study. *J Natl Canc Inst,* 84, 1491–500.

Toniolo, P. G., Levitz, M., Zeleniuch-Jacquotte, A., Banerjee, S., Koenig, K. L., Shore, R. E., Strax, P. & Pasternack, B. S. 1995. A prospective study of endogenous estrogens and breast cancer in postmenopausal women. *J Natl Cancer Inst,* 87, 190–7.

Trichopoulou, A., Katsouyanni, K., Stuver, S., Tzala, L., Gnardellis, C., Rimm, E. & Trichopoulos, D. 1995. Consumption of olive oil and specific food groups in relation to breast cancer risk in Greece. *J Natl Cancer Inst,* 87, 110–6.

Turpeinen, A. M., Mutanen, M., Aro, A., Salminen, I., Basu, S., Palmquist, D. L. & Griinari, J. M. 2002. Bioconversion of vaccenic acid to conjugated linoleic acid in humans. *Am J Clin Nutr,* 76, 504–10.

Visonneau, S., Cesano, A., Tepper, S. A., Scimeca, J. A., Santoli, D. & Kritchevsky, D. 1997. Conjugated linoleic acid suppresses the growth of human breast adenocarcinoma cells in SCID mice. *Anticancer Res,* 17, 969–73.

Watanabe, M., Koga, T. & Sugano, M. 1985. Influence of dietary cis- and trans-fat on 1,2-dimethylhydrazine-induced colon tumors and fecal steroid excretion in Fischer 344 rats. *Am J Clin Nutr,* 42, 475–84.

Welsch, C. W. 1992. Relationship between dietary fat and experimental mammary tumorigenesis: A review and critique. *Cancer Res,* 52, 2040s–48s.

WHO. 1990. *Cancer: Causes, Occurrence and Control.* Lyon: IARC.

WHO. 2013. What is cancer? *Cancer Glossary. cancer.org. [Online].* https://www.cancer.org/cancer/cancer-basics/what-is-cancer.html. Accessed April 08, 2016.

WHO. 2014. Cancer Fact sheet N°297. *Defining Cancer [Online].* http://www.afro.who.int/index.php?option=com_docman&task=doc_download&gid=6139. Accessed April 26, 2016.

WHO. 2016. *World Health Statistics Annual [Online].* Available: http://www.who.int/whosis/ [Accessed March 10 2016].

Willet, W. & Lenart, E. 1998. Reproducibility and validity of food-frequency questionnaires. *In:* Willet, W. (ed.) *Nutritional epidemiology.* 2nd ed. New York: Oxford University Press, p. 101–47.

Willett, W. C. 2000. Diet and cancer. *The Oncologist,* 5, 393–404.

Willett, W. C., Hunter, D. J., Stampfer, M. J., Colditz, G., Manson, J. E., Spiegelman, D., Rosner, B., Hennekens, C. H. & Speizer, F. E. 1992. Dietary fat and fiber in relation to risk of breast cancer. An 8-year follow-up. *Jama,* 268, 2037–44.

Willett, W. C., Stampfer, M. J., Colditz, G. A., Rosner, B. A. & Speizer, F. E. 1990. Relation of meat, fat, and fiber intake to the risk of colon cancer in a prospective study among women. *N Engl J Med,* 323, 1664–72.

Wynder, E. L., Cohen, L. A., Muscat, J. E., Winters, B., Dwyer, J. T. & Blackburn, G. 1997. Breast cancer: Weighing the evidence for a promoting role of dietary fat. *J Natl Cancer Inst,* 89, 766–75.

Yu, M. C. 1991. Nasopharyngeal carcinoma: Epidemiology and dietary factors. *IARC Sci Publ*, 105, 39–47.

Zeegers, M. P. A., Goldbohm, R. A. & Van Den Brandt, P. A. 2001. Consumption of vegetables and fruits and urothelial cancer incidence: A prospective study. *Canc Epidemiol Biomarkers Prev*, 10, 1121–8.

Zock, P. L. & Katan, M. B. 1998. Linoleic acid intake and cancer risk: A review and meta-analysis. *Am J Clin Nutr*, 68, 142–53.

Index

A

ACE, *see* Angiotensin-converting enzyme
ACL, *see* ATP-citrate lyase
Actinobacteria, 409
Acute lung injury (ALI), 129
Acute lymphocytic leukemia (ALL), 342
Acute phase reactants (APRs), 324
Acute respiratory distress syndrome (ARDS), 129
ADH1C, *see* Alcohol dehydrogenase 1C
Advanced glycation end products (ADEs), 195
Aging, nutrition and, 451–482
    antioxidants, 463–464
    B vitamins, 465–466
    calcium and vitamin D, 459–463
    carotenoids, 465
    coenzyme Q10, 473–474
    dietary fibers, 468–469
    disease concerns, 457–458
    formulation challenges, 474–475
    future opportunities, 475
    glucosamine, chondroitin quercetin, and collagen, 468
    healthy aging and nutrition issues, 454–457
    healthy nutrition, 453–454
    malnutrition, 457
    omega-3 fatty acids, 466–468
    plant polyphenols and catechins, 464–465
    plant stanols/sterols, 465
    potassium, 470–471
    prebiotics and probiotics, 469–470
    whey protein, 471
    zinc, 344, 471–473
Alcohol
    consumption, 172
    dehydrogenase 1C (ADH1C), 108
    effect on genes, 33–36
Aldehyde dehydrogenase 2 (ALDH2), 4
ALI, *see* Acute lung injury

ALL, *see* Acute lymphocytic leukemia
Alzheimer's disease, 67, 193, 298, 504
AMP-activated protein kinase (AMPK), 233
Amyloid precursor protein (APP), 194
Angiotensin-converting enzyme (ACE), 245, 391
Anticodon, 256
Antioxidants, 463–464, 505
Apoptosis, 293, 339–340
Apoptosis signal-regulating kinase 1 (ASK-1), 89
APP, *see* Amyloid precursor protein
APRs, *see* Acute phase reactants
AQUA (absolute quantification), 142
ARDS, *see* Acute respiratory distress syndrome
ASD, *see* Autism spectrum disorder
Asian–Indian phenotype, 71
ASK-1, *see* Apoptosis signal-regulating kinase 1
Ataxia-telangiectasia mutated (ATM), 351
Atherosclerosis, zinc and, 346–347
ATP-citrate lyase (ACL), 233
Attention deficient hyperactivity disorder, 67
Autism spectrum disorder (ASD), 302
Ayurvedic medicine, 72–73

B

BAT, *see* Brown adipose tissue
Betaine-homocysteine-*S*-methyltransferase (BHMT), 339
Bifidobacteria, 409
Biology and optimal health, 201–215
    applying systems biology to medicine, 208–211
    disease and health problems, using systems biology to understand, 209–210
    drugs and vaccines, using systems biology to develop, 210–211

systems biology, perspectives on, 203–206
top-down and bottom-up approaches to systems biology, 206–208
Bladder cancer, 172–174, 243, 431, 544
Brain function, gut microbiota and, 409
Breast cancer, 74–75, 171, 187, 235, 294, 359, 542
Breathomics, for lung disease prevention, 115, 126–129
Broad sense heritability model, 193
Brown adipose tissue (BAT), 384

C

Caffeine, effect on genes, 36–37
Calcium, aging and, 459–463
cAMP, *see* Cyclic adenosine monophosphate
Cancer
  individualized nutrition and, 440
  prevention, vitamins and, 299
  selenium and, 355–356
  therapeutic management of, 519
  zinc and, 342–343
Cancer, dietary fats and, 529–555
  bladder, 544
  breast, 542
  cancer process, 531–532
  cervix, 542–543
  colon and rectum, 540–541
  conjugated linoleic acid and cancer, 535–536
  diet and cancer, 533–534
  effects of dietary fats on carcinogenesis, 534
  endometrium, 542
  environmental factors, 532
  kidney, 543–544
  liver, 540
  lung, 539
  monounsaturated fatty acid and cancer, 536
  nasopharynx, 538
  opinions and outcomes, 544–548
  oral cavity, pharynx, and esophagus, 538
  ovary, 542
  pancreas, 540
  polyunsaturated fats, 534–535
  prostate, 543
  saturated fatty acids, 537–538
  stomach, 539–540
  trans fatty acids and cancer, 537
Cancer, facts and controversies based on diet, genomics, and, 169–189
  cancer, understanding risk reduction and prevention of, 171–173

CRC biology, improving clinical decisions through understanding of, 184–185
developing world, genomics and health in, 179–180
dietary fats and health, 177–178
fruit and vegetable consumption in adolescence and early adulthood, risk of breast cancer and, 178
homeostasis model assessment beta cell function and insulin resistance, 186–187
mitochondria organelle transplantation, 181–182
nutrients, 174–175
ovarian cancer, mesothelial signature of, 182
pheochromocytoma, current concepts of, 178–179
postmenopausal breast cancer in whites, decreased risk of, 187–188
preconditioning, 176
prostate cancer, composition and metabolism of PUFAs in, 185–186
retrograde axonal damage, 183–184
saccharin, toxicological aspects of, 173–174
saturated and omega-6 and omega-3 polyunsaturated fatty acids, 175–176
Cancer, nutrigenomics and, 74–79
  breast cancer, 74
  cervical cancer, 75
  HPV-related dysplasia, 75
  lipid metabolism pathway, 75
  methylene tetrahydrofolate reductase gene, 76
  prostate cancer, 77
  transcriptomic profiling, 75
Cap-binding protein complex (CBC), 249
Carbon nanotubes (CNTs), 116
Cardiovascular disease (CVDs), 162, 280, 346
  states, cutting-edge research in, 66–72
  therapeutic management of, 519–520
Cardiovascular health, individualized nutrition and, 440
Carotenoids, 465
Castration-resistant prostate cancer (CRPC), 77
Catechins, 464–465
CBC, *see* Cap-binding protein complex
Cellular retinol-binding proteins (CRBPs), 281
Central nervous system (CNS), 280

Cervical cancer, 542–543
CF transmembrane conductance regulator (CFTR), 119
CHARGE Consortium, *see* Cohorts for Heart and Aging Research in Genomic Epidemiology Consortium
Choline deficiency, 247
Chondroitin quercetin, aging and, 468
Chronic degenerative diseases, 191–199
  advanced glycation end products, 195
  Alzheimer's disease, 193–196
  amyloid precursor protein, 194
  broad sense heritability model, 193
  common and rare variants, 192–197
  infinitesimal model, 192
  rare allele hypothesis, 192
  rare-variant association studies, 193
  type 2 diabetes, 196–197
CID, *see* Collision-induced dissociation
Cigarette smoking, 170
CJD, *see* Creutzfeldt–Jakob disease
CLA, *see* Conjugated linoleic acid
Cleavage stimulation factor (CSF), 248
CNS, *see* Central nervous system
CNTs, *see* Carbon nanotubes
Cobalamin deficiency, 28, 148
Coenzyme Q10, 473
Cohorts for Heart and Aging Research in Genomic Epidemiology (CHARGE) Consortium, 66
Collagen, aging and, 468
Collision-induced dissociation (CID), 40
Colon cancer, 540–541
Colorectal cancer, 356–358
Common-disease–common-variant hypothesis, 192
Common diseases and diet intakes, genetic susceptibility to, 423–450
  alteration of gene expression or structure, 427–429
  approaches to demonstrate genetic susceptibility, 424–426
  balance between health and disease states, 438
  caloric restriction, 434–435
  carbohydrates, 433–434
  commercial interests, 441–442
  diet as risk factor for disease, 429–435
  fats, 433
  genetic susceptibility, 424
  individualized nutrition, dietary intervention based on, 438–440
  interface between the nutritional environment and genetic processes, 426–427

micronutrients, 431–433
population screening, 440–441
protein, 434
public health perspective, 442–443
role of diet-regulated genes in chronic diseases, 435–438
Conjugated linoleic acid (CLA), 535
COPD, *see* Lung disease prevention, trends in omics-based methods and techniques
COX-2 mRNA, 148
CpG dinucleotide, 8
CRBPs, *see* Cellular retinol-binding proteins
Creutzfeldt–Jakob disease (CJD), 46
CRISPR system, 10
Crohn's disease, 503
CRPC, *see* Castration-resistant prostate cancer
CSF, *see* Cleavage stimulation factor
C-terminal domain (CTD), 248
Cushing syndrome, 219
CVD, *see* Cardiovascular disease
Cyclic adenosine monophosphate (cAMP), 119
Cytokines, 71, 218

D

DASH diet, *see* Dietary Approaches to Stop Hypertension diet
DBD, *see* DNA-binding domain
Degenerative diseases, *see* Chronic degenerative diseases
Depression, 67
Developing world
  genomics and health in, 179–180
  nutrition problems in, 486
DHA, *see* Docosahexaenoic acid
Diabetes; *see also* Prenatal nutrition exposure (adult obesity, diabetes, and hypertension and)
  role of pro-inflammatory factors and metabolic stress in, 220–223
  therapeutic management of, 520–521
  type 2 diabetes, 196–197, 345
Dickkopf 1 (DKK1) promoter region, 240
Dietary advice and eating behavior, gene-based, 515–527
  cancer, 519
  cardiovascular disease, 519–520
  diabetes, 520–521
  gene–diet interaction in management of diseases, 521–523
  nutrigenetics, 517–518

Index   559

nutrigenomics and nutrigenetics (legal aspects), 523–524
prophylactic or therapeutic management of some diseases, 519–521
single nucleotide polymorphisms, 518–519
Dietary Approaches to Stop Hypertension (DASH) diet, 439
Dietary fats, *see* Cancer, dietary fats and
Dietary fiber, 468–469
Dietary health effects, molecular means to understand, *see* Proteomics, understanding dietary health effects using
Differential in-gel electrophoresis (DIGE), 47, 92
DiGeorge syndrome, 232
Diseases, genetic susceptibility to, *see* Common diseases and diet intakes, genetic susceptibility to
Diseases, pathogenesis of, *see* Pathogenesis of diseases, role of nutritional factors in
DNA
-binding domain (DBD), 250
-binding proteins, 137
damage response pathways, 317
methyltransferases (DNMTs), 230
mismatch repair, 357
Docosahexaenoic acid (DHA), 67, 245
Down's syndrome, 194
Dragon Estrogen Responsive Genes Database, 90
DRIP, *see* Vitamin D receptor interacting protein
Drug development, 210–211

E

Eating behavior, *see* Dietary advice and eating behavior, gene-based
ECP, *see* Eosinophil cationic protein
EGCG, *see* Epigallocatechin gallate
EGF, *see* Epidermal growth factor
Electron capture dissociation (ECD), 95
Electron transfer dissociation (ETD), 95
Electrospray interface (ESI), 40
Electrospray ionization–ion trap (ESI-IT), 95
Electrospray ionization–quadruple/time of flight (ESI-Q/TOF), 95
Elongation factors (EFs), 248
EMT, *see* Epithelial-to-mesenchymal transition
Endometrial cancer, 542
Engineered nanoparticles (ENMs), 115

Enteric nervous system (ENS), 146
Environmental effect, 2
Eosinophil cationic protein (ECP), 128
Epidermal growth factor (EGF), 429
Epigallocatechin gallate (EGCG), 239
Epigenetics, 228
Epigenomics, 8–10
Epithelial-to-mesenchymal transition (EMT), 243
ESI, *see* Electrospray interface
ESI-IT, *see* Electrospray ionization–ion trap
ESI-Q/TOF, *see* Electrospray ionization–quadruple/time of flight
Esophageal cancer, 538
ETD, *see* Electron transfer dissociation
Eukaryotic release factors (eRFs), 257
Exogenous food contaminants, 39–41
Exons, 248

F

FA, *see* Folic acid
Fast food, 170
Fat-free mass (FFM), 246, 474
Fats, *see* Cancer, dietary fats and
Fat-soluble vitamins, 280–297, 488
vitamin A, retinoids, and carotenoids, 280–289
vitamin D, 289–297
Fatty acid desaturase (FADS2) gene, 246
Fetal vitamin A deficiency syndrome, 281
Flavonoids, 413
Folate deficiency, 280, 289–299, 301, 543
Folic acid (FA), 297
Food allergens, 41–44
Food functions, novel approaches in, *see* Nutrigenomics research, novel approaches in food functions based on
Food insecurity, 506
Fourier transform ion cyclotron resonance (FTICR), 95, 139
Fruits and vegetables, effect on genes, 38–39
FTO locus, obesity and, 11–13

G

Galactose-1-phosphate uridyltransferase (GALT), 430
Gas chromatography (GC), 41
Gene editing, molecular biology tools for, 10–13
Gene expression, 227–277
bioactive food components, 238–242
DNA methylation, 230–231

560   Index

energy, carbohydrates, and lipids, 233–237
epigenetic control of, 229–247
histone modifications and chromatin structure, 231–232
housekeeping genes, 228, 247
micro RNAs, 232–233
miRNAs, nutritional regulation of, 242–243
nuclear receptor superfamily, 250–255
overview, 228
PPARs, 253–255
prenatal nutrition status, 243–247
protein and amino acid content of diet, 237–238
protein synthesis, role of energy and amino acids in, 257–258
protein synthesis, translational control of, 255–258
RAR/RXR nuclear receptor, 252
transcriptional control of, 247–255
transcription factors, 228
vitamin D nuclear receptor, 253
Gene Ontology database, 90
Genes, effect of food on, 32–39
alcohol, 33–36
caffeine, 36–37
dietary fat, 37
fruits and vegetables, 38–39
Gene set enrichment analysis (GSEA), 184
Genetically modified (GM) plants, 42
Genistein, 240
Genome-wide association studies (GWAS), 5, 61, 191
Genomics, 3–10, 25–26; *see also* Cancer, facts and controversies based on diet, genomics, and epigenomics, 8–10
genome-wide association studies, 5
nutrigenetics, 5
nutrigenomics, 5
single nucleotide polymorphisms, 3
transcriptomics, 5–7
Glucocorticoids, 394–395
Glucosamine, aging and, 468
Glutathione S-transferases (GSTs), 38
GM plants, *see* Genetically modified plants
GSEA, *see* Gene set enrichment analysis
GWAS, *see* Genome-wide association studies

H

HATs, *see* Histone acetyltransferases
HDACs, *see* Histone deacetylases
HDL, *see* High-density lipoprotein
"Healthy Plate," 170

Heat shock proteins (HSPs), 324
Hereditary hemochromatosis (HH), 323
Heritability, 2
Heterochromatin, 231
HFD, *see* High-fat diet
HGP, *see* Human Genome Project
HH, *see* Hereditary hemochromatosis
HHRA, *see* Human health risk assessment
hIECs, *see* Human intestinal epithelial cells
High-density lipoprotein (HDL), 33, 105, 177
High-fat diet (HFD), 381
High hydrostatic pressure (HHP) technology, 45
Histone acetyltransferases (HATs), 231
Histone deacetylases (HDACs), 231, 379
Histone methylation, 235
HIV/AIDS, *see* Human immunodeficiency virus/acquired immunodeficiency syndrome
Homeopathic medicine, 72–73
Hormone response element (HRE), 250
Housekeeping genes, 228, 247
HSPs, *see* Heat shock proteins
Human Genome Project (HGP), 61
Human health risk assessment (HHRA), 115
Human immunodeficiency virus/acquired immunodeficiency syndrome (HIV/AIDS), 205, 484
Human intestinal epithelial cells (hIECs), 146
Human Proteome Detection and Quantification Project, 142
Hypertension, 439; *see also* Prenatal nutrition exposure (adult obesity, diabetes, and hypertension and)

I

IBD, *see* Irritable bowel disease
IBS, *see* Inflammatory bowel syndrome
ICAT, *see* Isotope coded affinity tag
IECs, *see* Intestinal epithelial cells
IIDA, *see* Iron-deficiency anemia
Individualized nutrition, 26, 438
Infections, gut microbiota and, 406–407
Infinitesimal model, 192
Inflammation, nutritional mechanism of, 489–492
Inflammatory bowel syndrome (IBS), 146
Insulin-like growth factor 2 (IGF2), 243
Insulin resistance, 295, 300
Intestinal epithelial cells (IECs), 146
Intestinal regulation and dysregulation, 218–219
Intrauterine growth restriction (IUGR), 384, 486

Index 561

Introns, 248
Ion-exchange chromatography, 94
Iron, 317–329
    -deficiency anemia (IDA), 317
    functions, 319–322
    nutrigenomics and, 322–329
    regulation mechanisms, 318–319
    regulatory proteins (IRPs), 318
    -responsive elements (IREs), 318
Irritable bowel disease (IBD), 219, 496
Isotope coded affinity tag (ICAT), 141

J

Jumonji domain-containing histone
    demethylase (JHDM), 321
Junk food, 170
c-Jun N-terminal kinases (JNK), 79, 271, 387

K

Keshan disease (KD), 348
Kidney cancer, 543–544
Krishna tulsi, 72

L

Lactic acid bacteria (LAB), 410
LC, *see* Liquid chromatography
LC-MS, *see* Liquid chromatography–mass
    spectrometry
LDL, *see* Low-density lipoprotein
Lean body mass (LBM), 246, 454
Leptin gene promoter, 236
Limit of detection (LOD), 44
Lipidomics, 129–132
    phosphatidylcholine, 130
    phosphatidylglycerol, 130–131
    sphingolipids, 131–132
Liquid chromatography (LC), 140
Liquid chromatography–mass spectrometry
    (LC-MS), 27, 41, 124
Liver cancer, 540
Liver X receptor (LXR), 282
LOD, *see* Limit of detection
Low-density lipoprotein (LDL), 162, 492
Lung disease prevention, trends in omics-
    based methods and techniques
    for, 115–133
    breathomics, 126–129
    lipidomics, 129–132
    metabolomics, 123–126
    proteomics, 119–122
    transcriptomics, 115–119
LXR, *see* Liver X receptor

M

MALDI-FTMS, *see* Matrix-assisted laser
    desorption/ionization Fourier
    transform mass spectrometry
Mammalian target of Rapamycin
    (mTOR), 257
MAPK, *see* Mitogen-activated protein
    kinase
Massively parallel signature sequencing
    (MPSS), 89
Mass spectrometry (MS), 119, 138
Maternal diet, *see* Prenatal nutrition
    exposure (adult obesity, diabetes,
    and hypertension and)
Matrix-assisted laser desorption/
    ionization Fourier transform mass
    spectrometry (MALDI-FTMS), 46
Medicine, metabolomics in, 162
Mediterranean diet, 176
Medullary thyroid carcinoma (MTC), 179
Mesenchymal stem/stromal cells (MSCs), 182
Messenger RNA (mRNA), 256
Metabolic stress, *see* Pro-inflammatory
    factors and metabolic stress, role
    of in disease
Metabolic syndrome, 68, 151, 409
Metabolomics, 30–31, 96–98
    advances in, 97
    analytical techniques in metabolomics,
    98–100
    for lung disease prevention, 115123–126
    mass spectrometry approaches, 99
    NMR approaches, 99–100
    studies, 96
Metabolomics, application of, 159–168
    conceptual developments, 162
    dietetics, 163–164
    diet and gene expression, 162–163
    future of nutrigenomics, 165
    interindividual response to nutrients, 164
    medicine, metabolomics in, 162
    microbiome-related metabolome, 164–165
    nutritional epigenetics, 164
    nutrition and toxicology, 161
    personalized medicine, 161
    pharmacogenomics to nutrigenomics, 161
    risks of nutrigenomics and
    nutrigenetics, 163
    targeted metabolomics, 160
    untargeted metabolomics, 160–161
Metallothioneins (MTs), 317
Methane monooxygenase (MMO), 319
Methylene tetrahydrofolate reductase
    (MTHFR) gene, 76

Microbiological toxins, 44–47
Microbiome, 13–14, 218
Microbiome, diet, and health, 405–422
  brain function, 409
  diet and gut microbiota, 409–416
  fermented products, 410–411
  immune response and inflammation,
    407–408
  impact of malnutrition, impact of, 414–415
  infections, 406–407
  macronutrients, effect of, 411–412
  minerals and micronutrients, 414
  noncommunicable diseases, 408–409
  obesity, 408
  polyphenols and flavonoids, 413
  rebalancing the gut microbiota, 415–416
  vitamins, 413–414
Mitochondria organelle transplantation,
    181–182
Mitogen-activated protein kinase (MAPK),
    239, 282, 320
MMO, *see* Methane monooxygenase
Monounsaturated fatty acids (MUFA), 440, 501
MPO, *see* Myeloperoxidase
MPSS, *see* Massively parallel signature
    sequencing
MS, *see* Mass spectrometry
MSCs, *see* Mesenchymal stem/stromal cells
MTC, *see* Medullary thyroid carcinoma
MTHFR gene, *see* Methylene
    tetrahydrofolate reductase gene
MTs, *see* Metallothioneins
MUFA, *see* Monounsaturated fatty acids
Multiple-reaction monitoring, 142
Multiple sclerosis, 289, 296
Multiwalled carbon nanotubes
    (MWCNTs), 116
Myeloperoxidase (MPO), 128

N

NAD, *see* Nicotinamide adenine dinucleotide
Narrow-sense heritability, 2
NASH, *see* Nonalcoholic steatohepatitis
Nasopharyngeal cancer, 538
Neural tube defects (NTDs), 298
Neuropeptide Y (NPY), 244, 381
Nicotinamide adenine dinucleotide (NAD), 428
NLS, *see* Nuclear localizing sequence
NMR, *see* Nuclear magnetic resonance
Nonalcoholic steatohepatitis (NASH), 497
NPY, *see* Neuropeptide Y
NTDs, *see* Neural tube defects
Nuclear localizing sequence (NLS), 251
Nuclear magnetic resonance (NMR), 96

Nutrigenomics, 23–31, 61–81
  Asian–Indian phenotype, 71
  biomarkers, 65
  cancer, 74–79
  cardiovascular disease states, cutting-
    edge research in, 66–72
  classic targets, 65
  future of, 165
  genetic mutation, 62
  genomics (gene analysis), 25–26
  homeopathic and ayurvedic medicine,
    72–73
  inborn error of metabolism, 24
  metabolomics (metabolite profiling), 30–31
  omics, 63–66
  order-made nutrition, 26
  personalized diet management, 24
  proteomics (protein expression analysis),
    26–29
  risks of, 163
  transcriptomics (gene expression
    analysis), 29–30
Nutrigenomics, applications of, 1–17
  environmental effect, 2
  epigenomics, 8–10
  gene editing, molecular biology tools
    for, 10–13
  genome-wide association studies, 5
  genomics, primer on, 3–10
  heritability, 2
  microbiome, 13–14
  narrow-sense heritability, 2
  nutrigenomics, introduction to, 2–3
  nutrigenomics in the genomics and
    postgenomics age, 1–2
  obesity and the *FTO* locus, 11–13
  transcriptomics, 5–7
Nutrigenomics research, novel approaches in
    food functions based on, 83–114
  future prospects, 108–109
  measuring nutrition responsive genome
    activity, 84–100
  metabolomics, 96–100
  nutrition research, use of nutrigenomics
    approach in, 102–108
  proteomics, 90–95
  systems biology, 100–102
  transcriptomics, 84–90

O

Obesity; *see also* Prenatal nutrition
    exposure (adult obesity, diabetes,
    and hypertension and)
  FTO locus and, 11–13

Index   563

gut microbiota and, 408
zinc and, 344–345
O-GlcNAc transferase enzyme (OGT), 232
Omega-3 fatty acids, 175–176, 466–468
Omega-6 polyunsaturated fatty acids, 175–176
Omics-driven novel technologies, 19–59;
    see also Lung disease prevention,
    trends in omics-based methods
    and techniques for
  application in the field of nutrition, 23–31
  description of omics technology, 20–22
  effect of food on genes, 32–39
  food safety, quality, and traceability,
    39–48
  future trends, 48–49
  history of omics, 22
  nutrigenomics, 23–31
  primary function of omics
    technologies, 22
  systems biology, 23
Oral cavity, cancer of, 538
Orbitrap instruments, 139
Order-made nutrition, 26
Orthogonal projections to latent
    structures–discriminant analysis
    (O2PLS-DA), 128
Osteoporosis, 455
Ovarian cancer, 182, 542
Oxidative stress, 492

P

Pancreatic cancer, 540
Parathyroid hormone (PTH), 462
Parkinson's disease, 67, 504
Pathogenesis of diseases, role of nutritional
    factors in, 483–513
  assessment of criteria, 487–489
  chronic diseases, 492–493
  developing world, nutrition problems
    in, 486
  global burden of chronic disease, 483–486
  infection, interaction between nutrition
    and, 493–494
  inflammation, nutritional mechanism of,
    489–492
  macronutrients, 495–501
  malnutrition and infection, cycle of,
    494–495
  micronutrients, 502–506
  oxidative stress, 492
Pathogens, 44–47
PBMCs, *see* Peripheral blood mononuclear
    cells
PC, *see* Phosphatidylcholine

PCa, *see* Prostate cancer
PEITC, *see* Phenethyl isothiocyanate
PEPCK, *see* Phosphoenolpyruvate
    carboxykinase
Peptide mass fingerprinting, 144
Peptide mass sequencing, 144
Peripheral blood mononuclear cells
    (PBMCs), 146, 242
Peroxisome proliferator-activated receptor
    (PPAR), 7, 69, 341
Personalized medicine, 161
Phagocytes, 219
Pharynx, cancer of, 539
Phenethyl isothiocyanate (PEITC), 76
Phenylthiocarbamide (PTC), 38
Pheochromocytoma, current concepts of,
    178–179
Phosphatidylcholine (PC), 130
Phosphoenolpyruvate carboxykinase
    (PEPCK), 244
PKC, *see* Protein kinase
Plant stanols/sterols, 465
Polyphenols, 413
Polyunsaturated fatty acids (PUFA), 30, 37,
    175, 522
Post-translational modifications (PTMs), 91
PPAR, *see* Peroxisome proliferator-
    activated receptor
Preconditioning, 176
Prenatal nutrition exposure (adult obesity,
    diabetes, and hypertension and),
    377–404
  diabetes in adults, 386–390
  fetal growth and programmed obesity,
    384–386
  glucocorticoids and programmed
    hypertension, 394–395
  hypertension in adults, 391–395
  hypothalamo-pituitaryadrenal axis and
    programmed obesity, 380–383
  insulin and leptin and programmed
    obesity, 383–384
  insulin-like growth factor 2 and
    development of diabetes, 386–387
  insulin receptor and development of
    diabetes, 390
  intrauterine growth restriction and
    development of diabetes, 388–389
  low birth weight and programmed
    hypertension, 393–394
  mitochondrial function and
    development of diabetes, 390
  nuclear receptors, signaling molecules,
    and transcription factors and
    development of diabetes, 387–388

obesity in adults, 380–386
pancreatic β cell and development of
  diabetes, 389
renin–angiotensin system, structure
  and function of glomeruli, and
  programmed hypertension,
  391–392
respiratory system and sympathetic
  function and programmed
  hypertension, 393
vascular changes and programmed
  hypertension, 392–393
white adipose tissue and programmed
  obesity, 384
Pro-inflammatory factors and metabolic
  stress, role of in disease, 217–225
chronic inflammatory state and its
  effects, 220
diabetes, 220–221
diabetic nephropathy, 222–223
diabetic neuropathy, 223
inflammation and diabetes, 221–222
intestinal regulation and dysregulation,
  218–219
Prostate cancer (PCa), 171, 185, 358, 543
Protein kinase C (PKC), 341
Proteomics, 26–29, 90–95
advances in, 91
bottom-up approach, 92–94
for lung disease prevention, 115, 119–122
middle-down approach, 95
top-down approach, 94–95
Proteomics, understanding dietary health
  effects using, 135–157
application of proteomics in nutritional
  interventions, 146–150
data processing, 143–144
description of proteomics do, 136–138
food deficiency, 149
multiple-reaction monitoring, 142
new view of proteins (historical
  perspective), 135–136
peptide mass fingerprinting, 144
peptide mass sequencing, 144
perspectives for proteomics in
  nutrition, 145
protein identification, 138–140
protein quantification, 140–143
proteomics in nutritional intervention,
  145–146
proteotypic peptides, 142
target-decoy database, 144
Proteotypic peptides, 142
PSAQ (protein standard absolute
  quantification), 142

PTC, *see* Phenylthiocarbamide
PTH, *see* Parathyroid hormone
PTMs, *see* Post-translational modifications
PUFA, *see* Polyunsaturated fatty acids

Q

QConCat, 142
Quadrupole–time-of-flight (Q-TOF)
  analyzer, 124
Quantitative reverse transcription PCR
  (RT-qPCR), 118
Quantitative trait loci (QTL), 437

R

RAR, *see* Retinoic acid receptor
Rare allele hypothesis, 192
Rare-variant association studies, 193
RBP, *see* Retinol-binding protein
Reactive oxygen species (ROS), 79, 317
Real-time PCR, 85
Rearranged during transfection (RET)
  proto-oncogene, 179
Renin–angiotensin system, 391–392
Reproductive tract infections (RTIs), 406
Research (nutrigenomics), *see*
  Nutrigenomics research, novel
  approaches in food functions
  based on
Resveratrol, 241
Retinoic acid, 71
Retinoic acid receptor (RAR), 281
Retinoid X receptor (RXR), 251, 252, 382, 428
Retinol-binding protein (RBP), 281
Reversed-phase (RP) chromatography, 94
Rheumatoid arthritis, 296
Ribosomal RNA (rRNA), 256
Rice bran, 68
RNA
  -induced silencing complex (RISC), 233
  sequencing, 117
ROS, *see* Reactive oxygen species
RP chromatography, *see* Reversed-phase
  chromatography
RTIs, *see* Reproductive tract infections
RT-qPCR, *see* Quantitative reverse
  transcription PCR
RXR, *see* Retinoid X receptor

S

Saccharin, toxicological aspects of, 173–174
SAGE, *see* Serial analysis of gene
  expression

Saturated fatty acids (SFAs), 177, 537
SELDI-TOF MS, *see* Surface-enhanced laser desorption/ionization–time-of-flight MS
Selenium, 347–360
  age-related diseases and, 359–360
  cancer and, 355–358
  deficiency, 348–349
  diseases and, 354–360
  epigenetics and, 349–350
  genomic stability and, 352–354
  nutrigenomics and, 350–352
  toxicity, 349
Serial analysis of gene expression (SAGE), 89
SFAs, *see* Saturated fatty acids
SILAC, *see* Stable isotope labelling with amino acids in cellular culture
Silencing mediator of retinoid and thyroid receptors (SMRT), 251
Single nucleotide polymorphisms (SNPs), 3, 25, 63, 518
Small for gestational age (SGA), 384
Small nuclear ribonucleoprotein (snRNP), 249
SMIRT, *see* Silencing mediator of retinoid and thyroid receptors
SNPs, *see* Single-nucleotide polymorphisms
Sphingolipids, 131–132
Stable isotope labelling with amino acids in cellular culture (SILAC), 27, 141
Sterol regulatory element binding proteins (SREBPs), 177
Stomach cancer, 171, 539–540
Sulforaphane, 241
Surface-enhanced laser desorption/ionization–time-of-flight (SELDI-TOF) MS, 28
Systems biology, 23, 100–102
  bottom-up approach, 208
  development of drugs and vaccines using, 210–211
  perspectives on, 203–206
  top-down approach, 207–208
  understanding disease and health problems using, 209–210

T

TAC, *see* Total antioxidant capacity
Tandem mass tag (TMT), 141
Targeted metabolomics, 160
TBK, *see* Total body potassium
TFs, *see* Transcription factors

TGF-beta, *see* Transforming growth factor-beta
Thiazolidinedione antidiabetic drugs, 68
TLRs, *see* Toll-like receptors
TMT, *see* Tandem mass tag
TNF, *see* Tumor necrosis factor
Toll-like receptors (TLRs), 292, 354
Total antioxidant capacity (TAC), 336
Total body potassium (TBK), 470
Trace elements, 315–375
  future insights, 361–362
  iron, 317–329
  selenium, 347–360
  zinc, 330–347
Transcription factor IID (TFIID), 248
Transcription factors (TFs), 228
Transcriptomics, 5–7, 29–30, 84–90
  advances in, 85
  bioinformatics and gene ontology database, 89–90
  gene expression microarray technology, 85–86
  for lung disease prevention, 115–119
  real-time PCR, 85
  sequencing-based technologies, 89
Trans fatty acids, 537
Transfer RNA (tRNA), 256
Transforming growth factor-beta (TGF-beta), 67, 104
Transient receptor potential vanilloid (TRPV), 253
Translation elongation factors 256
Transmissible spongiform encephalopathy (TSE), 46
Trans-Proteomic Pipeline, 144
Trans-unsaturated fats, 501
Triglycerides, 530
TRPV, *see* Transient receptor potential vanilloid
TSE, *see* Transmissible spongiform encephalopathy
Tubeimoside-1, 78
Tumor necrosis factor (TNF), 104, 222
Two-dimensional gel electrophoresis (2DE), 90–91
Type 2 diabetes (T2D), 71, 196–197, 295, 345

U

Ultra-performance liquid chromatography (UPLC), 44
Untargeted metabolomics, 160–161
Urinary tract infections (UTIs), 406
Ursolic acid, 72

V

Vaccine development, 210–211
Vitamins, 279–314
    effect of on gut microbiota, 413–414
    fat-soluble, 280–297, 488
    folate and cobalamins, 297–303
    future insights, 304–305
    Vitamin A, 71, 280, 504
    Vitamin B, 466
    Vitamin D, 253, 282, 289, 459–463
    water-soluble, 297–303, 488
von Hippel–Lindau syndrome, 179, 350

W

Water-soluble vitamins, 297–303, 488
Whey protein, 471
White adipose tissue (WAT), 384

Z

Zein proteins, 47
Zinc, 330–347
    aging and, 344, 471–473
    apoptosis and, 339–340
    atherosclerosis and, 346–347
    cancer and, 342–343
    deficiency, 28, 331–332, 503
    epigenetics and, 337–339
    genome and, 332–337
    metabolism and, 341–342
    obesity and, 344–345
    overload, 332
    signaling and, 341
    type 2 diabetes and, 345–346